MULTISTAGE CARCINOGENESIS

Proceedings of the 22nd International Symposium of
The Princess Takamatsu Cancer Research Fund, Tokyo, 1991

MULTISTAGE CARCINOGENESIS

Edited by
CURTIS C. HARRIS, SETSUO HIROHASHI,
NOBUYUKI ITO, HENRY C. PITOT, TAKASHI SUGIMURA,
MASAAKI TERADA, and JUN YOKOTA

JAPAN SCIENTIFIC SOCIETIES PRESS, Tokyo
CRC PRESS, Boca Raton Ann Arbor London Tokyo

Published jointly by:
Japan Scientific Societies Press
Hongo 6-2-10, Bunkyo-ku, Tokyo 113, Japan
ISBN 4-7622-6717-1
and
CRC Press
2000 Corporate Blvd., N.W., Boca Raton, FL 33431, U.S.A.
ISBN 0-8493-7749-8

CIP Data available from Library of Congress

Distributed in all areas outside Japan and Asia between Pakistan and Korea by CRC Press.

Printed in Japan

Princess Takamatsu Cancer Research Fund

* The members of Board of Directors, Auditors, Councillors, and Scientific Advisors at the 22nd International Symposium are listed in alphabetical order.

Organizing Committee of the 22nd International Symposium

Curtis C. HARRIS
Laboratory of Human Carcinogenesis, National Cancer Institute, NIH, Bethesda, Maryland 20892, U.S.A.

Setsuo HIROHASHI
Pathology Division, National Cancer Center Research Institute, Tokyo 104, Japan

Nobuyuki ITO
Department of Pathology, Nagoya City University Medical School, Nagoya 467, Japan

Henry C. PITOT
Department of Oncology and Pathology, McArdle Laboratory for Cancer Research, University of Wisconsin-Madison Medical School, Madison, Wisconsin 53706, U.S.A.

Takashi SUGIMURA
National Cancer Center, Tokyo 104, Japan

Masaaki TERADA
Genetics Division, National Cancer Center Research Institute, Tokyo 104, Japan

Jun YOKOTA
Section of Studies on Metastasis, National Cancer Center Research Institute, Tokyo 104, Japan

Preface

The 22nd International Symposium of The Princess Takamatsu Cancer Research Fund was held November 19 to 21, 1991 in Tokyo. The subject, "Multistage Carcinogenesis", is a longstanding concept in the field of carcinogenesis. Initially, multiple events in human cancer development were suggested by the age distribution curve of cancer incidence. Studies of carcinogenesis in experimental animals have generated the concepts called tumor initiation and promotion. In addition, the concept of tumor progression was suggested when stepwise processes to acquire more malignant phenotypes were found by clinical observations of minute cancer lesions.

With the recent progress in the molecular understanding of genetic mechanisms of carcinogenesis, the concept of multistage carcinogenesis has again become a primary focus of cancer research. Molecular genetic analyses of human cancers as well as experimental model systems for tumor development have revealed that multiple genetic alterations are necessary to convert a normal cell into a malignant cell. Multiple genetic alterations in protooncogenes and tumor suppressor genes contribute to each step in multistage carcinogenesis.

Multistage carcinogenesis has significant implications for establishing new strategies of cancer prevention, diagnosis and treatment. Individuals, who are at high risk for cancer development but are not yet suffering from clinical cancer, carry preneoplastic lesions with some but an insufficient set of genetic alterations for cancer development. Molecular diagnosis of these genetic changes should improve cancer risk estimation and identify individuals who may most benefit from chemopreventive therapy. Therefore, genetic abnormalities of protooncogenes and tumor suppressor genes during each step of multistage carcinogenesis are potential molecular targets for cancer prevention and treatment.

The symposium covered correlation between multiple genetic alterations and multiple stages in experimental and human carcinogenesis, regulatory mechanisms of cell growth and differentiation, genetic instability, mechanisms of promotion, progression, invasion and metastasis. The most recent findings in broad areas of cancer research, especially those showing very rapid progress, were discussed in the context of multistage carcinogenesis and are presented in this Proceedings.

Curtis C. Harris
Setsuo Hirohashi
Nobuyuki Ito
Henry C. Pitot
Takashi Sugimura
Masaaki Terada
Jun Yokota

Contents

Experimental Observation of Multistage Carcinogenesis

Regulation of Cell Growth and Differentiation in Multistage Carcinogenesis

Genetic Instability and Multistage Carcinogenesis

Promotion, Progression, Invasion, and Metastasis

Contributors

Kari ALITALO	Department of Pathology, University of Helsinki, SF-00290 Helsinki, Finland
Allan BALMAIN	Beatson Institute for Cancer Research, Wolfson Laboratory for Molecular Pathology, Bearsden, Glasgow G61 1BD, Scotland
Mariano BARBACID	Department of Molecular Biology, Bristol-Myers Squibb, Pharmaceutical for Medical Research Institute, Princeton, New Jersey 08543-4000, U.S.A.
David BEACH	Cold Spring Harbor Laboratory, Cold Spring Harbor, New York 11724, U.S.A.
Maarten C. BOSLAND	Institute of Environmental Medicine, New York University Medical Center, Anthony J. Lanza Research, Laboratories, Tuxedo, New York 10987, U.S.A.
Vincent CASTRONOVO	Laboratory of Pathology, National Cancer Institute, NIH, Bethesda, Maryland 20892, U.S.A.
Eric R. FEARON	The Johns Hopkins University School of Medicine, Baltimore, Maryland 21205, U.S.A.
Judah FOLKMAN	Department of Surgery, Harvard Medical School, Children's Hospital Medical Center, Boston, Massachusetts 02115-5737, U.S.A.
Stephen H. FRIEND	Massachusetts General Hospital Cancer Center, Harvard Medical School, Charlestown, Massachusetts 02129, U.S.A.
Curtis C. HARRIS	Laboratory of Human Carcinogenesis, National Cancer Institute, NIH, Bethesda, Maryland 20892, U.S.A.
Steven H. HINRICHS	Department of Pathology and Microbiology, University of Nebraska Medical Center, Omaha, Nebraska 68198-6495, U.S.A.
Setsuo HIROHASHI	Pathology Division, National Cancer Center Research

	Institute, Chuo-ku, Tokyo 104, Japan
Peter M. HOWLEY	Laboratory of Tumor Virus Biology, National Cancer Institute, NIH, Bethesda, Maryland 20892, U.S.A.
Nobuyuki ITO	Department of Pathology, Nagoya City University Medical School, Mizuho-ku, Nagoya 467, Japan
Peter A. JONES	Kenneth Norris Jr. Comprehensive Cancer Center, University of Southern California, Los Angels, California 90033-0800, U.S.A.
Motoya KATSUKI	Department of DNA Biology, Tokai University School of Medicine, Isehara, Kanagawa 259-11, Japan
Tomoyuki KITAGAWA	Department of Pathology, Cancer Institute, Japanese Foundation for Cancer Research, Toshima-ku, Tokyo 170, Japan
Marc E. LIPPMAN	Vincent T. Lombardi Cancer Research Center, Georgetown University Medical School, Washington, D.C. 20007, U.S.A.
Lawrence A. LOEB	Department of Pathology—SM-30 School of Medicine, University of Washington, Seattle, Washington 98195, U.S.A.
Suresh H. MOOLGAVKAR	Division of Public Health Sciences, Fred Hutchinson Cancer Research Center, Seattle, Washington 98104, U.S.A.
Harold L. MOSES	Department of Cell Biology, Vanderbilt University School of Medicine, Nashville, Tennessee 37232, U.S.A.
Yusuke NAKAMURA	Department of Biochemistry, Cancer Institute, Japanese Foundation for Cancer Research, Toshima-ku, Tokyo 170, Japan
Paul NETTESHEIM	Laboratory of Pulmonary Pathobiology, National Institute of Environmental Health Sciences, Research Triangle Park, North Carolina 27709, U.S.A.
Hiroto OKAYAMA	Department of Molecular Genetics, Research Institute for Microbial Disease, Osaka University, Suita, Osaka 565, Japan
Chawalit PAIROJKUL	Department of Pathology, Faculty of Medicine, Khon Kaen University, Khon Kaen 40002, Thailand
Henry C. PITOT	Department of Oncology and Pathology, McArdle Laboratory for Cancer Research, University of Wisconsin-Madison Medical School, Madison, Wisconsin 53706, U.S.A.
Takashi SUGIMURA	National Cancer Center, Chuo-ku, Tokyo 104, Japan
Yoshimi TAKAI	Department of Biochemistry, Kobe University School of Medicine, Chuo-ku, Kobe 650, Japan
Noritoshi TAKEICHI	Laboratory of Pathology, Cancer Institute, Hokkaido University School of Medicine, Kita-ku, Sapporo 060, Japan
Masaaki TERADA	Genetics Division, National Cancer Center Research

Institute, Chuo-ku, Tokyo 104, Japan

I. Bernard WEINSTEIN — Comprehensive Cancer Center, College of Physicians and Surgeons, Columbia University, New York, New York 10032, U.S.A.

Tadashi YAMAMOTO — Department of Oncology, Institute of Medical Science, University of Tokyo, Minato-ku, Tokyo 108, Japan

Mitsuhiro YANAGIDA — Department of Biophysics, Faculty of Science, Kyoto University, Sakyo-ku, Kyoto 606, Japan

Jun YOKOTA — Section of Studies on Metastasis, National Cancer Center Research Institute, Chuo-ku, Tokyo 104, Japan

Opening Address

H.I.H. Princess Kikuko Takamatsu

It is my great pleasure to deliver the opening address at this 22nd International Symposium of the Princess Takamatsu Cancer Research Fund. To all of the participants, particularly those who have traveled from abroad to be with us here, I extend my hearty welcome.

I share the grief of many people who have lost loved ones to cancer. I myself suffered from the loss of my mother more than 50 years ago, then my husband, Prince Takamatsu, four years ago, and recently Emperor Showa, two years ago. However, I am very optimistic that progress in cancer research will eventually conquer this tragic disease.

The subject of this year's symposium is "Multistage Carcinogenesis". Most clinical cancers are considered to develop through multiple stages over a long period of time, and I understand that multiple genetic changes and causative factors in the environment are involved in human cancer development. I have heard from my scientific advisors that links among multiple genetic changes, multiple causative factors, and multiple stages of carcinogenesis are currently subjects of very active study in the field of cancer research. I hope that the presentations at this meeting by the world's leading scientists in this exciting field will lead to stimulating discussions and make a significant contribution to a better understanding of the mechanisms of carcinogenesis and progression, which is essential for the prevention and treatment of human cancers.

I would like to express my sincere gratitude to Dr. Curtis C. Harris of the National Cancer Institute and Dr. Henry C. Pitot of the McArdle Laboratory for Cancer Research, both from the United States, for their valuable assistance in organizing this symposium.

I hereby announce the opening of the 22nd International Symposium of the Princess Takamatsu Cancer Research Fund. I am confident that the symposium will be a great success.

Dr. Henry C. Pitot

Your Imperial Highness:

I am privileged, in speaking for both the organizers and participants of the 22nd International Symposium of the Princess Takamatsu Cancer Research Fund, to thank you for your opening address, for the gracious hospitality that has been extended to us all on this occasion, and for honoring us with your presence during these proceedings. Cancer is a disease that affects all of humanity either directly or indirectly. We especially empathize with you on experiencing the loss of your husband, your mother, and other members of your family to this disease. Many of us have similarly been affected.

This symposium is concerned with the nature of the development of cancer through a series of stages from the first contact of a cell with a carcinogenic agent to the appearance of malignant disease. The multistage nature of cancer development was inferred from the numerous studies over the last century and a half on human and animal materials, including the pioneering experiments reported by your countrymen, Drs. Yamagiwa and Ichikawa in 1914, and by Dr. Yoshida and his colleagues in 1933. It was only as a result of these basic animal experiments on the induction of skin and liver cancer that the demonstration and characterization of distinct stages in neoplastic development in these tissues could be realized. During the last 50 years, and particularly since 1980, our knowledge of the basic nature and development of cancer has increased exponentially. The genetic events in cancer development occur both at the first interaction of a carcinogen with a cell and again after the progeny of that carcinogen-altered or initiated cell have developed into a large colony. This second genetic event endows the affected cell with malignant or cancerous potential, and is termed progression. Between these two irreversible events in cancer development is the reversible stage of promotion, which consists of the replication of initiated cells but requires the continued presence of the promoting agent. The implications of this simple scheme are enormous. The inhibition of the promotion stage by the elimination of promoting agents from one's immediate environment occurs after the cessation of smoking, after the lowering of the fat and caloric content of one's diet, and with the moderation of alcoholic intake. The stage of promotion may also be actively prevented by chemicals such as retinoids and antioxidants. Since the duration of the stage of promotion is extended in the development of many human cancers, its modification or inhibition may lead to the prevention of many human cancers.

The development of cancer itself occurs during the final, irreversible stage of progression. Our knowledge of the basic processes active during this stage comprise many of the subjects that will be reported at this symposium by your countrymen and their international colleagues. The roles of the expression of dominant protooncogenes and the lack of expression of recessive tumor suppressor genes during this stage will be among the many exciting presentations. Genes potentially active in the development of metastases—the ultimate fatal event in progression—will be described, as will chromosomal changes occurring during this stage. A thorough understanding of the mechanisms involved in the stage of progression will ultimately lead to the most effective therapy of patients afflicted with this dread disease.

The fight against cancer is worldwide. This annual symposium, which bears your name and to which you have given so much of your time and effort, is an outstanding example of international cooperation in science. This can only lead to a more rapid and complete understanding and ultimate control of this scourge of the human race. You, yourself, are following in the footsteps of numerous Japanese scientists who have already made outstanding contributions to cancer research. Through this symposium and its continuance for years to come, you will play a major role in the ultimate control of cancer. We all congratulate you, thank you, and wish you every joy and happiness, Princess Takamatsu, for many years into the future.

LECTURES

MULTISTAGE CARCINOGENESIS, C. C HARRIS ET AL. (EDS.),
JAPAN SCI. SOC. PRESS, TOKYO/CRC PRESS, BOCA RATON, PP. 3–19, 1992

KEYNOTE LECTURE

Molecular Basis of Multistage Carcinogenesis

Curtis C. Harris

Laboratory of Human Carcinogenesis, National Cancer Institute, National Institutes of Health, Bethesda, Maryland 20892, U.S.A.

Abstract: Revealing the molecular basis of human disease including cancer will be viewed as one of the triumphs of biomedical research in the 20th Century. One successful strategy has been to analyze abnormalities in cancer-related genes occurring in preneoplastic and neoplastic lesions in humans and animal models. These gene abnormalities, *e.g.*, mutations, can be specifically linked in some cases to environmental carcinogens in molecular epidemiological studies of human populations and in more controlled experimental conditions using animal or *in vitro* models of carcinogenesis. A second successful strategy has been to capitalize on advances from basic research such as defining signal transduction pathways in mammalian cells and the genetic control of the cell cycle in yeast. Mutations in yeast cell division control genes can lead to genomic instability and aneuploidy which are hallmarks of cancer. Therefore, the role of these genes in human carcinogenesis is being intensely investigated. The involvement of the p53 gene in the majority of human cancers has focused attention on the molecular and biochemical mechanisms of this tumor suppressor gene. The analysis of the p53 mutational spectrum in human cancers has provided evidence that both exogenous and endogenous causes of mutation contribute to human carcinogenesis. The increased understanding of the molecular basis of carcinogenesis has important implications in the prevention, diagnosis and treatment of human cancer.

Physicians, epidemiologists, and cancer researchers studying animal models have long recognized through observation of cancer development and mathematical modeling of cancer mortality data that carcinogenesis is a multistage process (*1*).* In the last decade, the molecular basis of this complex disorder of cellular organization and recognition and of molecular control of growth and differentiation pathways is being discovered in part due to recent advances in biotechnology that now allow researchers to test hypotheses many of which were proposed decades ago. For example, Boveri's speculations of cell division promoting and inhibiting chromosomes can be viewed from the prospective of the 1990's as oncogenes and tumor suppressor genes.

* Due to space limitations and the breadth of this topic, comprehensive reviews will be frequently cited and are the source of additional citations. This review is adapted from a recent comprehensive review (*1*).

"The unlimited tendency to rapid proliferation in malignant tumor cells (could result) from a permanent predominance of the chromosomes that promote division .... Another possibility (to explain cancer) is the presence of definite chromosomes which inhibit division .... Cells of tumors with unlimited growth would arise if those "inhibiting chromosomes" were eliminated .... (Since) each kind of chromosome is represented twice in the normal cell, the depression of only one of these two might pass unnoticed ...." —Boveri, 1914; translation published in 1929 (*2*).

Cancer-related genes were first identified from the analysis of mammalian retroviruses (*2*). DNA transfection technology, identification of related genes by amplification of DNA sequences coding functional domains by the polymerase chain reaction, reverse genetics *etc.* have rapidly expanded the number of these cancer-related genes. Molecular analysis of preneoplastic lesions, tumors and their metastasis have provided probabilistic information in regard to frequency of occurrence of the mutated protooncogenes and tumor suppressor genes in the spectrum of preneoplastic and neoplastic lesions. Whereas the frequency various among these lesions and a linear sequence of mutagenic and epigenetic events can be proposed, a critical analysis of these data indicate that the composite of these genetic events is more important than their sequence in a tissue type and that the most probable sequence varies among tissue types (*1, 3*).

Multistage Carcinogenesis

Carcinogenesis is a multistage process driven by carcinogen-induced genetic and epigenetic damage in susceptible cells that gain a selective growth advantage and undergo clonal expansion as the result of activation of protooncogenes and/or inactivation of tumor suppressor genes. The traditional view of carcinogenesis (Fig. 1) is derived primarily from animal models. The first stage of the carcinogenic process, tumor initiation, involves exposure of normal cells to chemical, physical or microbial

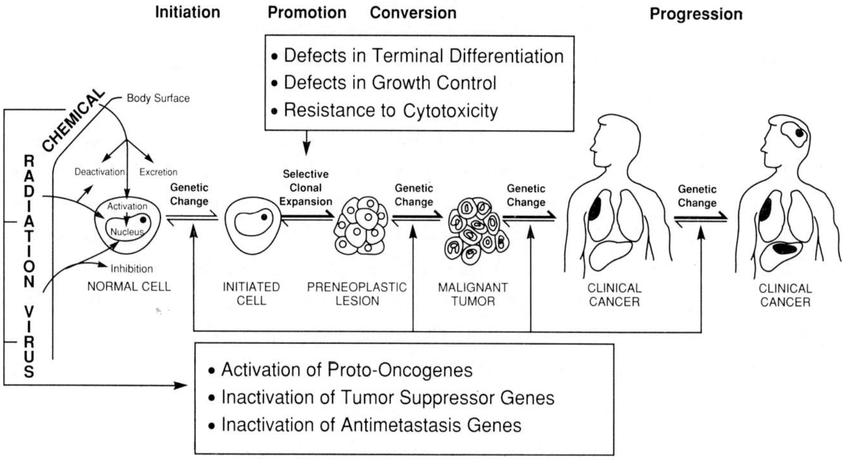

FIG. 1. Carcinogenesis is a multistage process involving multiple genetic and epigenetic events in protooncogenes, tumor suppressor genes, and anti-metastasis genes.

carcinogens that cause a genetic change(s) providing the initiated cells with both an altered responsiveness to their microenvironment and moreover exerts a selective clonal expansion advantage when compared to the surrounding normal cells (*4–6*). The initiated cells may have decreased responsiveness to the intercellular signals that maintain normal tissue architecture and regulate the homeostatic growth and maturation of cells. For example, initiated cells may be less responsive to negative growth factors and inducers of terminal cell differentiation (*4, 7–13*). Perturbation of the normal microenvironment by (a) physical means, *e.g.*, wounding of the mouse skin or partial hepatectomy in rodents, (b) chemical agents, *e.g.*, exposure of the mouse skin to certain phorbol esters or exposure of the rat liver to phenobarbital, (c) the inflammatory process, or (d) microbial agents, *e.g.*, influenza virus enhancement of rodent lung carcinogenesis or hepatitis viruses in human liver carcinogenesis, may also foster such selective clonal expansion of the initiated cells (*9, 14–16*).

Tumor promotion results in proliferation of the initiated cells to a greater extent than normal cells and enhances the probability of additional genetic damage including endogenous mutations accumulating in the expanding population of these cells. The probability of a subpopulation of initiated cells converting to malignancy can be substantially increased by their further exposure to DNA damaging agents (*17*–19) that may activate protooncogenes (*20*) and/or inactivate tumor suppressor genes. Malignant cells continue to exhibit progressive phenotypic changes during tumor progression (*21*), and may exhibit intrinsic genomic instability that is manifested by abnormal number and structure of chromosomes, gene amplification, and altered gene expression (*22–24*).

This classical view of two stage carcinogenesis involving a mutation, tumor initiation, and an epigenetic change, tumor promotion, has been conceptually important but is also considered to be simplistic in that the number of independent genetic and epigenetic events may be 6 or more in certain types of cancer (*3, 25, 26*). Furthermore, chemical carcinogens may: (a) not be considered mutagens, termed nongenotoxic carcinogens (*27*); (b) have both genetic and epigenetic effects such as the ability to induce mutations and the property of decreasing DNA methylation, respectively (*28*) or increase cellular proliferation; and (c) dose-response relationship with respect to tumor formation (*29, 30*). These and other observations have generated an active debate concerning both the contribution of endogenous mutagenic mechanisms, *e.g.*, oxy-radical DNA damage, DNA depurination, DNA polymerase infidelity and deamination of 5-methylcytosine, *versus* exogenous environmental mutagens and the value of animal bioassays to identify carcinogens and aid in human cancer risk assessment. This debate is not merely an academic one in that societal and regulatory decisions critical to public health are at issue.

1. Critical DNA targets: protooncogenes and tumor suppressor genes

Protooncogenes are normal cellular genes that, when inappropriately *activated* as oncogenes, cause dysregulation of growth and differentiation pathways and enhance the *probability* of neoplastic transformation. Carcinogens can cause the genetic changes that can lead to activation of protooncogenes, including base substitution mutations (*31*), chromosomal translocations (*32*), and gene amplification (*24, 33*). For example, *ras* protooncogenes are activated primarily at codons 12, 13, and 61 by base sub-

TABLE 1. Examples of Functions of Putative Tumor Suppressor Genes

Induce terminal differentiation
Maintain genomic stability
Trigger senescence
Induce programmed cell death
Regulate cell growth
Signal transducers of negative growth factors
Regulators, *e.g.*, protein tyrosine phosphatase γ (PTPase γ) of tyrosine kinases
Inhibit proteases
Alter DNA methylase activity
Modulate histocompatibility antigens
Regulate angiogenesis
Facilitate cell-cell communication

stitution mutations caused by chemical and physical carcinogens in both cultured mammalian cells and animal models (*34–37*) including transplacental exposure to chemical carcinogens (*38*). Mutation of the Ha-*ras* protooncogene is an early event in rodent models of skin and mammary carcinogenesis (*34, 39*). In addition, the v-Ha-*ras* transgene can substitute for the initiation step in mouse skin carcinogenesis in transgenic mice (*40, 41*). This animal model should be useful for investigating the molecular mechanisms of tumor promoters and antipromoters.

In contrast to protooncogenes, tumor suppressor genes are normal cellular genes that, when inappropriately *inactivated*, cause dysregulation of growth and differentiation pathways and enhance the *probability* of neoplastic transformation. Based on the multifunctional classes of tumor suppressor genes (Table 1) their number may equal that of the oncogenes. Loss of function of the products of both alleles is the basis of the 2-hit hypothesis and the recessive nature of the genetic process (*42*). In addition to inactivation of both alleles by mutational mechanisms (base substitution mutations, deletions, chromosomal nondisjunction, and recombination) (*43*), inactivation of a normal allele by genomic imprinting (*44*), and its gene product by an increased rate of proteolytic digestion (*45*) or dominant negative mechanisms (*46*) have been proposed. Based on target size theory, the inactivation of a single allele of a tumor suppressor gene should have an intrinsically higher probability than activation of a protooncogene, *e.g.*, one of the *ras* protooncogenes in which mutations in only a few specific codons will lead to activation. The requirement for inactivation of both alleles of a tumor suppressor gene counterbalances this probability except in those cases in which an inactivated allele is inherited or the mechanism of inactivation is *via* a dominant negative mechanism, as proposed for the p53 tumor suppressor gene (*46, 47*).

Ionizing irradiation and carcinogenic hormones, metals, aldehydes, or fibers such as asbestos are generally inefficient in the production of point mutations at the gene level, but are more efficient at causing chromosomal abnormalities and losses (*48*). Therefore, one would speculate that tumor suppressor genes would be targeted by these carcinogens more readily than protooncogenes. Whereas many electrophilic metabolites of chemical carcinogens form carcinogen-DNA adducts and cause point mutations, chemical carcinogens also cause chromosomal abnormalities and micronuclei. Thus, both cytogenetic and mutagenesis assays have been developed to assess these mutational changes (*23, 49–51*).

2. Mutational spectrum

The molecular analysis of mutationally-activated *ras* protooncogenes in animal models of carcinogenesis generally supports the concept of mutational spectrum reflecting the DNA adduct formation and mutagenic activities elicited by specific chemical carcinogens. For example, the mutations found in activated *ras* proto-oncogenes associated with tumors of rodents exposed to the methylating N-nitroso compounds are predominantly G: C→A: T base substitutions; these are likely due to methylation of guanine at the 0^6 position followed by mispairing with thymine during DNA synthesis (*39, 52–55*). Although there are several guanine residues in *ras* codons that would generate a transforming protein if substituted with adenine, the animal experiments have revealed that the mutations occur overwhelmingly at only one of the "possible" mutation sites. However, preferential mutation sites are within the admittedly narrow range of possibilities for activating *ras* genes. Unexplained mutational specificities have been observed in other experimental systems (*56–58*) and may reflect the differences in the spectrum of promutagenic carcinogen-DNA adducts, specificity of DNA repair enzymes (*59*) and/or the resultant amino acid changes are either silent or lethal.

TABLE 2. Nature of p53 Gene Base Substitution Mutations[a] by Cancer Type

Cancer location	Total mutations	Mutations at G: C			Transitions at CpG	Mutations at A: T		
		A: T	T: A	C: G		T: A	G: C	C: G
Somatic Mutations:								
Stomach	10	6 (60)[b]	2 (20)	0	5 (50)	1 (10)	0	1 (10)
Lung: SCLC	43	6 (60)[c]	20 (47)[c]	5 (12)	5 (12)[c]	2 (5)	6 (14)	2 (5)
non-SCLC	47	13 (28)[c]	24 (51)[c]	5 (11)	9 (19)[c]	2 (4)	2 (4)	1 (2)
Breast	63	27 (43)	12 (19)	9 (14)	14 (22)	3 (5)	10 (16)	2 (3)
Colon	48	36 (75)[c]	0†	2 (4)	30 (63)[c]	2 (4)	8 (17)	0
Esophagus	41	18 (44)	11 (27)	0	8 (20)	5 (12)	4 (10)	3 (7)
Liver	22	3 (14)	16 (73)[c]	1 (5)	0†	1 (5)	1 (5)	0
Bladder	15	7 (47)	2 (13)	3 (20)	5 (33)	0	2 (13)	1 (7)
Ovary	14	6 (43)	1 (7)	4 (29)	1 (7)	0	1 (7)	2 (14)
Sarcoma	12	8 (66)	2 (17)	2 (17)	7 (58)	0	0	0
Brain	24	17 (71)[c]	2 (8)	1 (4)	9 (38)	0	3 (13)	1 (4)
Skin	16[d]	11[d] (69)	4 (25)	1 (6)	1 (6)	0	0	0
All solid tumors	355	160 (45)	96 (27)	33 (9)	94 (26)	16 (5)	37 (10)	13 (4)
Lymphomas and leukemias	83	45 (54)	6 (7)[c]	7 (8)	35 (42)[c]	4 (5)	14 (17)	7 (8)
All tumors	438	205 (47)	102 (23)	40 (9)	129 (29)	20 (5)	51 (12)	20 (5)
Germline Mutations:								
Li-Fraumeni Syndrome	18	12 (67)	2 (11)	0	7 (39)	0	3 (17)	1 (86)

Other tumor types with ≤5 mutations reported thus far: endometrial (5); anal (3); thyroid (1); erythroleukemia (1); larnyx (1); cholangiocarcinoma (2); cervical (2); mesothelioma (2). Additional muatation studies on occupational/therapeutic drug exposure groups: Lung (radon) (6). SCLC: small cell lung cancer.

[a] Coding sequence mutations resulting in amino acid substitution. [b] Numbers in parentheses are percentage of mutations. [c] The difference between this value and corresponding number for all other solid tumors grouped together (χ^2, $p<0.01$ or less), calculated for tumors with total mutations >20. [d] Includes 3 double tandem mutations.

Although the mutational spectra of *ras* protooncogenes in rodent tumors caused by methylating carcinogens is consistent with the formation of the promutagenic 0^6-methyl-dG and mutational spectrum caused by N-nitroso-N′-methylurea in the *aprt* gene of CHO cells, an alternative hypothesis is that the mutant *ras* genes preexist in certain cells and exposure to the methylating agent facilitates clonal expansion of these mutant cells. This latter hypothesis has been indirectly tested by investigating the induction of rodent tumors by chemical carcinogens that form DNA adducts with differing chemical specificity. The mutational spectra can be highly correlated with each chemical carcinogen and reflected the predicted base substitution (*31*), *e.g.*, G: C→T: A transversion for benzo[a]pyrene which forms predominantly the N^2-BPDE-dG adduct (*60*) and A: T→T: A transversion for 7,12-dimethylbenzanthracene (DMBA) which forms predominantly the N^6-DMBA-diolepoide-dA adduct (*61*).

The mutational spectra of activated *ras* protooncogenes in tumors and preneoplastic lesions caused by chemical carcinogens in animal models may prove to be instructive in the interpretation of mutations in protooncogenes and tumor suppressor genes found in human cancers. The spectra of Ki-*ras* protooncogene mutations in human adenocarcinomas vary according to tissue site; for example, G: C→T: A transversions occur in lung tumors, whereas G: C→A: T transitions predominate in colonic tumors. The interpretation of these results, however, may be confounded by spontaneous mutations engendered by either endogenous mutagens or DNA polymerase errors. As two examples, 8-OH-dG, caused by oxy-radical damage (*62*) and DNA depurination can produce G: C→T: A transversions, and DNA polymerase infidelity will also produce G: C→T: A transversions as well as other changes (*63*).

The p53 tumor suppressor gene is ideally suited for analysis of mutational spectrum. First, p53 is well-conserved in evolution (*64*) and 5 domains are $>90\%$ homologous in DNA sequence among humans and rodents that are frequently used in animal models of carcinogenesis. Second, p53 is mutated in diverse types of human cancer (*65–69*). Third, a wide spectrum of mutational types and codon sites have been observed that presumably define regions of the p53 protein likely to be essential for its biological activity in cell cycle control, tumor suppression and for its interaction with other cellular and viral proteins. A recent review (*70*) has concluded that the majority of the mutations in human tumors occurs in the evolutionarily highly conserved domains in exons 5–8 of the p53 gene, and the missense mutations are predominantly transitions at G: C base pairs and are almost all ($>99\%$) at amino acids that are entirely conserved in mouse, rat, monkey and human. Mutational spectra also vary among cancer types (Table 2). The G: C→A: T transitions are the most frequent in colon tumors and 70% of the mutations occur at CpG dinucleotides. These findings are consistent with the endogenous mutational mechanism due to deamination of 5-methylcytosine residues found at CpG dinucleotides in the mammalian genome. More than half of the p53 mutations in colon tumors are at "hotspots", codons 175, 248 or 273, each of which is a CpG dinucleotide.

In contrast to colon tumors, CpG dinucleotides are less frequently sites of mutations in most other types of human cancers. Whereas G: C→T: A mutations are rare in colon tumors, these transversions are significantly more common in breast and lung cancers. The G: C→T: A mutations in Ki-*ras* protooncogene are also found in human lung adenocarcinomas (*71–73*) and in rodent lung cancers caused by benzo-[a]pyrene. Whereas CpG→TpG mutations occur with intermediate frequency in esophageal cancers, 36% of the mutations are at A: T pairs which may be due in part to DNA depurination and/or exposure to chemical carcinogens such as urethane, that is a contaminant of certain alcoholic beverages.

The most striking p53 mutational spectrum is found in hepatocellular carcinomas from either Qidong, People's Rebublic of China (*74*) or southern Africa (*75*). Eleven out of 12 base substitution mutations in 26 tumors were at a single site, the 3rd base position of codon 249, and all but one were G: C→T: A transversions. One additional mutation at codon 157 was also a G: C→T: A transversion. These tumors were from patients who live in geographic areas where aflatoxin B_1 and hepatitis B virus are major risk factors. Aflatoxin B_1 is a naturally-occurring hepatocarcinogen that forms N7dG promutagenic adducts and induces primarily G: C→T: A transversions and G: C→A: T transitions in experimental systems (*76*). Analysis of liver tumors from geographical areas where aflatoxin B_1 is considered not to be a significant risk factor will be instructive in determining whether exposure to this fungal carcinogen or another co-incident carcinogen may be responsible for these p53 mutations.

An analysis of mutational spectra in human tumors from populations with differing risk factors may provide insight in a manner similar to the studies in experimental animals described above. In addition to further studies of liver cancer, the mutational spectra of Ki-*ras* and/or the p53 gene could be compared to bronchogenic cancers, including the use of paraffin-embedded, fixed archival tissue, from cigarette smokers versus nonsmokers and from workers in high risk occupations, *e.g.*, uranium mining, mustard gas production, asbestos mining and chlormethyl ether production.

3. *Genomic instability*

Normal human somatic cells maintain a diploid karyotype and have a mutation frequency of about 10^{-8} for hemoglobin variants (point mutations), about 10^{-7}

TABLE 3. Examples of Gene Abnormalities Associated with Genomic Instability[a)]

Gene	Species	Genomic instability	
		Activation	Type
RAD 9	*S. cerevisiae*	Mutation	Chromosomal loss
RAD 18	*S. cerevisiae*	Mutation	Base substitution (G: C→T: A transversion)
$p34^{cdc2}$	*S. pombe*	Mutation	Aneuploidy
Topoisomerase II	*S. pombe*	Mutation	Abnormal chromosomal segregation
nod	*Drosophila*	Mutation	Abnormal chromosomal segregation
DNA polymerase α	Human	Mutation	Base substitution
p53	Human (Li-Fraumeni syndrome)	Mutation	Aneuploidy
RAG-1	Human	Mutation[b)]	Chromosomal rearrangements and deletions
scid	Murine	Mutation	Aberrant V-(D)-J recombination and double-strand break DNA repair
Unknown	Human (Bloom's syndrome)	Unknown	Hyperrecombination

[a)] Ref. *1* [b)] *In vitro* experimental studies.

for *hprt* variants (measures many classes of mutations, but the assay does not detect mitotic recombination) and about 10^{-5} for glycophorin A or major histocompatibility complex (HLA) variants (measures most classes of mutations including somatic recombination, gene conversion or chromosomal non-dysjunction) (*77–79*).

The potential sources for these observed mutation frequencies include exposure to "background" levels of environmental chemical and physical agents and endogenous mechanisms (*80*) such as: (a) the *chemical instability of DNA, e.g.*, depurination (one can calculate that cell undergoes 10^4 depurinations per day (*63*)) or deamination of 5-methylcytosine to yield thymidine (*81, 82*); (b) *free radicals of oxygen, e.g.*, hydroxyl ions (from measurements of 8-OHdG and thymine glycol in urine, about 10^4 oxy-radical induced DNA lesions occur in each human cell per day (*83*)); and (c) *DNA replication errors*. Imbalances in deoxynucleoside triphosphate pools (*84*) and mutations in DNA polymerase alpha (*85*) are examples of mechanisms leading to infidelity of DNA synthesis. Inactivation of RAD18, a putative DNA repair gene in *Saccharomyces cerevisiae*, leads to an increase in the frequency of G: C→T: A transversions (*86*). Therefore, examples of gene abnormalities associated with genomic instability are rapidly being identified (Table 3).

Considering the multiplicity of proteins involved in DNA synthesis, DNA repair, mitosis, and the cell cycle, the number of potential gene targets in somatic cells is large and could result in the mutator phenotype (*22, 87*) that could increase the probability of both neoplastic transformation and the generation of more malignant subclones during tumor progression (*21, 88*). If such mutations occur in germ cells and are nonlethal, they could lead to congenital abnormalities and increased cancer risk in an inherited manner. The hypothesis that genomic instability may have an inherited basis and be associated with increased cancer risk is supported by studies of Bloom's syndrome, where an increase in cytogenetic endpoints is observed (*89*) and of colonic carcinomas, where a significant increase in allelic deletions is found in tumors from patients who have first degree relatives with cancer (*90*).

Cytogenetic studies (*91, 92*) have provided the bulk of the indirect evidence supporting the hypothesis that genomic instability is a potential mechanism driving tumor progression. The evidence is less compelling (*93*) when the frequencies of either spontaneous point mutations (*94–101*) or drug-induced gene amplification (*102–106*) is compared in normal and neoplastic cells.

Recombinase infidelity (*107*), telomere reduction (*108*), and DNA hypomethylation (*3, 109*) are examples of additional mechanisms of genomic instability. The frequency of somatic recombinational events at certain loci, *e.g.*, immunoglobulin genes, is relatively high, but specific DNA sequences at these loci are recognized by the responsible V-(D)-J recombinases. Although the degree of infidelity of wild type and mutant recombinases is not known, a possible example of "illegitimate" V-(D)-J recombinase activity leading to interstitial deletion and rearrangements in a growth-regulatory gene has been recently described (*110*).

Hastie *et al.* (*108*) have shown that telomere reduction is common in both colorectal adenomas and carcinomas and have speculated that telomere reduction may be involved as an early event in carcinogenesis. Interestingly, studies of yeast (*111*) and maize (*112*) have shown that chromosomes without terminal repeats or telomeres are prone to rearrangements or loss. Studies in yeast have also identified genes involved in cell cycle control and mitosis, *e.g.*, RAD9 and cdc-2, that, when mutated, influence the fidelity of mitosis (*113, 114*). For example, certain mutations in RAD9 of *S. cerevisiae* increases the rate of chromosomal loss by 7- to 21-fold (*115*) and topoisomerase II mutants in *S. pombe* have abnormal segregation of the intertwined daughter chromosomes at the end of DNA replication (*116*) and abnormal chromosome condensation (*117*). Since human homologues of such genes are being identified, similar investigations could be conducted using cultured human cells, and human tumors could be examined for mutations in these genes.

Analogous to the yeast paradigm of a mutator phenotype associated with dysregulation of cell cycle control (*113*), certain activated protooncogenes or inactivated tumor suppressor genes could lead to genomic instability. The rapid appearance of aneuploidy and "spontaneous" immortalization of cultured human fibroblasts from donors with the Li-Fraumeni syndrome, who have an inherited mutant p53 allele (*118*), is consistent with this hypothesis. The genomic instability caused by certain DNA viruses such as SV40, adenovirus and papillomavirus could also be due to the inactivation of p53 and/or Rb.

As argued by Loeb (*80*), the impression of a high degree of genomic stability may be misleading when one considers that the human body contains about 10^{14} cells and, within the average human lifespan, the cells undergo a total of 10^{16} divisions. Therefore, spontaneous mutagenesis may significantly contribute to the prevalence of certain cancer types that have no apparent risk factors and minimal variations in incidence occur among different geographic areas. However, epidemiological studies have: (a) identified significant cancer risk factors, *e.g.*, tobacco smoke and hepatitis B virus; (b) found substantial geographic variation in the incidence of the most common types of human cancer; and (c) found that migrant populations frequently acquire the risk of cancer prevailing in their new geographic location of residence (*119–121*). Based on the above and other considerations (*120*), it has been estimated that about 80% of all cancer in the United States is due to environmental factors. Finally, one can speculate that the rates of spontaneous mutations, *e.g.*, deamination of 5-methylcytosine, may be altered by environmental chemicals directly and/or indirectly *via* generation of endogenous agents such as the intracellular signal transducer, nitric oxide.

Molecular Epidemiology of Human Cancer

Combined laboratory-epidemiological studies of human cancer have a long history and have been named metabolic (*122*), biochemical (*123*), and molecular epidemiology (*124*). Whereas classical epidemiology has been successful in identifying high cancer risk *populations*, *e.g.*, cigarette smokers, the primary goal of molecular epidemiology is to identify *individuals* in these populations who are at the highest cancer risk. The current strategy involves improved exposure assessment by measuring biologically effective doses of carcinogens and secondly, analysis of host susceptibility factors within the framework of well-desinged epidemiological studies (*125*).

The identification of inherited or acquired host susceptibility factors (Table 4) is also becoming an important factor in the risk assessment equation (*125*). Analogous

TABLE 4. Examples of Inherited Predisposition of Human Cancer[a)]

Candidate gene	Condition	Examples of cancer type
p53	Li-Fraumeni syndrome	Carcinomas of the breast and bladder; sarcomas
Rb	Familial retinoblastoma	Retinoblastoma
APC	Familial polyposis coli	Colon
CYP2D6	Extensive debrisoquine phenotype	Lung
XPAC	Xeroderma pigmentosum A	Skin

a) Ref. *1*.

to the confoundment of exposure assessment by complex mixtures, time course variables, *etc.*, generic problems concerning the use of data on host susceptibility factors in risk assessment are evident: (a) rank order of "potency or weight" of various host susceptibility factors influencing the cancer risk in individuals exposed to carcinogens; (b) "potency" impact of the degree of the interindividual variation in a specific host susceptibility factor; and (c) interactive effects among various host susceptibility factors. In addition, societal and ethical issues come to the forefront whenever individuals at high disease risk are identified. These issues are already being actively discussed (*126*). Finally, the conduct of well-designed and multifaceted molecular epidemiological studies will require the development of a new cadre of scientists that have knowledge and skills in both laboratory science and analytical epidemiology.

REFERENCES

1. Harris, C. C. Chemical and physical carcinogenesis: advances and perspectives. Cancer Res., *51*: 5023s–5044s, 1991.
2. Bishop, J. M. Molecular themes in oncogenesis. Cell, *64*: 235–248, 1991.
3. Fearon, E. R. and Vogelstein, B. A genetic model for colorectal tumorigenesis. Cell, *61*: 759–767, 1990,
4. Yuspa, S. H. and Harris, C. C. Molecular and cellular basis of chemical carcinogenesis. *In*; D. Schottenfeld and J. F., Fraumeni (eds.), Cancer Epidemiology and Prevention, pp. 23–43, W. B. Saunders, Philadelphia, 1982.
5. Cerutti, P. A. Prooxidant states and tumor promotion. Science, *227*: 375–381, 1985.
6. Weinstein, I. B., Borner, C. M., Krauss, R. S., O'Driscoll, K., Choi, P. M., Moritomi, M., Hoshina, S., Hsieh, L. L., Tchou-Wong, K. M., Guadagno, S. N., Ueffing, M., and Guillem, J. Pleiotropic effects of protein kinase C and the concept of carcinogenesis as a progressive disorder in signal transduction. *In*; J. Brugge, T. Curren, E. Harlow, and F. McCormick (eds.), Origins of Human Cancer, pp. 113–124, Cold Spring Harbor Laboratory Press, New York, 1991.
7. Willey, J. C., Moser, C. E., Jr., Lechner, J. F., and Harris, C. C. Differential effects of 12-O-tetradecanoylphorbol′-13-acetate on cultured normal and neoplastic human bronchial epithelial cells. Cancer Res., *44*: 5124–5126, 1984.
8. Parkinson, E. K. Defective responses of transformed keratinocytes to terminal differentiation stimuli. Their role in epidermal tumour promotion by phorbol esters and by deep skin wounding. Br. J. Cancer, *52*: 479–493, 1985.
9. Yuspa, S. H. and Poirier, M. C. Chemical carcinogenesis: from animal models to

molecular models in one decade. Adv. Cancer Res., *50*: 25–70, 1988.
10. Pfeifer, A., Lechner, J. F., Masui, T., Reddel, R. R., Mark, G. E., and Harris, C. C. Control of growth and squamous differentiation in normal human bronchial epithelial cells by chemical and biological modifiers and transferred genes. Environ. Health Perspect., *80*: 209–220, 1989.
11. Yuspa, S. H., Ben, T., Hennings, H., and Lichti, U. Divergent responses in epidermal basal cells exposed to the tumor promoter 12-O-tetradecanoylphorbol-13-acetate. Cancer Res., *42*: 2344–2349, 1982.
12. Parkinson, E. K., Grabham, P., and Emmerson, A. A subpopulation of cultured human keratinocytes which is resistant to the induction of terminal differentiation-related changes by phorbol, 12-myristate, 13-acetate: evidence for an increase in the resistant population following transformation. Carcinogenesis, *4*: 857–861, 1983.
13. Moses, H. L., Yang, E. Y., and Pietenpol, J. A. TGF-β stimulation and inhibition of cell proliferation: new mechanistic insights. Cell, *63*: 245–247, 1990.
14. Slaga, T. J. Overview of tumor promotion in animals. Environ. Health Perspect., *50*: 3–14, 1983.
15. Haugen, A. and Harris, C.C. Interactive effects between viruses and chemical carcinogens. *In*; C. S. Cooper and P. L. Grover (eds.), Carcinogenesis and Mutagenesis, Handbook of Experimental Pharmacology, pp. 249–268, Springer-Verlag, London, 1990.
16. Pitot, H. C. Principles of carcinogenesis: chemical. *In*; V. T. DeVita, Jr., S. Hellman, and S. A. Rosenberg (eds.), Cancer. Principles and Practice of Oncology, pp. 116–135, J. B. Lippincott, Philadelphia, 1990.
17. Hennings, H., Shores, R., Wenk, M. L., Spangler, E. F., Tarone, R., and Yuspa, S. H. Malignant conversion of mouse skin tumours is increased by tumour initiators and unaffected by tumour promoters. Nature, *304*: 67–69, 1983.
18. O'Connell, J. F., Klein-Szanto, A. J., Digiovanni, D. M., Fries, J. W., and Slaga, T. J. Malignant progression of mouse skin papillomas treated with ethylnitrosourea, N-methyl-N′-nitro-N-nitrosoguanidine, or 12-O-tetradecanoylphorbol-13-acetate. Cancer Lett., *30*: 269–274, 1986.
19. Hennings, H. Malignant conversion: the first stage in progression from benign to malignant tumors. *In*; T. J. Slaga, A. J. P. Klein-Szanto, R. K. Boutwell, D. E. Stevenson, H. L. Spitzer, and B. D'Motto (eds.), Skin Carcinogenesis, pp. 95–105, Alan R. Liss, New York, 1989.
20. Yuspa, S. H., Hennings, H., Roop, D., Strickland, J., and Greenhalgh, D. A. Genes and mechanisms involved in malignant conversion. *In*; C. C. Harris and L. A. Liotta (eds.), Genetic Mechanisms in Carcinogenesis and Tumor Progression, pp. 115–126, Wiley-Liss, New York, 1990.
21. Foulds, L. The experimental study of tumor progression: a review. Cancer Res., *14*: 317–339, 1954.
22. Nowell, P. C. The clonal evolution of tumor cell populations. Science, *194*: 23–28, 1976.
23. Rowley, J. D. Molecular cytogenetics: Rosetta stone for understanding cancer—Twenty-ninth G. H. A. Clowes Memorial Award Lecture. Cancer Res., *50*: 3816–3825, 1990.
24. Schimke, R. T. The search for early genetic events in tumorigenesis: an amplification paradigm. Cancer Cells, *2*: 149–151, 1990.
25. Peto, R., Roe, F. J., Lee, P. N., Levy, L., and Clack, J. Cancer and ageing in mice and men. Br. J. Cancer, *32*: 411–426, 1975.
26. Cairns, J. Mutation selection and the natural history of cancer. Nature, *255*: 197–

200, 1975.

27. Butterworth, B. E. and Slaga, T. J. (eds.). *In*; Nongenotoxic Mechanisms in Carcinogenesis—Banbury Report Vol. 25, Cold Spring Harbor Laboratory Press, New York, 1987.
28. Wilson, V. L., Smith, R. A., Longoria, J., Liotta, M. A., Harper, C. M., and Harris, C. C. Chemical carcinogen-induced decreases in genomic 5-methyldeoxycytidine content of normal human bronchial epithelial cells. Proc. Natl. Acad. Sci. U.S.A., *84*: 3298–3301, 1987.
29. Lutz, W. K. Dose-response relationship and low dose extrapolation in chemical carcinogenesis. Carcinogenesis, *11*: 1243–1247, 1990.
30. Swenberg, J. A., Richardson, F. C., Boucheron, J. A., Deal, F. H., Belinsky, S.A., Charbonneau, M., and Short, B. G. High- to low-dose extrapolation: critical determinants involved in the dose response of carcinogenic substances. Environ. Health Perspect., *76*: 57–63, 1987.
31. Singer, B. and Grunberger, D. Molecular Biology of Mutagens and Carcinogens, Plenum Press, New York, 1983.
32. Preston, R. J. Mechanisms of induction of specific chromosomal alterations. *In*; B. M. Sutherland and A. D. Woodhead (eds.), DNA Damage and Repair in Human Tissues, pp. 329–336, Plenum Press, New York, 1990.
33. Lavi, S. Carcinogen-mediated amplification of viral DNA sequences in simian virus 40-transformed Chinese hamster embryo cells. Proc. Natl. Acad. Sci. U.S.A., *78*: 6144–6148, 1981.
34. Brown, K., Buchmann, A., and Balmain, A. Carcinogen-induced mutations in the mouse c-Ha-ras gene provide evidence of multiple pathways for tumor progression. Proc. Natl. Acad. Sci. U.S.A., *87*: 538–542, 1990.
35. Barbacid, M. *ras* genes. Annu. Rev. Biochem., *56*: 779–827, 1987.
36. Newcomb, E. W., Diamond, L. E., Sloan, S. R., Corominas, M., Guerrero, I., and Pellicer, A. Radiation and chemical activation of *ras* oncogenes in different mouse strains. Environ. Health Perspect., *81*: 33–37, 1989.
37. Balmain, A. and Brown, K. Oncogene activation in chemical carcinogenesis. Adv. Cancer Res., *51*: 147–182, 1988.
38. Yamasaki, H., Hollstein, M., Martel, N., Cabral, J. R., Galendo, D., and Tomatis, L. Transplacental induction of a specific mutation in fetal Ha-ras and its critical role in post-natal carcinogenesis. Int. J. Cancer, *40*: 818–822, 1987.
39. Sukumar, S. An experimental analysis of cancer: role of *ras* oncogenes in multistep carcinogenesis. Cancer Cells, *2*: 199–204, 1990.
40. Bailleul, B., Surani, M. A., White, S., Barton, S.C., Brown, K., Blessing, M., Jorcano, J., and Balmain, A. Skin hyperkeratosis and papilloma formation in transgenic mice expressing a *ras* oncogene from a suprabasal keratin promoter. Cell, *62*: 697–708, 1990.
41. Leder, A., Kuo, A., Cardiff, R. D., Sinn, E., and Leder, P. v-Ha-*ras* transgene abrogates the initiation step in mouse skin tumorigenesis: effects of phorbol esters and retinoic acid. Proc. Natl. Acad. Sci. U.S.A., *87*: 9178–9182, 1990.
42. Knudson, A. G., Jr. Mutation and cancer: statistical study of retinoblastoma. Proc. Natl. Acad. Sci. U S.A., *68*: 820–823, 1971.
43. Cavenee, W. K., Dryja, T. P., Phillips, R. A., Benedict, W. F., Godbout, R., Gallie, B. L., Murphree, A. L., Strong, L. C., and White, R. L. Expression of recessive alleles by chromosomal mechanisms in retinoblastoma. Nature, *305*: 779–784, 1983.
44. Sapienza, C. Genome imprinting, cellular mosaicism and carcinogenesis. Mol. Carcinogen., *3*: 118–121, 1990.

45. Scheffner, M., Werness, B. A., Huibregtse, J. M., Levine, A. J., and Howley, P. M. The E6 oncoprotein encoded by human papillomavirus types 16 and 18 promotes the degradation of p53. Cell, *63*: 1129–1136, 1990.
46. Herskowitz, I. Functional inactivation of genes by dominant negative mutations. Nature, *329*: 219–222, 1987.
47. Green, M. R. When the products of oncogenes and anti-oncogenes meet. Cell, *56*: 1–3, 1989.
48. Barrett, J. C. The relationship between mutagenesis and carcinogenesis. *In*; J. Brugge, T. Curren, E. Harlow and F. McCormick (eds.), Origins of Human Cancer, pp. 101–112, Cold Spring Harbor Laboratory Press, New York, 1991.
49. Waldren, C., Correll, L., Sognier, M. A., and Puck, T.T. Measurement of low levels of x-ray mutagenesis in relation to human disease. Proc. Natl. Acad. Sci. U.S.A., *83*: 4839–4843, 1986.
50. Gray, J. W., Lucas, L., Kallioniemi, O., Kallioniemi, A., Kuo, W. L., Pinkel, D., Tkachuk, D., and Weier, U. Applications of fluorescence *in situ* hybridization in biological dosimetry. *In*; B. L. Gledhill and F. Mauro (eds.), Trends in Biological Dosimetry, Wiley-Liss, New York, in press.
51. Wolff, S. Biological dosimetry with cytogenetic endpoints. *In*; B. L. Gledhill and F. Mauro (eds.), Trends in Biological Dosimetry, pp. 351–362, Wiley-Liss, New York, 1991.
52. Loveless, A. Possible relevance of 0-6 alkylation of deoxyguanosine to the mutagenicity and carcinogenicity of nitrosamines and nitrosamides. Nature, *223*: 206–207, 1969.
53. Loechler, E. L., Green, C. L., and Essigmann, J. M. *In vivo* mutagenesis by 06-methylguanine built into a unique site in a viral genome. Proc. Natl. Acad. Sci. U.S.A., *81*: 6271–6275, 1984.
54. Zarbl, H., Sukumar, S., Arthur, A. V., Martin-Zanca, D., and Barbacid, M. Direct mutagenesis of Ha-*ras*-1 oncogenes by N-nitroso-N-methylurea during initiation of mammary carcinogenesis in rats. Nature, *315*: 382–385, 1985.
55. Basu, A. K. and Essigmann, J. M. Site-specifically alkylated oligodeoxynucleotides: probes for mutagenesis, DNA repair and the structural effects of DNA damage. Mutat. Res., *233*: 189–201, 1990.
56. Doniger, J., Notario, V., and DiPaolo, J. A. Carcinogens with diverse mutagenic activities initiate neoplastic guinea pig cells that acquire the same N-*ras* point mutation. J. Biol. Chem., *262*: 3813–3819, 1987.
57. Pelling, J. C., Neades, R., and Strawhecker, J. Epidermal papillomas and carcinomas induced in uninitiated mouse skin by tumor promoters alone contain a point mutation in the 61st codon of the Ha-*ras* oncogene. Carcinogenesis, *9*: 665–667, 1988.
58. Brookes, P. Chemical carcinogens and *ras* gene activation. Mol. Carcinogen., *2*: 305–307, 1989.
59. Topal, M. D. DNA repair, oncogenes and carcinogenesis. Carcinogenesis, *9*: 691–696, 1988.
60. Weinstein, I. B., Jeffrey, A. M., Jennette, K. W., Blobstein, S. H., Harvey, R. G., Harris, C. C., Autrup, H., Kasai, H., and Nakanishi, K. Benzo(a)pyrene diol epoxides as intermediates in nucleic acid binding *in vitro* and *in vivo*. Science, *193*: 592–595, 1976.
61. Dipple, A., Pigott, M., Moschel, R. C., and Costantino, N. Evidence that binding of 7,12-dimethylbenz(a)anthracene to DNA in mouse embryo cell cultures results in extensive substitution of both adenine and guanine residues. Cancer Res., *43*: 4132–4135, 1983.
62. Wood, M. L., Dizdaroglu, M., Gajewski, E., and Essigmann, J. M. Mechanistic

studies of ionizing radiation and oxidative mutagenesis: genetic effects of a single 8-hydroxyguanine (7-hydro-8-oxoguanine) residue inserted at a unique site in a viral genome. Biochemistry, *349*: 7024–7032, 1990.
63. Lindahl, T. and Nyberg, B. Rate of depurination of native deoxyribonucleic acid. Biochemistry, *11*: 3610–3618, 1972.
64. Soussi, T., Caron de Fromentel, C., and May, P. Structural aspects of the p53 protein in relation to gene evolution. Oncogene, *5*: 945–952, 1990.
65. Nigro, J. M., Baker, S. J., Preisinger, A. C., Jessup, J. M., Hostetter, R., Cleary, K., Bigner, S. H., Davidson, N., Baylin, S., Devilee, P., Glover, T., Collins, F. S., Weston, A., Modali, R., Harris, C. C., and Vogelstein, B. Mutations in the p53 gene occur in diverse human tumor types. Nature, *342*: 705–708, 1989.
66. Takahashi, T., Nau, M. M., Chiba, I., Birrer, M. J., Rosenberg, R. K., Vinocour, M., Levitt, M., Pass, H., Gazdar, A. F., and Minna, J. D. p53: a frequent target for genetic abnormalities in lung cancer. Science, *246*: 491–494, 1989.
67. Iggo, R., Gatter, K., Bartek, J., Lane, D., and Harris, A. L. Increased expression of mutant forms of p53 oncogene in primary lung cancer. Lancet, *335*: 675–679, 1990.
68. Mulligan, L. M., Matlashewski, G., Scrable, H. J., and Cavenee, W. K. Mechanisms of p53 loss in human sarcomas. Proc. Natl. Acad. Sci. U.S.A., *87*: 5863–5867, 1990.
69. Hollstein, M., Metcalf, R. A., Welsh, J., Montesano, R., and Harris, C. C. Frequent mutation of the p53 gene in human esophageal cancer. Proc. Natl. Acad. Sci. U.S.A., *87*: 9958–9961, 1990.
70. Hollstein, M., Sidransky, D., Vogelstein, B., and Harris, C. C. p53 mutations in human cancers. Science, *253*: 49–53, 1991.
71. Rodenhuis, S., Van de Wetering, M. L., Mooi, W. J., Evers, S. G., van Zandwijk, N., and Bos, J. L. Mutational activation of the K-*ras* oncogene. A possible pathogenetic factor in adenocarcinoma of the lung. N. Engl. J. Med., *317*: 929–935, 1987.
72. Slebos, R. J., Kibbelaar, R. E., Dalesio, O., Kooistra, A., Stam, J., Meijer, C. J., Wagenaar, S. S., Vanderschueren, R. G., van Zandwijk, N., Mooi, W. J., Bos, J. L., and Rodenhuis, S. K-*ras* oncogene activation as a prognostic marker in adenocarcinoma of the lung. N. Engl. J. Med., *323*: 561–565, 1990.
73. Bos, J. L. *Ras* oncogenes in human cancer: a review. Cancer Res., *49*: 4682–4689, 1989.
74. Hsu, I. C., Metcalf, R. A., Sun, T., Welsh, J., Wang, N. J., and Harris, C. C. p53 gene mutational hotspot in human hepatocellular carcinomas from Qidong, China. Nature, *350*: 427–428, 1991.
75. Bressac, B., Kew, M., Wands, J., and Ozturk, M. Selective G to T mutations of p53 gene in hepatocellular carcinoma from southern Africa. Nature, *350*: 429–431, 1991.
76. McMahon, G., Davis, E. F., Huber, L. J., Kim, Y., and Wogan, G. N. Characterization of c-Ki-*ras* and N-*ras* oncogenes in aflatoxin B_1-induced rat liver tumors. Proc. Natl. Acad. Sci. U.S.A., *87*: 1104–1108, 1990.
77. Albertini, R. J., Sullivan, L. M., Berman, J. K., Greene, C. J., Stewart, J. A., Silveira, J. M., and O'Neill, J. P. Mutagenicity monitoring in humans by autoradiographic assay for mutant T lymphocytes. Mutat. Res., *204*: 481–492, 1988.
78. Cole, J., Waugh, A. P. W., Beare, D. M., Sala-Trepat, M., Stephens, G. and Green, M. H. L. HPRT mutant frequencies in circulating lymphocytes: population studies using normal donors, exposed groups and cancer-prone syndromes. *In*; B. L. Gledhill and F. Mauro (eds.), Trends in Biological Dosimetry, pp. 319–328, Wiley-Liss, New York, 1991.
79. Menichini, P. and Abbondandolo, A. Somatic gene mutations in humans. *In*; B. L. Gledhill and F. Mauro (eds.), Trends in Biological Dosimetry, pp. 267–279, Wiley-

Liss, New York, 1991.

80. Loeb, L. A. Endogenous carcinogenesis: molecular oncology into the twenty-first century—presidential address. Cancer Res., *49*: 5489–5496, 1989.
81. Ehrlich, M. and Wang, R. Y. 5-Methylcytosine in eukaryotic DNA. Science, *212*: 1350–1357, 1981.
82. Ehrlich, M., Zhang, X. Y., and Inamdar, N. M. Spontaneous deamination of cytosine and 5-methylcytosine residues in DNA and replacement of 5-methylcytosine residues with cytosine residues. Mutat. Res., *238*: 277–286, 1990.
83. Ames, B. N. Endogenous DNA damage as related to cancer and aging. Mutat. Res., *214*: 41–46, 1989.
84. Phear, G., Nalbantoglu, J., and Meuth, M. Next-nucleotide effects in mutations driven by DNA precursor pool imbalances at the aprt locus of Chinese hamster ovary cells. Proc. Natl. Acad. Sci. U.S.A., *84*: 4450–4454, 1987.
85. Liu, P. K., Chang, C. C., Trosko, J. E., Dube, D. K., Martin, G. M., and Loeb, L. A. Mammalian mutator mutant with an aphidicolin-resistant DNA polymerase alpha. Proc. Natl. Acad. Sci. U.S.A., *80*: 797–801, 1983.
86. Kunz, B. A., Kang, X., and Kohalmi, L. The yeast *rad18* mutator specifically increases G: C-> T: A transversion without reducing correction of G-A or C-T mismatches to G: C pairs. Mol. Cell. Biol., *11*: 218–225, 1991.
87. Loeb, L. A., Springgate, C. F., and Battula, N. Errors in DNA replication as a basis of malignant changes. Cancer Res., *34*: 2311–2321, 1974.
88. Chorazy, M. Sequence rearrangements and genome instability. A possible step in carcinogenesis. J. Cancer Res. Clin. Oncol., *109*: 159–172, 1985.
89. German, J. Bloom's syndrome, X. The cancer proneness points to chromosome mutation as a crucial event in human neoplasia. *In*; J. German (ed.), Chromosome Mutation and Neoplasia, pp. 347–357, Alan R. Liss, New York, 1983.
90. Kern, S. E., Fearon, E. R., Tersmette, K. W., Enterline, J. P., Leppert, M., Nakamura, Y., White, R., Vogelstein, B., and Hamilton, S. R. Allelic loss in colorectal carcinoma. JAMA, *261*: 3099–3103, 1989.
91. Nowell, P. C. Mechanisms of tumor progression. Cancer Res., *46*: 2203–2207, 1986.
92. Wolman, S. R. Karyotypic progression in human tumors. Cancer Metast. Rev., *2*: 257–293, 1983.
93. Barrett, J. C., Tsutsui, T., Tlsty, T., and Oshimura, M. Role of genetic instability in carcinogenesis. *In*; C. C. Harris and L. A. Liotta (eds.), Genetic Mechanisms in Carcinogenesis and Tumor Progression, pp. 97–114, Wiley-Liss, New York, 1990.
94. Seshadri, R., Kutlaca, R. J., Trainor, K., Matthews, C., and Morley, A. A. Mutation rate of normal and malignant human lymphocytes. Cancer Res., *47*: 407–409, 1987,
95. Elmore, E., Kakunaga, T., and Barrett, J. C. Comparison of spontaneous mutation rates of normal and chemically transformed human skin fibroblasts. Cancer Res., *43*: 1650–1655, 1983.
96. Cifone, M. A. and Fidler, I. J. Increasing metastatic potential is associated with increasing genetic instability of clones isolated from murine neoplasms. Proc. Natl. Acad. Sci. U.S.A., *78*: 6949–6952, 1981.
97. Kendal, W. S. and Frost, P. Metastatic potential and spontaneous mutation rates: studies with two murine cell lines and their recently induced metastatic variants. Cancer Res., *46*: 6131–6135, 1986.
98. Frost, P., Kendal, W., Hunt, B., and Ellis, M. The prevalence of ouabain-resistant variants after mutagen treatment. Lack of correlation between the frequency of variant expression and the metastatic phenotype. Invasion Metast., *8*: 73–86, 1988.
99. Sager, R. Mutation rates and mutational spectra in tumorigenic cell lines. Cancer

Surv., *7*: 325–333, 1988.

100. Goldberg, S. and Defendi, V. Increased mutation rates in doubly viral transformed Chinese hamster cells. Somatic Cell. Genet., *5*: 887–895, 1979.
101. Yamashina, K. and Heppner, G. H. Correlation of frequency of induced mutation and metastatic potential in tumor cell lines from a single mouse mammary tumor. Cancer Res., *45*: 4015–4019, 1985.
102. Chambers, A. F., Harris, J. G., and Grundy, J. S. Rates of generation of MTX-resistant variants in cells temperature sensitive for malignant transformation. Somatic Cell Mol. Genet., *14*: 253–259, 1988.
103. Sager, R., Gadi, I. K., Stephens, L., and Grabowy, C. T. Gene amplification: an example of accelerated evolution in tumorigenic cells. Proc. Natl. Acad. Sci. U.S.A., *82*: 7015–7019, 1985.
104. Tlsty, T. D., Margolin, B. H., and Lum, K. Differences in the rates of gene amplification in nontumorigenic and tumorigenic cell lines as measured by Luria-Delbruck fluctuation analysis. Proc. Natl. Acad. Sci. U.S.A., *86*: 9441–9445, 1989.
105. Tlsty, T. D. Normal diploid human and rodent cells lack a detectable frequency of gene amplification. Proc. Natl. Acad. Sci. U.S.A., *87*: 3132–3136, 1990.
106. Wright, J. A., Smith, H. S., Watt, F. M., Hancock, M. C., Hudson, D. L., and Stark, G. R. DNA amplification is rare in normal human cells. Proc. Natl. Acad. Sci. U.S.A., *87*: 1791–1795, 1990.
107. Croce, C. M. Molecular biology of leukemias and lymphomas. *In*; J. Brugge, T. Curren, E. Harlow and F. McCormick (eds.), Origins of Human Cancer, pp. 527–543, Cold Spring Harbor Laboratory Press, New York, 1991.
108. Hastie, N. D., Dempster, M., Dunlop, M. G., Thompson, A. M., Green, D. K., and Allshire, R. C. Telomere reduction in human colorectal carcinoma and with ageing. Nature, *346*: 866–868, 1990.
109. Schmid, M., Haaf, T., and Grunert, D. 5-Azacytidine-induced undercondensations in human chromosomes. Hum. Genet., *67*: 257–263, 1984.
110. Aplan, P. D., Lombardi, D. P., Ginsberg, A. M., Cossman, J., Bertness, V. L., and Kirsch, I. R. Disruption of the human SCL locus by "illegitimate" V-(D)-J recombinase activity. Science, *250*: 1426–1429, 1990.
111. Lundblad, V. and Szostak, J. W. A mutant with a defect in telomere elongation leads to senescence in yeast. Cell, *57*: 633–643, 1989.
112. McClintock, B. Cold Spring Harbor Symp. Quant. Biol., *16*: 13–49, 1951.
113. Hartwell, L. H. and Weinert, T. A. Genetic control of mitotic fidelity in yeast and its relation to cancer. *In*; J. Brugge, T. Curren, E. Harlow, and F. McCormick (eds.), Origins of Human Cancer, Cold Spring Harbor Laboratory Press, New York, in press.
114. Bischoff, J. R. and Beach, D. Model systems for the study of p53 function. *In*; J. Brugge, T. Curren, E. Harlow, and F. McCormick (eds.), Origins of Human Cancer, Cold Spring Harbor Laboratory Press, New York, in press.
115. Weinert, T. A. and Hartwell, L. H. Characterization of RAD9 of *Saccharomyces cerevisiae* and evidence that its function acts posttranslationally in cell cycle arrest after DNA damage. Mol. Cell Biol., *10*: 6554–6564, 1990.
116. Uemura, T. and Yanagida, M. Isolation of type I and II DNA topoisomerase mutants from fission yeast: single and double mutants show different phenotypes in cell growth and chromatin organization. EMBO J., *3*: 1737–1744, 1984.
117. Uemura, T., Ohkura, H., Adachi, Y., Morino, K., Shiozaki, K., and Yanagida, M. DNA topoisomerase II is required for condensation and separation of mitotic chromosomes in *S. pombe*. Cell, *50*: 917–925, 1987.

118. Bischoff, F. Z., Yim, S. O., Pathak, S., Grant, G., Siciliano, M. J., Giovanella, B. C., Strong, L. C., and Tainsky, M. A. Spontaneous abnormalities in normal fibroblasts from patients with Li-Fraumeni cancer syndrome: aneuploidy and immortalization. Cancer Res., *50*: 7979–7984, 1990.
119. Higginson, J. and Muir, C. S. Environmental carcinogenesis: misconceptions and limitations to cancer control. J. Natl. Cancer Inst., *63*: 1291–1298, 1979.
120. Doll, R. and Peto, R. The Causes of Cancer. Oxford Press, New York, 1981.
121. Muir, C. S. Epidemiology, basic science, and the prevention of cancer: implications for the future. Cancer Res., *50*: 6441–6448, 1990.
122. Wynder, E. L. and Reddy, B. S. Metabolic epidemiology of colorectal cancer. Cancer, *34*: 801–806, 1974.
123. Harris, C. C., Vahakangas, K., Autrup, H., Trivers, G. E., Shamsuddin, A. K. M., Trump, B. F., Boman, B. M., and Mann, D. L. Biochemical and molecular epidemiology of human cancer risk. *In*; D. Scarpelli, J. Craighead, and N. Kaufman (eds.). The Pathologist and the Environment, pp. 140–167, Williams and Wilkins, Baltimore, 1985.
124. Perera, F. P. and Weinstein, I. B. Molecular epidemiology and carcinogen-DNA adduct detection: new approaches to studies of human cancer causation. J. Chronic Dis., *35*: 581–600, 1982.
125. Harris, C. C. Molecular epidemiology of human cancer in the 1990's. *In*; B. L. Gledhill and F. Mauro (eds.), Trends in Biological Dosimetry, pp. 543–558, Wiley-Liss, New York, 1991.
126. Proceedings of the American Academy of Arts and Sciences, "Risk", AAAS, Cambridge, MA, 1990.

MULTISTAGE CARCINOGENESIS, C. C. HARRIS ET AL. (EDS.),
JAPAN SCI. SOC. PRESS, TOKYO/CRC PRESS, BOCA RATON, PP. 21–33, 1992

NAKAHARA MEMORIAL LECTURE

Pathways of Carcinogenesis—Genetic and Epigenetic

Henry C. PITOT, Yvonne DRAGAN, Yi-hua XU, Jodi PETERSON, James HULLY, and Harold CAMPBELL

McArdle Laboratory for Cancer Research, Departments of Oncology and Pathology, The Medical School, University of Wisconsin, Madison, Wisconsin 53706, U.S.A.

Abstract: Considerable experimental evidence has developed to argue that carcinogenesis occurs in a series of stages whose characteristics allow division into the distinct stages of initiation, promotion, and progression. The stage of initiation results from subtle genetic alterations in individual target cells caused both by experimental perturbations as well as by ambient environmental factors. Initiation of a cell may result from the mutation of one or a few key genes whose expression is modified by many other genes. Promoting agents induce the clonal development of initiated cells susceptible to the proliferative effects of the specific promoting agent. The stage of progression is characterized by evolving karyotypic instability and may be induced by specific clastogenic effects and/or agents, the latter termed progressor agents. Carcinogens may induce cancer by an action at all three stages or selectively by an action at any one or two of the individual stages of carcinogenesis. Cancer then develops as a result of fortuitous, endogenous, or ambient environmental factors, thus accounting for the action of both genotoxic and non-genotoxic agents as carcinogens.

It is both a privilege and a humbling experience in presenting this lecture dedicated to the memory and honor of Dr. Waro Nakahara, one of the international leaders in cancer research of this century. After receiving his doctorate in biology from Cornell University in 1918, he began his scientific career at the Rockefeller Institute and returned to Japan in 1925, becoming Director and then President of the National Cancer Center during the last two decades of his life. On his death in January 1976, he left a legacy of scientific contributions to our understanding of the cancer problem that has been surpassed by very few. His discovery of the carcinogenic action of 4-nitroquinoline 1-oxide, which is an excellent mutagen, added greatly to our early understanding of the molecular biology of chemical carcinogenesis. The report by his group of a circulating factor in tumor-bearing animals which alters liver catalase represented one of the earliest demonstrations of the role of hormones and hormone-like factors in the host-tumor relationship, the ultimate cause of death in the cancer patient.

Of special significance to this Symposium was the awareness of Professor

Nakahara of the quantitative actions of two or more carcinogens administered simultaneously as occurs so frequently with human experience. While he distinguished such experiments from the process of multistage carcinogenesis, he studied the effects of low doses of physical or chemical carcinogens followed by low-level exposure to another carcinogenic agent. Thus, it is altogether fitting that we honor the life of this great experimental oncologist in this symposium, paying tribute to his career and his contributions, so many of which paved the way for a number of the reports already presented at this meeting.

Malignant neoplasia is recognized as developing as a consequence of and in concert with a variety of genetic alterations. However, there are several examples of cancer arising from non-DNA reactive chemicals (*1, 2*), inert substances (*3*), and developmental processes (4, *5*). For each of these examples, there is no indication of any direct irreversible interaction with the genome of the target cell, yet the evidence for the role of structural genomic alterations in cancer development is otherwise overwhelming (*6*). This review addresses the reconciliation of the induction of cancer by these means with the well-documented genetic basis for this induction and for progression through an analysis of the pathogenesis of neoplasia.

The stages of neoplastic development. The neoplastic process can be divided into the distinct stages of initiation, promotion, and progression on the basis of experimental evidence from mouse epidermis (*7, 8*), rat liver (*9, 10*), and other multistage models of carcinogenesis (*11–13*). In addition, epidemiological studies of human cancer support the multistage nature of cancer development (*14, 15*). The properties of multistage carcinogenesis have been previously detailed (*16*); characteristics of the individual stages are summarized in Table 1. The initial and final stages—initiation and progression—involve alterations in the genome. The types of alterations that result in initiation may include base transitions and transversions due to point mutations or small deletions without overt structural chromosomal changes (*17, 18*). In contrast, progression is characterized by an evolving karyotypic instability (*19*). In experimental systems (*2, 17, 20*), but rarely if ever in the human (*21*), the stages of initiation and progression may be simultaneously induced, thus eliminating the intermediate stage of promotion, which does not involve structural genetic changes (*18, 19*). The reversible stage of promotion has been well characterized in models of multistage carcinogenesis (*16, 22*) and can be identified as relevant to the development of a number of human cancers (*14, 15, 20*). This review provides some of the experimental evidence for the presence or absence of genetic changes in each of the three stages that occur during neoplastic development.

TABLE 1. Evidence for a Genetic Basis for the Stage of Initiation[a]

The genotoxicity of all known initiating agents.
Clonal growth of papillomas in mouse skin and altered hepatic foci and nodules in rat liver.
Specific mutations in proto-oncogenes in mouse liver and skin as well as rat mammary gland.
The demonstration of DNA damage following administration of initiating doses of complete carcinogens.
Quantitative correlation between mutagenesis and initiation *in vivo*.

[a] See text for specific references for each example given.

Initiation

Studies performed during the 1940s, which provided the basis for multistage mouse epidermal studies, first suggested that initiation results in the alteration of the genome (*23–25*). When initiation was effected by the administration of a subcarcinogenic dose of a polycyclic hydrocarbon, a long latency between administration of this carcinogen and of the promoting regimen could ensue without altering the yield of tumors compared with tumors resulting when no intermission was imposed between initiation and the start of promotion. Since the epidermis sustains a constant rate of replication, the property of initiation must be inherited and transmitted to daughter cells arising during the interval between initiation and promotion. More recently, Van Durren *et al.* (*26*) have confirmed this irreversible property of initiation in the mouse skin after a 1-year latency between carcinogen exposure and the beginning of promotion. Further studies on the rat liver (*27*) have extended to this second histogenic system the finding in the mouse epidermis that initiation is irreversible. Recent evidence for the genetic basis of the initiation stage is summarized in Table 1.

Initiating agents and/or their metabolites are ubiquitously mutagenic (*16*). Therefore, subcarcinogenic doses of genotoxic carcinogens are able to initiate cells in experimental models of multistage carcinogenesis (*17, 22*) and induce substantial DNA damage, which can be detected with a variety of techniques (*28–30*). The clonality of the early lesions that develop from single initiated cells has been observed in the mouse and rat liver, as well as in other systems (*31, 32*). Although discrete mutations have been observed in proto-oncogenes (*33–35*), generally the mutations have been observed only in the resulting neoplasms, with the inference that the mutation occurred during the stage of initiation, a point not yet proven (*35, 36*). Changes in oncogenes have not been observed in all of the models of multistage carcinogenesis (*37–39*), and even in the mouse liver only one-third of the early lesions exhibit alterations in one or more proto-oncogenes (*33*). The frequency of such mutations can be modified by hormonal (*36*) and dietary (*40*) factors. While specific gene mutations common to all initiated cells have not been identified, the finding of mutations in some but not all initiated cell populations may indicate our inability to detect changes in all of the potentially relevant genes.

Additional evidence for the genetic basis of the stage of initiation could be provided by the demonstration of a high degree of correlation between mutagenicity and initiation by a single agent following *in vivo* administration. Putatively initiated hepatocytes which arise spontaneously and those which occur following carcinogen administration can be detected by their aberrant expression of the placental isozyme of glutathione S transferase (PGST; *41, 42*). Most of these putatively initiated hepatocytes maintain a stable expression of PGST after withdrawal from carcinogen administration or on chronic carcinogen administration. This laboratory has used an F_1 cross of the Nagase analbuminemic rat (*43*) with the wild-type Sprague-Dawley rat to quantitate mutation at the albumin locus, scored as loss of albumin expression in hepatocytes of the F1 progeny. Because a previous study on the effect of chronic carcinogen administration in the analbuminemic rat indicated a high reversion rate of the mutation (*44*), we have examined the forward mutation in the F_1 progeny. Additionally, unpublished studies (Dragan *et al.*) with the analbuminemic

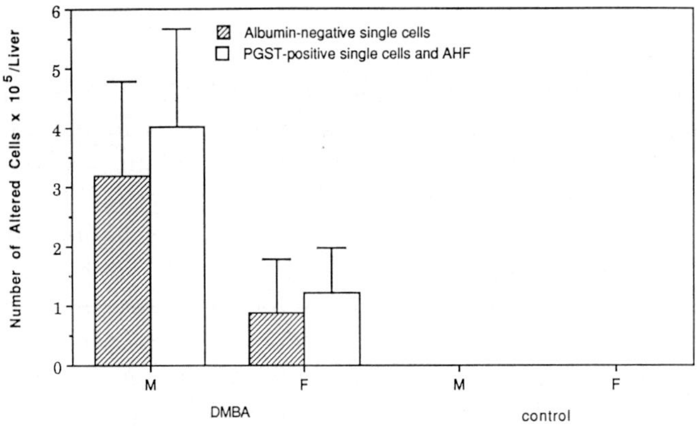

FIG. 1. The number of albumin-deficient hepatocyte foci and the number of foci of hepatocytes (single cells combined with AHF) expressing the placental isozyme of glutathione S transferase in the F_1 cross of a male Sprague-Dawley with a female Nagase analbuminemic rat. The F_1 progeny were treated once with 30 mg dimethylbenzanthracene (DMBA)/kg body weight following a partial hepatectomy. The rats were sacrificed 16 weeks later. The number of hepatic foci of altered protein expression was identified by immunohistochemical techniques and scored with a light microscope. The number of single cells per liver was determined by the method of Laird and Barton (*79*) and the number of foci per liver in DMBA and phenobarbital treated rats was determined by quantitative stereology (*80*).

rat had demonstrated that altered hepatic foci (AHF) developed less frequently than did albumin-positive hepatocytes in a similar experimental design. In these studies, dimethylbenzanthracene (DMBA) was used as the initiating agent, since previous experiments had shown its effectiveness in this capacity in rat hepatocarcinogenesis (*45*). Since PGST is the most effective single marker for AHF that develops after phenobarbital (PB) promotion (*46*), single hepatocytes and AHF-expressing PGST were compared with albumin-negative cells and foci. In both male and female rats, the number of PGST-positive and albumin-negative single hepatocytes was essentially equivalent in the DMBA-initiated animals (Fig. 1). While promotion with PB did not alter the total number of single hepatocytes and AHF-expressing PGST, some effect of promotion alone on altered PGST and albumin expression in single hepatocytes was noted in male rats. The altered expression of albumin in single hepatocytes of uninitiated rats exposed to PB could have been influenced by the known inhibitory effect of PB on albumin gene expression (*47*). Because the number of albumin-negative hepatocytes (which reflect mutation at presumably a single genetic locus) and the number of PGST-positive hepatocytes (which indicate putatively initiated hepatocytes) were the same, these two processes may follow single hit kinetics, and hence initiation may result from mutation at a single genetic locus to give rise to a large population of initiated cells. Thus, the experimental data suggest that initiation is the result of subtle, permanent, and heritable genetic damage that alters the cell such that it possesses the potential to develop clonally *in vivo* under specific circumstances.

Promotion

The characteristics of the process of promotion were not well defined in early studies of the multistage nature of carcinogenesis in the mouse epidermis. These studies were rather linked to those of Foulds (*48*), who described the process following initiation as a continuous evolution that he termed progression. It is only in the last decade that a clear distinction between the processes involved in initiation and promotion has been described. The separation of carcinogenesis into three distinct stages is based on the demonstration that promotion is operationally reversible, unlike the stages of initiation and progression, and that promotion does not involve structural genetic changes, whereas progression is characterized by an evolving karyotypic instability (*19*).

The experimental evidence for a lack of any direct involvement of structural chromosomal damage during the stage of promotion is provided in Table 2. The primary characteristic of promotion is the unstable and reversible nature of the lesions promoted by such agents, further emphasizing the nonheritable nature of the induced changes. Evidence for the reversible nature of some preneoplastic lesions has been obtained in mouse skin (*23*), rat liver (*16*), and in the human (*49*). In addition, alteration of the format of administration of the promoting agent by change of the frequency of administration can inhibit (*23*) or markedly decrease (*50*) the development of preneoplastic lesions in experimental systems. A similar pattern of a diminished response to a promoting stimulus after intermittent exposure has been detailed in human lung cancer (*51*), which is known to require a long period of promotion (*52*). Although the mechanism for the regression of preneoplastic lesions after cessation of administration of the promoting stimulus is unknown, apoptosis or single-cell death may be at least partially responsible for this action in the rat liver (*53*).

Unlike the majority of initiating agents, the best-studied promoting agents are effective without being metabolized (*7, 16, 22*). In addition, many promoting agents interact with specific receptors of the target cell to reversibly activate a number of genes (*54*). Each promoting agent may act selectively on a subset of the initiated cell population to alter gene expression and to promote their growth, as can be seen by the different phenotypic populations of AHF that arise when animals are initiated with the same initiating agent and promoted with different agents (*55*). Thus, promoting agents may enhance the growth of a relatively small number of the initiated

TABLE 2. Evidence for the Epigenetic Basis of the Stage of Promotion[a]

Unstable or reversible nature of lesions developing during the stage of promotion.
Lack of requirement for metabolism of promoting agents for them to be effective.
Necessity for interaction of most promoting agents with specific receptors to be effective.
Reversible gene activation in both normal and preneoplastic cells by promoting agents.
Lack of induction of structural DNA alterations by promoting agents.

[a] See text for specific references for each example given.

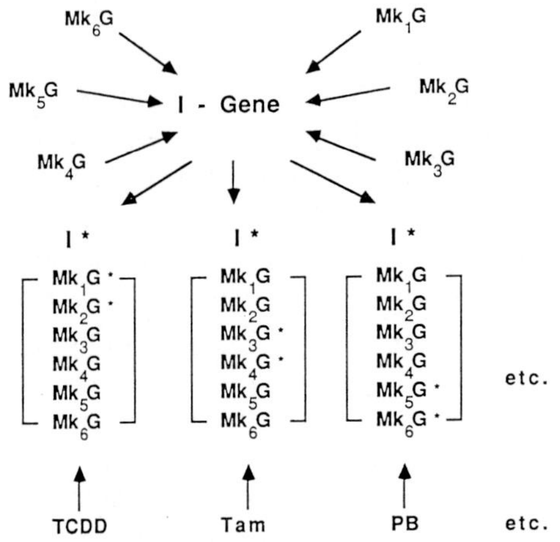

FIG. 2. Model for the effect of promoter-dependent marker gene (MkG) expression on one or a few initiation genes (I-genes). Individual promoting agents may selectively promote the growth of a subset of the initiated cell population.

cell population, as seen in Fig. 1. As predicated by the data of Fig. 1, Fig. 2 provides a theoretical depiction of the effect of individual promoting agents on the entire population of initiated cells. This type of data, in conjunction with the dose-response curves for initiators in hepatocarcinogenesis, is compatible with the possibility that one or a few genes are involved in the initiation process. The expression of this putative I-gene may then be modulated by other genes that may or may not have sustained a mutation and which may impinge on the action of the I-gene. This model can explain the data presented in Fig. 1 and the selective promotion of specific phenotypes (reflective of their respective phenotypes) of initiated cell populations. This theory can be partially tested by examining the phenotypic complexity of AHF promoted by specific agents and by the study of combinations of promoting agents.

Although promoting agents are incapable of direct induction of structural genetic changes, they may induce metabolic changes that can secondarily result in mutations. Specifically, the formation of active oxygen radicals that occurs with chronic treatment with a number of promoting agents can result in hydroxylation of some DNA bases (*56*), DNA strand breaks (*57*), and chromosomal alterations (*58*). These secondary effects of promoting agents may involve the increased rate of transition of cells from the state of promotion to that of progression, in which the genetically altered preneoplastic cell population may develop structural chromosomal changes (*19*).

Progression

The constant evolution of the neoplastic cell toward increased growth rate, aggressiveness, and metastatic capability encompasses the progression of neoplastic disease as defined by Foulds (*48*) and as observed in multistage carcinogenesis models (*19*). The basis for the constant evolution during progression reflects the karyotypic changes that accompany malignant neoplasia, as discussed by Boveri (*59*). Thus, the stage of progression is a direct result of the genomic alterations reflected in the karyotype. Unlike the stages of initiation and promotion, the process of progression parallels and is a consequence of genetic changes. Several characteristics of progression to consider include the contribution of karyotypic instability to the development of malignant neoplasia and its relationship to the stages of initiation and progression.

Gene activation and inactivation during the stage of progression. The evolving karyotypic instability of progression provides extensive ramifications for the genetic basis of malignant neoplasia. Roles in cancer development for the increased expression of dominant oncogenes (*60*), as well as for the altered expression of recessive tumor suppressor genes (*61*), have been established. The altered expression of these genes has been linked to karyotypic changes (*62*). The presence of malignant cells with amplified genes (*63, 64*), especially within those cells developing resistance to specific drugs (*65*), is a further consequence of such karyotypic instability, since cells with normal karyotypes rarely show endogenous or induced gene amplification (*66*). Even an increase in mitotic activity such as that provided by exposure to endogenous or exogenous promoting agents can lead to an increased risk for the occurrence of an occasional abnormality in karyotype (*67*). The relevance of such "spontaneous progression", which has been attributed in the development of neoplasia to the induction of high rates of mitotic activity, has been emphasized in an epigenetic model of carcinogenesis (*68*). Further changes in the promoted cell population that may result from increased mitotic activity and that may lead to the process of progression include the selection of cells exhibiting spontaneous mutations in critical genes and altered methylation patterns (*69*), which have been suggested as important in that cancer development process (*70*).

The relation of promotion to progression-progressor agents. The multistage concept of neoplastic development involves three stages: two of the stages, initiation and progression, have a genetic basis; the intermediate stage of promotion involves alterations in gene expression but apparently not in gene structure. These considerations imply that the two stages of cancer development involving genetic alterations need not result from identical structural changes. In addition, it is conceivable and experimentally demonstrable that exposure to a complete carcinogen administered once (*71*) or continually (*72*) induces the development of cancer without discernible stages, as has been described by Foulds (*48*). Thus, for the experimental demonstration of the stage of promotion, subcarcinogenic doses of initiating agents must be employed. Furthermore, the dose-response curves of hepatocarcinogens for altered hepatic foci that are linear at low doses demonstrate no further increase in AHF at higher doses, yet malignant neoplasms appear even in the absence of further promotion (*71*).

Since karyotypic alterations are the hallmark of progression, those chemicals capable of inducing karyotypic alterations are the best candidates for potential progressor agents. Progressor agents can be defined as those agents capable of inducing the transition of cells from the stage of promotion to that of progression (*19*). While complete carcinogens have progressor activity, several human carcinogens not generally considered to be complete carcinogens may also have progressor activity. These human carcinogens may include arsenic, asbestos, and benzene. With the

TABLE 3. The Incidence of Hepatocellular Carcinoma (HCC) in Animals Treated on an Initiation-promotion-initiation Model of Multistage Hepatocarcinogenesis

Treatment	Incidence HCC	
	IPI	IPI (P)
DEN/PB–	3/14	1/8
DEN/PB/HU	1/12	6/9
DEN/PB/ENU	2/17	8/9
DEN/PB/300 rad	5/10	6/11
DEN/PB/benzene	NT	8/9

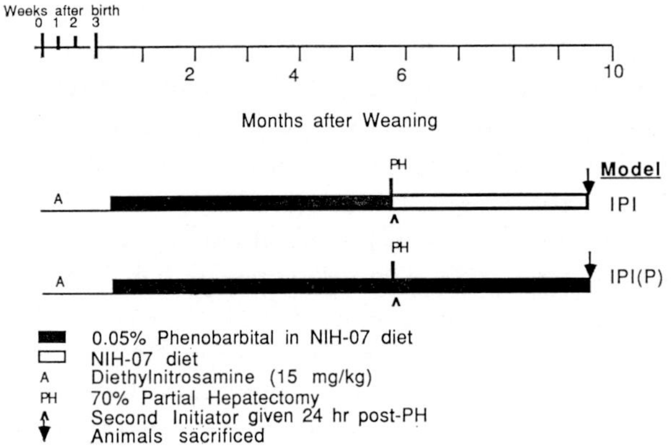

FIG. 3. The format for an initiation-promotion-initiation model of multistage hepatocarcinogenesis. See text for further details.

initiation-promotion-initiation protocol (*73–75*), we have tested whether several agents possess the capacity to convert cells from the stage of promotion to that of progression while being relatively inefficient for complete carcinogenesis (Fig. 3). The results of such studies with hydroxyurea, benzene, and gamma radiation as the progressor agents are provided in Table 3. A substantial increase in yield of malignant neoplasms is obtained with these agents when administered after initiation and promotion compared with the yield when given alone or when compared with appropriate controls.

These preliminary results suggest that some agents exert their carcinogenic potential by acting primarily on cells already in the stage of promotion. As discussed above and reinforced by the effects of gamma radiation, provided in Table 3, active oxygen radicals which have been suggested to be important during promotion (*56–58*), may also exert carcinogenic effects during progression.

Conclusions

The multistage nature of the development of malignant neoplasia permits the classification of carcinogenic agents as acting primarily at one, two, or all of the stages of initiation, promotion, and progression. Complete carcinogens by definition exhibit properties of initiating, promoting, and progressor agents (*16*, *76*). Few if any agents serve only to initiate cells, but many complete carcinogens given at sub-carcinogenic doses function as incomplete carcinogens or initiating agents. Many agents with a promoting action (phenobarbital, 12-O-tetradecanoylphorbol-13-acetate (TPA), 2,3,7,8-tetrachlorodibenzo-*p*-dioxin (TCDD), and peroxisome-proliferating agents) may also act through indirect mechanisms to stimulate the transition of cells from promotion to progression (*56–58, 77, 78*). One mechanism may be their shared ability to increase active radical formation. Progressor agents without significant initiating or promoting activity may be more common than previously recognized. Several human carcinogens that are effective clastogens, including arsenic, benzene, and asbestos, may be examples of carcinogenic agents for which whole-animal bioassays are not yet available. The model and techniques used to generate the data in Table 3 are a step in this direction, but require further refinement before they are generally applicable. The realization of the importance of the multistage nature of cancer development and the nature of the action of specific agents on these stages permits a better understanding of the role of permanent and transient genetic changes on the genesis of cancer in animals.

REFERENCES

1. Ashby, J. Origins of current uncertainties in carcinogen/mutagen screening. Environ. Mol. Mutag., *16*: 51–59, 1989.
2. Ashby, J. and Tennant, R. W. Definitive relationships among chemical structure, carcinogenicity and mutagenicity for 301 chemicals tested by the U.S. NTP. Mutat. Res., *257*: 229–306, 1991.
3. Brand, K. G. Diversity and complexity of carcinogenic processes: conceptual inferences from foreign-body tumorigenesis. J. Natl. Cancer Inst., *57*: 973–976, 1976.
4. Markert, C. L. Neoplasia: A disease of cell differentiation. Cancer Res., *28*: 1908–1914, 1968.
5. Damjanov, I., Bagasra, O., and Solter, O. Genetic and epigenetic factors regulate the evolving malignancy of embryo-derived teratomas. Cold Spring Harbor Conf. Cell Prolif., *10*: 501–517, 1983.
6. Miller, E. C. Some current perspectives on chemical carcinogenesis in humans and experimental animals: presidential address. Cancer Res., *38*: 1479–1496, 1978.
7. Slaga, T. J., Fischer, S. M., Weeks, C. E., Klein-Szanto, A. J. P., and Reiners, J. Studies on the mechanisms involved in multistage carcinogenesis in mouse skin. J. Cell. Biochem., *18*: 99–119, 1982.
8. Marks, F. and Fürstenberger, G. Experimental evidence that skin carcinogenesis is a multistep phenomenon. Br. J. Dermatol., *115* (Suppl. 31): 1–8, 1986.
9. Schulte-Hermann, R. Tumor promotion in liver. Arch. Toxicol., *57*: 147–158, 1985.
10. Farber, E. aud Sarma, D. S. R. Biology of disease. Hepatocarcinogenesis: a dynamic cellular perspective. Lab. Invest., *56*: 4–22, 1987.
11. Cohen, S. M. Multistage carcinogenesis in the urinary bladder. Fd. Chem. Toxic., *23*: 521–528, 1985.
12. Chang, W. W. L. Morphological basis of multistep process in experimental colonic carcinogenesis. Virchows Arch. Cell Pathol., *41*: 17–37, 1982.
13. Medina, D. Initiation and promotion in mouse mammary tumorigenesis. Prog. Clin. Biol. Res., *132B*: 187–203, 1983.
14. Moolgavkar, S. H., Day, N. E., and Stevens, R. G. Two-stage model for carcinogenesis: epidemiology of breast cancer in females. J. Natl. Cancer Inst., *65*: 559–569, 1980.
15. Day, N. E. Time as a determinant of risk in cancer epidemiology: the role of multi-

stage models. Cancer Surveys, *2*: 577–594, 1983.
16. Pitot, H. C. Mechanisms of chemical carcinogenesis: theoretical and experimental bases. *In*; C. S. Cooper and P. L. Grover (eds.), Handbook of Experimental Pharmacology, Vol. 94/I, pp. 3–29, Springer-Verlag, Berlin-Heidelberg, 1990.
17. Sargent, L., Xu, Y.-H., Sattler, G. L., Meisner, L., and Pitot, H. C. Ploidy and karyotype of hepatocytes isolated from enzyme-altered foci in two different protocols of multistage hepatocarcinogenesis in the rat. Carcinogenesis, *10*: 387–391, 1989.
18. Boyd, J. A. and Barrett, J. C. Genetic and cellular basis of multistep carcinogenesis. Pharmacol. Ther., *46*: 469–486, 1990.
19. Pitot, H. C. Progression: the terminal stage in carcinogenesis. Jpn. J. Cancer Res., *80*: 599–607, 1989.
20. Doll, R. and Peto, R. (eds.) The Causes of Cancer, Oxford University Press, Oxford, 1981.
21. Sontag, J. M. Aspects in carcinogen bioassay. *In*; H. Hiatt, J. Watson, and J. Winsten (eds.), Origins of Human Cancer, pp. 1327-1338, Cold Spring Harbor Laboratory, Cold Spring Harbor, 1977.
22. Boutwell, R. K. Some biological aspects of skin carcinogenesis. Prog. Exp. Tumor Res., *4*: 207–240, 1964.
23. Rous, P. and Kidd, J. G. Conditional neoplasms and subthreshold neoplastic states: a study of the tar tumors of rabbits. J. Exp. Med., *73*: 369–390, 1941.
24. Berenblum, I. The cocarcinogenic action of croton resin. Cancer Res., *1*: 44–50, 1941.
25. Mottram, J. C. A developing factor in experimental blastogenesis. J. Pathol. Bacteriol., *56*: 181–187, 1944.
26. Van Duuren, B. L., Sivak, A., Katz, C., Seidman, I., and Melchionne, S. The effect of aging and interval between primary and secondary treatment in two-stage carcinogenesis on mouse skin. Cancer Res., *35*: 502–505, 1975.
27. Xu, Y.-H., Campbell, H. A., Sattler, G. L., Hendrich, S., Maronpot, R., Sato, R., and Pitot, H. C. Quantitative stereological analysis of the effects of age and sex on multistage hepatocarcinogenesis in the rat by use of four cytochemical markers. Cancer Res., *50*: 472–479, 1990.
28. Pegg, A. E. and Perry, W. Alkylation of nucleic acids and metabolism of small doses of dimethylnitrosamine in the rat. Cancer Res., *41*: 3128–3132, 1981.
29. Brambilla, G., Carlo, P., Finollo, R., Bignone, F. A., Ledda, A., and Cajelli, E. Viscometric detection of liver DNA fragmentation in rats treated with minimal doses of chemical carcinogens. Cancer Res., *43*: 202–209, 1983.
30. Ward, E. J. Persistent and heritable structural damage induced in heterochromatic DNA from rat liver by *N*-nitrosodimethylamine. Biochemistry, *26*: 1709–1717, 1987.
31. Weinberg, W. C. and Iannaccone, P. M. Clonality of preneoplastic liver lesions: histological analysis in chimeric rats. J. Cell Sci., *89*: 423–431, 1988.
32. Tanooka, H. Monoclonal growth of cancer cells: experimental evidence. Jpn. J. Cancer Res., *79*: 657–665, 1988.
33. Büchmann, A., Mahr, J., Bauer-Hofmann, R., and Schwarz, M. Mutations at codon 61 of the Ha-*ras* proto-oncogene in precancerous liver lesions of the B6C3F1 mouse. Mol. Carcinogen., *2*: 121–125, 1989.
34. Brown, K., Buchmann, A., and Balmain, A. Carcinogen-induced mutations in the mouse c-Ha-*ras* gene provide evidence of multiple pathways for tumor progression. Proc. Natl. Acad. Sci. U.S.A., *87*: 538–542, 1990.
35. Zarbl, H., Sukumar, S., Arthur, A., Martin-Zanca, D., and Barbacid, M. Direct mutagenesis of Ha-*ras*-1 oncogenes by *N*-nitroso-*N*-methylurea during initiation of mammary carcinogenesis in rats. Nature, *315*: 382–385, 1985.

36. Zhang, R., Haag, J. D., and Gould, M. N. Quantitating the frequency of initiation and cH-*ras* mutation in *in situ* *N*-methyl-*N*-nitrosourea-exposed rat mammary gland. Cell Growth Diff., *2*: 1–6, 1991.
37. Stowers, S. J., Wiseman, R. W., Ward, J. M., Miller, E. C., Miller, J. C., Anderson, M. W., and Eva, A. Detection of activated proto-oncogenes in *N*-nitrosodiethylamine-induced liver tumors: a comparison between $B6C3F_1$ mice and Fischer 344 rats. Carcinogenesis, *9*: 271–276, 1988.
38. Schaeffer, B. K., Zurlo, J., and Longnecker, D. S. Activation of c-Ki-*ras* not detectable in adenomas or adenocarcinomas arising in rat pancreas. Mol. Carcinogen., *3*: 165–170, 1990.
39. Fujimoto, Y., Ishizaka, Y., Tahira, T., Sone, H., Takahashi, H., Enomoto, K., Mori, M., Sugimura, T., and Nagao, M. Possible involvement of c-*myc* but not *ras* genes in hepatocellular carcinomas developing after spontaneous hepatitis in LEC rats. Mol. Carcinogen., *4*: 269–274, 1991.
40. Llor, X., Jacoby, R. F., Teng, B.-B., Davidson, N. O., Sitrin, M. D., and Brasitus, T. A. K-*ras* mutations in 1,2-dimethylhydrazine-induced colonic tumors: effects of supplemental dietary calcium and vitamin D deficiency. Cancer Res., *51*: 4305–4309, 1991.
41. Moore, M. A., Nakagawa, K , Satoh, K., Ishikawa, T., and Sato, K. Single GST-P positive liver cells—putative initiated hepatocytes. Carcinogenesis, *8*: 483–486, 1987.
42. Satoh, K., Hatayama, I., Tateoka, N., Tamai, K., Shimizu, T., Tatematsu, M., Ito, N., and Sato, K. Transient induction of single GST-P positive hepatocytes by DEN. Carcinogenesis, *10*: 2107–2111, 1989.
43. Nagase, S., Shimamune, K., and Shumiya, S. Albumin-deficient rat mutant. Science, *205*: 590–591, 1979.
44. Makino, R., Sato, S., Esumi, H., Negishi, C., Takano, M., Sugimura, T., Nagase, S., and Tanaka, H. Presence of albumin-positive cells in the liver of analbuminemic rats and their increase on treatment with hepatocarcinogens. Jpn. J. Cancer Res. (Gann), *77*: 153–159, 1986.
45. Pitot, H. C., Goldsworthy, T. L., Moran, S., Kennan, W., Glauert, H. P., Maronpot, R. R., and Campbell, H. A. A method to quantitate the relative initiating and promoting potencies of hepatocarcinogenic agents in their dose-response relationships to altered hepatic foci. Carcinogenesis, *8*: 1491–1499, 1987.
46. Hendrich, S., Campbell, H. A., and Pitot, H. C. Quantitative stereological evaluation of four histochemical markers of altered foci in multistage hepatocarcinogenesis in the rat. Carcinogenesis, *8*: 1245–1250, 1987.
47. Hardwick, J. P., Gonzalez, F. J., and Kasper, C. B. Transcriptional regulation of rat liver epoxide hydratase, NADPH-cytochrome P-450 oxidoreductase, and cytochrome P-450b genes by phenobarbital. J. Biol. Chem. *258*: 8081–8085, 1983.
48. Foulds, L. Tumour progression and neoplastic development. *In*; O. Mühlbock and P. Emmelot (eds.), Cellular Control Mechanisms and Cancer, pp. 242–258, Elsevier Science Publishers, Amsterdam, 1964.
49. Edmondson, H. A., Reynolds, T. B., Henderson, B., and Benton, B. Regression of liver cell adenomas associated with oral contraceptives. Ann. Int. Med., *86*: 180–182, 1977.
50. Xu, Y.-D., Dragan, Y. P., Young, T., and Pitot, H. C. The effect of the format of administration and the total dose of phenobarbital on altered hepatic foci following initiation in female rats with diethylnitrosamine. Carcinogenesis, *12*: 1009–1016, 1991.
51. Zatonski, W., Becher, H., and Lissowska, J. Smoking cessation: intermediate non-smoking periods and reduction of laryngeal cancer risk. J. Natl. Cancer Inst., *82*: 1427–1428, 1990.

52. Reif, A. E. Effect of cigarette smoking on susceptibility to lung cancer. Oncology, *38*: 76–85, 1981.
53. Schulte-Hermann, R., Timmermann-Trosiener, I., Barthel, G., and Bursch, W. DNA synthesis, apoptosis, and phenotypic expression as determinants of growth of altered foci in rat liver during phenobarbital promotion. Cancer Res., *50*: 5127–5135, 1990.
54. Pitot, H. C. Fundamentals of Oncology, 3rd ed., pp. 149–150, Marcel Dekker, Inc., New York, 1986.
55. Pitot, H. C., Dragan, Y., Sargent, L., and Xu, Y.-H. Biochemical markers associated with the stages of promotion and progression during hepatocarcinogenesis in the rat. Environ. Health Perspect., *93*: 181–189, 1991.
56. Wei, H. and Frenkel, K. *In vivo* formation of oxidized DNA bases in tumor promoter-treated mouse skin. Cancer Res., *51*: 4443–4449, 1991.
57. Birnboim, H. C. Importance of DNA strand-break damage in tumor promotion. *In*; O. F. Nygaard, M. G. Simic, and J. N. Hauber (eds.), Radioprotectors and Anticarcinogens, pp. 539–556, Academic Press, New York, 1983.
58. Kinzel, V., Färber, B., Petrusevska, R. T., and Fusenig, N. Cytogenetic effects of phorbol ester tumor promoters: possible role in multistep tumorigenesis. Prog. Clin. Biol. Res., *340D*: 133–141, 1990.
59. Boveri, T. Zur Frage der Entstehung maligner Tumoren, Gustav-Fishcer, Jena, 1914.
60. Field, J. K. and Spandidos, D. A. The role of *ras* and *myc* oncogenes in human solid tumours and their relevance in diagnosis and prognosis (review). Anticancer Res., *10*: 1–22, 1990.
61. Marshall, C. J. Tumor suppressor genes. Cell, *64*: 313–326, 1991.
62. Rowley, J. D. Molecular cytogenetics: Rosetta stone for understanding cancer—Twenty-ninth G. H. A. Clowes Memorial Award Lecture. Cancer Res., *50*: 3816–3825, 1990.
63. Mäkelä, T. P. and Alitalo, K. Proto-oncogene amplification: role in tumour progression. Ann. Clin. Res., *18*: 290–296, 1986.
64. Fukumoto, M., Shevrin, D. H., and Roinson, I. B. Analysis of gene amplification in human tumor cell lines. Proc. Natl. Acad. Sci. U.S.A., *85*: 6846–6850, 1988.
65. Schimke, R. B. Gene amplification in cultured cells. J. Biol. Chem., *263*: 5989-5992, 1988.
66. Tlsty, T. D. Normal diploid human and rodent cells lack a detectable frequency of gene amplification. Proc. Natl. Acad. Sci. U.S.A., *87*: 3132–3136, 1990.
67. Ames, B. N. and Gold, L. S. Chemical carcinogenesis: too many rodent carcinogens. Proc. Natl. Acad. Sci. U.S.A., *87*: 7772–7776, 1990.
68. Cohen, S. M., Purtilo, D. T., and Ellwein, L. B. Pivotal role of increased cell proliferation in human carcinogenesis. Modern Pathol., *4*: 371–382, 1991.
69. Dizik, M., Christman, J. K., and Wainfan, E. Alterations in expression and methylation of specific genes in livers of rats fed a cancer promoting methyl-deficient diet. Carcinogenesis, *12*: 1307–1312, 1991.
70. Jones, P. A. DNA methylation and cancer. Cancer Res., *46*: 461–466, 1986.
71. Scherer, E. and Emmelot, P. Kinetics of induction and growth of precancerous liver-cell foci, and liver tumour formation by diethylnitrosamine in the rat. Eur. J. Cancer, *11*: 689–696, 1975.
72. Bannasch, P. and Zerban, H. Pathogenesis of primary liver tumors induced by chemicals. Tumor Biol., *100*: 1–15, 1986.
73. Potter, V. R. Alternative hypotheses for the role of promotion in chemical carcinogenesis. Environ. Health Perspect., *50*: 139–148, 1983.
74. Moolgavkar, S. H. Carcinogenesis modeling: from molecular biology to epidemiology.

Annu. Rev. Public Health, *7*: 151–169, 1986.

75. Hennings, H., Spangler, E. F., Shores, R., Mitchell, P., Devor, D., Shamsuddin, A. K. M., Elgjo, K. M., and Yuspa, S. H. Malignant conversion and metastasis of mouse skin tumors: a comparison of SENCAR and CD-1 mice. Environ. Health Perspect., *68*: 69–74, 1986.
76. Pitot, H. C. and Dragan, Y. P. Facts and theories concerning the mechanisms of carcinogenesis. FASEB J., *5*: 2280–2286, 1991.
77. Reddy, J. K. and Rao, M. S. Oxidative DNA damage caused by persistent peroxisome proliferation: its role in hepatocarcinogenesis. Mutat. Res., *214*: 63–68, 1989.
78. Al-Bayati, Z. A. F., Murray, W. J., and Stohs, S. J. 2,3,7,8-Tetrachlorodibenzo-*p*-dioxin-induced lipid peroxidation in hepatic and extrahepatic tissues of male and female rats. Arch. Environ. Contam. Toxicol., *16*: 159–166, 1987.
79. Laird, A. K. and Barton, A. D. Cell proliferation in precancerous liver: relation to presence and dose of carcinogens. J. Natl. Cancer Inst., *27*: 827–838, 1961.
80. Campbell, H. A., Xu, Y.-D., Hanigan, M. H., and Pitot, H. C. Application of quantitative stereology to the evaluation of phenotypically heterogeneous enzyme-altered foci in the rat liver. J. Natl. Cancer Inst., *76*: 751–767, 1986.

CLINICAL OBSERVATION OF MULTISTAGE CARCINOGENESIS

MULTISTAGE CARCINOGENESIS, C. C. HARRIS ET AL. (EDS.),
JAPAN SCI. SOC. PRESS, TOKYO/CRC PRESS, BOCA RATON, PP. 37–48, 1992

A Genetic Basis for the Multi-step Pathway of Colorectal Tumorigenesis

Eric R. FEARON

The Oncology Center, The Johns Hopkins University School of Medicine, Baltimore, Maryland 21205, U.S.A.

Abstract: Colorectal tumors provide an excellent system in which to search for and study the genetic alterations involved in the development of a common human cancer. Data from many clinical and histopathological studies suggest that most carcinomas arise from preexisting adenomas. In addition, colorectal tumors of various stages of development can be obtained for studies of genetic alterations, unlike the situation in many other common human cancers in which only the most advanced lesions can be studied. A current view is that colorectal tumor development and progression results from the accumulation of somatic genetic alterations (mutations) in both oncogenes and tumor suppressor genes. Mutations in four to five genes may be necessary for the development of a malignant tumor; fewer changes may suffice for benign tumor formation. Although the genetic alterations often occur in a preferred sequence, the total accumulation of changes, rather than their order with respect to one another, appears to be a critical determinant of the biological properties of the tumor. Study of the genes targeted by somatic mutation in these tumors may provide insights, not only into the pathogenesis of the disease, but also into the mechanisms of origin of mutations and the potential environmental and dietary factors underlying colorectal tumor development.

It is now apparent that the development of common human tumors, such as those of the colon and rectum, is a highly complex process with many potential causes, including environmental and dietary factors and both inherited and somatic mutations. Over the past decade a great deal of progress has been made towards the elucidation of some of the genetic factors that underlie colorectal tumor development. A present view is that human cancer in general, and colon and rectal cancer in particular, results, at least in part, from mutations in two different classes of genes —oncogenes and tumor suppressor genes (*1–3*). In general terms, wild-type alleles of cellular oncogenes are thought to function in a positive fashion in the normal growth regulatory circuits of the cell. Somatic mutations or deregulated expression of the alleles of these cellular oncogenes can result in loss of proper growth regulation, and resultant tumor initiation or tumor progression events. In contrast, the normal function of tumor suppressor genes is to act as a negative regulator of cell growth, or perhaps to transduce negative growth regulatory signals. Mutations that inactivate the wild-type function of tumor suppressor alleles promote tumorigenesis. Such inactivating mutations can be the result of either inherited or somatic mutations.

In this manuscript, the natural history of colorectal tumors as a multi-step process will be considered with respect to the inherited and somatic mutations identified at specific stages of tumor development. Mutations in a member of the *ras* oncogene family and in several tumor suppressor genes appear to be crucial to cancer development. Although there appears to be a preference for the relative time of occurrence of specific mutations, several lines of evidence suggest that the accumulation of multiple genetic alterations, rather the specific order of their occurrence, may be of primary importance. While much progress has been made toward identifying some of the inherited mutations that underlie the predisposition to colorectal cancer and, as well, a number of the genes targeted by somatic mutations during colorectal tumorigenesis, many questions remain to be addressed before a full understanding of the molecular basis of colorectal tumor development will be achieved. Some of these questions concerning the possible mechanisms by which somatic mutations arise and contribute to the initiation and progression of colorectal tumors will be highlighted.

Natural History of Colorectal Tumors Suggests a Multi-step Pathway

A variety of clinical and histopathological studies have provided strong support for the present view that the majority of colorectal cancers arise from pre-existing adenomatous polyps over a period of years to decades (*4*, *5*). In this process of tumor development and progression, a small adenoma of low malignant potential may arise from the colonic mucosa. A number of studies suggest that adenomas do not arise directly from normal mucosal cells; rather adenomas may arise from areas of hyperproliferative mucosa (*6*) or from regions with dysplastic crypt formation (*7*). Subsequent progression of the small adenoma to a larger adenoma with increased malignant potential may then occur in some cases. Finally, a percentage of tumors may progress to invasive and metastatic cancer. Although some discrete stages of tumor formation can be discerned by histopathological and clinical criteria, the biological process is likely to be continuous. This multi-step pathway of tumor progression can be seen in either sporadic or inherited cases of colorectal tumors.

In perhaps ten percent of colorectal cancer cases, an inherited genetic factor(s) may be a primary determinant of cancer development (*8*). One syndrome which strongly predisposes to colorectal cancer development is familial adenomatous polyposis (FAP). In this autosomal dominant syndrome, estimated to affect nearly 1 in 8,000 individuals in the U.S., affected individuals develop hundreds to even several thousand adenomas in their colon and rectum by the end of the second to third decades of life (*9*, *10*). Only a small fraction of the adenomas progress to cancers in patients with FAP or the related variant Gardner syndrome; thus, the predominant predisposition is adenoma formation. The gene responsible for this syndrome was mapped to chromosome 5q in 1987 (*11–13*), and recent studies have resulted in the identification and cloning of the predisposition gene, now referred to as the adenomatous polyposis coli (APC) gene (*14–17*). The role of, and alterations in, the APC gene in both inherited and sporadic colorectal tumors will be discussed below. In addition, several forms of inherited colorectal cancer, not associated with extensive polyposis, have been described by Lynch and his colleagues (*8*). Presumably, cancers in these cases also arise through a multi-step process, although more rapid progression from the small adenoma stage to carcinoma may be a feature of this syndrome.

In the majority of cases, however, no obvious inherited genetic component can be documented; thus, these cases are termed "sporadic." Some investigators have suggested that even the majority of these "sporadic" colorectal cancer cases may not arise in a truly sporadic fashion. Rather, it has been proposed that the development of colorectal cancer in the general population may be attributed, in part, to a dominantly-inherited predisposition to the development of adenomas in affected individuals (*18*). A fraction of these adenomas may then progress to cancer.

Somatic Mutations and Tumor Initiation

The specific molecular mechanisms underlying the initiation of human colorectal tumors are only incompletely understood, however several lines of evidence support the proposal that colorectal adenomas and carcinomas arise as the result of somatic mutational events. Of note, studies of the clonality of adenomas from patients with either inherited or sporadic tumors suggest that each adenoma arises from a single intestinal crypt (*19*). This observation is consistent with the hypothesis that a mutational event causes one or a small number of cells from within the crypt to initiate the neoplastic process by clonal expansion (*20, 21*). Therefore, even in FAP patients who have inherited mutations in the APC gene, the data suggest that additional somatic mutations are necessary for adenoma formation, and it is likely that additional mutations are necessary for further progression to carcinoma.

FAP and the APC Gene

As noted above, the gene linked to the development of polyposis in individuals affected by FAP or Gardner syndrome (GS) was mapped to chromosome 5q21. Recent studies have led to the identification of the APC gene, which is mutated in the germline of patients with FAP or GS (*14–17*). The inherited mutations identified in the APC gene, thus far, appear to result in inactivation of the gene, and include gross deletions of the gene, and more localized mutations that cause frameshifts or create stop codons or missense mutations in the gene product (*15–17*). Although FAP and related polyposis syndromes are relatively uncommon, the potential importance of alterations of the APC gene in the development of the majority of colorectal tumors has been highlighted by the demonstration that loss of heterozygosity (LOH) events involving 5q are present in 35–50% of tumors of patients with no obvious inherited tendency to colorectal cancer (22–25). LOH involving 5q can only rarely be noted in patients with polyposis; however, these 5q LOH events are the most common genetic alteration so far described in small, early adenomas from patients without polyposis (*23, 24*). Moreover, with regard to the relative temporal occurrence of LOH involving 5q in tumors of patients without polyposis, the frequency of 5q LOH is nearly identical in both small adenomas and carcinomas (*23*). Therefore, the data, in toto, suggest that the APC gene is a tumor suppressor gene that may contribute to the development of some colorectal tumors as a result of germline inactivation. In the majority of colorectal tumors, the gene may be inactivated by somatic mutations, and perhaps inactivation may occur at an early stage of tumor development.

Somatic Mutations in Both Oncogenes and Multiple Tumor Suppressor Genes Underlie Colorectal Tumor Progression

Mutations in one of the three *ras* genes have been found to be present in about 50% of colorectal carcinomas (*23, 26, 27*), and in a similar percentage of adenomas over 1 cm in size (*23*). Adenomas of this size are thought to have an increased risk of malignant transformation (*4, 5*). In contrast, *ras* mutations have been identified in fewer than 10% of adenomas under 1 cm. Over 85% of the mutations detected are present at codons 12 or 13 of the K-*ras* gene (*23*). The difference in relative prevalence of *ras* mutations in small compared to large adenomas suggests two alternative hypotheses for the role of *ras* gene mutations in colorectal tumorigenesis. Mutations in a *ras* gene may be an early/initiating event in only a fraction of tumors, but these adenomas may then have a higher likelihood of progressing to a larger size than adenomas without *ras* mutations. Alternatively, *ras* mutations may arise in one cell of a small, pre-existing adenoma and result in clonal expansion of cells with increased malignant potential. Presently, it is not possible to distinguish between these two hypotheses. Further studies of adenomas of various sizes and histopathological types, as well as studies of classical or transgenic animal models of colorectal neoplasia, may help to identify the role of *ras* gene mutations in colorectal tumor initiation, progression, or both.

In general, allelic losses are thought to be selected for during tumorigenesis by the unmasking of either somatic or inherited mutations in tumor suppressor genes in the affected chromosomal region (*28–30*). In colorectal tumors, the regions most frequently affected by LOH events are chromosomes 17p and 18q (*31*), and thus these regions were suspected to contain novel tumor suppressor genes. Allelic losses involving chromosome 18q can be observed in over 70% of colorectal carcinomas, in almost 50% of late adenomas, and very infrequently in earlier stage adenomas (*23*). A common region of allelic loss centered around chromosome band 18q21 has been identified, and a candidate tumor suppressor gene from this region has been identified (*32*). This gene, termed deleted in colorectal carcinoma (DCC), encodes a protein that has significant homology with the NCAM (neural cell adhesion molecule) family (*33*). The DCC cDNAs identified to date encode a putative transmembrane gene product with four immunoglobulin-like domains, multiple repeats of a fibronectin type III-related domain and a cytoplasmic domain not highly related to any previously identified gene product (ref. *32*, K. R. Cho and B. Vogelstein, personal communication). The DCC gene is highly conserved in other mammalian species, and a *Xenopus* homologue has recently been identified that has over 80% identity at the amino-acid level with the human sequence, over virtually the full-length of the predicted amino acid sequence (E. R. Fearon, unpublished results).

Although the normal function of the DCC gene is unknown, alterations or inactivation of the gene could perhaps account, at least in part, for some of the altered properties of adhesion and invasion noted in colorectal tumor cells. In this regard, a limited number of examples of somatic mutations at the DCC locus that might inactive the gene's function have been identified in colorectal tumors thus far. These mutations include a homozygous deletion of the 5′ portion of the gene in one case, mutations in intron sequences in about 15% of cases, and two cases with somatic point mutations affecting coding sequences or splice elements (ref. *32*, J. W. Simons and B. Vogelstein, personal communication). In addition, in over 80% of the colorectal cell lines studied to date, DCC gene expression has been found to be greatly reduced or absent, compared to the level of DCC gene expression in normal mucosa or in colorectal tumor cell lines with detectable DCC transcripts (*32*). Studies are underway to demonstrate that a wild-type copy of the DCC gene will suppress some aspect of the tumorigenic phenotype when introduced into colorectal tumor cells with defects in its endogenous DCC alleles.

The chromosomal region identified as most frequently affected by LOH events in colorectal carcinomas is chromosome 17p, which is affected in over 75% of cases (*31*). In contrast, LOH on 17p is detected infrequently in adenomas of any stage, including large, high grade adenomas with foci of carcinoma (*23*). In several cases, LOH of 17p has been found to be associated with the progression of individual tumors from adenoma to carcinoma (*23*, *34*, *35*). The common region of allelic loss on 17p includes the p53 gene, and a number of lines of evidence suggest that the tumor suppressor gene targeted by these allelic losses in colorectal tumors is the p53 gene (*35–37*). Sequence analysis of a large number of p53 alleles from colorectal carcinomas that had suffered LOH for 17p revealed that a single missense mutation could be detected in the remaining p53 allele in 20 of the 22 cases (*35*). Similar analyses of p53 alleles from carcinomas with no LOH on 17p (two p53 alleles present) and adenomas, both with one and two p53 alleles, also have been carried out (*35*). These data on the relative frequency of p53 mutations in adenomas and carcinomas are summarized in Fig. 1. The majority of the mutations are in the most highly

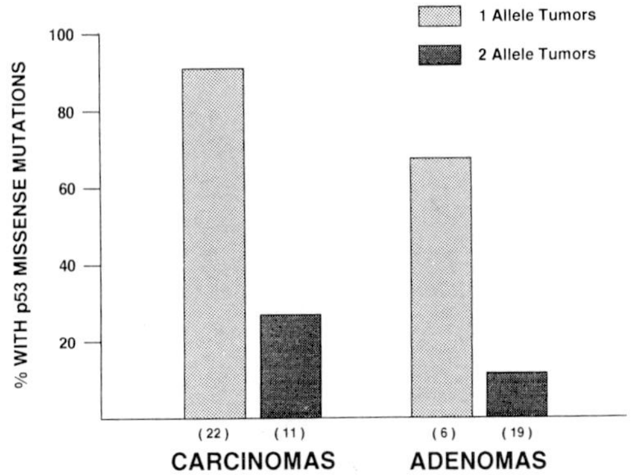

FIG. 1. The frequency of p53 mutations in colorectal adenomas and carcinomas. This figure summarizes the data on the prevalence of p53 mutations in colorectal tumors as presented in Baker *et al.* (ref. *35*). The percentage of each tumor type with base substitutions in the p53 gene that result in missense mutations is indicated. One allele tumors have suffered LOH for 17p sequences, including the region containing the p53 gene. Two allele tumors have retained heterozygosity for 17p sequences. The number of tumors of each type for which p53 alleles were studied by sequence analysis is indicated in parentheses.

conserved regions of the gene, similar to the findings in other tumor types. In particular, the codons most frequently affected by these missense mutations in colorectal tumors are 175, 248, and 273 (*35, 38*). In addition, as noted by Hollstein et al., the majority of the mutations are transition mutations, and predominantly transitions at CpG sites (*38*). This observation will addressed below.

Point mutation of one p53 allele coupled with loss of the remaining wild-type allele appears to occur very frequently during the development of colorectal carcinoma. The data obtained thus far are consistent with the proposal that point mutation of one p53 allele precedes the loss of the wild-type allele (*3*). Presumably, the point mutated allele may arise be selected for, because it can function in a dominant negative fashion to inactivate the wild-type p53 gene product in the cell; further growth and progression results in selection for loss of the remaining wild-type allele. Both mutation of one p53 allele and loss of the wild-type allele appear to occur relatively late in tumor development in the majority of colorectal tumors (*35*). The molecular basis for this apparent selection of mutated p53 alleles only in late stages of colorectal tumor development is unknown. It is intriguing to consider the hypothesis that other genes expressed in colorectal cells may significantly modify or abrogate the effects of a mutated p53 allele. Perhaps these interacting or modifying

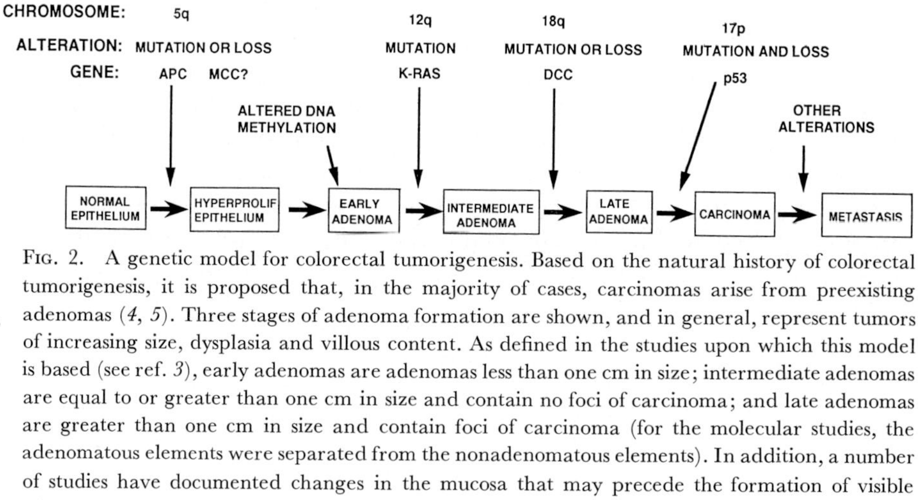

FIG. 2. A genetic model for colorectal tumorigenesis. Based on the natural history of colorectal tumorigenesis, it is proposed that, in the majority of cases, carcinomas arise from preexisting adenomas (*4, 5*). Three stages of adenoma formation are shown, and in general, represent tumors of increasing size, dysplasia and villous content. As defined in the studies upon which this model is based (see ref. *3*), early adenomas are adenomas less than one cm in size; intermediate adenomas are equal to or greater than one cm in size and contain no foci of carcinoma; and late adenomas are greater than one cm in size and contain foci of carcinoma (for the molecular studies, the adenomatous elements were separated from the nonadenomatous elements). In addition, a number of studies have documented changes in the mucosa that may precede the formation of visible adenomas and that can be characterized as hyperproliferative (*not* hyperplastic polyps) (see ref. *6*). The relative timing of the genetic events is indicated with respect to the various stages of colorectal tumor development shown. The chromosome regions most frequently affected, the particular gene believed to be targeted by mutation, and the type of mutation at the oncogene or tumor suppressor gene (point mutation, LOH, *etc.*) are indicated. In patients with FAP, germline mutation in the APC gene is believed to be responsible for the hyperproliferative epithelium seen in these patients (ref. *6*). In tumors arising in patients without polyposis, somatic mutation of the APC or MCC (ref. *44*) genes may play a role in early stages of tumorigenesis, although this is not yet fully established. Alterations in DNA methylation (reviewed in ref. *3*) can be seen in very small adenomas of patients both with and without polyposis. Loss of chromosomes 18q and 17p usually occurs at a later stage of tumorigenesis than does chromosome 5q loss or *ras* gene mutation. However, the order of these changes is not invariant, and it seems most likely that the accumulation of multiple genetic alterations in both oncogenes and tumor suppressor genes is most important, not the order *per se*. Figure modified with permission (*3*).

genes may need to be inactivated before mutated p53 alleles can exert a phenotypic effect.

A Genetic Model of Colorectal Tumorigenesis

As review above, somatic mutations in a member of an oncogene family and multiple tumor suppressor genes are believed to be, at least in part, the basis for the development and progression of colorectal tumors. A model incorporating these genetic alterations with respect to different stages of tumorigenesis has been proposed (*3*) and is illustrated in Fig. 2. There appears to be a preference for a specific genetic alteration to be present at a high frequency only at particular stages of colorectal tumorigenesis, and this is the basis for assigning a relative order to the genetic alterations in the multi-step pathway. However, even though these mutations that presumably underlie the progressive waves of clonal expansion tend to arise in a certain order, this order is not invariable (*3, 23*). Therefore, it seems most likely that the accumulation and interaction of the specific genetic alterations present in a cell may determine its phenotype. Although the model depicted in Fig. 2 accurately reflects much of the data obtained to date from studies of colorectal tumors in both patients with sporadic and inherited forms of the disease (*23, 25, 39, 40*), it is likely to be incomplete and overly simplistic.

Mechanisms of Mutation—ras vs. p53

In colorectal tumors, as in the majority of most common human types, p53 base substitution mutations are the most frequent specific genetic alteration identified to date. Hollstein *et al.* have reviewed the p53 gene mutational spectrum in human tumors and have found that it differs among cancers of different types, including colon, lung, esophagus, breast, liver, brain, and others (*38*). In particular, transition mutations were predominant in the thirty-nine p53 mutations observed in colorectal tumors, with 79% of the mutations resulting in G: C to A: T transitions and 15% of the mutations resulting in A: T to G: C transitions (see Fig. 3A). Over two-thirds of the G: C to A: T transitions were at CpG sites. The mutability of CpG dinucleotides in the human genome has been documented and attributed to the presence of 5-methylcytosine residues found at these dinucleotides in the mammalian genome (*41*). Indeed, Rideout *et al.* have shown that several of these CpG sites within the p53 gene are methylated in human peripheral blood cells (*42*). Thus, it is possible that mutations in the p53 gene in many tumors might result from spontaneous deamination of methylated cytosine residues that then goes unrepaired.

It is interesting to contrast these findings on the mutational spectrum of the p53 gene in colorectal tumors with the mutations observed in the *ras* genes of these tumors. As noted above, mutation of the p53 gene appears to occur only at later stages of colorectal tumorigenesis, while *ras* gene mutation may be an early/initiating event in at least some tumors. In addition, while a large number of mutations could conceiveably inactivate the normal function of the p53 gene, only a limited range of mutations are known to activate the oncogenic function of the three *ras* genes (*43*). These mutations include amino acid substitutions at positions 12, 13, and 61 of the

p53 Gene Base Substitutions

Mutations at G:C			
-> A:T	-> T:A	-> C:G	Transitions at CpG
79%	0%	3%	67%

Mutations at A:T		
-> T:A	-> G:C	-> C:G
3%	15%	0%

(A)

GENE	SEQUENCE 11	12	13	14	% of ras mutations at: CODON 12	CODON 13
K-*ras*	GCT	GGT	GGC	GTA	69%	19%
N-*ras*	GCA	GGT	GGT	GTT	3%	3%
H-*ras*	GCC	GGC	GGT	GTG	0%	N.S.

(B)

***ras* Gene Base Substitutions at Codons 12 and 13**

Mutations at G:C			
-> A:T	-> T:A	-> C:G	Transitions at CpG
61%	30%	9%	0%

(C)

FIG. 3. Comparison of the nature of base substitutions in the p53 and *ras* genes. A) The nature of bases substitutions in the p53 gene in a large number of tumor types has previously been summarized by Hollstein *et al.* (ref. *38*), and the data presented in that manuscript for p53 gene base substitutions in a total of 39 colorectal tumors with base substitutions is shown here. The percentage of each type of base substitution is indicated in the figure. B) The nucleotide sequence of codons 11–14 of the three human *ras* genes is shown. In addition, the percentage of *ras* mutations at each of the codons studied in a panel of 192 colorectal tumors, with 68 total *ras* mutations at codons 12 or 13 is indicated (data from ref. *23*). Codon 13 of the H-*ras* gene was not studied (N.S.) for mutation. C) The percentage of each type of base substitution in the 64 colorectal tumors with mutations at codon 12 or 13 of the K-*ras* and *N-ras* genes is indicated.

K-*ras* and N-*ras* genes, and substitutions at positions 12 and 61 of the H-*ras* gene. In a study of 192 colorectal tumors, and in which 68 total *ras* gene mutations were identified, no H-*ras* mutations were observed (*23*). Mutations at codon 61 of the K-*ras* and N-*ras* genes also were infrequent, with only 3% of the observed *ras* mutations present at each of these codons. As noted in Fig. 3B, over 94% of the *ras* gene mutations were present at codons 12 and 13 of the K-*ras* and N-*ras* genes. Mutations that would result in amino acid substitution would alter one of the first two nucleotide positions of the codons (G in all four cases). While transition mutations were predominant (70%, see Fig. 3C), 30% of the mutations observed were transversions. Also of interest was the observation that no H-*ras* mutations were noted, even though the H-*ras* gene is the only *ras* gene that contains CpG dinucleotides in this target region for mutations that can activate the oncogenic function of *ras*. The basis for the absence of H-*ras* mutations in colorectal tumors (and many other tumor types) is presently unknown, but several explanations can be proposed. First, the H-*ras* gene may have little or no oncogenic potential when mutated at position 12 in colorectal cells, although *in vitro* transformation studies suggest both H-*ras* and K-*ras* have similar transforming activities (*43*). Second, although the *ras* gene might have oncogenic potential if mutated, the CpG dinucleotides in this region of the H-*ras* gene might not be methylated in colorectal cells and therefore would not be a target for spontaneous deamination events. Lastly, given the already noted difference in the relative time of occurrence of *ras* mutations and p53 mutations, the failure to observe transition mutations at the CpG dinucleotides of H-*ras* might be due to possible differences in the mechanisms of mutation at different stages of colorectal tumorigenesis.

Future Studies

The studies of genetic alterations in colorectal tumors have provided thus far a preliminary understanding of the multi-step natural history of colorectal tumors; however, much work remains before the pathogenesis of colorectal adenomas and carcinomas will be fully understood. Very little is known about the normal function of the oncogenes and tumor suppressor genes that are implicated in colorectal tumor development. In addition, many questions remain regarding the environmental and dietary influences on the origin of the somatic mutations, and the relative contribution of the various inherited and somatic mutations to different stages of tumor development. Lastly, it is presently unknown which of the mutations are rate-limiting for tumor development, whether any one mutation is sufficient for the development of a particular tumor stage, and whether all of the mutations identified are, in fact, necessary for tumorigenesis. Nevertheless, future studies undoubtedly will begin to address these questions and will provide fundamental insights into the pathogenesis of colorectal neoplasia.

REFERENCES

1. Weinberg, R. A. Oncogenes, antioncogenes, and the molecular bases of multistep carcinogenesis. Cancer Res., *49*: 3713–3721, 1989.
2. Bishop, J. M. The molecular genetics of cancer. Science, *235*: 305–311, 1987.
3. Fearon, E. R. and Vogelstein, B. A genetic model for colorectal tumorigenesis. Cell, *61*: 759–767, 1990.
4. Muto, T., Bussey, H. J. R., and Morson, B. C. The evolution of cancer of the colon and rectum. Cancer, *36*: 2251–2270, 1975.
5. Sugarbaker, J. P., Gunderson, L. L., and Wittes. *In*; V. T. DeVita, S. Hellman, and S. A. Rosenberg (eds.), Cancer: Principles and Practices of Oncology, pp. 800–803, Lippincott, Philadelphia, 1985.
6. Lipkin, M. Biomarkers of increased susceptibility of gastrointestinal cancer: new application to studies of cancer prevention in human subjects. Cancer Res. *48*: 235–245, 1988.

7. Tudek, W. R., Bird, R. P., and Bruce, W. R. Foci of aberrant crypts in the colon of mice and rats exposed to carcinogens associated with foods. Cancer Res., *49*: 1236–1240, 1989.
8. Utsunomiya, J. and Lynch, H. T. (eds.). Hereditary Colorectal Cancer, Springer-Verlag, New York, 1990.
9. Burt, R. W. and Samowitz, W. S. The adenomatous polyp and the hereditary polyposis syndromes. Gastroenterol. Clinics North Am., *17*: 657–678, 1988.
10. Bussey, H. J. R. Familial Polyposis Coli: Family studies, Histopathology, Differential Diagnosis, and Results of Treatment. Johns Hopkins University Press, Baltimore, 1975.
11. Herrera, L., Kakati, S., Gibas, L., Pietrzak, E., and Sandberg, A. Brief clinical report: Gardner syndrome in a man with an interstitial deletion of 5q. Am. J. Med. Genet., *25*: 473–476, 1986.
12. Bodmer, W. F., Bailey, C., Bodmer, J., Bussey, H. J. R., Ellis, A., Gorman, P., Lucibello, F. C., Murday, V., Rider, S. H., Scambler, P., Sheer, D., Solomon, E., and Spurr, N. K. Localization of the gene for familial polyposis on chromosome 5. Nature, *328*: 614–616, 1987.
13. Leppert, M., Dobbs, M., Scambler, P., O'Connell, P., Nakamura, Y., Stauffer, D., Woodward, S., Burt, R., Hughes, J., Bardner, E., Lathrop, M., Wasmuth, J., Lalouel, J.-M., and White, R. The gene for familial polyposis coli maps to the long arm of chromosome 5. Science, *238*: 1411–1413, 1987.
14. Kinzler, K. W., Nilbert, M. C., Su, L.-K., Vogelstein, B., Bryan, T. M., Levy, D. B., Smith, K. J., Preisinger, A. C., Hedge, P., McKechnie, D., Finniear, R., Markham, A., Groffen, J., Bogusi, M. S., Altshul, S. F., Horii, A., Ando, H., Miyoshi, Y., Miki, Y., Nishisho, I., and Nakamura, Y. Identification of FAP locus genes from chromosome 5q21. Science, *253*: 661–665, 1991.
15. Nishisho, I., Nakamura, Y., Miyoshi, Y., Miki, Y., Ando, H., Horii, A., Koyama, K., Utsunomiya, J., Baba, S., Hedge, P., Markham, A., Krush, A. J., Petersen, G., Hamilton, S. R., Nilbert, M. C., Levy, D. B., Bryan, T. M., Preisinger, A. C., Smith, K. J., Su, L.-K., Kinzler, K. W., and Vogelstein, B. Mutations of chromosome 5q21 genes in FAP and colorectal cancer patients. Science, *253*: 665–669, 1991.
16. Joslyn, G., Carlson, M., Thliveris, A., Albertsen, H., Gelbert, L., Wamowitz, W., Groden, J., Stevens, J., Spirio, L., Robertson, M., Sargeant, L., Krapcho, K., Wolff, E., Burt, R., Hughes, J. P., Warrington, J., McPherson, J., Wasmuth, J., LePaslier, D., Abderrahim, H., Cohen, D., Leppert, M., and White, R. Identification of deletion mutations and three new genes at the familial polyposis locus. Cell, *66*: 601–613, 1991.
17. Groden, J., Thliveris, A., Samowitz, W., Carlson, M., Gelbert, L., Albertsen, H., Joslyn, G., Stevens, J., Spirio, L., Robertson, M., Sargeant, L., Krapcho, K., Wolff, E., Burt, R., Hughes, J. P., Warrington, J., McPherson, J., Wasmuth, J., LePaslier, D., Abderrahim, H., Cohen, D., Leppert, M., and White, R. Identification and characterization of the familial adenomatous polyposis coli gene. Cell, *66*: 589–600, 1991.
18. Cannon-Albright, L. A., Skolnick, M. H., Bishop, D. T., Lee, R. G., and Burt, R. W. Common inheritance of susceptibility to colonic adenomatous polyps and associated colorectal cancers. N. Engl. J. Med., *319*: 533–537, 1988.
19. Fearon, E. R., Hamilton, S. R., and Vogelstein, B. Clonal analysis of human colorectal tumors. Science, *238*: 193–197, 1987.
20. Ponder, B. A. J. and Wilkinson, M. M. Direct examination of the clonality of carcinogen-induced colonic epithelial dysplasia in chimeric mice. J. Natl. Cancer Inst., *77*: 967–976, 1986.

TABLE 3. Cell Growth Inhibition Induced by gp30

	SK-Br-3	MDA-453	CHO/*erb*B-2	CHO/DHFR	MDA-468	MCF-7
gp30	31±3.1	24±2.8	20±2.5	99±10.5	18± 1.2	100± 1.0
4D5 antibody	32±6.0	34±8.1	22±1.9	98± 8.0	104± 8.3	92± 4.5
TGFα	73±4.3	91±2.8	89±8.4	95±14.5	79±10.1	105±14.6
Control antibody	87±4.0	91±1.2	87±7.2	94± 8.8	92±12.5	99± 6.8

SKBr-3, MDA 453, MDA 468, and MCF-7 cells were plated in 24 well plates in IMEM (Biofluids) supplemented with 5% FCS. Parental CHO cells and CHO cells transfected with the DHFR gene or the erbB-2 gene were in 24 well plates (Costar) in α-MEM (Biofluids) supplemented by 10% dialyzed FCS, 0.75 mg/ml G418 and Methotrexate (MTX) 50 nM for the CHO parental and CHO-DHFR cells or 250 nM for the CHO-erbB-2 cells. After 24 hr the medium was removed and replaced with control serum free medium (SFM) containing fibronectin, transferrin, hepes, glutamine, trace elements, and bovine serum albumin (BSA), or SFM with the addition of 2.0 ng/ml gp30, 10 ng/ml recombinant TGF-α (Genentech), or with 25 μg/ml 4D5 specific anti-p185^{erbB-2} monoclonal antibody. Cells were grown to 90% confluence of control and counted. Each group was assayed in triplicate. Results are shown as growth relative to control. The experiments were performed three times and the results were reproducible.

by gp30 ligand was reversed by an EGFR blocking antibody in MDA-468 cells, but not in SKBr-3 or MDA-453 cells. In addition, EGF and TGF-α inhibited the growth of MDA-468 cells and SKBr-3 cells but not that of MDA-453 or MCF-7 cells. Cell growth inhibition of SKBr-3 and MDA-468 cells by EGF was reversed by an anti-EGFR blocking antibody. Although these results were partially surprising, since we did not expect cell growth inhibition, the observed cellular effects in the different cell lines correlated with the results obtained in the tyrosine kinase experiments. We speculated that the effects of gp30 on cells with very high levels of erbB-2 or EGFR were either an inhibitory ligand effect or the effect was of the same nature than those observed with EGF on cells overexpressing EGFR. High levels of EGF will inhibit cell proliferation in cells that overexpress EGFR, such as MDA-468 cells or A431 cells (*22, 23*).

4. *Effect of gp30 on colony formation of human breast cancer cells*

In an anchorage-independent growth assay, gp30 ligand prevented colony formation of SKBr-3 and MDA-453 cells. The anchorage-independent growth of SKBr-3 and MDA-453 cells were inhibited 60%–70% by the novel gp30 although not by EGF or TGF-α. This inhibition was not reversed by an anti-EGF receptor blocking antibody in SKBr-3 cells. Therefore, these results correlated with those on anchorage-dependent conditions.

5. *Growth of SKBr-3 cells treated with low doses of gp30*

We wondered whether gp30 was an inhibitory ligand, or the inhibitory function of gp30 resulted from hyperstimulation of the erbB-2 receptor. Since gp30 and 4D5 have similar antagonistic effects, we hypothesized that the two molecules might have a similar mechanism of action. Although doses of gp30 larger than 0.5 ng/ml are growth inhibitors for SKBr-3 cells, we observed in separate experiments that 0.15 ng/ml of gp30 had a slight stimulatory effect on these erbB-2 cell line, which was against the possibility that gp30 is an inhibitory ligand. Furthermore, treatment of SKBr-3 cells with 4D5 antibody, which induces growth inhibition by itself could be reversed by low concentrations of gp30. Paradoxical effects of growth factors interacting with their receptors have been described previously. Our data support that gp30 and 4D5 bind to $p185^{erbB-2}$ at the same or close binding sites and/or that the affinity of 4D5 for $p185^{erbB-2}$ is lower than that of gp30.

Binding Properties of gp30

At this point, an iodinated monoclonal antibody that binds to the N-glycosylated portion of erbB-2 and acts partially as a ligand by allosteric interaction with the ligand-binding domain of the receptor became available. If 4D5 and gp30 have similar biological effects on erbB-2 overexpressing cells, they may bind to the same or a very close binding site. By iodinating 4D5, we developed a competition binding assay on SKBr-3 cells. We used unlabelled 4D5 to determine a standard curve. By performing radio receptor competition assays in whole cells and antibody cross-linking experiments, we could directly address the question of whether gp30 actually binds to p185/erbB-2.

1. erbB-2 radio receptor competition assay

In order to determine whether gp30 binds specifically to the erbB-2 receptor, purified gp30 was used as a competitor to iodinated anti-erbB-2 antibody (4D5 kindly provided by Michael Shepard, Genentech, Inc., CA.). Iodinated 4D5 monoclonal antibody was used for radio receptor binding experiments, in the presence of increasing concentrations of unlabelled antibody or gp30-ligand. The antibody binds specifically to erbB-2 in SKBr-3 cells and MDA-453 cells with an optimal K_d of about 5 nM. gp30 ligand displaced the binding of 4D5 anti-erbB-2 antibody to its receptor in intact cells (SKBr-3 or MDA-453 cells), to a greater extent than unlabeled antibody, whereas the binding of a control iodinated 6E9 anti-erbB-2 antibody was not altered.

The inhibition of 4D5 binding to erbB-2 by gp30 appeared to be specific, since the binding was not affected by excess levels of EGF or TGF-α.

2. erbB-2 receptor cross-linking competition assay

To further verify that the results obtained from the radio receptor competition was specific, iodinated 4D5 was covalently cross-linked to $p185^{erbB-2}$, in the presence and absence of unlabeled 4D5 antibody and gp30-ligand. The autoradiogram showed a specific high molecular weight (330–340 kDa) 4D5 binding site, that was blocked by the inclusion of 5 nM unlabelled 4D5 antibody, and the inclusion of 2 ng of unlabelled gp30. No inhibition was obtained in the presence of 30 nM unlabelled EGF. Therefore, we concluded from these experiments that gp30 binds to erbB-2 oncoprotein.

3. Characterization and purification of a different erbB-2 ligand derived from SKBr-3 cells

Since 4D5 and gp30 were able to compete in binding to $p185^{erbB-2}$, we speculated that this assay could be used as a detection assay for putative erbB-2 ligands. To identify possible additional erbB-2 ligands, we used the RRA we had developed, using iodinated 4D5 antibody, and a control anti-erbB-2 antibody. The control was primarily used to rule out the possibility of shed erbB-2 that can compete with 4D5 binding.

4. Characterization of additional erbB-2 ligands

Conditioned media from different human breast cancer cell lines were tested and two were determined to possess erbB-2 ligand activity. One from MDA-231 cells and from SKBr-3 cells. Conditioned media from SKBr-3 cells also showed a dramatic inhibition of colony formation and cell proliferation of SKBr-3 cells.

5. Purification of a putative erbB-2 ligand in SKBr-3 cells (the p75 ligand)

Since SKBr-3 seemed to secrete a putative erbB-2 ligand, our next step was to isolate this factor in order to obtain its N-terminal sequence and to determine the degree of homology with gp30 and members of the TGF-α family. The purification was facilitated by using purified extracellular domain from erbB-2 (ECD-kindly provided by Dr. M. Shepard, Genetech, CA). Since iodinated 4D5 bind to purify ECD (data not shown), we decided to utilize these techniques to purify different ligands. ECD was coupled to polyacrylamide-hydrazide sepharose. Concentrated SKBr-3 conditioned media was run through the beads. Elution of the putative erbB-2 ligands was performed stepwise with 1.0 M citric acid at pH: 3.0. All fractions were desalted and then used in a biological assay. We then studied the effects of the putative ligand on the proliferation of breast carcinoma cell lines.

The homogeneity of the sample was further confirmed by analysis on an SDS-PAGE with silver staining, which showed a single band with a molecular weight of 75 kDa. This preparation was used for further analyses.

Biological Properties of the erbB-2 Ligand Secreted by SKBr-3 Cells (p75)

To explore the possibility of identifying a ligand for erbB-2 we used two independent assays: erbB-2 RRA and the effect on cell proliferation of cells with erbB-2 overexpression.

1. Binding of p75 to erbB-2 oncoprotein

To determine whether p75 binds specifically to the erbB-2 receptor, purified p75 was used as a competitor to iodinated anti-erbB-2 antibody (4D5) in SKBr-3 cells. Iodinated 4D5 was used for radio receptor binding experiments, in the presence of increasing concentrations of unlabelled antibody, p75-ligand, or gp30. p75 displaced the binding of 4D5 anti-erbB-2 antibody to its receptor in intact cells (SKBr-3 cells), to a greater extent than the unlabeled antibody, whereas the binding of a control iodinated 6E9 anti-erbB-2 antibody was not alrered.

2. Binding of p75 to EGFR

Since gp30 was identified as a growth factor with binding to both EGFR and erbB-2 receptor, we speculated that p75 might also bind to both molecules. We performed an EGFR radio receptor competition assay in MDA-468 cells. Purified p75 was used as a competitor to iodinated EGF (Amersham). Iodinated EGF was used in the presence of increasing concentrations of unlabelled EGF, gp30-ligand or p75-ligand. p75-ligand did not displace the binding of either gp30 or EGF to EGFR in intact MDA-468 cells. The same result was obtained in the assay described previously on A431 membranes. EGF and gp30, used as controls, displaced the binding of iodinated EGF.

3. Effects of p75 on cell proliferation of erbB-2 overexpressing cells

We wished to determine the effect of p75 on cell proliferation. Since p75 binds to the erbB-2 oncoprotein and does not bind to EGFR, it was relevant to study p75 biological effects. The effects that p75 may have specifically for cells that overexpress erbB-2 is significantly important for the development of therapeutic agents. The effect of p75 on cells that express or overexpress erbB-2 receptor and EGFR was determined as follows:

Cells were treated with p75, gp30 using EGF control. Exposure of SKBr-3 and MDA-453 to p75 and gp30 inhibited their growth by 60–70%. MDA-468 cells were not inhibited by p75 and were growth inhibited by gp30. The effects of p75 on cells with very high levels of erbB-2 were similar to the effects of gp30. However, p75 appears specific for erbB-2.

From these data our conclusions are:

1) MDA-231 cells secrete a gp30 size glycoprotein with some TGF-α properties; this is not the result of post-translational modification of authentic TGF-α. gp30 binds to heparin sepharose in contrast to EGF and TGF-α. Purified gp30 has been fully characterized as a ligand that binds directly and independently to erbB-2 or EGFR.
2) SKBr-3 cells secrete a p75 with some of gp30 properties. Purified p75 has been partially characterized as a biologically active ligand for erbB-2 receptor with no apparent affinity to EGFR.
3) Purified gp30 and p75 inhibit cell proliferation of cells overexpressing erbB-2-receptor in a dose-dependent manner. However, low doses of gp30 slightly stimulate cell proliferation of SKBr-3 cells.
4) gp30 and p75 displace the binding of a specific anti-erbB-2 antibody to erbB-2 receptor.
5) gp30 is a ligand for erbB-2 and EGFR, whereas p75 is a specific erbB-2 ligand.

We believe that manipulation of these ligands may turn out to have important biological effects on growth of human neoplasia. Our studies in the near future will explore these possibilities.

REFERENCES

1. Coffey, R. J., Jr., Derynk, R., Wolcox, J. N., Bringman, T. S., Goustin, A. S., Moses, H. L., and Pittelkow, M. R. Production and auto-induction of transforming growth factor α in human keratinocytes. Nature, *328*: 817–820, 1987.
2. Carpenter, G. and Cohen, S. Epidermal growth factor. Annu. Rev. Biochem., *48*: 193, 1979.
3. Rizzino, A. Growth factor beta: multiple effects on cell differentiation and extracellular matrices. Dev. Biol., *130*: 411–422, 1988.
4. Bano, M., Salomon, D. S., and Kidwell, W. R. Purification of a mammary-derived growth factor from human milk and human mammary tumors. J. Biol. Chem., *260*:

5745–5752, 1988.
5. Spitzer, E., Grosse, R., Kunde, D., and Schmidt, H. E. Growth of mammary epithelial cells in breast cancer biopsies correlates with EGF binding. Int. J. Cancer, *39*: 279–282, 1987.
6. Sainsbury, J. R. C., Frandon, J. R., Needham, G. K., Malcolm, A. J., and Harris, A. L. Epidermal growth factor receptors and oestrogen receptors in human breast cancers. Lancet, *i*: 1398–1402, 1987.
7. Slamon, D., Clark, G. M., Wong, S. G., Levin, W. J., Ullrich, A., and McGuire, W. L. Human breast cancer: Correlation of relapse and survival with amplification of the Her-2/neu oncogene. Science, *235*: 177–182, 1987.
8. Yarden, Y., Kwang, W. J., Yang-Feng, T., Coussens, L., Munemitzu, S., Dull, T. J., Chem, E., Schlessinger, J., Froncke, U., and Ullrich, A. Human proto-oncogene c-kit: a cell surface receptor tyrosine kinase for an unidentified ligand. EMBO J., *6*: 3341–3351, 1987.
9. Bargmann, C. I. and Weinberg, R. A. Oncogene activation of the neu-encoded receptor protein by point mutation and deletion. EMBO J., *7*: 2043–2050, 1988.
10. Van Zoelen, E. J. J., van Rooijen, M. A., van Oostwaard, T. M. J., and de Laat, S. W. Production of transforming growth factors by Simian sarcoma virus-transformed cells. Cancer Res., *47*: 1582–1587, 1987.
11. Kawamoto, T., Sato, J. D., Le, A., Polikoff, J., Sato, G. H., and Mendelsohn, J. Growth stimulation of A431 cells by epidermal growth factor: identification of high affinity receptors for epidermal growth factor by an anti-receptor monoclonal antibody. Proc. Natl. Acad. Sci. U.S.A., *80*: 1337–1341, 1983.
12. King, C. R., Borello, I., Bellot, F., Comoglio, P., and Schlessinger, J. EGF binding to its receptor triggers a rapid tyrosine phosphorylation of the erbB2 protein in the mammary tumor cell line SKBR3. EMBO J., *7*: 1647–1651, 1988.
13. Stern, D. F. and Kamps, M. P. EGF-stimulated tyrosine phosphorylation of p185neu: a potential model of receptor interactions. EMBO J., *7*: 995–1001, 1988.
14. Kraus, M. H., Popescu, N. C., Amsbaugh, S. C., and King, R. C. Overexpression of the EGF-receptor-related proto-oncogene erbB2 in human mammary tumor cell lines by different molecular mechanisms. EMBO J., *6*: 605–610, 1987.
15. Van de Vijver, M., Van de Bersselaar, R., Devilee, P., Cornelisse, C., Peterse, J., and Nusse, R. Amplification of the new (c-erbB2) oncogene in human mammary tumors is relatively frequent and is often accompanied by amplification of the linked c-erbA oncogene. Mol. Cell. Biol., *7*: 2019–2023, 1987.
16. Slamon, D., Godolphin, W., Jones, L. A., Holt, J. A., Wong, S. G., Keith, D. E., Levin, W. J., Stuart, S. G., Udove, J., Ullrich, A., and Press, M. F. Studies of the Her-2/neu proto-oncogene in human breast and ovarian cancer. Science, *244*: 707–712, 1989.
17. Kraus, M., Issing, W., Miki, T., Popescu, N., and Aaronson, S. Isolation and characterization of erbB3, a third member of the erbB epidermal growth factor receptor family: evidence for overexpression in a subset of human mammary tumors. Proc. Natl. Acad. Sci. U.S.A., *186*: 9193–9197, 1989.
18. Lupu, R., Wellstein, A., Sheridan, J., Ennis, B., Zugmaier, G., Katz, D., Lippman, M. E., and Dickson, R. B. A novel breast cancer-like growth factor: purification and characterization. J. Biol. Chem., in press.
19. Lupu, R., Colomer, R., Zugmaier, G., and Lippman, M. E. A candidate ligand of the erbB-2 protooncogene interacts directly with both EGF receptor and erbB-2. Science, *249*: 1552–1555, 1990.
20. Chen, C. and Okayama, H. High efficiency transformation of mammalian cells by

plasmid DNA. Mol. Cell. Biol., *8*: 2745–2752, 1987.
21. Campbell, V. and Slamon, D. J. Personal communication.
22. Kawamoto, T., Mendelsohn, J., Le, A., Sato, G. H., Lazar, C. S., and Gill, G. N. Relation of epidermal growth factor receptor concentration to growth of human epidermal carcinoma A431 cells. J. Biol. Chem., *259*: 7761–7766, 1984.
23. Ennis, B. W., Valverius, E. M., Bates, S. E., Lippman, M. E., Bellot, F., Kris, R., Schlessinger, J., Masui, H., Goldenberg, A., Mendelsohn, J., and Dickson, R. B. Anti-EGF receptor antibodies inhibit the autocrine stimulated growth of MDA-468 human breast cancer cells. Mol. Endocr., *3*: 1830–1838, 1989.

MULTISTAGE CARCINOGENESIS, C. C. HARRIS ET AL. (EDS.),
JAPAN SCI. SOC. PRESS, TOKYO/CRC PRESS, BOCA RATON, PP. 61–70, 1992

Cancer Risks from Germ Line Tumor Suppressor Gene Mutations

Thierry FREBOURG,*[1] David MALKIN,*[1] and Stephen FRIEND*[1],*[2]

Molecular Genetics, MGH Cancer Center, Charlestown, Massachusetts 02129,[1] and Department of Pediatrics, The Children's Hospital, Boston, Massachusetts 02115,*[2] U.S.A.*

Abstract: It has been well established that sometimes cancer clusters within specific families. This has suggested the possibility that some of those families might carry genetic defects which provide susceptibility to specific cancers. Retinoblastoma, an embryonal tumor of the eye represents an extreme example of a tumor which has a dramatic genetic component. Several studies have shown that inactivation at the retinoblastoma gene is probably both necessary and sufficient to initiate retinoblastoma formation. Patients who survive the inherited form of the disease are at risk of developing mesenchymal tumors, melanoma and brain tumors in as high as 10% of the patients before they are 40 years old. Because the product of the retinoblastoma gene, p105Rb, is expressed in all cell types, the obvious question is what accounts for these tissue specific differences in the role of p105Rb. Small cell lung carcinomas virtually all have associated mutations in the Rb gene and yet those tumors do not occur at a significantly increased frequency in patients with the hereditary form of retinoblastoma.

In order to identify genes which might predispose to some of the more common adult malignancies, we have focused on one form of hereditary breast cancer. We chose a rare form of hereditary breast cancer which occurs in families with sarcomas (Li-Fraumeni Syndrome). By use of the candidate gene approach we tested which germ line p53 mutations were found in affected family members with Li-Fraumeni Syndrome (LFS). We have found that virtually all of the families with LFS have germ line p53 mutations, and that these tumors have undergone inactivation of the remaining wild-type p53 allele.

In order to investigate the role of germ line p53 mutations outside of these rare families, we have begun to investigate other high risk groups. These results indicate that *de novo* germ line p53 mutations certainly occur in these high risk groups. These findings along with the recognition of the germ line p53 mutations in families with LFS provide clues about the importance of uncovering hidden susceptibilities from germ line tumor suppressor genes not only for the care of patients, but also for understanding the primary events that normally regulate the growth of cells in various tissue.

In the heyday of dominant oncogenes a decade ago, they held close to a sole billing on the Marquee of Transformation. It was easy to conceptualize how inappropriate activations of growth stimulating genes alone might result in a cancer. The

GTP activating protein, *ras*, seemed likely to be at the root of many malignancies. We now know that although the role of dominant oncogenes is clearly a vital one, and although the dominant oncogenes have provided multiple clues about altered signalling pathways, that there are also other important events which are necessary in order to transform normal human cells. Clues regarding these other events come from numerous experiments. Early experiments by Henry Harris showed that fusion of normal and malignant cells almost always resulted in a suppression of tumorigenicity (*1*). Another indication that dominant oncogenes were not the sole alterations responsible for most cancers came from the fact that alterations in dominant oncogenes are primarily clustered in the later stages of cancer, and in the more aggressive malignancies. Furthermore, if one examines the nature of chromosome changes found in malignancies, most detectable cytogenetic alterations are deletions. Deletions are not what one would expect to activate dominant oncogenes. Other clues about an alternate class of genes involved in transformation came from epidemiologic studies. Virtually all cancers that usually occur in a sporadic form, also occasionally cluster in families. It was the contrast between sporadic and familial forms of cancer that led Al Knudson to postulate the seminal "two hit hypothesis". This hypothesis suggested that one mechanism for tumor formation might be the inactivation of both copies of a growth limiting gene (*2*). The familial forms of cancer could therefore be due to the presence of one inactivated tumor suppressor gene in the constitutional cells of affected family members. He successfully applied this two hit model to explain frequencies of two embryonal tumors, retinoblastoma and Wilms' tumor. This paper will focus on our efforts to understand the cancer risks generated by inactivation of two tumor suppressor genes, the retinoblastoma (Rb) gene and the p53 gene. We will show evidence that individuals who carry germ line mutations in these genes are a risk for a diverse but overlapping set of both pediatric and adult tumors.

Clues from the Rb Gene

The cloning of the Rb gene on chromosome 13q14 allowed a direct test of Dr. Alfred Knudson's two hit model (*3*). When DNA was examined from sporadic retinoblastomas, both copies of the Rb gene could be shown to have suffered alterations. These alterations ranged from mutations which resulted in missense or nonsense mutations to deletions of all sizes. The common theme was that it appeared as if both wild type Rb genes had to be inactivated. Analysis of tumors from patients with hereditary retinoblastoma also revealed inactivation of both wild type Rb alleles. The important difference was that the constitutional cells of the patients with the hereditary form of the disease also had an inactivation of one of the two alleles. This meant that a single alteration in the solitary remaining wild-type allele could release the cell from its normal regulated growth.

Beyond confirming of the two hit hypothesis for retinoblastoma, the isolation of the Rb gene allowed us to look at whether the inactivation of this gene had a role in the development of other malignancies. The ubiquitous expression of the retinoblastoma protein led us to survey a large group of tumors for Rb gene inactivations (*4*). Inactivations were found in osteosarcomas and soft tissue sarcomas which frequently develop as second primary malignancies in retinoblastoma survivors. John Minna's group next found alterations in small cell lung carcinoma (*5*). Since then, the Rb gene has been found inactivated in a wide range of tumors that also include: breast, brain, prostate and bladder cancer and several leukemias (*6*). The important fact is that the inactivation of the same Rb gene which appears sufficient to uncouple the regulated growth of retinal cells, is neither sufficient nor rate limiting for the development of small cell lung carcinoma. This suggests that a single tumor suppressor gene may play a different role in controlling the growth of cells in various tissues.

Finding that a Tumor Suppressor Gene Inactivation Correlates with Risk of Cancer in Families with Li-Fraumeni Syndrome

Breast cancer is one of the most prevalent cancers in American women. Close to 1 in 10 American women develop this cancer. Breast cancer is also one of the cancers in which family history is one of the strongest risk factors. It has been estimated that as many as 1% of American women may carry an inactivated tumor suppressor gene which sets them at very high risk to develop breast cancer. If one studies families with breast cancer, it quickly becomes evident that there are a multitude of different types of hereditary breast cancer. Breast cancer in some families occurs clustered with tumors of the gastrointestinal tract. In other families it appears clustered with brain tumors. In still other families it can either occur as the only type of cancer or it can be clustered with a diversity of other tumors (*7*). Our interest was in identifying a gene which provided susceptibility to one of these diverse forms of breast cancer. Hence we chose an odd, but importantly thereby a recognizable form of inherited breast cancer called Li-Fraumeni Syndrome (LFS). These families were first identified as sarcoma patients in which cancers clustered under the age of 45. When Fred Li and Joseph Fraumeni noted this peculiar clustering, they decided to classify families containing a child with sarcoma and two other close relatives with cancer under the age of 45 as having, "LFS" (*8*). Because there was no chromosome localization of this gene, we sought a potential candidate gene. Because

TABLE 1. Cancers in 43 Families with LFS

Tumor type	Age at diagnosis (years)[a]			
	0–14	15–44	>44	All ages
Component tumors of LFS:				
Breast carcinoma*	0	49	11	60
Soft tissue sarcoma*	13	12	4	29
Brain tumors	12	15	1	28
Osteosarcoma*	6	6	2	14
Leukemia*	8	4	2	14
Adrenocortical carcinoma	5	0	0	5
Possible component tumors of LFS:				
Lung carcinoma*	0	7	12	19
Prostate carcinoma	0	0	8	8
Pancreas carcinoma	0	1	6	7
Melanoma	0	1	2	3

[a] Only first cancer was counted in patients with multiple tumors. (Malkin *et al.*, Science, 1990).
* Somatic mutations of p53 have been described in the sporadic forms of these tumors.

almost all other cloned genes which provided cancer risk as their primary inactivation had been tumor suppressor genes, we searched for a tumor suppressor gene which had not already had a specific embryonal tumor already associated with it. The obvious candidate gene to test was the p53 gene, not only because it had not been linked to any familial cancers, but also because it had already been noted to be inactivated in sporadic forms of many of the component LFS. Table 1 shows the six most common tumors which occur in LFS and the ages at which they presented in a series of over 28 families with the syndrome. Breast cancer is the most frequent malignancy in these families followed by soft tissue sarcomas. The asterisk are placed next to the tumors of which, at the time of our investigation, the sporadic forms of these tumors had already been noted to undergo p53 alterations. This correlation was strong enough that we decided to test if p53 alterations could be found in the constitutional cells of affected family members. We used the polymerase chain reaction to clone a region of genomic DNA encoding exons 5 through 8 from peripheral lymphocytes. This allowed us to initially identify germ line p53 mutations in five families with LFS. It was possible to show that the mutations resulted in missense mutations in highly conserved regions of the protein previously only found altered in tumors. Furthermore, the tumors which were able to be tested had lost the remaining wild type p53 allele. This work suggested that germ line p53 mutations might provide one explanation for the LFS (*9*). This then allowed us to identify relatives of affected individuals in those families who by virtue of having a germ line p53 mutation carried a high but unsuspected risk of developing cancer. Since that time numerous groups including ours have found many germ line p53 mutations in other families with LFS (*10*, *11*). Importantly, there are also some families in which it has not been possible to detect any p53 mutations. This suggests that there may be more than one form of LFS.

Search for Germ Line p53 Mutations outside of LFS

The original definition of LFS stated that there should be a proband with a sarcoma, and two other first degree relatives who developed cancer under the age of 45. If, as is true with some genetic disorders, there were few *de novo* mutations, it might be that there would be few individuals outside the families with LFS who have germ line p53 mutations. On the other hand, there are some genetic disorders where *de novo* mutation are quite frequent. For example, over 80% of the germ line retinoblastoma mutations are *de novo* (*12*). In order to determine the importance of germ line p53 mutations outside of the LFS, we decided to test groups of individuals who might be likely to carry such mutations. One striking feature of the affected members in families with LFS is the high frequency at which they develop second malignancies, almost 50% of the affected members develop more than one malignant neoplasm. If there were patients with *de novo* germ line mutations, until they transmitted the trait and two others first degree relatives subsequently cancer, they could not be recognized by the original clinical definition. However, they should be at a high risk to develop a second primary malignant neoplasm and therefore, they should be able to be ascertained by screening individuals with multiple primary malignant neoplasms.

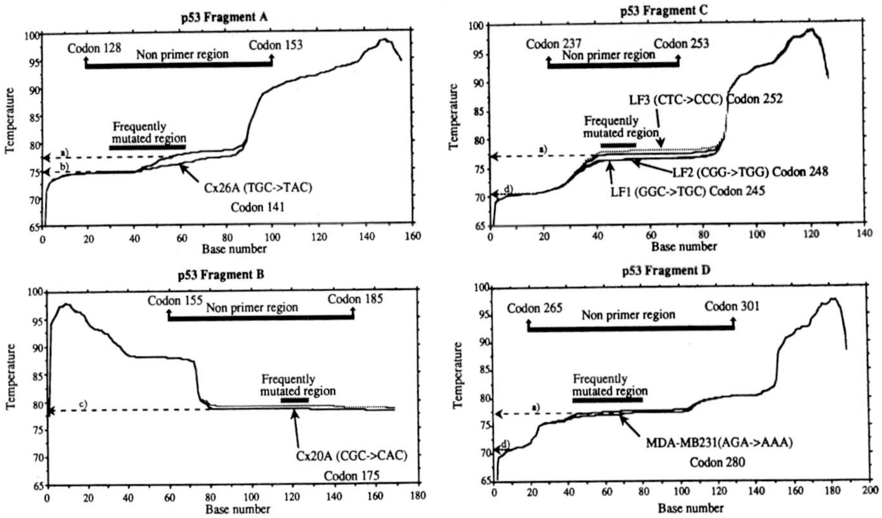

FIG. 1. Theoretical melting profiles of the four PCR-amplified fragments of the p53 gene at temperatures (°C) giving a 50% chance of the base pair being in the double stranded state.

The original screening for germ line p53 mutations was performed by subcloning polymerase chain reaction amplified genomic DNA, and sequencing six independent subclones. Whereas this technique is quite reliable, it is also very time consuming. Since we wanted to survey many DNA samples for germ line p53 mutations, we felt the need to develop a rapid screening test. There were several DNA based techniques including hydroxylamine modification and single stranded confirmational polymorphisms. Because of an uncertainty about the ease and sensitivity of these techniques, we began a collaboration with Anne-Lise Børresen to modify gradient gel electrophoresis techniques to detect mutations in the p53 gene. The underlying concept of this DNA screening technique is that single base pair changes will result in variations in how that fragment will migrate through an acrylamide gel when electrophoresed under partially denaturing conditions. This technique originally developed as a denaturing gradient gel electrophoresis by Leonard Lehrman takes advantage of the fact that a single base pair change alters intrastrand and interstrand hydrogen bonding significantly enough to lead to a variation in local unfolding under partially denaturing conditions. The use of a G-C clamp of 30–40 nucleotides can act to anchor one end of the fragment and computer programs have been developed to analyze the largest fragment of any specific DNA sequence which would still enable detection of any mutation within the region. Figure 1 shows an example of a melting profile for a DNA fragment of p53 which spans the conserved region A where mutations have been noted to be clustered. It can be seen that at a denaturant concentration of 77% which is labelled as "a" there is an obvious difference between the forces stabilizing the wild type p53 fragment and the forces stabilizing a p53 fragment containing a mutation from G>A in codon 141. Similar fragments were designed which could be directly amplified from lymphocyte DNA for three other regions of p53. We then tested the sensitivity of this technique termed, "constant denaturant gel electrophoresis" (CDGE), to detect mutations by analyzing eight

TABLE 2. Characteristics of Patients with Germ Line p53 Gene Mutations

Patient No.	Sex	Age at diagnosis (years)		Tumor histiotype		Location of mutation				Inherited mutation
		Primary	Secondary	Primary	Secondary	Exon	Codon	Base change	Amino acid switch	
6	F	1	32	Neuroblastoma	Breast carcinoma	7	248	CGG-TGG	Arg-Trp	Yes
15	F	7	12	Liposarcoma	Osteosarcoma	8	282	CGG-TGG	Arg-Trp	Yes
38	M	22	30	Soft-tissue sarcoma	Gastric carcinoma	8	273	CGT-CAT	Arg-His	Not analyzed
49	M	17	26	Non-Hodgkin's lymphoma	Colon carcinoma	9	325	GGA-GTA	Gly-Val	Yes

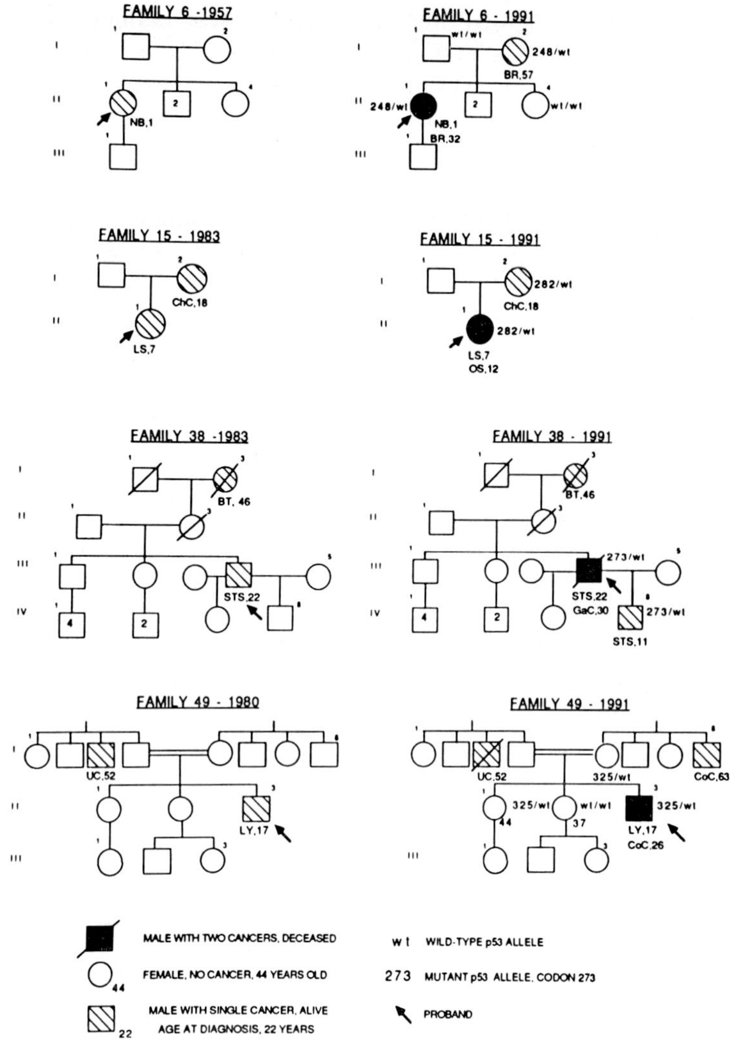

FIG. 2. Pedigrees of four patients with multiple primary malignancies who carry a germ line p53 mutation. On the left the families are shown at the time the proband developed the first malignancy. The families as they existed at the end of the study in 1991 are shown on the right.

fragments containing single base pair mutations which had been identified by sequence analysis. All eight mutations were able to be detected by the CDGE technique. This allowed us to have some confidence that the technique might be helpful in screening large numbers of DNA samples for p53 mutations. Therefore, we began to screen constitutional cells (lymphocytes) from patients with multiple primary malignancy neoplasms.

We analyzed DNA from 59 patients with multiple primary malignancies who did not have any history consistent with LFS. Four of these individuals (6.7%) were found to have germ line p53 mutations. As is shown in Table 2 these patients had a diverse set of malignancies. Whereas breast cancer, soft tissue sarcoma and osteosarcomas are classic component tumors of LFS, these patients also developed gastric CA and neuroblastoma which had never been seen in families with LFS. These data suggest that germ line p53 mutations are clearly found at relatively high frequencies outside LFS, and that germ line p53 mutations may predispose to some malignancies not previously considered to be part of LFS. Figure 2 shows the pedigrees for the four patients with germ line p53 mutations. The pedigrees have been drawn twice. Once at the time of presentation of the first malignancy, and secondly at the time that we performed this study. Three of the four individuals had a first degree relative with cancer when they developed their first malignancy. In two of the cases in the time interval after the presentation of the first malignancy, other family members developed cancer. These facts suggest that individuals with a first degree relative with cancer may be especially prone to develop a second malignancy because they carry a germ line tumor suppressor gene mutation. Furthermore, if germ line p53 mutations could be detected in patients when they first presented with a cancer, it might be possible to screen other family members and identify family members who were also at a high risk to develop cancer.

In the past year since the original detection of the first germ line p53 mutations, a multitude of germ line p53 mutations have been ascertained. Some of these mutations have occurred in patients who have little, if any, remarkable family history. We therefore felt, that it might be helpful to develop an independent series of tests to determine if the mutations had any detectable biological function which might be associated with providing a risk for developing cancer.

Although there are many characteristics about the wild type and mutant p53 which have been previously noted, the functions of p53 remain unclear. Therefore, we decided to assay the p53 proteins resulting from the various germ line p53 mutations in several different ways. Each of seven different p53 mutations was first synthesized in a p53 expression construct by the use of oligo-directed mutagenesis. These mutant p53 containing expression constructs were then introduced into sarcoma cell lines by standard calcium phosphate transfection techniques. The presence of DNA, RNA, and protein could easily by analyzed in these recipient cell lines. As is shown in Table 3 we characterized several parameters. We analyzed whether the transfected p53 protein could bind to SV40 large T antigen, or bind to antibody PAb 240 which recognizes many mutant p53 proteins found in sporadic tumors. We also tested whether the hsc-70 proteins bound to the germ line mutant p53 proteins. As is clear there is much heterogeneity among these proteins. The restrictions on what mutant p53 proteins might be tolerated in the germ line initially noted by ourselves do not seem to apply to many of these germ line p53 mutant proteins. We have found that the most unifying characteristics of the germ line p53 proteins is whether reintroduction of them on these very high expression level constructs blocks the growth of osteosarcomas. All but one of the germ line p53 mutations have lost the vital cell growth limiting function of wild type p53. In fact, the single exception at codon 181 is the exception which proves the rule. When we went back and analyzed many affected relatives of the patients in a family with breast cancer, the mutation at codon 181 did not segregate with the risk for cancer. This fact addresses a very important point. There are likely to be several rare mutations found in the p53 gene distinct from common polymorphisms which will be found in con-

TABLE 3. Biological Properties of Germ Line p53 Mutants

Mutant	Amino acid switch	Conserved region	Observed in	Inhibition of Saos-2 growth	Ab240	hsc70 binding	T binding
181	Arg-His	III	BC	+	−	−	+
245	Gly-Cys	IV	LFS	−	+	+	+
248[a]	Arg-Trp	IV	LFS, SMN	−	−	−	−
252	Leu-Pro	IV	LFS	−	++	++	−
258	Glu-Lys	IV	LFS	−	++	++	+
273[a]	Arg-His	V	SMN	−	−	−	−
282[a]	Arg-Trp	V	SMN	−	+	+	+
Wild type				+	−	−	+

BC, breast carcinoma; LFS, Li-Fraumeni syndrome; SMN, second malignant neoplasm.

[a] The mutation has been previously reported in sporadic tumors.

served domains, which will not necessarily lead to an increased risk of cancer. Hence, we recommend that if questions arise about the significance of a given p53 mutation, assays should be performed before risk assessment is presented in a clinical context.

In summary, we have found germ line mutations in the p53 and Rb gene both provide unique spectra of cancer susceptibilities in different tissues. Several high risk patient groups have been identified which warrant screening for these mutations. Rapid DNA based screening methods such as CDGE are evolving to where large-scale testing will soon be widely used. The mutations found in various tumor suppressor genes are likely to be numerous and biological assays should help complement the detection of the mutations so as to provide useful risk assessment data.

Acknowledgments

S.H.F. is a Lucille P. Markey Foundation Scholar. This work was made possible by partial support from the Lucille P. Markey Foundation, the American Cancer Society and the Canadian MRC (D.M.).

REFERENCES

1. Harris, H. Cell fusion and the analysis of malignancy. The croonian lecture. Proc. R. Soc. Land. B, *179*: 1–20, 1971.
2. Knudson, A. G., Jr. Mutation and cancer. Statistical Analysis of retinoblastoma. Proc. Natl. Acad. Sci. U.S.A., *68*: 820–823, 1971.
3. Friend, S. H., Bernards, R., Rogelj, and Weinberg, R.A. A human DNA segment with properties of the gene that predispose to retinoblastoma and osteosarcoma. Nature, *323*: 643–646, 1986.
4. Friend, S. H., Horowitz, J. M., Gerber, M. R. *et al.* Deletion of a DNA sequence in retinoblastomas and mesenchymal tumors. Proc. Natl. Acad. Sci. U.S.A., *84*: 9059–9063, 1987.
5. Harbour, J. W., La, S. H., Whang-Peng, J., Gasder, A. F., Minna, J. D., and Kaye, F. J. Abnormalities in structure and expression of the human retinoblastoma gene in SCLC. Science, *24*: 353–357, 1988.
6. Lee, E., Y.-H, P., To, H., Shew, J.-Y., Scully, P., and Lee, W. H. Inactivation of the retinoblastoma susceptibility gene in human breast cancers. Science, *241*: 218–221, 1988.

7. Li, F. P. Cancer families. Cancer Res., *45*: 5381–5386, 1988.
8. Li, F. P., Fraumeni, J. F., Jr. A cancer family syndrome in twenty-four kindreds. Cancer Res., *48*: 5358, 1988.
9. Malkin, D., Li, F. P., Strong, L. C., Fraumeni, J. F., Nelson, C. E. *et al.* Germ line p53 mutations in a familial syndrome of breast cancer sarcomas and other neoplasms. Science, *250*: 1233–1238, 1990.
10. Sivastava, S., Zou, Z. Q., Pirolla, K., Blattner, W., and Chang, E. H. Germ line transmission of a mutated p53 gene in a family with Li-Fraumeni Syndrome. Nature, *348*: 747–749, 1990.
11. Law, J. C., Strong, L. C., Chidamberan, A., and Ferrell, R. E. A germ line mutation in exon 5 of the p53 gene in an extended cancer family. Cancer Res., *51*: 6385–6387, 1991.
12. Friend, S. H. The genetic basis of cancer Ch 3. *In* Cossman (ed.), Molecular Genetics in Cancer Diagnosis, Elsevier Science Publishers, New York, 1990.
13. Børresen, A. L., Hovig, E., Smith-Sørresen, B. *et al.* Constant denaturant gel electrophoresis as a rapid screening technique for p53 mutations. Proc. Natl. Acad. Sci. U.S.A., *88*: 8405–8409, 1991.

MULTISTAGE CARCINOGENESIS, C. C HARRIS ET AL. (EDS.),
JAPAN SCI. SOC. PRESS, TOKYO/CRC PRESS, BOCA RATON, PP. 71–76, 1992

Tumor Suppressor Genes Involved in Metastasis of Lung and Colorectal Carcinomas

Jun YOKOTA, Keizo OOKAWA, Ryo NISHIKAWA, and Yuichi SAMESHIMA
Section of Studies on Metastasis, National Cancer Center Research Institute, Tokyo 104, Japan

Abstract: Inactivation of tumor suppressor genes is now believed to play an important role in various progression stages of human cancers. To clarify the possible involvement of tumor suppressor gene inactivation in the acquisition of metastatic potential in lung and colorectal carcinoma cells, we examined various genetic alterations in both primary tumors and metastases obtained from patients with lung and colorectal carcinomas. In lung carcinoma, loss of heterozygosity on chromosomes 3p, 13q, and 17p is a common genetic alteration, and both *RB* and *p53* genes are inactivated as a result of chromosome 13q and 17p losses. In some cases, allelic loss on chromosome 11p and amplification of *myc* family oncogenes occur during tumor progression. In colorectal carcinoma, *p53* and *DCC* alterations were detected in 100% of metastases, and sequential accumulation of allelic losses on chromosomes 13q, 14q, and 18q in the process of metastasis was observed. These results indicate that a subset of tumor suppressor genes is involved in metastasis of lung and colorectal carcinomas.

Recent advances in molecular genetics of human cancer have revealed that inactivation of the tumor suppressor gene plays an important role in the development of human cancer. Allelic chromosomal losses as well as mutations of tumor suppressor genes are common genetic events in a variety of human cancers. Colorectal carcinoma and lung carcinoma are two of the most common adult cancers, and several genetic alterations associated with the development of these cancers have been identified. However, because there has been no systematic study on genetic alterations in metastatic tumors, it is still unknown whether or not there are specific tumor suppressor genes involved in the metastasis of these cancers. To identify tumor suppressor genes involved in metastasis, we have started comparative studies of genetic alterations between primary tumors and metastases on the following assumption. If inactivation of specific tumor suppressor genes is associated with the acquisition of metastatic potential in tumor cells, the incidence of those genetic alterations in metastases would be higher than that in primary tumors. Accumulation of these genetic alterations in the process of metastasis could be recognized if both primary tumors and metastases from the same patients were analyzed for several genetic alterations. Although we have not yet identified a tumor suppressor gene(s) responsible for the metastatic ability in tumor cells, several pieces of unique information have been obtained from this study. Here, we summarize the results of our molecular genetic studies on these cancers and offer genetic models for tumor progression especially in association with metastasis.

Genetic Alterations in Lung Carcinoma

We previously reported that simultaneous allelic losses on chromosomes 3p, 13q, and 17p occur in nearly 100% of small cell lung carcinomas (SCLC) (*1–3*). In addition to these genetic alterations, other genetic changes, such as chromosome 11p loss and N-*myc* amplification, in the process of metastasis was also observed in SCLC (*1*). In non-small cell lung carcinoma (non-SCLC), although incidence of allelic losses for chromosomes 3p, 13q, and 17p in primary tumors was 30–40%, it was 70–80% in brain metastases (Nishikawa *et al.*, unpublished data). As in the case of SCLC, chromosome 11p losses and c-*myc* amplification further accumulate during the progression of non-SCLC. Target tumor suppressor genes inactivated as a result of allelic losses on chromosomes 13q and 17p are the *RB* and *p53* genes, respectively (*4–7*). The *WT* gene is a candidate tumor suppressor gene inactivated as a result of 11p loss, although no mutation of the *WT* gene in lung carcinoma has been reported to date. No tumor suppressor gene(s) on chromosome 3p has yet been identified. Although we do not have any data on *ras* mutations in our samples, association of these mutations with poor prognosis of patients was reported (*8*). These results suggest that 6 genetic alterations causing inactivation of 3 tumor suppressor genes, *RB*, *p53*, and the gene on 3p, would be necessary for the conversion of a normal lung epithelial cell into a fully malignant tumor cell with metastatic ability. Amplification of *myc* family oncogenes, point mutations of *ras* family oncogenes, and inactivation of tumor suppressor gene(s) on chromosome 11p may further enhance the metastatic ability of tumor cells *in vivo* (Fig. 1).

Our results indicate that the same subset of genes is involved in the development of SCLC and non-SCLC. Although the histological features of SCLC are different from those of non-SCLC, both types of tumors are believed to originate from lung

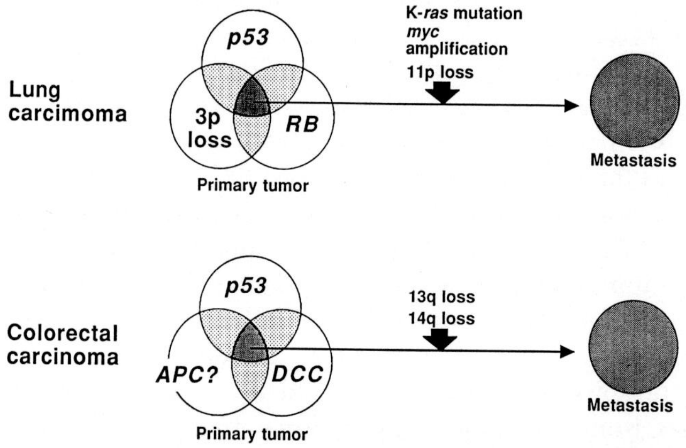

FIG. 1. Genetic models for human lung and colorectal carcinoma progression.

epithelial cells. SCLC is the most aggressive lung cancer showing a high incidence of metastases at the time of diagnosis, but the clinical features of non-SCLC take on a similarity to those of SCLC during progression. Thus, it is likely that the molecular mechanisms of SCLC progression are similar to those of non-SCLC progression.

Genetic Alterations in Colorectal Carcinoma

Inactivation of the *p53* gene on chromosome 17p, the *DCC* gene on chromosome 18q and the *APC* and *MCC* genes on chromosome 5q, in addition to activation of the K-*ras* gene, have been considered critical events for the development of colorectal carcinoma (*9–14*). The hypothesis that stepwise accumulation of defective tumor suppressor genes is involved in the genesis and progression of colorectal carcinoma has emanated from molecular genetic studies on various progressive stages of tumors, from small adenomas to carcinomas (*9*, *15*). However, it is still unknown whether or not there are specific tumor suppressor genes involved in metastasis of colorectal carcinoma, due to the lack of any systematic studies on genetic alterations in metastatic colorectal carcinomas. To identify tumor suppressor genes involved in metastasis of colorectal carcinoma, we performed restriction fragment length polymorphism (RFLP) analysis on both primary tumors and liver metastases to search for chromosomal loci which are frequently and specifically lost in metastases (*16*). In some cases, we were able to compare the patterns of LOH individually in the tumors and metastases from the same patient.

At the *TP53* locus on chromosome 17p, LOH was detected in 10 of 17 (59%) primary tumors and 9 of 10 (90%) liver metastases, respectively. Rearrangement was observed in one primary tumor with allelic loss of the *p53* gene and in one liver metastasis which did not show allelic *p53* loss. In the latter case, the presence of *p53* mutation in the other allele was also detected by polymerase chain reaction-single strand conformation polymorphism (PCR-SSCP) analysis. In total, alterations of the *p53* gene were detected in 59% (10/17) of primary tumors and in 100% (10/10) of liver metastases. As far as determined by PCR-SSCP analysis of exons 5–8 in the *p53* gene, mutations were detected in 17 of 38 (45%) primary tumors and 16 of 31 (52%) liver metastases. On chromosome 18q, the *DCC* locus showed LOH in 100% (19/19) of liver metastases, while the incidence of LOH at the *DCC* locus was 75% (18/24) in primary tumors. These results indicate that concordant alterations of the *DCC* and *p53* genes are necessary for colorectal tumor cells to acquire metastatic ability.

In addition to the *TP53* and *DCC* loci, a higher incidence of LOH in liver metastases than in primary tumors was also observed on chromosomes 1p, 13q, and 14q. Furthermore, sequential accumulation of LOH or rearrangement in the process of metastasis was observed on chromosomes 13q, 14q, and 18q, while alterations at the *TP53* locus were always detected in both primary tumors and metastases from the same patient. These results suggest that inactivation of several tumor suppressor genes, especially those on chromosomes 13q and 14q, plays an important role in the acquisition of metastatic potential in colorectal carcinoma (Fig. 1).

Tumor Suppressor Genes Involved in Metastasis

To identify tumor suppressor genes involved in metastasis, we looked for LOH at various chromosomal loci and mutations in several tumor suppressor genes in primary tumors and in metastases of lung and colorectal carcinomas. Our results, in combination with several other molecular genetic studies on these tumors, suggest that multiple genetic alterations are necessary to convert a normal cell to a fully malignant tumor cell. Further accumulation of genetic alterations occurs secondarily in tumor cells during progression. We speculate that genetic alterations occurring secondarily in tumor cells may control the clinical and biological behavior rather than being critical for tumorigenesis. Therefore, it is very likely that a subset of those genes plays an important role in the acquisition of metastatic ability in tumor cells. Based on the hypothesis described above and the result of our molecular genetic studies, we have drawn genetic models for lung and colorectal carcinoma progression (Fig. 1).

Since we do not have data on genetic changes in precancerous lesions such as adenomas, the initial critical genetic event for malignant conversion is still unknown. However, it was concluded that alterations of the *RB*, *p53*, and 3p genes play a central role in the genesis as well as progression of lung carcinoma, while the *p53* and *DCC* genes (and possibly the *APC* gene) are the critical genes for the development of colorectal carcinoma. Inactivation of these tumor suppressor genes correlates with more malignant behavior of the tumor. Thus, inactivation of two to three tumor suppressor genes is apparently necessary for tumor cells to acquire metastatic ability.

It is still unknown, however, whether these genetic changes are adequate to cause metastasis of tumor cells. For this reason, we searched further for several other genetic alterations which are frequently observed in metastases. In lung carcinoma, amplification of *myc* family oncogenes often occurs secondarily *in vivo* during progression and *in vitro* during cultivation (*17*). LOH on chromosome 11p is also a frequent genetic event in lung cancer (*18*), and sequential accumulation of 11p loss in the process of metastasis was observed in a case of SCLC (*1*). In colorectal carcinoma, allelic losses on chromosomes 13q and 14q in metastases were significantly higher than those in primary tumors, and sequential accumulation during metastasis was also observed. These results indicate that at least four to five genes are mutated when tumor cells form metastatic nodules in the distant organ. Most of the target genes for mutations are tumor suppressor genes. Thus, it is very likely that a subset of tumor suppressor genes has the critical function of controlling metastatic ability in tumor cells. We believe that this approach will enable us to identify metastasis suppressor genes.

Acknowledgments

This study was supported in part by Grants-in-Aid from the Princess Takamatsu Cancer Research Fund and from the Ministry of Health and Welfare for a Comprehensive 10-Year Strategy for Cancer Control, Japan. K. Ookawa and Y. Sameshima are recipients of a Research Resident Fellowship from the Foundation for Promotion of Cancer Research.

REFERENCES

1. Yokota, J., Wada, M., Shimosato, Y., Terada, M., and Sugimura, T. Loss of heterozygosity on chromosomes 3, 13, and 17 in small-cell carcinoma and on chromosome 3 in adenocarcinoma of the lung. Proc. Natl. Acad. Sci. U.S.A., *84*: 9252–9256, 1987.
2. Mori, N., Yokota, J., Oshimura, M., Cavenee, W. K., Mizoguchi, H., Noguchi, M., Shimosato, Y., Sugimura, T. S., and Terada, M. Concordant deletions of chromosomes 3p and loss of heterozygosity for chromosomes 13 and 17 in small cell lung carcinoma. Cancer Res., *49*: 5130–5135, 1989.
3. Yokota, J., Mori, N., Akiyama, T., Shimosato, Y., Sugimura, T., and Terada, M. Multiple genetic alterations in small-cell lung carcinoma. *In*; A. G. Knudson, Jr. *et al.* (eds.), Genetic Basis for Carcinogenesis: Tumor Suppressor Genes and Oncogenes. pp. 43–48, Japan Sci. Soc. Press, Tokyo/Taylor & Francis, Ltd., London, 1990.
4. Yokota, J., Akiyama, T., Fung, Y.-K. T., Benedict, W. F., Namba, Y., Hanaoka, M., Wada, M., Terasaki, T., Shimosato, Y., Sugimura, T., and Terada, M. Altered expression of the retinoblastoma (*RB*) gene in small-cell carcinoma of the lung. Oncogene, *3*: 471–475, 1988.
5. Mori, N., Yokota, J., Akiyama, T., Sameshima, Y., Okamoto, A., Mizoguchi, H., Toyoshima, K., Sugimura, T., and Terada, M. Variable mutations of the *RB* gene in small-cell lung carcinoma. Oncogene, *5*: 1713–1717, 1990.
6. Sameshima, Y., Akiyama, T., Mori, N., Mizoguchi, H., Toyoshima, K., Sugimura, T., Terada, M., and Yokota, J. Point mutation of the *p53* gene resulting in splicing inhibition in small cell lung carcinoma. Biochem. Biophys. Res. Commun., *173*: 697–703, 1990.
7. Sameshima, Y., Matsuno, Y., Hirohashi, S., Shimosato, Y., Mizoguchi, H., Sugimura, T., Terada, M., and Yokota, J. Alterations of the *p53* gene are common and critical events for the maintenance of malignant phenotypes in small-cell lung carcinoma. Oncogene, *7*: 451–457, 1992.
8. Slebos, R. J. C., Kibbelaar, R. E., Dalisio, O., Kooistra, A., Stam, J., Meijer, C. J. L. M., Wagenaar, S. S., Vanderschueren, G. J. R. A., van Zandwijk, N., Moor, W. J., Bos, J. L., and Rodenhuis, S. K-*ras* oncogene activation as a prognostic marker in adenocarcinoma of the lung. N. Engl. J. Med., *323*: 561–565, 1990.
9. Fearon, E. R. and Vogelstein, B. A genetic model for colorectal tumorigenesis. Cell, *61*: 759–767, 1990.
10. Kinzler, W. K., Nilbert, M. C., Vogelstein, B., Bryan, T. M., Levy, D. B., Smith, K. J., Preisinger, A. C., Hamilton, S. R., Hedge, P., Markham, A., Carlson, M., Joslyn, G., Groden, J., White, R., Miki, Y., Miyoshi, Y., Nishisho, I., and Nakamura, Y. Identification of a gene located at chromosome 5q21 that is mutated in colorectal cancers. Science, *251*: 1366–1370, 1991.
11. Kinzler, K. W., Nilbert, M. C., Su, L. K., Vogelstein, B., Bryan, T. M., Levy, D. B., Smith, K. J., Preisinger, A. C., Hedge, P., McKechnie, D., Finniear, R., Markham, A., Groffen, J., Boguski, M. S., Altschul, S. F., Horii, A., Ando, H., Miyoshi, Y., Miki, Y., Nishisho, I., and Nakamura, Y. Identification of *FAP* locus genes from chromosome 5q21. Science, *253*: 661–664, 1991.
12. Nishisho, I., Nakamura, Y., Miyoshi, Y., Miki, Y., Ando, H., Horii, A., Koyama, K., Utsunomiya, J., Baba, S., Hedge, P., Markham, A., Krush, A. J., Peterson, G., Hamilton, S. R., Nilbert, M. C., Levy, D. B., Bryan, T. M., Preisinger, A. C., Smith, K. J., Su, L. K., Kinzler, K. W., and Vogelstein, B. Mutations of chromosome 5q21 genes in *FAP* and colorectal cancer patients. Science, *253*: 665–669, 1991.
13. Groden, J., Thliveris, A., Samowitz, W., Carlson, M., Gelbert, L., Albertsen, H.,

Joslyn, G., Stevens, J., Spirio, L., Robertson, M., Sargeant, L., Krapcho, K., Wolff, E., Burt, R., Hughes, J. P., Warrington, J., McPherson, J., Wasmuth, J., Paslier, D. L., Abderrahim, H., Cohen, D., Leppert, M., and White, R. Identification and characterization of the familial adenomatous polyposis coli gene. Cell, *66*: 589–600, 1991.

14. Joslyn, G., Carlson, M., Thliveris, A., Alvertsen, H., Gelbert, L., Samowitz, W., Groden, J., Stevens, J., Spirio, L., Robertson, M., Sargeant, L., Krapcho, K., Wolff, E., Burt, R., Hughes, J. P., Warrington, J., McPherson, J., Wasmuth, J., Paslier, D. L., Abderrahim, H., Cohen, D., Leppert, M., and White, R. Identification of deletion mutations and three new genes at the familial polyposis locus. Cell, *66*: 601–613, 1991.
15. Vogelstein, B., Fearon, E. R., Hamilton, S. R., Kern, S. E., Preisinger, A. C., Leppert, M., Nakamura, Y., White, R., Smits, A. M. M., and Bos, J. L. Genetic alterations during colorectal-tumor development. N. Engl. J. Med., *319*: 525–532, 1988.
16. Ookawa, K., Sakamoto, M., Hirohashi, S., Yoshida, Y., Sugimura, T., Terada, M., and Yokota, J. Concordant p53 and DCC alterations and allelic losses on chromosomes 13q and 14q associated with liver metastasis of colorectal carcinoma. Int. J. Cancer, in press.
17. Yokota, J., Wada, M., Yoshida, T., Noguchi, M., Terasaki, T., Shimosato, Y., Sugimura, T., and Terada, M. Heterogeneity of lung cancer cells with respect to the amplification and rearrangement of *myc* family oncogenes. Oncogene, *2*: 607–611, 1988.
18. Weston, A., Willey, J. C., Modali, R., Sugimura, H., McDowell, E. M., Resau, J., Light, B., Hausen, A., Mann, D. L., Trump, B. F., and Harris, C. C. Differential DNA sequence deletions from chromosomes 3, 11, 13, and 17 in squamous-cell carcinoma, large-cell carcinoma, and adenocarcinoma of the human lung. Proc. Natl. Acad. Sci. U.S.A., *86*: 5099–5103, 1989.

MULTISTAGE CARCINOGENESIS, C. C. HARRIS ET AL. (EDS.),
JAPAN SCI. SOC. PRESS, TOKYO/CRC PRESS, BOCA RATON, PP. 77–86, 1992

Multistage Carcinogenesis of Liver-fluke-associated Cholangiocarcinoma in Thailand

Chawalit PAIROJKUL,*1 Tomoyuki SHIRAI,*2 Setsuo HIROHASHI,*3 Witaya THAMAVIT,*4 Watcharabhong BHUDHISAWAT,*5 Thongueb UTTARAVICIEN,*5 Makoto ITOH,*6 and Nobuyuki ITO*2

*Department of Pathology and Department of Surgery, Faculty of Medicine, Khon Kaen University, Khon Kaen 40002, Thailand,**1, *5 *First Department of Pathology and Department of Medical Zoology, Nagoya City University Medical School, Nagoya 467, Japan,**2, *6 *Pathology Division, National Cancer Center Research Institute, Tokyo 104, Japan**3, *and Department of Pathobiology, Faculty of Science, Mahidol University, Bangkok 10400, Thailand**4

Abstract: In northeast Thailand, the traditional habit of eating ground, raw freshwater and salt-fermented fish on a daily basis results in a local population repeatedly exposed to both liver fluke (*Opisthorchis viverrini*) infection and consuming nitrosamine-contaminated food from early in life. Epidemiological studies have revealed a coincident high prevalence of cholangiocarcinoma in this region and we have demonstrated in animal models that dietary contamination with nitrosamines and Opisthorchiasis are strong predisposing factors for cholangiocarcinogenesis. Thus all Syrian golden hamsters receiving a combination of subcarcinogenic doses of dimethylnitrosamine (DMN) and infection with flukes developed cholangiocarcinomas, while chemical administration or fluke infection alone did not cause cancer. Synergistic induction by chemical carcinogens and liver fluke infection was found to be related to levels of exposure to both. In this two-stage carcinogenesis model, nitrosamines are considered to act as genotoxicants exerting carcinogenic effects, while the liver flukes are assumed to play epigenetic roles. In our studies of biliary pathology related to worm burden in humans we found that while most of the subjects had worms, only a minority (25%) demonstrated a pathology of adenomatous hyperplasia, which is believed to predispose bile ducts to subsequent development of carcinomas, indicating the possible role of flukes as promoters. Biliary changes in nontumorous areas of hepatectomy specimens, including fibrosis (with or without adenomatous hyperplasia) which is found in most cases, and dysplasia in the fibrotic ducts indicate a conversion event in carcinogenesis: other factors may be required to aggravate the simple proliferation lesion so that they subsequently change to carcinomas. Furthermore, commonality in tumor phenotypes and expressions of *ras* p21 in both fluke related and non-fluke-related cholangiocarcinomas suggest that some similar mechanisms might be operating, at least in the relatively late stages of this multistage carcinogenesis involving the bile ducts.

Cholangiocarcinoma (CCA), a primary carcinoma of the intrahepatic biliary tree, is infrequently encountered worldwide, with an annual incidence of about 2 cases per 100,000 in Western countries (*1*). In contrast, the prevalence rates are high among the oriental populations who are endemically infected with the liver fluke species, *Clonochis sinensis* or *Opisthorchis viverrini* (OV), in parts of China, Korea, and Thailand (*2–5*). Northeast Thailand has the highest risk of all, with an estimated annual incidence rate of 135.4/100,000 in males and 43.8/100,000 in females (*6*).

In northeast Thailand about 7 million people are estimated to be infected with liver fluke, OV (*7*). Among village communities, a prevalence rate of 70–90% is common (*7, 8*). Humans become infected by consuming uncooked freshwater fish which contain infective encysted metacercariae in their muscles. In the duodenum the larvae excyst and ascend the common bile duct to establish chronic infection, mainly in the segmental bile ducts and their branches. The infections are related to secondary hepatobiliary infections, including recurrent suppurative cholangitis, and also cholelithiasis (*9*).

An association between chronic trematode infection and CCA was first proposed by Katsurada (1897) in his report of primary liver cancer occurring with clonochiasis in Japan (*10*). One of the key findings suggesting that flukes might be involved in carcinogenesis is their longevity: a survival span of over 20 years in human hosts was recorded (*11*). Chronic infection results in bile duct epithelial changes including adenomatous hyperplasia, goblet cell metaplasia and periductal fibrosis. Dysplasia as well as carcinoma *in situ* arising in conjunction with fluke-induced non neoplastic duct lesions has been demonstrated (*2, 3, 9*). In Thailand both experimental and epidemiological studies suggest that dietary contamination with carcinogens might be an essential causative factor of cholangiocarcinogenesis. Analysis of foodstuffs consumed daily among the local people, including vegetables and water, in fact revealed contamination with N-nitroso compounds and nitrosamines (*12, 13*). In addition, a study of geographical variation of liver cancers found that the frequency of CCA varies more than 12-fold between regions of Thailand, with occurrence primarily relating to the endemic nature of Opisthorchiasis and also possibly to differences in the nature of foods containing nitrosamines (*4*). A statistical investigation of potential risk factors for CCA indicated an association with Opisthorchiasis and a habit related to nitrosamine exposure, with odds ratios of 5 and 6, respectively (*14*). We and other groups have also found clear synergistic effects of nitrosamines and Opisthorchiasis in inducing CCA in Syrian Golden hamsters, under conditions whereby the administration of chemical carcinogens or fluke infection alone do not cause cancer (*15, 16*). Epidemiological studies have demonstrated that endogenous nitrosation occurs at a significantly higher level in northeastern subjects than in individuals from other regions. The results for people suffering from Opisthorchiasis were about 10 times greater than the control groups (*17, 18*). Clinicopathological observation has verified that biliary cancers associated with liver flukes occur not only at the sites where the flukes have established chronic infection but in the peripheral parts of the liver and the extrahepatic bile duct (*19, 20*). This fact raises the question of whether the fluke might be the sole promoting factor. In this context it is interesting that associated chronic biliary infections and bile stasis have also been found to be risk factors for CCA (*21–23*). In this article we present an overview of our studies aimed at understanding the various stages of carcinogenesis in the case of fluke-related CCAs. The different approaches adopted include animal model experiments and pathological studies in tumor and non-tumor cases. Our findings support the hypothesis that contamination with dietary carcinogens and fluke infection are involved in carcinogenesis. Bile stasis also could be a factor promoting an environment favorable to carcinogenesis, since it was previously found in Japan that *ras* oncogenes may be activated during cholangiocarcinogenesis (*24*). We also investigated *ras* p21 expression in CCAs in Thailand, the findings suggesting that the bile duct might proceed to malignancy by some similar pathways independent of fluke involvement.

Dietary Carcinogens and Fluke Infection

Natural infection by liver flukes in animals rarely causes cancer, and the observation that CCA develops only in a small percentage of chronic cases implies that other factors must be required for malignant transformation (*25*). Since OV-associated-CCA is confined to a restricted group of people, environmental carcinogenic factors are likely contributors. In Thailand exogenous or endogenous nitrosamines have been demonstrated to be formed from nitrates and nitrites in local foods (*12*, *13*), and it is known that secondary amino compounds can react with nitrites to give rise to potent carcinogens, including dimethylnitrosamine (DMN) (*26*). This consideration first led us to investigate the interactions between liver fluke infestation and nitrosocompounds or their precursors. Syrian hamsters respond to OV infection with proliferative changes in the intrahepatic bile duct similar to those observed in man (*27*). In a first experiment, a subcarcinogenic dose of DMN (25 ppm, 10 weeks) was administered in drinking water to animals receiving 100-metacercariae. After only 8 weeks CCAs were found in all hamsters receiving both treatments, while at the end of the 22nd week no tumors were observed in the respective control groups given either carcinogen or parasites alone (*15*). Evaluation of the relationship between carcinogen dose and the level of OV infection revealed that 40% of the hamsters developed carcinomas even with as few as 12 metacercariae, with a DMN dose of 6.25 ppm. The necessity of parasitic infection for tumor induction was evidenced by the fact that no tumors developed in the group receiving DMN at 6.25 ppm alone (*28*). The underlying enhancement of neoplasia by OV remains unclear: whether direct physical trauma, parasitic obstruction, chemical mediators, or immunological reactions are responsible for enhancement of tumor development as well as the observed damage and regenerative lesions (*2*, *3*, *27*). Theoretical considerations do suggest that proliferation within the duct epithelia could act during both the initiation and promotion stages of neoplasia (*29*). Early epithelial proliferation during the period of DMN administration could result in enhanced first-stage initiation, and the continued presence of parasites causing chronic increase in cell turnover might act as a second stage, promoting stimulus to cholangiocarcinogenesis. Even though the 12 metacercariae in hamsters are estimated to be equivalent to the 2,000–3,000 flukes sometimes found in man, the DMN dose used in the experiment is still very high compared to the level of human exposure. However, since the peak age for CCA in Thailand is around 50 years (*6*), a cumulative effect operating over a long period of years is possible (*30*). The hypothesis that the combined effects of dietary carcinogens and parasitic infection could be responsible for CCA development is further substantiated by comparative studies in populations in different regions using a N-nitrosoproline test (*31*). Significantly higher endogenous nitrosation among northeastern people than among those of other low-risk regions was found. Individuals with liver fluke infection had levels of nitrosation about 10 times higher than people in the same region without infection, indicating that parasitic infection could lead to a strong increase in endogenous nitrosamine synthesis in the cancer prone site (*18*). The underlying mechanism by which parasites lead to endogenous nitrosation is still under investigation.

Fluke as a Promoter

Even though various studies have clearly indicated OV infection and dietary carcinogens to be risk factors for CCA, the identification of high risk groups in endemic communities is still very difficult, since eating habits ensure a relatively homogeneous exposure to both risk factors. Most of the infected individuals have subclinical symptoms (*32*). In studying the worm burden in relation to biliary pathology in 50 accident victims we found that 80% of the cases were infected with flukes, and the number of worms per individual ranged from 1–1,693. Adenomatous hyperplasia (Fig. 1), which is characterized by invaginated proliferation with coiling and branching of the surface epithelium, was found mainly in segmental ducts and the proximal parts of regional ducts in 10 cases, with different levels of worm burden: individuals younger than 40 years of age had 280 worms or more while those older than 40 had lower worm burdens (1–126). Accompanying findings in individuals with worm burdens

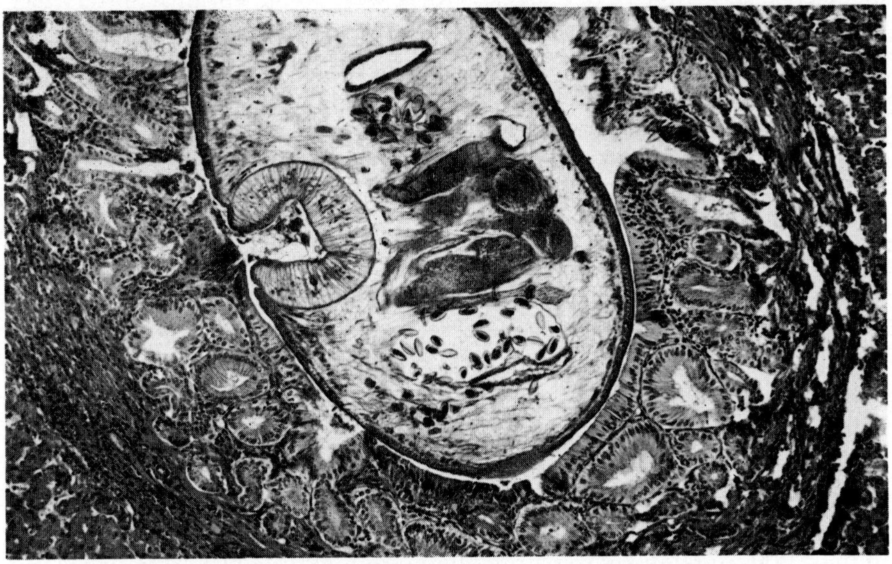

FIG. 1. Adenomatous hyperplasia at a branch of the segmental duct. Also illustrated: worm uses ventral sucker to bite the surface epithelium to anchor itself against the bile flow. Note inflammatory reaction at the injury site and periductal area. (Haematoxylin & Eosin, ×100)

over 150 included periductal fibrosis, scattered goblet cell metaplasia and 15 cases of focal subcapsular bile duct dilatation, indicative of bile stasis. Direct observation revealed adenomatous hyperplasia to be related to both intensity and chronicity of infection (*33*). Its pathogenesis is still unknown, and whether chemical metabolite products from parasites or from the cell-mediated immune response, or both, are involved requires elucidation (*2*, *3*, *27*). Persistent adenomatous hyperplasia suggests that the fluke has the potential to propagate clones of altered cells which are active in the transitional stages leading to carcinoma. While both experimental and pathological evidence of the histogenetic role of this lesion has been established (*2*, *3*, *7*), however, tumor incidence data clearly indicate that the phenomenon of malignant development occurs only in a minority of cases. Other exogenous or endogenous factors, such as genetic and interindividual variation in carcinogen metabolism and DNA repair processes are considered to be important determinants of cancer susceptibility (*34*).

Bile Stasis: A Promoting Environment

Biliary carcinomas associated with Opisthorchiasis are found to arise in both the extra and intrahepatic bile ducts (*19*, *20*). The most common form is the hilar type (41%), that is, tumors originating in the main intrahepatic bile duct or proximal extrahepatic ducts which invade deep into the hepatic parenchyma at the hepatic hilum. The peripheral type, tumors confined to within the liver itself, is less common (17%). The primary sites can be either the segmental ducts or their branches, the regional ducts. Tumors occur most frequently in the posterior segment of the right lobe (83%) (*19*). There is still no explanation for this. We studied the distribution of worms in 87 accident cases and found no significant differences between worm

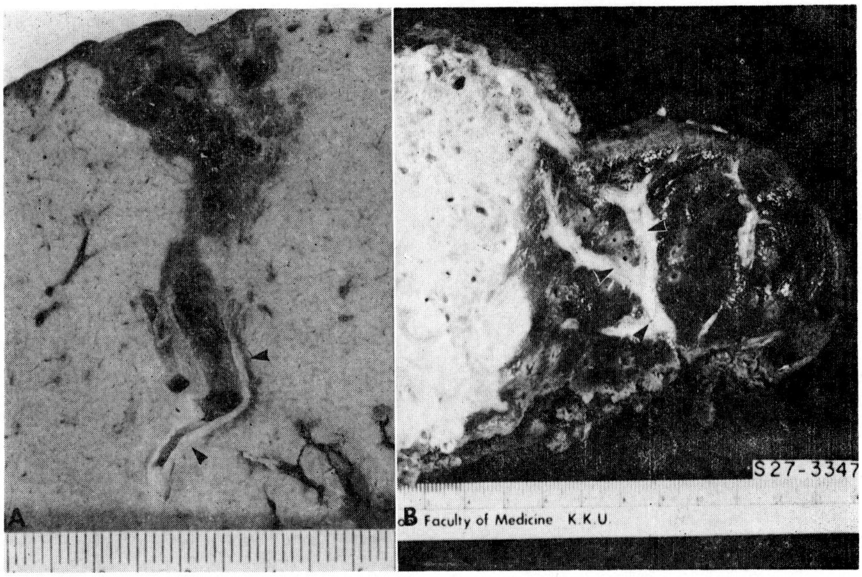

FIG. 2. Fibrotic intrahepatic bile ducts (arrow) of peripheral cholangiocarcinomas: (A) early case (B) late case. Note that both are located at the posterior aspect of the livers.

loads in any sectors (right posterior, right anterior, left median and left lateral sectors) when considering worms/gm of liver (*35*). An indirect correlation with worm burden in cases of CCA was also found in a case-controlled prospective study (*36*). These findings suggest that worm burden alone cannot explain tumor predominant sites. We examined the biliary tract pathology of peripheral type CCAs in 22 hepatectomy specimens from patients for which there was evidence of Opisthorchiasis (ova in stool or bile). All cases had biliary changes with predominant underlying fibrosis (Fig. 2): fibrosis with and without adenomatous hyperplasia was respectively found in 12/22 (56%) and 8/22 (36%) of the segmental ducts, and in 9/22 (41%) and 13/22 (59%) of the regional ducts. Adenomatous hyperplasia alone was found in 2 cases. Dysplasia over the surface epithelium was apparent in 6 cases, and in 3 cases it was demonstrated in association with regression epithelium of the fibrotic ducts. This suggests that the bile ducts in tumor cases are mostly fibrotic and could cause bile stasis. These pathological changes could result either from chronic OV infestation or a sequelae of associated chronic infections (*37*). In fact, in both a community survey by ultrasonography and in autopsy cases Opisthorchiasis-linked bile stasis was found (*37, 38*). Chronic biliary infection and bile stasis were found to be risk factors for malignant change in cases of intrahepatic lithiasis, and choledochal cysts infecting bile and bile constituent are suspected to be carcinogenic factors (*21–23, 39*). A recent study found N-nitroso compounds in bile not only in gallstone patients but in normal people, presumably from local endogenous gastric nitrosation (*40*). This could account for the excess risk from carcinogenic effects in cases with bile stasis. Bile stasis indirectly caused by the fluke could be producing an environment in which repeated bacterial infection results in continued cell death and compensatory regeneration which, in turn, might act as a nonspecific enhancing stimulus and more susceptible to carcinogens in bile. This might be one possible explanation for the fact that tumors are commonly found in the hilar region, the portal route of bile and the anatomically dominant portion, the posterior aspect of the liver.

Genetic Factor

Tumor phenotypes of CCA with or without a relationship to fluke are basically

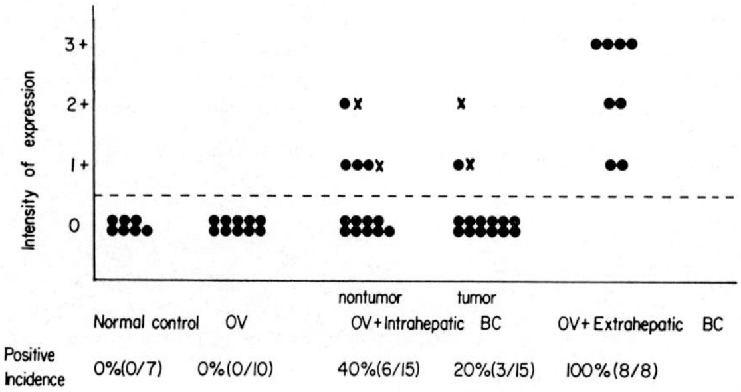

FIG. 3. Positive incidence and scores for intensity of immunoperoxidase staining of *ras* p21 in relation to OV-infection group (OV) and OV-associated biliary cancer groups (BC). Score for staining from 1+ (definite but weak staining) to 3+ intense staining; 0 represents a negative reaction. × indicates a case with positive staining in both tumor and nontumor areas.

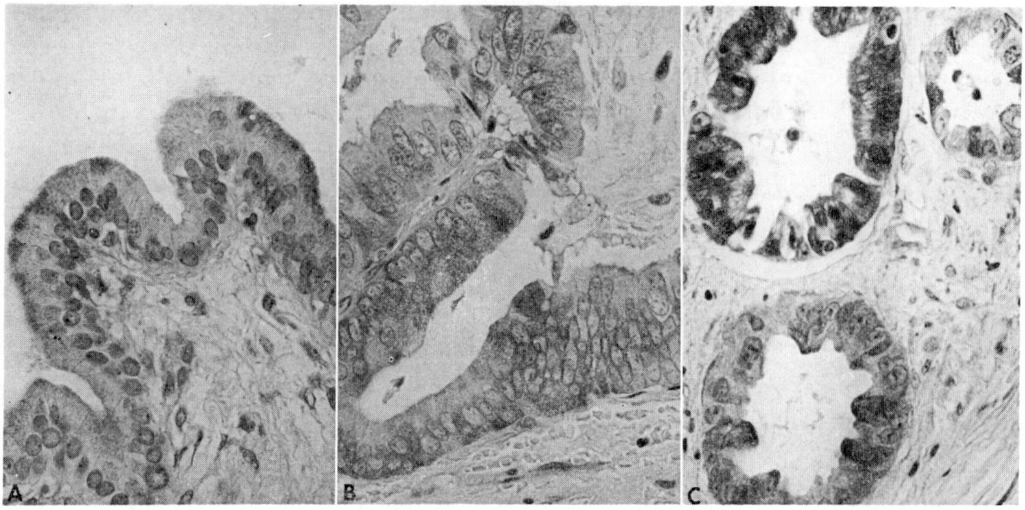

FIG. 4. Immunoperoxidase staining for *ras* p21, showing submembranous expression of the antigens in the segmental duct epithelial of the non-tumor area (A), diffuse weak cytoplasmic expression on papillary mucinous adenocarcinoma of the intrahepatic bile duct (B), the same case as (A), and intensive expression of *ras* p21 on tubular adenocarcinoma of the extrahepatic bile duct (C). (ABC staining for *ras* p21 with Haematoxylin, ×400)

similar, the majority of lesions are mucin-producing adenocarcinomas of variable grades of differentiation. Well-differentiated CCA accounts for 66% of cases in Japan (*24*) and 58% in Thailand (*41*), and carcinoembryonic antigens have been detected in nearly all such tumors from both places (*24, 41*). An immunohistochemical study demonstrated that there was *ras* p21 expression in 39/42 (88%) of the cases of CCA in Japan, suggesting that the *ras* oncogene is probably involved in cholangiocarcinogenesis (*24*). We studied p21 expression using immunohistochemical staining (Avidin-Biotin-Peroxidase Complex method with mouse monoclonal antibody to normal human *ras* p21, NCC, Tokyo) in OV-associated biliary cancers, and compared bile ducts in nontumor areas of cancer patients with bile ducts in the liver of accident cases with OV infection. The results are summarized in (Fig. 3). Whereas no bile ducts in the OV group had positive expression, both bile ducts in nontumor areas ($p<0.03$, Fischer's exact test) and intrahepatic tumors demonstrated enhanced p21 expression. This suggests that *ras* p21 expression might not be caused by the process of parasites but might rather be related to the neoplastic process. In two cases, p21 were exhibited in both tumor and nontumor areas (Fig. 4), implying that *ras* p21 might be involved in the initial phase of the transformation event. Obviously more case studies are needed to confirm this notion. Regarding the observed difference between frequency of cases in which expression of p21 antigens in the intra- and extrahepatic cancers could have been caused by variation of phenotypes, we found that all 6 cases (6/15) which showed negative staining in the intrahepatic cancer group were the undifferentiated tubular type. It has been reported that the expression of p21 antigens is lost with increasing dedifferentiation of tumor cells (*24*). Enhanced p21 antigen expression occurs in cancer cells, especially those of the extrahepatic bile duct type (Fig. 4), of which all our extrahepatic cases are evidence.

This expression could be an effect of the neoplastic process; alternatively, it may be involved in the transformation event. Although the activation of the *ras* gene has been demonstrated in a wide variety of human tumors, gene activation by point mutation has been found in only about 15% (*42*). There are observations indicating that not only qualitative alteration of proteins by somatic mutation of cellular *ras* gene but also quantitative changes are important in carcinogenesis (*42, 43*). Whether overexpression of *ras* gene is the underlying mechanism in transformation in our cases requires further study.

In conclusion, our findings add support to the concept that carcinogenesis is a multistage process involving both genetic and epigenetic changes. Further studies comparing the molecular basis of *ras* gene alteration and identifying other oncogenes and tumor suppressor genes are warranted to aid our understanding of cholangiocarcinogenesis.

Acknowledgments

This work was supported, in part, by grants from the Faculty of Medicine, Khon Kaen University, the Mahidol Foundation, Thailand, and the Monbusho International Scientific Research Program, Japan. We also thank Dr. Malcolm Moore and Mr. David Narot for comments and help in preparation of the manuscript.

REFERENCES

1. Muir, C., Waterhouse, J., Mack, T., Powell, J., and Whelan, S. (eds.). Cancer Incidence in Five Continents, vol. 5, pp. 791–856, IARC, Lyon, 1987.
2. Hou, P. C. The relationship between primary carcinoma of the liver and infestation with *Clonorchis sinensis*. J. Pathol. Bacteriol., *72*: 239–246, 1956.
3. Kim, Y. Liver carcinoma and liver fluke infection. Arzneim Forsch., *34*: 1121–1126, 1984.
4. Srivatanakul, P., Sontipong, S., Chotiwan, P., and Parkin, D. M. Liver cancer in Thailand: temporal and geographic variations. J. Gastroenterol. Hepatol., *3*: 413–420, 1988.
5. Vatanasapt, V., Uttaravichien, T., Mairiang, E., Pairojkul, C., Chartbanchachai, V., and Haswell-Elkins. M. R. Northeast Thailand: A region with a high incidence of cholangiocarcinoma. Lancet, *335*: 116, 1990.
6. Green, A., Uttaravichien, T., Bhudhisawasdi, V., Chartbanchachai, W., Elkins, D., Marieng, E. M., Pairojkul, C., Dhiensiri, T., Kanteekaew, N., and Haswell-Elkins, M. Cholangiocarcinoma in Northeast Thailand: a hospital-based study. Trop. Geogr. Med., *43(2)*: 193–198, 1991.
7. Preuksaraj, S. Public health aspects of opisthorchiasis in Thailand. Drug Res., *34*: 1119, 1984.
8. Upatham, E. S., Brockelman, W. Y., Viyanant, V., Lee, P., Kraengraeng, R., and Prayoonwinat, B. Incidence of endemic *Opisthorchis viverrini* infection in a village in northeast Thailand. Am. J. Trop. Med. Hyg., *34*: 903–906, 1985.
9. Tansurat, P. Opisthorchiasis. *In*; P. A. Marcial-Rojas (ed.), Pathology of Protozoal and Helminthic Diseases with Clinical Correlation, pp. 536–545, Williams & Wilkins, Baltimore, 1971.
10. Katsurada, F. Beitrag zur kenntnis des distomum spatulatum. Beit Pathol. Anat., *28*: 479–505, 1900.
11. Atwood, H. D. and Chou, S. T. The longevity of *Clonorchis sinensis*. Pathology, *10*:

153–156, 1978.

12. Migasena, P., Reansuwan, W., and Changbungrung, S. The nitrates and nitrites in local Thai preserved protein foods. J. Med. Assoc. Thailand, *63*: 500–505, 1980.
13. Migasena, P. and Changbumrung, S. The role of nitrosamines in the causation of primary carcinoma. J. Med. Assoc. Thailand, *57*: 75–178, 1974.
14. Parkin, D. M., Srivatanakul, P., Khlat, M., Chenvidthya, P., Chotiwan, P., Insiripong, S., Labbe, K. A., and Wild, C. P. Liver Cancer in Thailand: a case-control study of cholangiocarcinoma. Int. J. Cancer, *48(3)*: 323–328, 1991.
15. Thamavit, W., Bhamarapravati, N., Sahaphong, S., Vajarasthira, S., and Angsubhakorn, S. Effects of dimethylnitrosamine on induction of cholangiocarcinoma in *Opisthorchis viverrini* infected Syrian golden hamsters. Cancer Res., *38*: 4634–4639, 1978.
16. Flavell, D. and Lucas, S. B. Promotion of N-nitrosodimethylamine initiated bile duct carcinogenesis in the hamster of the human liver fluke, *Opisthorchis viverrini*. Carcinogenesis, *4*: 927–930, 1983.
17. Srianujata, S., Tonbuth, S., and Bunyaratvej, S. High urinary excretion of nitrate and N-nitrosoproline on Opisthorchiasis subjects. *In*; H. Bartsch, I. K. O'Neill, and R. Schulte-Hermann, (eds.), The Relevance of N-nitroso Compounds to Human Cancer: Exposures and Mechanisms, pp. 544–546, IARC, Lyon, 1987.
18. Srivatanakul, P., Ohshima, H., Khlat, M., Parkin, M., Sukarayodhin, S., Bronet, I., and Bartch, H. Endogenous nitrosation and liver fluke as risk factors for cholangiocarcinoma in Thailand. *In*; I. K. O'Neill, J. Chen, and H. Bartsch, (eds.), Relevance of Human Cancer of N-nitroso Compounds, Tobacco and Mycotoxin, pp. 88–94, IARC, Lyon, 1991.
19. Dhiensiri, T., Wibulpolprasert, B., Mairiang, E., Chaiyakam, J., and Mairiang, P. Detection of cholangiocarcinoma by multiple image modalities. *In*; S. Santasiri, (ed.), Proceedings of the Workshop on Development of Early Diagnosis and Management of Cholangiocarcinoma Associated with Opisthorchiasis, pp. 48–57, Mahidol University Press, Bangkok, 1989.
20. Juttijudata, P., Chiemchaisri, C., and Palavatana, C. Causes of cholestasis in Thailand. A study of 276 consecutive patients. Am. J. Surg., *147*: 360–365, 1984.
21. Falchuk, K. R., Lesser, P. B., Galdabini, J. J., and Isselbacher, K. J. Cholangiocarcinoma as related to chronic intrahepatic cholangitis and hepatolithiasis. Am. J. Gastroenterol., *66*: 57–61, 1976.
22. Koga, A., Ichimiya, H., Yamaguchi, K., Miyazaki, K., and Nakayama, F. Hepatholithiasis associated with cholangiocarcinoma: possible etiologic significance. Cancer, *55*: 2826–2829, 1985.
23. Bloustein, P. A. Association of carcinoma with congenital cystic conditions of the liver and bile ducts. Am. J. Gastroenterol., *67*: 40–46, 1977.
24. Nonomura, A., Ohta, G., Hayashi, M., Izumi, R., Watanabe, K., Takayanagi, N., and Matsubara, F. Immunohistochemical localization of *ras* p21 and carcinoembryonic antigens (CEA) in cholangiocarcinoma. Liver, *7*: 142–148, 1987.
25. Flavell, D. J. Liver fluke infection as an aetiological factor in bile-duct carcinoma of man. Trans. R. Soc. Trop. Med. Hyg., *75*: 814–824, 1981.
26. Lijinsky, W. and Greeblatt, M. Carcinogen dimethylnitrosamine produced *in vivo* from nitrite and aminopyrine. Nature New Biol., *236*: 177–178, 1972.
27. Bhamarapravati, N., Thammavit, W., and Vajrasthira, S. Liver changes in hamsters infected with a liver fluke of man, *Opisthorchis viverrini*. Am. J. Trop. Med. Hyg., *27*: 787–794, 1978.
28. Thamavit, W., Kongkanuntn, R., Tiwawech, D., and Moore, M. A. Level of Opisthor-

chis infestation and carcinogen-dose dependence of cholangiocarcinoma induction in Syrian golden hamsters. Virch. Arch., Abt. B., *54*: 52–58, 1987.
29. Pitot, H. C. and Scirica, A. E. The stages of initiation and promotion in hepatocarcinogenesis. Biochim. Biophys. Acta, *605*: 191–215, 1984.
30. Druckrey, H., Schildbach, A., Schmahl, D., Preussmann, R., and Ivankovic, S. Quantitative analysis of the carcinogenicity of diethylnitrosamine. Arzneim Forsch., *10*: 841–851, 1963.
31. Ohshima, H. and Bartsch, H. Urinary N-nitrosamino acids as an index of exposure to N-nitroso compounds. *In*; H. Bartsch, K. Hemminki, and I. K. O'Neil, (eds.), Method for Detecting DNA Damaging Agents in Humans: Applications in Cancer Epidemiology and Prevention, pp. 83–91, IARC, Lyon, 1988.
32, Upatham, E. S., Viyanant, V., Kurathong, S., Brockelman, W. Y., Menaruchi, A., Saowakontha, S., Intarakhao, C., Vajarashthira, S., and Warren, K. S. Morbidity in *Opisthorchiasis viverrini*: study of a community in Khon Kaen, Thailand. Am. J. Trop. Med. Hyg., *31(6)*: 1156–1163, 1982.
33. Pairojkul, C., Sithithaworn, P., Sripa, B., Thamawit, W., Ito, N., and Itoh, M. Risk groups for opisthorchiasis-associated cholangiocarcinoma: indicated by a study of worm burden related biliary pathology. Kan Tan Sui, *22*: 393–403, 1991.
34. Harris, C. Interindividual variation among humans in carcinogen metabolism, DNA adduct formation and DNA repair. Carcinogenesis, *10*: 1563–1566, 1990.
35. Sithithaworn, P., Tesana, S., Pipitgool, V., Kaewkes, S., Thaiklar, K., Pairojkul, C., Sripa, B., Paupairoj, A., Sanpitak. P., and Aranyanat, C. Quantitative post mortem study of *Opisthorchis viverrini* in man in Northeast Thailand. Trans. Roy. Soc. Trop. Med. Hyg., *85*: 765–768, 1991.
36. Kurathong, S., Lerdverasirikul, P., Wongpatoon, V., Pramoolsinsap, C., Kanjanapitak, A., Varawithaya, W., Phupradit, P., Bunyaratvej, S., Upatham, S., and Brockelman, W. Y. *Opisthorchis viverrini* infection and cholangiocarcinoma: a prospective, case-control study. Gastroenterology, *89*: 151–156, 1985.
37. Evans, H., Bourgeois, C. H., Comer, D. S., and Keschamrus, N. Biliary tract changes in opisthorchiasis. Am. J. Trop. Med. Hyg., *20*: 667–671, 1971.
38. Elkins, D. B., Haswell-Elkins, M. R., Mairiang, E., Mairiang, P., Sithithaworn, P., Kaewkes, S., Bhudhisawasdi, V., and Uttaravichien, T. A high frequency of hepatobiliary disease and suspected cholangiocarcinoma associated with heavy *Opisthorchis viverrini* infection in a small community in Northeast Thailand. Trans. R. Soc. Trop. Med. Hyg., *84*: 715–719, 1990.
39. Tabata, M. and Nakayama, F. Bacteria and gallstones: etiological significance. Dig. Dis. Sci., *26*: 218–224, 1981.
40. Caygill, C. P. J., Leach, S. A., Fernandez, F., Duncan, S., Hill, M. J., Massey, R., and Hall, R. Endogenous N-nitrosation and cancer of the biliary tract. *In*; I. K. O'Neill, J. Chen, and H. Bartsch (eds.), Relevance of Human Cancer of N-nitroso Compounds, Tobacco and Mycotoxin, pp. 137–138, IARC, Lyon, 1991.
41. Sripa, B., Pairojkul, C., Thamavit, W., Moore, M. A., and McKenzie, I. F. C. Immunohistochemical study of CEA, AFP, and GST–II. Abstracts of the Second National Congress of Pathology, p. 12, Bangkok, 1990.
42. Tanaka, T., Slamon, D. J., Bathora, H., and Cune, M. J. Expression of p21 *ras* oncoproteins in human cancer. Cancer, *46*: 1465–1470, 1986.
43. Kurzrock, R., Gallik, G. E., and Gutterman, J. U. Differential expression of p21 *ras* gene products among histologic subtypes of fresh primary human lung tumors. Cancer Res., *46*: 1530–1534, 1986.

MULTISTAGE CARCINOGENESIS, C. C. HARRIS ET AL. (EDS.),
JAPAN SCI. SOC. PRESS, TOKYO/CRC PRESS, BOCA RATON, PP. 87–93, 1992

Pathology and Molecular Mechanisms of Multistage Human Hepatocarcinogenesis

Setsuo HIROHASHI

Pathology Division, National Cancer Center Research Institute, Tokyo 104, Japan

Abstract: Recent fundamental research has disclosed the presence of multiple genetic alterations including activation of oncogenes and inactivation of tumor suppressor genes in various human cancers. These multiple genetic alterations are thought to be correlated with multiple stages of carcinogenesis and further progression. Hepatocellular carcinoma (HCC) is a typical example. The majority of HCCs are associated with infection by hepatitis virus B or C. In the damaged liver, small nodular lesions develop due to clonal expansion of hepatocytes. Some of these nodules are diagnosed as early HCC of the well differentiated type and correspond to *in situ* or microinvasive carcinoma. Within these nodules, moderately or poorly differentiated HCCs often emerge as nodule-in-nodule lesions when the diameter of the nodules exceeds 1.5 cm. Ordinary HCCs formed by progression show highly increased cell proliferation, neovascularization, production of high-molecular-mass forms of basic fibroblast growth factor and aneuploidy in some tumors. Corresponding to this stage of malignant progression, HCCs show loss of heterozygosity for multiple chromosomes including chromosomes 4, 16q and 17p. Tumor suppressor gene *p*53, located on 17p, is frequently mutated in high-grade, but not in early, HCCs. Thus, it is strongly suggested that inactivation of multiple tumor suppressor genes plays an important role in progression, and probably directly or indirectly causes chromosome instability, enhanced cell proliferation and neovascularization.

The recent remarkable progress in imaging diagnosis has made it possible to detect an increasing number of minute hepatocellular carcinomas (HCCs), some of which can be removed successfully by surgery. In addition, lesions intermediate between regenerative nodules and minute HCCs, *i.e.* borderline lesions, can also be detected. Analysis of these lesions has revealed the natural course of human hepatocarcinogenesis (*1–3*). Simultaneously, over the last decade, there has been rapid progress in our fundamental understanding of carcinogenesis. A number of oncogenes as well as some tumor suppressor genes have been identified, and their roles in carcinogenesis and tumor progression are becoming clearer.

In these studies, all the surgical specimens of HCCs were examined macroscopically by pathologists soon after removal, and samples for DNA extraction were taken from each grossly distinct area. DNA samples extracted from the tissues were analyzed by the Southern blot technique and the polymerase chain reaction (PCR). The integration pattern of hepatitis B virus DNA was used as a marker of tumor cell clonality, and loss of heterozygosity of chromosomes was examined using various polymorphic probes corresponding to each chromosome. Oncogenes and tumor suppressor genes were analyzed by PCR amplification and subsequent dot-blot analysis or single-strand conformation polymorphism (SSCP) analysis combined with direct sequencing to elucidate the base changes of the mutations. Morphological features of HCCs and related lesions were studied using not only conventional histopathological techniques but also immunohistochemistry for several markers of cell proliferation and angiogenesis. DNA ploidy of tumor cells was also analyzed. Thus, we had an opportunity to study the genetic alterations and other molecular features that form the basis of hepatocarcinogenesis, and to correlate the results with clinicopathological findings.

Pathology of Multistage Human Hepatocarcinogenesis

One of the unique features of advanced HCC is the morphologic heterogeneity existing within a single tumor nodule. This heterogeneity is now considered to result from stepwise tumor progression (*1, 2, 4*). When the tumors are smaller, less than 1.5 cm in diameter in most cases, they are usually homogeneous in morphology and composed of very well differentiated tumor cells resembling hepatocytes. The tumor cells are small and crowded, indicating that their proliferative activity is higher than that of hepatocytes in the surrounding non-tumorous liver. Some of these tumors show abnormal features, such as acinar or irregular cord structures, and these are diagnosed as well differentiated HCC. Since portal triads containing portal veins and bile ducts are still preserved in these tumors, the lesions are considered to correspond to *in situ* carcinomas or those at an early invasive stage in other organs. Thus, we previously proposed the term early HCC for these lesions (*1, 2*) (Fig. 1). When the tumors become larger, around 2 cm in diameter, they often show a nodule-in-

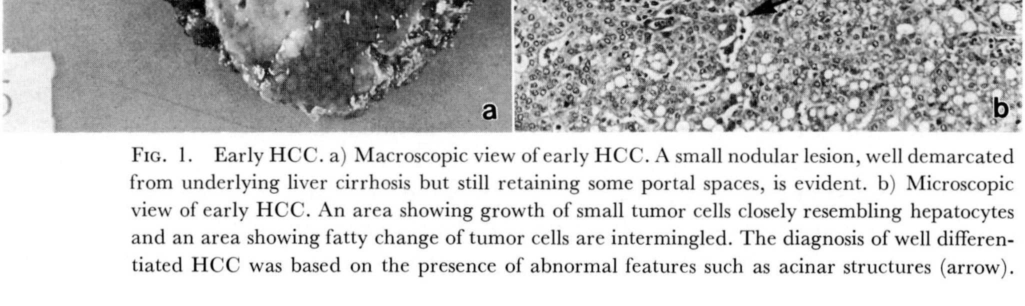

FIG. 1. Early HCC. a) Macroscopic view of early HCC. A small nodular lesion, well demarcated from underlying liver cirrhosis but still retaining some portal spaces, is evident. b) Microscopic view of early HCC. An area showing growth of small tumor cells closely resembling hepatocytes and an area showing fatty change of tumor cells are intermingled. The diagnosis of well differentiated HCC was based on the presence of abnormal features such as acinar structures (arrow).

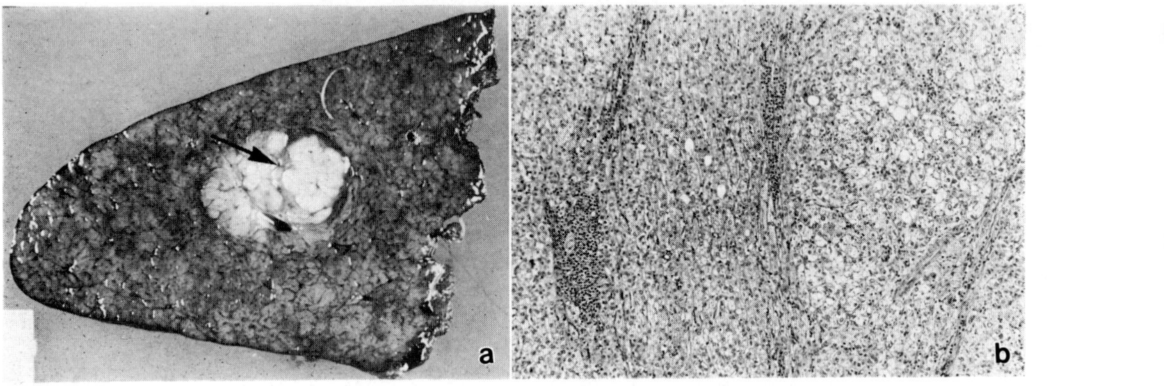

FIG. 2. Nodule-in-nodule lesion of HCC indicating stepwise progression from early to ordinary HCC. a) Macroscopic view. A nodule of ordinary HCC (arrow) showing destructive growth is evident within a tumor of early HCC. b) Microscopic view of the boundary between the well differentiated early HCC component in the center and the less differentiated ordinary HCC component at right.

nodule appearance (*5*). The peripheral areas of the tumors show a histology identical to that of early HCC, and the inner nodule shows the histology of ordinary HCC of Edmondson grade II or III (Fig. 2). These lesions are considered to represent a stage of stepwise progression. Portal vein tumor thrombi and intrahepatic metastasis are rarely detected in or surrounding early HCCs, whereas they become more frequent in nodule-in-nodule lesions and advanced HCCs as the tumor diameter increases. These findings indicate that early HCCs are different from usual HCCs of high-grade malignancy, and are the lesions which correspond to the early stage of hepatocarcinogenesis, being precursors of advanced HCCs.

Clonal Expansion and Subclonal Progression in Human Hepatocarcinogenesis

Viral DNA is a useful marker of clonality when the virus is integrated randomly into the cellular DNA of host cells. Hepatitis B virus fulfills this requirement, but no information on the integration of hepatitis C virus has yet been reported. We analyzed a few small nodular lesions including early HCCs, nodule-in-nodule lesions and advanced HCCs. The DNAs were extracted, and the integration patterns of hepatitis B virus were analyzed by Southern blotting using several restriction enzymes. A clonal integration pattern indicating the clonal origin of the lesion was detected not only in advanced HCCs but also in early HCCs, their precursors and nodule-in-nodule lesions (*6, 7*). Most interestingly, the early HCC component and advanced HCC component of one nodule-in-nodule lesion showed an identical pattern of integration, indicating that one of the tumor cells of early HCC had progressed to advanced HCC (*6*). When multiple lesions, suggested morphologically to be independent in origin, were analyzed by the same technique, the integration patterns of hepatitis B virus differed among the lesions, clearly indicating their multicentric origin (*7*).

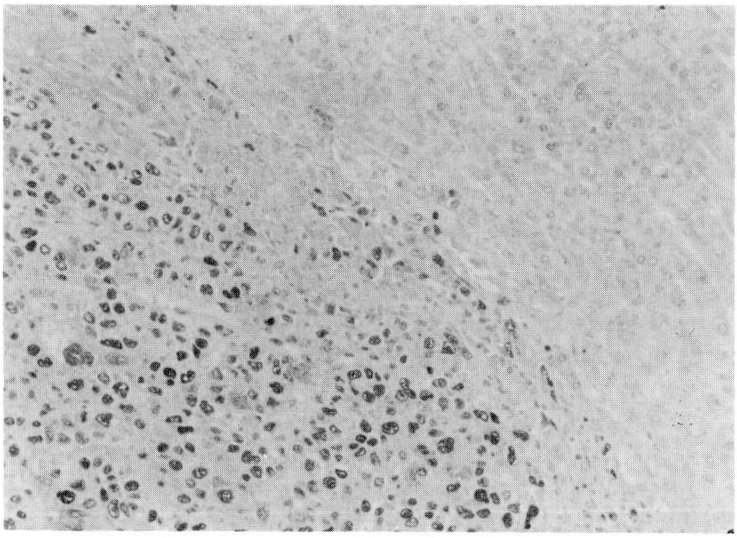

FIG. 3. Immunohistochemical demonstration of PCNA in a nodule-in-nodule HCC. Many tumor cells of the inner nodule (lower left) are stained positively for PCNA, indicating acquisition of marked proliferative activity at this stage of progression.

Alteration of Tumor Cell Proliferative Activity during Human Hepatocarcinogenesis

Proliferating cell nuclear antigen (PCNA), also known as cyclin, is an auxiliary protein of DNA polymerase-delta and shows prominent accumulation in S-phase nuclei of proliferating cells. Small HCCs showing a nodule-in-nodule appearance were analyzed in terms of cell proliferative activity. The analysis was carried out by successful immunohistochemical staining of PCNA in formalin-fixed paraffin-embedded tissue sections. In all cases, the PCNA labeling index of the inner nodule, showing the histology of ordinary HCC, was much higher than that of the peripheral area of early HCC, which in turn was slightly higher than that of the non-cancerous liver of the patient (*8*) (Fig. 3). The data presented here provide supporting evidence that the successive emergence and expansion of a more rapidly proliferating subclone within a nodule result in the stepwise progression of malignancy of human HCC.

Alteration of Tumor DNA Ploidy during Human Hepatocarcinogenesis

DNA cytophotometry was performed in 12 cases of small HCC with a nodule-in-nodule appearance, in which the early HCC component, ordinary HCC component and non-tumorous liver tissue showing chronic hepatitis or cirrhosis were analyzed separately. Isolated cell smears were prepared from formalin-fixed paraffin-embedded tissues, stained with propidium iodide, and the amount of nuclear DNA was measured by the two-wavelength method using microspectrophotometry (AH2-QRFL, Olympus, Tokyo). The early HCC component showed a diploid pattern in 8 of the 12 cases. The ordinary HCC component showed an aneuploid peak in 7 cases, of which 3 exhibited the aneuploid peak only in the ordinary HCC component. The mean nuclear DNA content showed a significant increase from the non-tumorous liver to the early HCC component and from the early HCC component to the ordinary HCC component. Polyploid cells were exceptional in the non-tumorous liver, but were detected in the early HCC component and were increased in number in the ordinary HCC component. These findings suggest that chromosomal and DNA instability may play an important role in the subclonal progression of human HCC.

Role of Angiogenesis in Human Hepatocarcinogenesis

The characteristic feature of HCC in imaging analysis by angiography is that the tumor becomes hypervascular with an increase in size. Correspondingly, small tumor vessels equipped with a wall of smooth muscle are often seen in the area of ordinary HCC but rarely in the area of early HCC. Angiogenesis is considered to play an important role in tumorigenesis. Various angiogenic factors have been identified, and their possible role in the growth of malignant tumors has been suggested. Among these factors, basic fibroblast growth factor (bFGF) is possibly one of the most important, since it strongly stimulates both the proliferation and locomotion of endothelial cells *in vitro* and angiogenesis *in vivo*. Expression of bFGF in HCCs was therefore investigated by RNA blot analysis (*9*). All of the examined hepatocellular carcinoma cells expressed bFGF, and the degree of expression was higher in surgically resected HCCs than in the corresponding adjacent non-cancerous liver tissue. Transcripts of bFGF were not detected in normal liver. Immunohistochemical analysis of bFGF also revealed that this growth factor is more strongly localized in areas of ordinary HCC than in areas of early HCC (Fig. 4). Acquisition by cancer cells of the capacity to produce bFGF could therefore be a key event in the stepwise progression of HCCs.

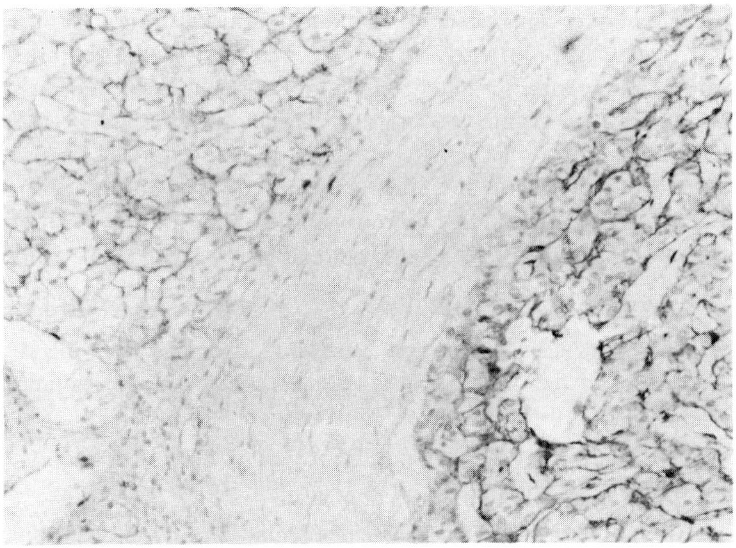

FIG. 4. Immunohistochemical demonstration of basic FGF in a nodule-in-nodule HCC. Basic FGF is more strongly localized in the inner nodule of the more progressed HCC at right.

Multiple Genetic Alterations in Human Hepatocarcinogenesis

In HCCs, only a small proportion of tumors have been shown to carry activated oncogenes. Point-mutational activation of the *ras* gene is rare; only 1 of 30 cases was shown to have mutation of the c-ki-*ras* gene (*10*). Coamplification of the *hist*-1 and *int*-2 genes, which are located on chromosome 11, has been found, but again only in 10% of cases. In contrast to this paucity of knowledge on oncogene activation, a considerable body of evidence indicates that inactivation of tumor suppressor genes plays an important role in hepatocarcinogenesis. Tumor suppressor genes are usually inactivated by mutation in one allele and by loss of the other allele on chromosomes. Thus, loss of a chromosome, when this is observed non-randomly in a particular tumor, is considered to represent the process of inactivation of a tumor suppressor gene. In HCCs, we have found that loss of heterozygosity of chromosomes 4, 16q and 17p is very frequent (*11, 12*). Loss of heterozygosity of chromosomes 5 and 11 has also been reported by other investigators (*13*). Thus, in HCCs, multiple chromosomes or portions of them are lost, indicating the involvement of inactivation of multiple tumor suppressor genes in hepatocarcinogenesis. Consistent with these findings, one of the tumor suppressor genes, p53, located on the short arm of chromosome 17, has been shown to be frequently mutated in HCCs (*14*). When these alterations, loss of heterozygosity and mutation of tumor suppressor genes, were correlated with the pathological features of HCCs, it was found that inactivation of tumor suppressor genes occurred at the stage of tumor progression, relatively late in hepatocarcinogenesis. Many well differentiated tumors, especially those of early HCCs, did not show inactivation of known tumor suppressor genes including p53, whereas poorly differentiated tumors showed these alterations very frequently. Especially in the loss of heterozygosity of chromosome 16q, the incidence reached 90% in poorly differentiated HCCs, and was correlated with the presence of metastasis, recurrence and poor prognosis (*12*). Taking these findings together with the pathological features of HCC progression, it is suggested that inactivation of tumor suppressor genes may be related directly or indirectly to highly increased cell proliferation, tumor neovascularization, and genetic and chromosomal instability of HCCs. At present, the genetic alterations responsible for the early process of hepatocarcinogenesis are not known. Extensive studies on the integration sites of hepatitis B virus DNA have shown that except for a few cases the sites are random, and integration of hepatitis C virus has not been demonstrated. The question of why and how clonal expansion of hepatocytes occurs in liver injured by viral infection remains to be studied.

Acknowledgments

This study was supported in part by Grants-in-Aid from the Princess Takamatsu Cancer Research Fund and the Ministry of Health and Welfare for a Comprehensive 10-Year Strategy for Cancer Control, Japan.

REFERENCES

1. Kanai, T., Hirohashi, S., Upton, M. P., Noguchi, M., Kishi, K., Makuuchi, M., Yamasaki, S., Hasegawa, H., Takayasu, K., Moriyama, N., and Shimosato, Y. Pathology of small hepatocellular carcinoma: a proposal for a new gross classification.

Cancer, *60*: 810–819, 1987.
2. Sakamoto, M., Hirohashi, S., and Shimosato, Y. Early stages of multistep hepatocarcinogenesis: adenomatous hyperplasia and early hepatocellular carcinoma. Hum. Pathol., *22*: 172–178, 1991.
3. Takayama, T., Makuuchi, M., Hirohashi, S., Sakamoto, M., Okazaki, N., Takayasu, K., Kosuge, T., Motoo, Y., Yamazaki, S., and Hasegawa, H. Malignant transformation of adenomatous hyperplasia to hepatocellular carcinoma. Lancet, *336*: 1150–1153, 1990.
4. Yuki, K., Hirohashi, S., Sakamoto, M., Kanai, T., and Shimosato, Y. Growth and spread of hepatocellular carcinoma: a review of 240 consecutive autopsy cases. Cancer, *66*: 2174–2179, 1990.
5. Watanabe, H., Hirohashi, S., Sakamoto, M., Hasegawa, H., Yamazaki, S., Makuuchi, M., Moriyama, N., and Takayasu, K. New macroscopic subtype of small hepatocellular carcinoma-common type in early type- and histological consideration of the multistep progression of HCC. Kanzo, *31*: 1267–1273, 1990 (in Japanese).
6. Tsuda, H., Hirohashi, S., Shimosato, Y., Terada, M., and Hasegawa, H. Clonal origin of atypical adenomatous hyperplasia of the liver and clonal identity with hepatocellular carcinoma. Gastroenterology, *95*: 1664–1666, 1988.
7. Sakamoto, M., Hirohashi, S., Tsuda, H., Shimosato, Y., Makuuchi, M., and Hosoda, Y. Multicentric independent development of hepatocellular carcinoma revealed by analysis of hepatitis B virus integration pattern. Am. J. Surg. Pathol., *13*: 1064–1067, 1989.
8. Matsuno, Y., Hirohashi, S., Furuya, S., Sakamoto, M., Mukai, K., and Shimosato, Y. Heterogeneity of proliferative activity in nodule-in-nodule lesions of small hepatocellular carcinoma. Jpn. J. Cancer Res., *81*: 1137–1140, 1990.
9. Shimoyama, Y., Gotoh, M., Ino, Y., Sakamoto, M., Kato, K., and Hirohashi, S. Characterization of high-molecular-mass forms of basic fibroblast growth factor produced by hepatocellular carcinoma cells: possible involvement of basic fibroblast growth factor in hepatocarcinogenesis. Jpn. J. Cancer Res., *82*: 1263–1270, 1991.
10. Tsuda, H., Hirohashi, S., Shimosato, Y., Ino, Y., Yoshida, T., and Terada, M. Low incidence of point mutation of c-Ki-*ras* and N-*ras* oncogenes in human hepatocellular carcinoma. Jpn. J. Cancer Res., *80*: 196–199, 1989.
11. Zhang, W., Hirohashi, S., Tsuda, H., Shimosato, Y., Yokota, J., Terada, M., and Sugimura, T. Frequent loss of heterozygosity on chromosomes 16 and 4 in human hepatocellular carcinoma. Jpn. J. Cancer Res., *81*: 108–111, 1990.
12. Tsuda, H., Zhang, W., Shimosato, Y., Yokota, J., Terada, M., Sugimura, T., Miyamura, T., and Hirohashi, S. Allele loss on chromosome 16 associated with progression of human hepatocellular carcinoma. Proc. Natl. Acad. Sci. U.S.A., *87*: 6791–6794, 1990.
13. Fujimori, M., Tokino, T., Hino, O., Kitagawa, T., Imamura, T., Okamoto, E., Mitsunobu, M., Ishikawa, T., Nakagama, H., Harada, H., Yagura, M., Matsubara, K., and Nakamura, Y. Allelotype study of primary hepatocellular carcinoma. Cancer Res., *51*: 89–93, 1991.
14. Murakami, Y., Hayashi, K., Hirohashi, S., and Sekiya, T. Aberrations of the tumor suppressor p53 and retinoblastoma genes in human hepatocellular carcinomas. Cancer Res., *51*: 5520–5525, 1991.

EXPERIMENTAL OBSERVATION OF MULTISTAGE CARCINOGENESIS

MULTISTAGE CARCINOGENESIS, C. C. HARRIS ET AL. (EDS.),
JAPAN SCI. SOC. PRESS, TOKYO/CRC PRESS, BOCA RATON, PP. 97–108, 1992

Functional Loss of Tumour Suppressor Genes in Multistage Chemical Carcinogenesis

Allan BALMAIN,*[1] Christopher J. KEMP,*[1] Philip A. BURNS,*[1]
Andrea B. STOLER,*[1] Deborah J. FOWLIS,*[2] and Rosemary J. AKHURST*[2]

CRC Beatson Laboratories, Glasgow[1] and Department of Medical Genetics,
University of Glasgow Yorkhill Hospital, Glasgow,*[2] Scotland*

Abstract: Studies of multistage carcinogenesis in mouse skin have provided many of the early concepts of tumour initiation, promotion and progression. Genetic approaches have led to the identification of a number of mutational alterations in proto-oncogenes and tumour suppressor genes which take place at specific stages of carcinogenesis in this particular system. Initiation involves, at least in a proportion of tumours, mutational activation of the cellular H-*ras* proto-oncogene. Trisomy of chromosome 7, which develops during the premalignant clonal expansion phase, possibly as a consequence of tumour promoter treatment, is followed by further alterations on chromosome 7 which lead to a relative increase in the expression of mutant *ras* alleles. The p53 tumour suppressor gene undergoes mutational alteration and loss of heterozygosity in a proportion of squamous carcinomas but this particular gene does not appear to be involved in the further transition of squamous carcinomas to highly undifferentiated spindle cell tumours. The latter transition appears to be a recessive event which can be complemented by fusion with cells at earlier stages of malignancy. Mouse skin carcinogenesis therefore continues to provide invaluable information on the nature of the genetic and biological transitions which occur during the step-wise progression of normal cells to malignancy.

It is now generally accepted that the growth of a malignant tumour by clonal expansion from a single normal cell requires the participation of a number of different classes of gene products. Some of these products exert a positive effect on cell growth and are frequently found to be activated constitutively in tumours as a result of mutation, gene amplification or other mechanisms which lead to deregulated expression. A different class of gene product is thought to be involved in negative growth regulation. Genes of this family, the tumour suppressor genes, are frequently deleted or in some other way functionally inactivated in a wide variety of tumour types. Multistage carcinogenesis is thought to involve a series of genetic events involving both of these classes of gene products. The purpose of this article is to review the current state of knowledge of the genetic and biological alterations which take

TABLE 1. Tumour Suppressor Genes in Human Tumours

Gene	Locus	Neoplasm
RBI	13q	Retinoblastoma, osteosarcoma, carcinomas of breast, lung, bladder
P53	17p	Almost all tumour types
WT1	11p13	Wilms tumour
?	11p15	Wilms tumour, carcinomas, Rhabdomyosarcoma
DCC	18q22	Colon carcinoma
NF1	17q11	Neurofibromatosis
FAP	5q21-22	Colon carcinoma
MEN-1	11q13	Parathyroid, pituitary, adrenal tumours
?	3p21	Lung carcinoma
?	3p12-14	Kidney carcinoma
?	1p36	Neuroblastoma

place during the development of both benign and malignant tumours in mouse skin.

A number of tumour suppressor genes have now been identified (Table 1) and in certain cases a functional role in the suppression of tumour cell growth has been demonstrated (*1*). Almost all of the genes shown in Table 1 have been identified as a consequence of the application of sophisticated molecular genetic approaches. These approaches were based initially on the Knudson two-hit model of carcinogenesis by which recessive mutations in tumour suppressor genes are revealed by loss of the corresponding normal allele by a variety of different genetic mechanisms (*2*). This was particularly successfully applied in the early studies of Cavenee *et al.* (*3*) who demonstrated the existence of multiple mechanisms by which loss of heterozygosity can occur in human tumours. This approach was initially not applied to studies of multistage carcinogenesis in animal model systems because of the inbred nature of strains of rodent used in the laboratory. We have attempted to overcome these difficulties by generating F1 hybrid mice, either between different inbred mouse strains carrying distinct genetic polymorphisms (*4*) or, more recently, by the use of interspecific hybrid mice derived by crossing *Mus musculus* inbred strains with *M. spretus* (*5*). Such interspecific hybrids are particularly informative because of the divergence of these species some two to three million years ago (*6*). As a consequence, hybrids display restriction fragment length polymorphisms at multiple genetic loci, making this an ideal system for the study of tumour suppressor gene losses during chemical carcinogenesis (Fig. 1).

The experimental model we have chosen for studies on genetic events in carcinogenesis is the classical mouse skin model, the main features of which are depicted in Fig. 2. In this model, initiation takes place by a single treatment of the skin with a chemical carcinogen giving rise to a population of initiated cells which remain dormant until they are stimulated to expand clonally by treatment with a tumour promoter such as 12-0-tetradecanoyl-phorbol-13-acetate (TPA) (*7*). A proportion of the resultant papillomas then undergo further genetic changes and progress to squamous carcinomas. Recently, an additional progression event has been identified in this classical model system, in that the squamous carcinomas have been shown to undergo a further change during progression to a highly invasive type of undifferentiated or spindle cell carcinoma (*5, 8, 9*).

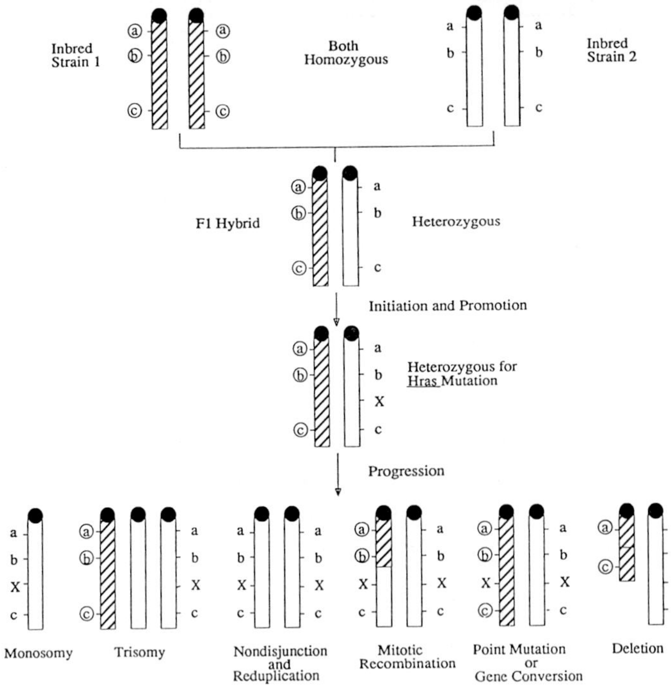

FIG. 1. The example shown is for chromosome 7 from inbred strain 1 (hatched columns) or inbred strain 2 (open columns). The letters a, b and c (or ⓐ, ⓑ, ⓒ) denote the different alleles on chromosome 7. F1 hybrid mice are heterozygous at each locus. The x indicates a mutation in the H-*ras* gene in initiated cells, which can become hemizygous or homozygous by a variety of different genetic mechanisms, as shown.

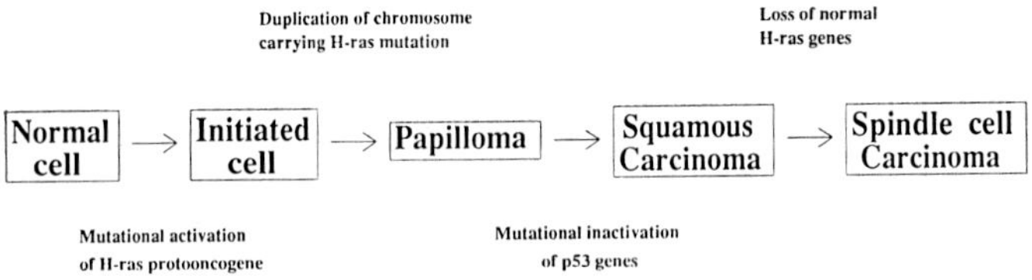

FIG. 2. The figure shows the sequence of biological events known to occur during development of skin tumours, and the genetic changes detected at different stages.

The mouse cellular Harvey-*ras* (H-*ras*) proto-oncogene is thought to be a major target for the initiating event caused by chemical carcinogens. This is based on evidence showing that particular chemical carcinogens which have a propensity to form adducts with specific nucleotides give rise ultimately to tumours carrying carcinogen-specific mutations in the H-*ras* gene. This is depicted in Fig. 3 which summarises the mutational spectrum seen in tumours induced by a variety of different chemical initiators (*10*). The polycyclic hydrocarbon dimethylbenzanthracene (DMBA) gives rise to papillomas and carcinomas, a very high proportion of which show the same A→T mutation at codon 61 of the H-*ras* gene. Work by a number of other groups has shown that DMBA efficiently forms adducts with the adenosine

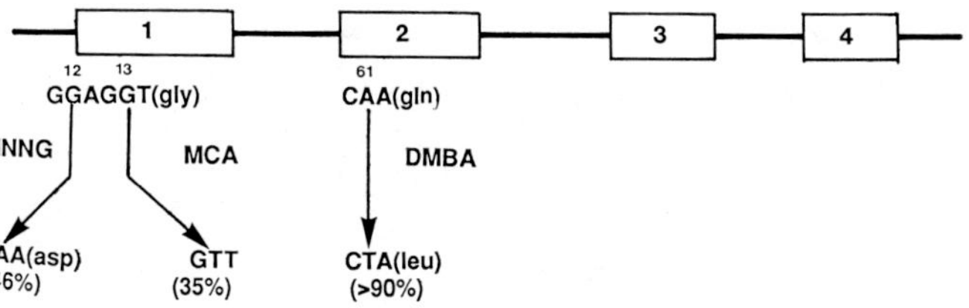

FIG. 3. The open boxes numbered 1–4 represent the H-*ras* coding exons. Mutations found in tumours induced by the carcinogens MNNG, MCA, and DMBA at codons 12, 13, and 61 are indicated.

residues, although the mechanism by which misrepair gives rise to transversion mutations of this kind is not yet known. Initiation with methylating agents such as methyl-nitro-nitrosoguanidine (MNNG) or methyl-nitrosourea (MNU) generates a proportion of tumours carrying G→A mutations at codon 12 of the H-*ras* gene. Such mutations have been observed in a number of other systems (*11*), and are thought to be the direct consequence of methylation of the guanosine residue by the carcinogen, inducing misrepair during subsequent rounds of DNA replication (*12*). Interestingly, the carcinogen methylcholanthrene (MCA) induces tumours carrying yet another kind of mutation, a G→T transversion mutation at codon 13 of the same target gene. The fact that the structurally different mutagenic agents give rise to tumours several months later which, nevertheless, carry the typical imprint of the initiating chemicals, lends a great deal of support to the idea that the mutations in fact occurred at the time of treatment with the chemical initiator (*13, 14*). The causal nature of these mutations in initiation of skin tumorigenesis has been supported by experiments involving treatment of mouse skin or cells in culture with retroviruses carrying mutant H-*ras* genes (*15, 16*) and by more recent experiments showing that transgenic mice harbouring mutant *ras* oncogenes which are expressed under the control of skin specific promoters induce the formation of benign tumours (*17*). Interestingly, in these latter experiments the *ras* gene was under the control of a keratin promoter which is normally switched on only after the commitment of cells to terminal differentiation. The fact that papillomas developed in such transgenic mice suggests that it is not essential that oncogene expression should take place in stem cells to induce tumour development. It is in fact conceivable that post-commitment cells in the basal layer or even cells within the suprabasal compartment can constitute a population of target cells for mutation during chemical initiation and are capable of giving rise at least to benign tumours. It is noteworthy that human keratinocytes which are committed to terminal differentiation can be rescured by the immortalising EIA adenovirus gene product (*18*) and are potentially capable of further transformation.

The function of a mutant H-*ras* gene in skin carcinogenesis is, however, not restricted to the initiation stage. Further changes either in mutant gene copy number and/or the relative expression levels of normal and mutant H-*ras* alleles are observed both during the development of the benign tumours and the transition to malignancy (*4, 19*; B. Jandrig, S. Haddow, and A. Balmain, unpublished observations). It would therefore appear that *ras* expression levels alter in a stepwise fashion, progressively in favour of the mutant allele during the development of malignancy.

It is tempting to correlate these changes in threshold expression levels of mutant *ras* with alterations in the differentiation pattern exhibited by cells at different stages of the process. For example, the keratin 13 gene is normally expressed only in some internal epithelia but can be switched on in papillomas harbouring mutant *ras* alleles (*20, 21*). Further changes involving the expression of the simple keratins K8 and 18 are observed both *in vitro* in cells expressing mutant *ras* alleles (*22, 23*) and *in vivo* (M. Quintanilla *et al.*, personal communication). Yet another stage is seen during the progression of squamous cell carcinomas to spindle cell carcinomas, at which point the synthesis of most of the epithelial keratins appears to be switched off, and in some cases even the simple keratins K8 and 18 are also undetectable (*22*). These spindle cells represent the extreme end of the spectrum of malignancy of epidermal keratinocytes, the development of which is associated with complete loss of normal *ras* alleles and/or over representation of mutant alleles. Other genes are however obviously also involved in this process (see below) the identification of which remains an important goal of future experimentation.

Loss of Tumour Suppressor Genes during Skin Tumour Progression

We have adapted the genetic approaches used for the identification of tumour suppressor gene loci in human tumours to studies of genetic events in mouse skin tumour progression. The interspecific *M. spretus*/*M. musculus* hybrids described above show a very high degree of heterozygosity at many loci distributed throughout the genome and loss of heterozygosity is therefore easily detected by the use of restriction fragment length polymorphism (RFLP) markers. The speed with which such analysis can be carried out has recently been greatly increased by the use of microsatellite polymorphisms which can be detected using the polymerase chain reaction (*24*). This general strategy promises to be extremely useful for the detection and identification of tumour suppressor genes in a number of different tumour types. Using a combination of these approaches we have looked for loss of heterozygosity at many different loci in a panel of chemically induced skin tumours. Markers on chromosomes 7 and 11 were frequently imbalanced or lost whereas at least one marker on chromosomes 2, 4, 9, 12, 14, 17, and 18 retained heterozygosity in the great majority of tumours (C. Kemp, F. Fee, and A. Balmain, in preparation). Allelic imbalance at a number of markers on chromosome 7 was the most frequent change observed, being detected in almost all papillomas and carcinomas which carried mutant *ras* genes. The H-*ras* allele is in fact carried on chromosome 7 and the chromosome bearing the mutant H-*ras* allele was always that which was over represented in the tumours. These results confirm and extend previous observations that nondisjunction leading to trisomy of chromosome 7 is a very common and early event in skin carcinogenesis, presumably serving to increase the dosage of mutant H-*ras* (*4, 25*).

Trisomy of chromosome 7 detected in early papillomas has also been found cytogenetically (*26*). Since TPA has been shown to induce a number of apparently random chromosomal changes in cells in culture and also in mouse epidermis *in vivo* (*27*), we propose that the induction of trisomy may take place as a direct consequence of TPA treatment. Interestingly, the non-tumour-promoting hyperplasiogenic agent RPA (retinoyl-phorbol-acetate) does not induce chromosome alterations and also does not give rise to papillomas after treatment of initiated mouse skin (*27*). This numerical chromosomal alteration may therefore be the equivalent of the so-called conversion step which has been postulated to be an important early event in the clonal selection of initiated cells to form papillomas (*27*, *28*).

Another chromosome showing frequent loss of heterozygosity in carcinomas but not in pre-malignant papillomas, was chromosome 11. Since the p53 tumour suppressor gene is located on this chromosome, a series of experiments was initiated to determine whether mutational alterations of the p53 gene could be found in skin tumours. Complete loss of chromosome 11 including the p53 allele was found in a total of four out of thirteen mouse skin carcinomas. The p53 alleles of these tumours have been sequenced by polymerase chain reaction (PCR) amplification and direct sequencing and it has been shown that all four carcinomas which were homozygous at the p53 locus had suffered mutational alterations (*5*). Three of these exhibited frameshift mutations resulting in severely truncated proteins, whereas the others showed a mis-sense mutation. On the basis of this relatively small number of tumours analysed, it would therefore appear that complete loss of p53 function is more common than the acquisition of a mutant p53 with novel functional properties. A larger number of tumours will have to be investigated to confirm this point.

Mutational alteration of p53 therefore plays an important role in the development and progression of mouse skin tumours (*5*; A Klein-Szanto, personal communication). The evidence to date suggests that complete loss of p53 function occurs at the transition between benign and malignant tumours and may therefore represent an important step in the acquisition of infinite self-renewal capacity by the tumour cells. It is interesting that in a number of analyses now carried out on human tumour systems, mutational alterations at the p53 locus also appear to correlate with the benign-malignant transition. This mouse skin model system may therefore provide an ideal opportunity to investigate the true function of the p53 gene in malignant progression.

Undifferentiated Spindle Cell Carcinomas Are Directly Derived from Squamous Carcinoma cells In Vivo

The origin of spindle cell tumours has been the subject of a great deal of controversy, with some pathologists claiming that they arise from pre-existing squamous lesions, whereas others categorise them as independently arising tumours of fibroblastic origin. We have previously shown (*9*) that alteration of the ratio of mutant to normal H-*ras* alleles on chromosome 7 is associated with an apparent change in the morphology of tumours from the squamous to the spindle cell type. These tumours were however all initiated with carcinogens which can cause the A→T mutation at codon 61 of the H-*ras* gene. It could therefore be argued that the mutations occurred independently in cells of epithelial or fibroblastic origin. A cell line has now been derived which has enabled us to provide the first direct demonstration of the squamous-spindle conversion. This cell line derived from a tumour induced in a *spretus/musculus* F1 mouse by multiple treatment with DMBA, clearly showed the presence of both epithelial cells and fibroblastic spindle-shaped cells *in vitro*. Each of these populations was isolated by single cell cloning. Upon subsequent reinjection into nude mice the epithelial cell clone (B9) gave rise to well differentiated squamous cell carcinomas whereas two independent spindle cell clones gave rise to undifferentiated or spindle cell tumours with a short latency period. Southern blotting analysis showed that the clones of both types carried the same H-*ras* mutation in the *M. musculus* allele. However more importantly, both cell types exhibited the same pattern of mutations in the p53 gene. Two mutations were present in the *musculus* allele, one of which was silent, and one in the *spretus* allele. The presence of this panel of four independent mutations in two genes detected in both the squamous and spindle cell types unequivocally shows that the two cell types have the same clonal origin. Furthermore it would appear that the mutant p53 gene is not crucial for this conversion event since both cell populations carried the same mutations. An investigation of the nature of the genetic alterations between these particular squamous and spindle cells is in progress. The derivation of the original tumour from a *spretus/musculus* F1 mouse provides ample opportunity to investigate loss of heterozygosity using multiple genetic markers in the spindle cells. Preliminary experiments have shown that chromosome 7 alterations can be detected in the spindle cell clones which lead to an alteration of the mutant to normal H-*ras* gene ratio. However, it has not been possible to date to reverse the spindle cell phenotype by expression of a transfected normal H-*ras* gene in a variety of spindle cells (S. Haddow, R. Crombie, and A. Balmain, unpublished results).

Loss of the Epithelial Phenotype in Spindle Cell Carcinomas Is Caused by a Recessive Mechanism

The results described above showed that a distinct genetic alteration can be associated with the progression of squamous to spindle cells. However, it was not possible from these results to determine whether this event was dominant, indicative of a gain of function, for example, mutation of a proto-oncogene to an activated form, or recessive, *i.e.* caused by loss or inactivation of a putative tumour suppressor gene. We have consequently investigated this question by carrying out cell fusions between spindle cells and a variety of epidermal cells at different stages of carcinogenesis (A. B. Stoler and A. Balmain, in preparation). A variety of cell lines have been derived from mouse skin tumours at various stages along the pathway towards malignancy. These include immortalised keratinocytes which are non-tumorigenic on subcutaneous injection into nude mice, papillomas which are either sensitive or resistant to the growth regulatory effects of transforming growth factor β (TGF-β), squamous cell carcinomas and spindle cell carcinomas. All of the cell lines apart from the spindle cell tumours retain clear evidence of the expression of epithelial cell markers.

Using a spindle cell carcinoma (carB) as the transformed parent, cells from these different points of the progression pathway have been used to form cell hybrids. The results indicated that both immortalised cells and papillomas possess the capacity to suppress transformation in a spindle cell carcinoma. Some tumours did arise after a long latency period. On histological analysis these proved to be either benign epithelial cysts or well differentiated (stage I) carcinomas. More importantly, the phenotype of all of these cell hybrids *in vitro* was that of epithelial cells rather than the spindle morphology of the tumorigenic parent. Even when squamous cell carcinomas were used as fusion parent with the spindle cells, the resulting hybrids resembled the squamous epithelial cells *in vitro*. On the other hand, fusion of the spindle cell carB with itself, or with another spindle cell carcinoma which was derived independently, gave rise to hybrids with a clear spindle morphology and short latency for tumour formation *in vivo*.

It thus appears that the suppression of malignancy in these hybrids is clearly associated with the re-establishment of the pattern of terminal differentiation (*1*). We conclude that a gene or genes which control the epithelial differentiation phenotype is lost or functionally inactivated at a very late stage of carcinogenesis in the skin. One of our most important future goals is therefore to focus on the nature of this gene and the elucidation of its possible role in control of epidermal differentiation.

Loss of Negative Growth Control by Transforming Growth Factor β during Tumour Progression

TGF-β is a potent negative growth regulator of epidermal cells, the response to which can frequently be lost during the development of squamous cell carcinomas. However, the stage of carcinogenesis at which the response to TGF-β is lost and the mechanistic relationships between loss of growth control and mutational alterations in proto-oncogenes or tumour-suppressor genes remains completely unclear. In previous experiments we have shown that TGF-β negatively regulates the growth of immortalised or normal mouse keratinocytes and that this down-regulation is not abrogated by expression of a mutant *ras* oncogene (*29*). Immortal keratinocytes transfected with a mutant human H-*ras* gene and also lines derived from papillomas harbouring mutant H-*ras* genes still showed a complete inhibition of growth on treatment with TGF-β. However some papilloma lines, even although they remained non-tumorigenic, had lost the response to this negative growth regulator, as had the majority of carcinoma lines tested.

An apparent paradox which emerged from these studies was that initiated cells and at least early papillomas appeared to respond to TGF-β but nevertheless underwent clonal expansion in response to treatment with the tumour promoter TPA which was previously shown to induce high levels of TGF-β mRNA in mouse epidermis (*30*). Further investigations of the synthesis of TGF-β mRNA and protein were carried out using a combination of *in situ* hybridisation and immunocytochemistry using isoform specific antibodies to TGF-β1 (*31*). Following TPA treatment of adult mouse skin there was a rapid induction of TGF-β1 protein. The intracellular protein was located mainly in suprabasal keratinocytes, *i.e.* that subpopulation of epidermal cells which had previously been shown to produce the highest levels of TGF-β1 mRNA (*30*). The extracellular or processed form of TGF-β1 was, on the other hand, predominantly found in the dermis, suggesting that this regulatory protein was produced in the epidermis in response to tissue damage but has its main site of action and/or storage in the underlying dermis. This is indicative of a paracrine type of regulatory communication between epidermal and mesodermal tissues in a manner similar to that proposed to exist in several mouse epithelia during foetal development (*32*).

The situation observed in papillomas and carcinomas induced by initiation with DMBA and promotion with TPA *in vivo* was somewhat different. Both papillomas and carcinomas had elevated levels of TGF-β1 mRNA in the basal keratinocytes but did not appear to contain significant levels of protein within the epithelial cells of the tumour or in the underlying stromal cells. It is therefore possible that since at least early tumours apparently still respond to negative growth regulation by TGF-β they may evade down-regulation by altered translational and/or post translational processing of the newly synthesised factor. It is in fact well known from other studies that TGF-β is subject to regulation at a number of different levels and that mRNA concentrations do not invariably correlate with levels of protein (*33, 34*). We conclude that developing papilloma cells must have evolved a means of evading the negative effects of this growth regulator and that one component of this evasion involves minimising production of bioactive TGF-β protein. However the situation in tumours is undoubtedly extremely complex and a number of other factors including the possible production of positive growth regulators such as TGF-α must also be taken into consideration. We have also not yet tested the possibility that other proteins of the TGF-β family, *e.g.*, TGF-β2 and TGF-β3, are produced by the tumours.

It is intriguing that loss of growth response to TGF-β appears to occur during the development of papillomas but precedes the acquisition of fully malignant properties. It has recently been proposed that the Rb gene product is a mediator of negative growth regulation by TGF-β in epithelial cells (*35, 36*). However, in the skin system there is as yet no evidence either in mouse or human tumours for deletions or other mutational inactivation mechanisms of the Rb gene. On the other hand, a significant proportion of malignant squamous carcinomas have been shown to harbour mutations in the p53 tumour suppressor gene (*5,* 37). It is therefore possible that in some circumstances negative growth regulation may be mediated by the p53 gene rather than the Rb gene product (*38*), although further experimentation will be necessary to confirm or refute this possibility.

Conclusions and Future Prospects

It is now apparent that multistage carcinogenesis in mouse skin, as in the human colon (*39*), involves a series of genetic events which can be correlated with altered biological properties of the developing tumour cells (Fig.2). The ability to manipulate the mouse model system however has made it possible to attain a greater degree of certainty as to the staging of these genetic events and, more importantly, to test their causal effects in the induction of tumorigenic properties. It is therefore possible to conclude that mutational activation of *ras* can be an initiating event in skin carcinogenesis in the mouse. Genetic studies involving inter-specific hybrid mice have allowed the further conclusion that numerical chromosomal alterations take place during the promotion phase of carcinogenesis and may be a direct consequence of chromosomal instability induced by tumour promoters, possibly due to the production of DNA-damaging active oxygen species. Further chromosomal alterations take place during the progression of benign tumours to squamous carcinomas, including point mutations and loss of heterozygosity at the murine p53 tumour suppressor gene. Possible biological consequences of this change at this particular stage of carcinogenesis include the loss of growth control by TGF-β or the acquisition of the immortal phenotype, both of which would undoubtedly lead to further clonal outgrowth of the developing tumour cells. Finally, squamous cell carcinomas can undergo yet additional transitions and give rise to highly invasive metastatic tumour types in which many of the typical features of epidermal differentiation are completely lost. This is a particularly interesting transition, the elucidation of which could have important consequences for our understanding of mechanisms of tumour invasion and metastasis. The fact that development of the spindle cell phenotype appears to be a recessive change offers new avenues to the cloning of the crucial gene(s) involved by a variety of different genetic approaches.

Acknowledgments

We are grateful to many colleagues for their help and co-operation in carrying out the work which is summarised in this article. The Beatson Institute is supported by generous grants from the Cancer Research Campaign of Great Britain. C.J.K. was the recipient of a Fellowship from the International Agency for Research on Cancer.

REFERENCES

1. Stanbridge, E. J. Human tumor suppressor genes. Annu. Rev. Genet., *24*: 615–657, 1990.
2. Knudson, A. G. Epidemiology of genetically determined cancer. *In*; G. Bock and J. Marsh (eds.), Genetic Analysis of Tumour Suppression, pp. 3–11, Chichester, Wiley and Sons, Ltd. 1989.
3. Cavenee, W. K., Dryja, T. P., Phillips, R. A., Benedict, W. F., Godbout, R., Gallie, B. L., Murphree, A. L., Strong, L. C., and White, R. L. Expression of recessive alleles by chromosomal mechanisms in retinoblastoma. Nature, *305*: 779–784, 1983.
4. Bremner, R. and Balmain, A. Genetic changes in skin tumour progression: correlation between presence of a mutant ras gene and loss of heterozygosity on mouse chromosome 7. Cell, *61*: 407–417, 1990.
5. Burns, P. A., Kemp, C. J., Gannon, J. V., Lane, D. P., Bremner, R., and Balmain, A. Loss of heterozygosity and mutational alterations of the p53 gene in skin tumors of interspecific hybrid mice. Oncogene, *6*: 2363–2370, 1991.
6. Robert, B., Barton, P., Minty, A., Daubas, P., Weydert, A., Bonhomme, F., Catalan, J., Chazottes, D., Guenet, J. L., and Buckingham, M. Investigation of genetic linkage between myosin and actin genes using an interspecific mouse back-cross. Nature, *314*: 181–183, 1985.
7. Boutwell, R. K. The function and mechanism of promoters of carcinogenesis. CRC Crit. Rev. Toxicol., *2*: 419–443, 1974.
8. Klein-Szanto, A. J. P., Larcher, F., Bonfil, R. D., and Conti, C. J. Multistage chemical carcinogenesis protocols produce spindle cell carcinomas of the mouse skin. Carcinogenesis, *10*: 2169–2172, 1989.
9. Buchmann, A., Ruggeri, B., Klein Szanto, A. J., and Balmain, A. Progression of squamous carcinoma cells to spindle carcinomas of mouse skin is associated with an imbalance of H-ras alleles on chromosome 7. Cancer Res., *51*: 4097–4101, 1991.
10. Brown, K., Buchmann, A., and Balmain, A. Carcinogen-induced mutations in the mouse c-Ha-ras gene provide evidence of multiple pathways for tumour progression. Proc. Natl. Acad. Sci. U.S.A., *87*: 538–542, 1990.
11. Zarbl, H., Sukumar, S., Arthur, A. V., Martin-Zanca, D., and Barbacid, M. Direct

mutagenesis of Ha-ras-1 oncogenes by N-nitroso-N-methylurea during initiation of mammary carcinogenesis in rats. Nature, *315*: 382–385, 1985.

12. Toorchen, D. and Topal, M. D. Mechanisms of chemical mutagenesis and carcinogenesis: effects on DNA replication of methylation at the O^6-guanine position of dGTP. Carcinogenesis, *4*: 1591–1597, 1983.
13. Balmain, A. and Brown, K. Oncogene activation in chemical carcinogenesis. Adv. Cancer Res., *51*: 147–182, 1988.
14. Barbacid, M. ras genes. Annu. Rev. Biochem., *56*: 779–827, 1987.
15. Brown, K., Quintanilla, M., Ramsden, M., Kerr, I.B., Young, S., and Balmain, A. v-ras genes from Harvey and BALB murine sarcoma viruses can act as initiators of two-stage mouse skin carcinogenesis. Cell, *46*: 447–456, 1986.
16. Roop, D. R., Lowy, D. R., Tambourin, P. E., Strickland, J., Harper, J. R., Balaschak, M., Spangler, E. F., and Yuspa, S. H. An activated Harvey ras oncogene produces benign tumours on mouse epidermal tissue. Nature, *323*: 822–854, 1986.
17. Bailleul, B., Surani, M. A., White, S., Barton, S. C., Brown, K., Blessing, M., Jorcano, J., and Balmain, A. Skin hyperkeratosis and papilloma formation in transgenic mice expressing a ras oncogene from a suprabasal keratin promoter. Cell, *62*: 697–708, 1990.
18. Barrandon, Y., Morgan, J. R., Mulligan, R. C., and Green, H. Restoration of growth potential in paraclones of human keratinocytes by a viral oncogene. Proc. Natl. Acad. Sci. U.S.A., *86*: 4102-4106, 1989.
19. Quintanilla, M., Brown, K., Ramsden, M., and Balmain, A. Carcinogen-specific mutation and amplification of Ha-ras during mouse skin carcinogenesis. Nature, *322*: 78–80, 1986.
20. Nischt, R., Roop, D. R., Mehrel, T., Yuspa, S. H., Rentrop, M., Winter, H., and Schweizer, J. Aberrant expression during two-stage mouse skin carcinogenesis of a type I 47-kDa keratin, K13, normally associated with terminal differentiation of internal stratified epithelia. Mol. Carcinogen., *1*: 96–108, 1988.
21. Gimenez Conti, I., Aldaz, C. M., Bianchi, A. B., Roop, D. R., Slaga, T. J., and Conti, C. J. Early expression of type I K13 keratin in the progression of mouse skin papillomas. Carcinogenesis, *11*: 1995–1999, 1990.
22. Diaz-Guerra, M., Haddow, S., Bauluz, C., Jorcano, J. L., Cano, A., Balmain, A., and Quintanilla, M. Expression of simple epithelial keratins in mouse epidermal keratinocytes harbouring Harvey-ras gene alterations. Cancer Res., in press.
23. Cheng, C., Kilkenny, A. E., Roop, D., and Yuspa, S. H. The v-ras oncogene inhibits the expression of differentiation markers and facilitates expression of cytokeratins 8 and 18 in mouse keratinocytes. Mol. Carcinogen., *3*: 363–373, 1990.
24. Love, J. M., Knight, A. M., McAleer, M. A., and Todd, J. A. Towards construction of a high resolution map of the mouse genome using PCR-analysed microsatellites. Nucl. Acids Res., *18*: 4123–4130. 1990.
25. Bianchi, A. B., Aldaz, C. M., and Conti, C. J. Non-random duplication of the chromosome bearing a mutated Ha-ras-1 allele in mouse skin tumours. Proc. Natl. Acad. Sci. U.S.A., *87*: 6902–6906, 1990.
26. Aldaz, C. M., Trono, D., Larcher, F., Slaga, T. J., and Conti, C. J. Sequential trisomization of chromosomes 6 and 7 in mouse skin premalignant lesions. Mol. Carcinogen., *2*: 22–26, 1989.
27. Furstenberger, G., Schurich, B., Kaina, B., Petrusevska, R. T., Fusenig, N. E., and Marks, F. Tumor induction in initiated mouse skin by phorbol esters and methyl methanesulfonate: correlation between chromosomal damage and conversion ('stage I of tumor promotion') *in vivo*. Carcinogenesis, *10*: 749–752, 1989.

28. Slaga, T. J. Mechanisms involved in multistage skin tumorigenesis. Carcinogen. Comp. Surv., *10*: 189–199, 1985.
29. Haddow, S., Fowlis, D. J., Parkinson, E. K., Akhurst, R. J., and Balmain, A. Loss of growth control by TGF-β occurs at a late stage of mouse skin carcinogenesis and is independent of ras gene activation. Oncogene, *6*: 1465–1470, 1991.
30. Akhurst, R. J., Fee, F., and Balmain, A. Localized production of TGF-beta mRNA in tumour promoter-stimulated mouse epidermis. Nature, *331*: 363–365, 1988.
31. Fowlis, D. J., Flanders, K. C., Duffie, E., Balmain, A., and Akhurst, R. J. Discordant TGF-β1 RNA and protein localisations during chemical carcinogenesis of the skin. Cell Growth Diff., in press.
32. Lehnert, S. A. and Akhurst, R. J. Embryonic expression pattern of TGF-beta 1 mRNA suggests both paracrine and autocrine mechanisms of action. Development, *104*: 263–273, 1988.
33. Glick, A. B., Sporn, M. B., and Yuspa, S. H. Altered regulation of TGF-beta 1 and TGF-alpha in primary keratinocytes and papillomas expressing v-Ha-ras. Mol. Carcinogen., *4:* 210–219, 1991.
34. Knabbe, C., Lippman, M. E., Wakefield, L. M., Flanders, K. C., Kasid, A., and Dickson, R. B. Evidence that transforming growth factor-beta is a hormonally regulated negative growth factor in human breast cancer cells. Cell, *48*: 417–428, 1987.
35. Pietenpol, J. A., Stein, R. W., Moran, E., Yaciuk, P., Schlegel, R., Lyons, R. M., Pittelkow, M. R., Munger, K., Howley, P. M., and Moses, H. L. TGF-beta 1 inhibition of c-myc transcription and growth in keratinocytes is abrogated by viral transforming proteins with pRB binding domains. Cell, *61*: 777–785, 1990.
36. Laiho, M., DeCaprio, J. A., Ludlow, J. W., Livingston, D. M., and Massague, J. Growth inhibition by TGF-β linked to suppression of retinoblastoma protein phosphorylation. Cell, *62*: 175–185, 1990.
37. Field, J. K., Spandidos, D. A., Malliri, A., Gosney, J. R., Yiagnisis, M., and Stell, P. M. Elevated p53 expression correlates with a history of heavy smoking in squamous cell carcinoma of the head and neck. Br. J. Cancer, *64*: 573–577, 1991.
38. Wyllie, F. S., Dawson, T., Bond, J. A., Goretzky, P., Game, S., Prime, S., and Wynford-Thomas, D. Correlated abnormalities of transforming growth factor-β1 response and p53 expression in thyroid epithelial cell transformation. Mol. Cell Endocrinol., *76*: 13–21, 1991.
39. Fearon, E. R. and Vogelstein, B. A genetic model for colorectal tumorigenesis. Cell, *61*: 759–767, 1990.

MULTISTAGE CARCINOGENESIS, C. C. HARRIS ET AL. (EDS.),
JAPAN SCI. SOC. PRESS, TOKYO/CRC PRESS, BOCA RATON, PP. 109–123, 1992

Multistage Prostate Carcinogenesis: The Role of Hormones

Maarten C. BOSLAND,[*1,*2] Henriette C. DREEF-VAN DER MEULEN,[*2] Saraswati SUKUMAR,[*3] Peter OFNER,[*4] Irwin LEAV,[*5] Xueliang HAN,[*6] and Joachim G. LIEHR[*6]

*Institute of Environmental Medicine, NYU Medical Center, Tuxedo, New York 10987, U.S.A.,[*1] Department of Biological Toxicology, TNO Toxicology and Nutrition Institute, Zeist, The Netherlands,[*2] The Salk Institute of Biological Studies, La Jolla, California 92037, U.S.A.,[*3] Departments of Anatomy & Cellular Biology,[*4] Urology[*4] and Pathology,[*5] Tufts University Schools of Medicine and Veterinary Medicine, Boston, Massachusetts 02111, U.S.A., Department of Pharmacology & Toxicology, University of Texas Medical Branch, Galveston, Texas 77550, U.S.A.[*6]*

Abstract: Prostate cancer is the most frequently occurring non-skin cancer in men in the U.S.A. and other Western countries, but its etiology is poorly understood. Human prostate carcinogenesis has been viewed as a multi-step process involving progression from low histologic grade, small latent carcinoma, to large, higher grade, metastasizing carcinoma. However, recent data suggest that a variety of pathogenetic pathways exist. The precise role of hormones in the genesis of human prostate cancer remains largely undefined. It is difficult to investigate stages in the development of human prostate cancer, but some animal models provide opportunities in this regard. Short-term treatment of rats with chemical carcinogens will produce a low incidence (5–15%) of prostate cancer, provided that prostatic cell proliferation is enhanced during carcinogen exposure. A high carcinoma incidence can only be produced by chronic treatment with testosterone following administration of carcinogens such as *N*-methyl-*N*-nitrosourea (MNU). Testosterone markedly enhances prostate carcinogenesis even at doses that do not measurably increase circulating testosterone. Thus, testosterone is a strong tumor promotor for the rat prostate. All such MNU-initiated, testosterone-promoted tumors are adenocarcinomas mostly originating from the dorsolateral and anterior, but not ventral, prostate lobes. A high frequency (70%) of activation of the K-*ras* gene by a G^{35} to A mutation occurs in these carcinomas. A variable frequency of activation of H-*ras* and K-*ras* genes occurs in human prostate carcinomas. Another rat model, representing a different pathogenetic pathway, involves chronic administration of estradiol-17β in combination with low-dose testosterone. The resulting carcinomas are low-grade and originate exclusively from periurethral ducts of the dorsolateral and anterior prostate. We recently found a major adduct by ^{32}P postlabeling analysis in the tissue region that includes these ducts, but not in, *e.g.*, the ventral prostate, of rats treated for 16–24 weeks. While it is unknown whether testosterone is a tumor promoter in this system, the presence of a DNA adduct suggests that estradiol-17β acts as a tumor-initiating agent in this system.

Cancer of the prostate is at present the single most frequently diagnosed cancer in males in the U.S.A. and many west European countries (not counting non-melanoma skin cancer), and it is the fourth most frequent cause of death due to cancer (*1*, *2*). Notwithstanding the clinical importance of prostate cancer, its etiology is not understood (*2*, *3*). Environmental factors are strongly suspected to be critical determinants of prostate cancer risk because of the following observations in studies of migrant populations (*2*, *4–7*). Prostate cancer incidence and mortality varies greatly world-wide. Japanese men, for example, are a typical low-risk population, and the U.S.A. is a high-risk country. The difference in risk between Japanese men and Afro-American men, who have the highest prostate cancer risk in the world, is more than 25-fold. Japanese migrants to the U.S.A. have acquired a risk that is close to, but not quite the same as, that among U.S. men. The change of environment, particularly dietary habits, is suspected to have caused this drastic, more than 10-fold, change in risk. Further, endogenous factors are probably not major determinants of prostate cancer risk.

A variety of epidemiological studies have yielded consistent evidence for rather strong positive correlations or associations between the intake of animal or saturated fats and prostatic cancer risk, as summarized elsewhere (*2*, *8*). Less strong and/or not fully consistent positive correlations or associations with prostate cancer risk have been found for intake of edible fats and oils, total fat, and total protein. Other positive or negative associations observed were either weak or inconsistent. Data on prostate cancer risk and intake of vitamin A and carotenes are conflicting, since both positive and negative associations have been reported (see ref. *2*). Although one study on testosterone-induced rat prostate cancer showed an enhancing effect of adding 20% (by weight) corn oil to a natural ingredient diet (*9*), two independent studies using semipurified diets in rat models have not found any effect of amount (*10*, *11*) or type of dietary fat (*10*), and type and amount of protein (*12*). Nevertheless, the epidemiological data strongly suggest that dietary factors, particularly fat, influence prostate cancer risk, perhaps by interacting with other critical risk determinants that were not tested in the animal model studies.

A major determinant of prostate cancer risk may be hormone action. In the following we describe a number of studies in rat model systems that have addressed this question against the background of a new concept about the natural history and multistage nature of human prostate cancer.

Natural History of Human Prostatic Cancer

Early studies on the natural history of human prostate cancer have suggested a multistep process that initially involves the formation of small, microscopic-size, carcinomas which are not clinically evident. These so-called latent carcinomas are a very prevalent incidental autopsy finding in aged men (*7*, *13*, *14*). Some of these carcinomas subsequently progress to clinically evident cancer with distant metastases. Populations that widely differ in risk for clinically evident prostate cancer exhibit a comparable prevalence of these latent prostate cancers, particularly those carcinomas that are small and histologically not very invasive (*4–7*). The international distribution of the prevalence of latent carcinomas that are larger and more invasive

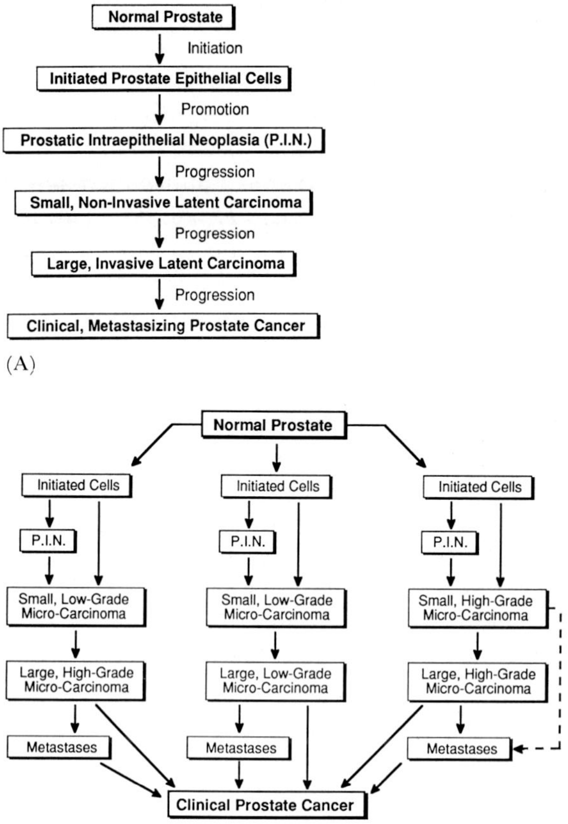

(B)

FIG. 1. A working hypothesis of the natural history of human prostatic cancer. A) A single pathogenetic pathway, multistage model of human prostatic carcinogenesis, including an initiation step, a promotion stage, and several steps in the progression toward clinical prostate cancer. This model comprises a major pathway in the natural history of human prostatic cancer established by McNeal and co-workers (*15, 17, 20, 21, 26, 29*). B) A multiple pathogenetic pathway model of human prostatic carcinogenesis. In this speculative hypothesis, formation of microscopic cancer may or may not involve a stage of PIN development, and development of clinical prostate cancer may or may not be preceded by formation of distant metastases. The interrupted line indicates that it is imaginable that high-grade carcinomas may metastasize even if they are still small.

parallels to some degree the geographic differences in clinically evident prostate cancer incidence (*2, 4–7*). Although it has been suggested that non-invasive latent cancer and invasive cancer, either latent or clinically evident, are different diseases (*14*), the current thinking is that they are different stages of the same process (*2, 15, 16*). In this view, the environmental factors that are likely responsible for the large geographic variation in prostate cancer occurrence would enhance progression from small, non-invasive latent carcinoma to larger, invasive cancer (*2, 4–7*). A comparison of age-specific latent cancer prevalence and clinical cancer incidence between Japan and the U.S.A. suggests that (i) in both populations the same number of carcinogenic events is required for the development of latent prostate cancer, (ii) a similar number of additional events is needed in both populations for progression from latent to clinically evident cancer, and (iii) the prevalence of factors causing these events differs between the two countries (*13*).

These data can be combined in the multistage model of human prostatic carcinogenesis depicted in Fig. 1A. This model has recently been refined by the identification of a premalignant lesion, ductacinar dysplasia (*17*), also known as prostatic intraepithelial neoplasia (PIN) (*18*), that is multicentric and occurs with high frequency in prostates that harbor a carcinoma (*17, 19, 20*). This lesion, particularly its high-grade variety, has been shown to be continuous with frank carcinoma in many cases, which strongly suggests that it can be a direct precursor of prostatic carcinoma (*17, 18, 20*). However, not all PINs will ultimately progress to carcinoma and not all prostate carcinomas may originate from PINs as discussed later.

The multistage model depicted in Fig. 1A is further complicated by some recent findings. First, McNeal, who has conducted pioneering work on the natural history of prostatic cancer (*15, 17, 20, 21*), has found a strong correlation between tumor volume and histological grade (using the Gleason system) and has proposed a slow, linear growth (=volume increase) for human prostatic cancer (*21*). A similar strong correlation between volume and grade was found in a Japanese study (*16*). However, other investigators have not found as consistent or as strong a correlation between these parameters (*19, 22–24*), and small high-grade carcinomas and large low-grade carcinomas do occur (*19, 23, 25*). Second, prostate carcinoma has been considered to arise predominantly from the peripheral zone (*21*) of the gland, but rarely from its center (*4, 5, 7, 21*). Newer data, however, indicate that a third zone in the human prostate, the transition zone (*26*), also frequently harbors carcinomas, which initially are often of lower histologic grade than those in the peripheral zone (*19, 26*). High-grade PIN is very often associated with peripheral zone cancers, but not as frequently with these transition zone carcinomas (*19, 27, 28*). Although these transition zone carcinomas may present as histologically distinct from peripheral zone cancers, it has been proposed that they are biologically similar (*26, 29*).

Based on these observations, we developed the working hypothesis of multistage human prostate carcinogenesis depicted in Fig. 1B. This model does not pretend to summarize all current knowledge derived from research on the natural history of human prostate cancer, a field that is rapidly changing. Rather, it attempts to capture the speculative new concept that clinically evident prostatic cancer may develop via a variety of pathogenetic pathways. Although one of the pathways in Fig. 1B is largely similar to that shown in Fig. 1A, the three pathways shown are hypothetical. All three have in common that they involve tumor growth and that they may or may not involve a stage of PIN. They differ in their pattern of progression: some cancers are high-grade early on, whereas other tumors remain low-grade. This model is probably an overt simplification. It does not take into account that carcinoma of the prostate is frequently multicentric, with often a large variation in histologic grade within one prostate (*7, 16, 19, 26, 29*), that different pathways probably occur predominantly in the peripheral or in the transition zone of the human prostate gland, and that the involvement of PIN as an early stage is common for peripheral zone carcinomas but not as frequent for transition zone cancers. Nevertheless, this model may explain several unresolved issues in human prostate carcinogenesis. Different pathways may be associated with different etiologies, which could in part explain why the epidemiology of prostate cancer is so complex, and why no major causes of prostate cancer have been identified thus far (*2*). The often reported considerable variation among clinically evident prostate carcinomas in histomorphology and biological behavior (*23, 30*) might be explained by different pathways leading to carcinomas that differ in grade and other characteristics. This multiple-pathway model is also consistent with a previously proposed two-disease model of prostate cancer (*2*). Obviously, this model greatly complicates the interpretation of the earlier mentioned latent cancer studies in high- and low-risk populations. It is, for example, not clear whether environmental factors can affect every pathway or just one or two, and whether the prevalence of the various pathways is similar or different in high- and low-risk populations. Further, if this model holds up, it will impede attempts to identify sequential genetic alterations associated with the multistage progression of prostate cancer, because they may differ greatly between pathways.

Animal Models of Prostatic Carcinogenesis

Epidemiologic research on human prostate carcinogenesis is impeded by the old age of most prostate cancer patients, the probably very long latent period of this cancer, and the apparent complexity of its etiology. As surrogates, several model systems of prostatic carcinogenesis have been developed during the past decade, all with the rat as experimental animal. The rodent prostate consists of four paired lobes that have, unlike in man, not merged into one anatomic structure. Three of these lobes are embryologically homologous to zones in the human prostate, but one lobe, the ventral prostate, does not have a human homologue (*31*). This is important because some of the animal models involve tumor development selectively in the ventral lobe. These models have in common that they depend on ventral lobe-selective metabolism of the carcinogens used, and that the neoplasms induced are not comparable to those found in men: 3,2′-dimethyl-4-aminobiphenyl (DMAB) produces non-invasive intra-acinar carcinomas or hyperplasias (*32, 33*), and nitrosobis(2-oxopropyl)amine (BOP) induces squamous cell carcinomas (*34*). More relevant are prostate carcinomas induced by a single exposure to variety of chemical carcinogens, such as *N*-methyl-*N*-nitosourea (MNU), provided that prostatic cell proliferation is stimulated by hormonal manipulation during administration (*35–37*). These tumors originate in the dorsolateral or anterior (=coagulating gland) lobes of the rat prostate and share some important characteristics with human prostate carcinomas. They are adenocarcinomas that metastasize *via* the hematogenic and lymphatic routes, vary considerably in degree of histologic differentiation, elevate serum acid phosphatase, and have a long latent period (*37*). Early, microscopic-size carcinomas and putative preneoplastic lesions have been identified in this system (*37, 38*). However, bony metastases have not been described, androgen sensitivity of these carcinomas is uncertain at present, and the incidence is only 5–15% after one year. Spontaneous prostate cancer incidence in rats, however, is very low, between 0.3 and 0.05% at 2.5–3 years of age (*39*). A high incidence of metastasizing adenocarcinomas of the rat prostate can only be obtained by combined treatment of rats with carcinogens and testosterone or with testosterone and estrogens as is discussed in the following sections.

Testosterone Is a Tumor Promoter of Rat Prostatic Carcinogenesis

The prostate is the classical target organ for androgenic hormones, which are essential for prostate development, and regulate cell death and renewal rates and cellular differentiation in the prostate. Most human prostate carcinomas are androgen sensitive and respond to androgen deprivation therapy, although relapse to a hormone-insensitive state always occurs sooner or later. Thus, a causal relation between androgens and prostate carcinoma development is biologically very plausible (see ref. *2* for references). However, there are no human data that directly link androgen exposure to the development of prostate cancer.

Production of prostate cancer by long-term testosterone treatment has been reported in many, but not all, rat strains (*38, 40–43*). The prostate cancer incidence found in these studies ranged from approximately 5 to 50%. Chronic administration of testosterone after a single or short-term treatment with three different chemical carcinogens that can target the prostate resulted in prostate cancer incidences of between 35 and 70% in several rat strains (*38, 42–45*). These carcinogens, MNU, DMAB, and BOP, by themselves produced either no prostate cancer or a low (3–10%) prostate cancer incidence. All thus induced prostate cancers were adenocarcinomas and they occurred exclusively in the dorsolateral prostate. Interestingly, DMAB and BOP also produced neoplastic lesions in the ventral prostate, but the androgen treatment did not influence this effect (*38, 42*). Thus, testosterone when administered chronically is, by definition, a weak complete carcinogen and a strong tumor promoter for the rat prostate, and chemical carcinogens such as MNU and testosterone act synergistically in producing prostate carcinomas.

Most of the studies that demonstrated the carcinogenic and tumor promoter activity of testosterone involved only one testosterone dose, and circulating testosterone levels were supra-physiological (*5–20* times control values) (*38, 44, 45*). However, we demonstrated that even a slight elevation of circulating testosterone,

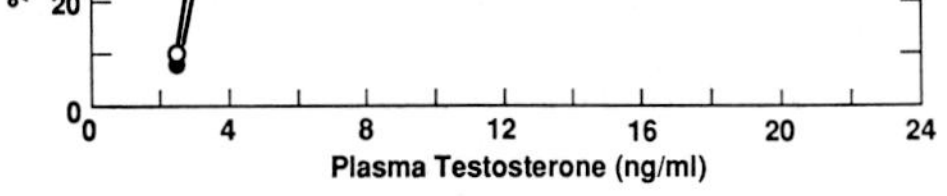

FIG. 2. Incidence of adenocarcinomas of the dorsolateral prostate and of all male accessory sex glands combined (dorsolateral prostate, coagulating gland, and seminal vesicle) *versus* plasma testosterone concentration in Wistar rats treated from 2 weeks after *i.v.* injection with MNU (40–45 mg/kg) with 0, 1, 2, or 4 Silastic implants (Dow Corning Silastic tubing, no. 602–305) containing a 3 cm-long filling of testosterone, which were replaced once after 6 months (*53*). The plasma testosterone concentrations for the four groups shown here are means of 2–8 groups of 5–10 rats each.

2- to 3-fold higher than control values, results in a 10–15% prostate cancer incidence, and that a 6- to 9-fold testosterone elevation produced a comparable incidence (*43*). Both of these testosterone doses given after a single injection with MNU increased carcinoma incidence in the dorsolateral prostate to 50–60% (80–90% in all accessory sex glands combined), while MNU treatment alone yielded a 5–10% incidence (Fig. 2). An even lower dose of testosterone did not produce a significant testosterone elevation, but still induced prostate cancer in approximately 45% of MNU-treated rats (Fig. 2). This very low testosterone dose probably only smoothed the circadian rhythm of circulating testosterone.

Human male populations that are at high risk for prostate cancer often, but not always, have slightly higher circulating testosterone levels than populations that have a lower risk (*2, 46, 47*). For example, total and free testosterone levels in young U.S. black men have been shown to be approximately 20% higher than in age-matched white males, in the absence of differences in sex-hormone-binding-globulin levels (*46*). Circulating total testosterone was approximately 13% higher in aged Dutch men that are at high risk for prostate cancer than in age-matched low-risk Japanese (*47*). However, more research is required to confirm these few studies and to determine the strength and magnitude of the association between exposure to endogenous testosterone and prostate cancer risk. Exposure to exogenous androgenic substances occurs in a significant number of males. Serum testosterone concentrations as high as 1.5- to 3-fold normal levels may result from medical applications such as testosterone replacement therapy and chronic testosterone administration as a form of male contraception (*48–50*). Furthermore, non-medical use of anabolic steroids with androgenic activity in males in the U.S. and probably other countries is considerable, but the exact magnitude of anabolic steroid abuse remains uncertain presently (*51*).

The mechanism of the carcinogenic/tumor promoting effect of testosterone on the rat prostate remains unknown. The hormone probably acts *via* a receptor-mediated mechanism, as suggested by the apparent absence of a threshold below which testosterone has no effect on prostate carcinogenesis, and by the very steep dose-response curve for the carcinogenic and tumor promoting activities of testosterone in rats, which reaches a maximum at low circulating testosterone levels. Thus, a very slight elevation of circulating testosterone increased prostate cancer risk in rats at least 10-fold, irrespective of prior carcinogen treatment. Such a dose-response relationship would explain the large differences in prostate cancer incidence observed among human populations in the absence of equally large variations in circulating testosterone levels. The apparent weak complete carcinogenic activity of testosterone in rats may well be due to its very strong tumor promoting properties.

These findings have implications for carcinogenic risk assessment of androgen exposure. Testosterone and other androgenic substances should be regarded as probable human prostate carcinogens (*52*). Consequently, testosterone substitution therapy should be used with reluctance, and with as low a dose as clinically possible, and human studies on testosterone as a male contraceptive method should be halted until more information about long-term risks of medical use of testosterone is available.

Oncogene Activation in MNU-induced Rat Prostatic Carcinomas

Rat neoplasms induced by methylating carcinogens frequently contain *ras* genes activated by a single point mutation. We have therefore examined prostate carcinomas induced in rats by a combination of a single injection of MNU and long-term treatment with testosterone for the presence of such activating *ras* gene point mutations (*53*). Activating mutations in codon 12 of the K-*ras* gene were found in 7/10 prostate carcinomas, using selective oligonucleotide hybridization analysis of DNA amplified by the polymerase chain reaction (PCR) (Fig. 3). No mutations were detected in codon 12 or 61 of H-*ras* oncogenes. The presence of PCR-engineered *Hph*I restriction sites created by the existence of a $G^{35} \rightarrow A$ mutation in the rat K-*ras* oncogene (*53*) defined the mutation as a GC→AT transition at the second position codon 12; no mutations at the first position were found. Production of O^6-methylguanine adducts in the K-*ras* 12th codon, followed by base mispairing during replicative DNA synthesis is thus the likely molecular mechanism of one of the first steps of the multi-stage process of MNU-induced prostatic carcinogenesis in this rat model system (*53*). While the mechanism responsible for the earlier-mentioned synergism between MNU and testosterone in producing rat prostate carcinomas remains to be defined, we postulate that prostatic epithelial cells with the activated oncogene have a selective growth advantage over other cells in the presence of protracted exposure to androgens.

These data in rat prostate carcinomas are consistent with the similar high frequency of activating $G^{35} \rightarrow A$ mutations in *ras* genes found in MNU-induced rat mammary carcinomas (*54–57*). The frequency of activating *ras* gene mutations in human prostate carcinomas described by others is variable. Three U.S. studies (*58–60*) found activated *ras* oncogenes in 1/8, 1/24, and 1/15 clinically evident carcinomas, respectively, whereas in a Japanese study of latent prostate cancers (*61*) 6/23 tumors had $G^{35} \rightarrow A$ mutations in the K-*ras* gene. The earlier-proposed multiple pathogenetic pathway model of human prostate carcinogenesis could explain this

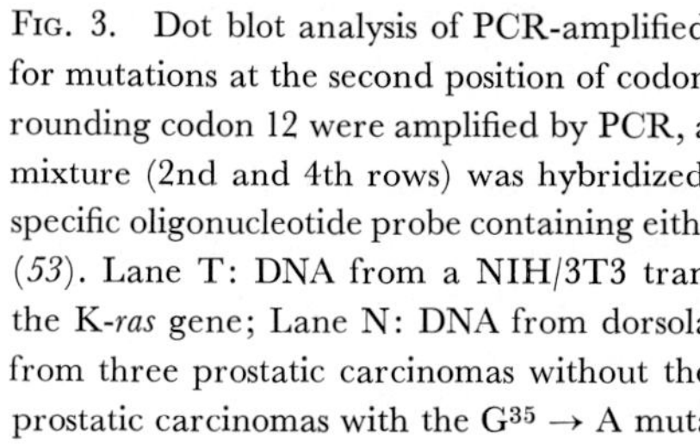

FIG. 3. Dot blot analysis of PCR-amplified DNA of rat prostate carcinomas induced by MNU for mutations at the second position of codon 12 of the K-*ras* gene. The K-*ras* gene sequences surrounding codon 12 were amplified by PCR, and 25 μl (1st and 3rd rows) and 2.5 μl PCR reaction mixture (2nd and 4th rows) was hybridized on Nytran membranes to a ^{32}P-end-labeled, allele-specific oligonucleotide probe containing either the wild-type sequence (G^{35}) or an A^{35} substitution (*53*). Lane T: DNA from a NIH/3T3 transformant homozygous for the $G^{35} \rightarrow A$ mutation in the K-*ras* gene; Lane N: DNA from dorsolateral prostate of an untreated rat; lanes 1–3: DNA from three prostatic carcinomas without the K-*ras* mutations (−); lanes 4–6: DNA from three prostatic carcinomas with the $G^{35} \rightarrow A$ mutation (+).

difference in *ras* gene activation. Multiple genetic alterations are likely to be involved in prostatic carcinogenesis analogous to the findings in human colon carcinogenesis (*62*), and they may occur not only in the epithelial cells of the prostate but also in the mesenchyme. Thompson and coworkers (*63, 64*) have infected v-H-*ras* and v-gag-*myc* into mouse fetal prostate epithelial and mesenchymal cells, followed by recombination of the two cell types and their implantation under the kidney capsule of syngeneic hosts. These elegant studies have demonstrated that only infection of both cell types with both oncogenes leads to subsequent carcinoma development in the transplants.

Loss or inactivation of tumor suppressor genes almost certainly plays some role in human prostate carcinogenesis, because a variety of cytogenetic abnormalities and allelic losses, particularly on chromosomes 6q and 10p, have been reported (*65, 66*). Allelic loss at 13q also occurs (*65*), and loss of heterozygosity of the retinoblastoma (RB) gene and a deletion in the promotor region of that gene have been found in 1/7 human prostate cancers (*67*). Introduction of the wild-type RB gene into the human prostate cancer cell line DU145 that carries a mutated RB gene has been shown to result in suppression of the neoplastic phenotype (*68*).

Estrogen-androgen-induction of Carcinogenesis in the Rat Prostate

Prostatic epithelial dysplasia is consistently induced by treatment of intact NBL rats for 16 weeks with slow-release implants containing estradiol-17β and testosterone which prevents estrogen-induced prostate atrophy (*69–71*). This putative preneoplastic lesion is multifocal and predominantly limited to prostate ducts, and it occurs exclusively in the dorsolateral prostate, but not in other rat accessory sex glands (*69, 70*). Prostate carcinoma induction in NBL rats by protracted treatment with estradiol and testosterone has been reported (*72*), but the precise incidence and prostate lobe of origin of these tumors was uncertain. Treatment of NBL rats with both these hormones for 16 weeks induces the type II estrogen receptor selectively in the dorsolateral prostate (*73*). The type II estrogen receptor is a cell proliferation marker, which has been implicated as a key factor in normal and abberant growth regulation in female estrogen-target tissues. Although this observation suggests that protracted stimulation of cell proliferation is involved in the formation of prostate dysplasia, the exact mechanism(s) whereby exposure to estradiol and testosterone leads to prostate carcinomas is unknown.

We treated NBL rats with estradiol in combination with testosterone *via* Silastic implants (*71*). All rats receiving this treatment developed dysplasia exclusively in the dorsolateral prostate within 16 weeks, and carcinomas in the dorsolateral prostate and/or the anterior prostate (=coagulating gland) after 42–52 weeks of treatment (unpublished data). All tumors were invasive, well differentiated, adenocarcinomas microscopic in size, that appeared to develop from the periurethral ducts of the dorsolateral and/or anterior prostate lobes. Thus, prostate carcinomas induced by this treatment probably represent a pathogenetic pathway of prostatic cancer formation distinct from that of the earlier-mentioned carcinomas induced by MNU and testosterone which often develop in the periphery of the glands and vary considerably in histologic grade. Since testosterone treatment *per se* does not induce

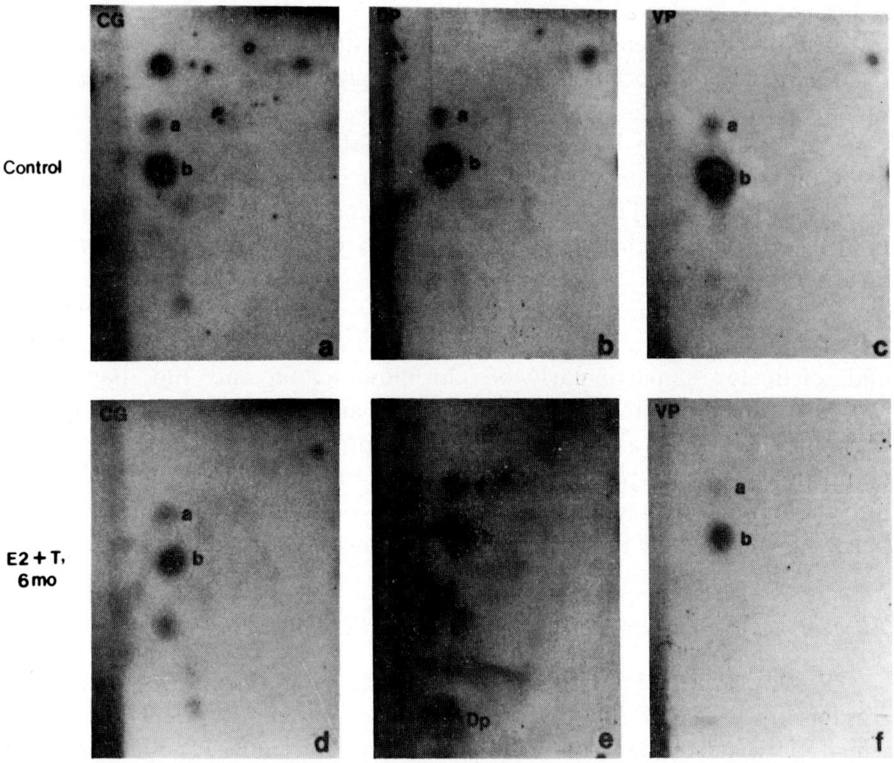

FIG. 4. ^{32}P-postlabeling analysis of prostate DNA of rats treated with estradiol-17β and testosterone for 24 weeks. DNA from coagulating gland (=anterior prostate; CG), dorsolateral prostate (DP), and ventral prostate (VP) was isolated and analyzed separately by the nuclease P1 enhancement procedure of the ^{32}P-postlabeling assay as described elsewhere (*76*). Adducts are lettered to the right of each spot. One major adduct (spot Dp) was induced in the dorsolateral prostate (panel e), but not in the ventral prostate (panel f) or the coagulating gland (panel d). This adduct spot was also found in this tissue at comparable intensity after 16 weeks of treatment as determined by Cherenkov counting (*76*), but it was not detectable after 8 weeks (data not shown). Adduct spots a and b are apparently indigenous adducts present in all prostate lobes, regardless of treatment; their intensities decreased for unknown reasons after 24 weeks of hormone treatment, but not after 8 or 16 weeks (data not shown).

dysplasia in NBL rats, these data suggest that the estrogen component of the combined hormone treatment can induce carcinomas in the rat prostate. This estrogen effect is not limited to the NBL rat and to estradiol-17β, because we have also observed dysplasia and carcinoma development in Sprague-Dawley rats and with diethylstilbestrol given in combination with testosterone. Interestingly, this diethylstilbestrol plus testosterone treatment also caused dysplasia (*71*) and carcinomas *in situ* in the ventral prostate. The mechanism for this shift in location of dysplasia is as yet incompletely understood, but may be related to differences in bioavailability of the estrogens in the different prostate lobes (*71*).

Induction of DNA adducts by structurally unrelated estrogens has been demonstrated by ^{32}P-postlabeling in the male hamster kidney (*74*), a classical target organ for estrogen-induced tumorigenesis. Therefore, we examined DNA adduct formation in DNA isolated (*75*) from prostate lobes of rats treated with estradiol and testosterone, using the nuclease P1-enhanced version of the ^{32}P-postlabeling assay (*76*). One major adduct was detected in DNA of dorsolateral prostate tissue (which included the ducts of these lobes and those of the anterior prostate and the seminal vesicle) after 16 or 24 weeks of hormone treatment (Fig. 4). This adduct could not be detected in DNA isolated from the ventral prostate or the distal portion of the anterior prostate of sex steroid-treated rats, or in DNA from any prostate lobe of rats treated for only 8 weeks or control rats (Fig. 4). This adduct was unique with respect to its chromatographic location, and it has not been observed before in any tissue of control or hormone-treated animals. At present, neither the nature of this major hormone-induced adduct, nor the mechanism of its formation is known. However, the selective occurrence of this adduct in the tissue of origin of the carcinomas coinciding with the appearance of putative preneoplastic focal lesions (dysplasias) suggests a causal relationship between DNA adduct formation and hormone-induced prostate cancer development. While it is unknown whether testosterone is a tumor promotor in this system, the presence of a DNA adduct may suggest that estradiol-17β acts as a tumor initiating agent.

Acknowledgments

The studies described in this paper were supported in part by Grants No. CIVO 80-3 and CIVO 84-3 from the Dutch Cancer Society, US PHS Grants No. CA13343, CA15776, CA43151, CA43233, CA48084, and CA48943, and US EPA Grant No. CR 813481. The authors want to thank all scientific and technical staff that have contributed to these studies.

REFERENCES

1. Carter, H. B. and Coffey, D. S. The prostate: An increasing medical problem. Prostate, *16*: 39–48, 1990.
2. Bosland, M. C. The etiopathogenesis of prostatic cancer with special reference to environmental factors. Adv. Cancer Res., *51*: 1–106, 1988.
3. Carter, B. S., Carter, H. B., and Isaacs, J. T. Epidemiologic evidence regarding predisposing factors to prostate cancer. Prostate, *16*: 187–197, 1990.
4. Akazaki, K. and Stemmermann, G. N. Comparative study of latent carcinoma of the prostate among Japanese in Japan and Hawaii. J. Natl. Cancer Inst., *50*: 1137–1144, 1973.
5. Breslow, N., Chan, C. W., Dhom, G., Drury, R. A. B., Franks, L. M., Gellei, B., Lee, Y. S., Lunberg, S., Sparke, B., Sternby, N. H., and Tulinius, H. Latent carcinoma of the prostate at autopsy in seven areas. Int. J. Cancer, *20*: 680–688, 1977.
6. Yatani, R., Chigusa, K., Akazaki, K., Stemmermann, G. N., Welsh, R. A., and Correa, P. Geographic pathology of latent prostatic carcinoma. Int. J. Cancer, *29*: 611–616, 1982.
7. Yatani, R., Kusano, I., Shiraisi, T., Akazaki, K., Hiyashi, T., and Stemmermann, G. N. Latent prostatic carcinoma: Pathological and epidemiological aspects. Jpn. J. Clin. Oncol., *19*: 319–326, 1989.
8. Bosland, M. C. Diet and cancer of the prostate: epidemiologic and experimental evidence. *In*; B. S. Reddy and L. A. Cohen (eds.), Diet, Cancer, and Nutrition: A Critical Evaluation, Vol. 1, pp. 125–149, CRC Press, Boca Raton, 1986.
9. Pollard, M. and Luckert, P. H. Promotional effects of testosterone and dietary fat on the development of autochthonous prostate cancer in rats. Cancer Lett., *32*: 223–227,

1986.

10. Bosland, M. C., Dreef-van der Meulen, H. C., and Scherrenberg, P. M. Effect of dietary fat on rat prostate carcinogenesis induced by *N*-methyl-*N*-nitrosourea and testosterone. Proc. Am. Assoc. Cancer Res., *31*: 144, 1990.
11. Pour, P. M., Groot, K., Kazakoff, K., Anderson, K., and Schally, A. V. Effects of high-fat diet on the patterns of prostatic cancer induced in rats by *N*-nitrosobis(2-oxopropyl) amine and testosterone. Cancer Res., *51*: 4757–4761, 1991.
12. Bosland, M. C., Dreef-van der Meulen, H. C., Scherrenberg, P. M., and Roverts, G. Effect of dietary protein on rat prostate cancer induction by *N*-methyl-*N*-nitrosourea and testosterone. Proc. Am. Assoc. Cancer Res., *321*: 148, 1991.
13. Carter, H. B., Piantadosi, S., and Isaacs, J. T. Clinical evidence for and implications of multistep development of prostate cancer. J. Urol., *143*: 742–746, 1990.
14. Franks, L. M. Latent carcinoma of the prostate. J. Pathol. Bacteriol., *68*: 603–613, 1954.
15. McNeal, J. E., Bostwick, D. G., Kindrachuk, R. A., Redwine, E. A., Freiha, F. S., and Stamey, T. A. Patterns of progression in prostate cancer. Lancet, *i*: 60–63, 1986.
16. Yatani, R., Shiraisi, T., Akazaki, K., Hiyashi, T., Heilbrun, L. K., and Stemmermann, G. N. Incidental prostatic carcinoma: morphometry correlated with histological grade. Virchows Arch. [A], *409*: 395–405, 1986.
17. McNeal, J. E. and Bostwick, D. G. Intraductal dysplasia: A premalignant lesion of the prostate. Human Pathol., *17*: 64–71, 1986.
18. Bostwick, D. G. and Brawer, M. K. Prostatic intra-epithelial neoplasia and early invasion in prostate cancer. Cancer, *59*: 788–794, 1987.
19. Greene, D. R., Egawa, S., Neehut, G., Flanagan, W., Wheeler, T. M., and Scardino, P. T. The distribution of residual cancer in radical prostatectomy specimens in stage A prostate cancer. J. Urol., *145*: 324–329, 1991.
20. McNeal, J. E., Villers, A., Redwine, E. A., Freiha, F. S., and Stamey, T. A. Microcarcinoma in the prostate: Its association with duct-acinar dysplasia. Human Pathol., *22*: 644–652, 1991.
21. McNeal, J. E. Origin and development of carcinoma in the prostate. Cancer, *23*: 24–34, 1969.
22. Christensen, W. N., Partin, A. W., Walsh, P. C., and Epstein, J. I. Pathologic findings in clinical stage A2 prostate cancer. Relation of tumor volume, grade, and location to pathologic stage. Cancer, *65*: 1021–1027, 1990.
23. Miller, G. J. Histopathology of prostate cancer: prediction of malignant behavior and correlation with ultrasonography. Urology, *33* (Suppl.): 18–26, 1989.
24. Partin, A. W., Epstein, J. I., Cho, K. R., Gittelsohn, A. M., and Walsh, P. C. Morphometric measurement of tumor volume and percent of gland involvement as predictors of pathological stage in clinical stage B prostate cancer. J. Urol., *141*: 341–348, 1989.
25. Stamey, T. A., McNeal, J. E., Freiha, F. S., and Redwine, E. Morphometric and clinical studies on 68 consecutive radical prostatectomies. J. Urol., *139*: 1235–1241, 1988.
26. McNeal, J. E., Redwine, E. A., Freiha, F. S., and Stamey, T. A. Zonal distribution of prostatic adenocarcinoma. Correlation with histologic pattern and direction of spread. Am. J. Surg. Pathol., *12*: 897–906, 1988.
27. Epstein, J. I., Cho, K. R., and Quinn, B. D. Relationship of severe dysplasia to stage A (incidental) adenocarcinoma of the prostate. Cancer, *65*: 2321–2327, 1990.
28. Quinn, B. D., Cho, K. R., and Epstein, J. I. Relationship of severe dysplasia to stage B adenocarcinoma of the prostate. Cancer, *65*: 2328–2337, 1990.

29. McNeal, J. E., Price, H. M., Redwine, E. A., Freiha, F. S., and Stamey, T. A. Stage A versus stage B adenocarcinoma of the prostate: Morphological comparison and biological significance. J. Urol., *139*: 61–65, 1988.
30. Miller, G. J. New developments in grading of prostate cancer. Sem. Urol., *8*: 9–18, 1990.
31. Price, D. Comparative aspects of development and structure in the prostate. Natl. Cancer Inst. Monogr. *12*: 1–25, 1963.
32. Shirai, T., Fukushima, S., Ikawa, E., Tagawa, Y., and Ito, N. Induction of prostate carcinoma *in situ* at high incidence in F344 rats by a combination of 3,2′-dimethyl-4-aminobiphenyl and ethinyl estradiol. Cancer Res., *46*: 6423–6426, 1986.
33. Shirai, T., Namakura, A., Fukushima, S., Tada, M., Morita, T., and Ito, N. Immunohistochemical demonstration of carcinogen-DNA adducts in target and non-target tissues of rats given a prostate carcinogen 3,2′-dimethyl-4-aminobiphenyl. Carcinogenesis, *11*: 653–658, 1990.
34. Pour, P. M. Prostate cancer induced in MRC rats by *N*-nitrosobis(2-oxopropyl)amine and *N*-nitrosobis(2-hydroxypropyl)amine. Carcinogenesis, *4*: 49–55, 1983.
35. Bosland, M. C., Prinsen, M. K., and Kroes, R. Adenocarcinomas of the prostate induced by *N*-nitroso-*N*-methylurea in rats pretreated with cyproterone acetate and testosterone. Cancer Lett., *18*: 69–78, 1983.
36. Bosland, M. C. and Prinsen, M. K. Induction of adenocarcinomas of the dorsolateral prostate induced in Wistar rats by *N*-methyl-*N*-nitrosourea, 7,12-dimethylbenz[a] anthracene, and 3,2′-dimethyl-4-aminobiphenyl following sequential treatment with cyproterone acetate and testosterone propionate. Cancer Res., *50*: 691–699, 1990.
37. Bosland, M. C., Prinsen, M. K., Dirksen, T. J. M., and Spit, B. J. Characterization of adenocarcinomas of the dorsolateral prostate induced in Wistar rats by *N*-methyl-*N*-nitrosourea, 7,12-dimethylbenz[a]anthracene, and 3,2′-dimethyl-4-aminobiphenyl following sequential treatment with cyproterone acetate and testosterone propionate. Cancer Res., *50*: 700–709, 1990.
38. Shirai, T., Tamano, S., Kato, T., Iwasaki, S., Takahashi, S., and Ito, N. Induction of invasive carcinomas in the accessory sex organs other than the ventral prostate of rats given 3,2′-dimethyl-4-aminobiphenyl and testosterone propionate. Cancer Res., *51*: 1264–1269, 1991.
39. Bosland, M. C. Adenocarcinoma, prostate, rat. *In*; T. C. Jones, U. Mohr, and R. D. Hunt (eds.), Genital System. pp. 252–260, Springer-Verlag, Berlin, 1987.
40. Noble, R. L. Prostate carcinoma in the Nb rat in relation to hormones. Int. Rev. Exp. Pathol., *23*: 113–159, 1982.
41. Pollard, M. P., Luckert, P. H., and Schmidt, M. A. Induction of prostate adenocarcinomas in Lobund Wistar rats by testosterone. Prostate, *3*: 563–568, 1982.
42. Pour, P. M. and Stepan, K. Induction of prostatic carcinomas and lower urinary tract neoplasms by combined treatment of intact and castrated rats with testosterone propionate and *N*-nitrosobis(2-oxopropyl)amine. Cancer Res., *47*: 5699–5706, 1987.
43. Bosland, M. C., Scherrenberg, P. M., Ford, H., and Dreef-van der Meulen, H. C. Promotion by testosterone of *N*-methyl-*N*-nitrosourea-induced prostatic carcinogenesis in rats. Proc. Am. Assoc. Cancer. Res., *30*: 272, 1989.
44. Pollard, M. and Luckert, P. H. Production of autochthonous prostate cancer in Lobund Wistar rats by treatment with *N*-nitroso-*N*-methylurea and testosterone. J. Natl. Cancer Inst., *77*: 583–587, 1986.
45. Hoover, D. M., Best, K. L., McKenney, B. K., Tamura, R. N., and Neubauer, B. L. Experimental induction of neoplasia in the accessory sex organs of male Lobund-Wistar rats. Cancer Res., *50*: 142–146, 1990.

46. Ross, R., Bernstein, L., Judd, H., Hanisch, R., Pike, M., and Henderson, B. Serum testosterone levels in healthy young black and white men. J. Natl. Cancer Inst., *76*: 45–48, 1986.
47. Schröder, F. H. Androgen and carcinoma of the prostate. *In*; E. Nieschlag and H. M. Behre (eds.), Testosterone-Action, Deficiency, Substitution, pp. 245–260, Springer-Verlag, Berlin, 1990.
48. Nieschlag, E. and Behre, H. M. Pharmacology and clinical uses of testosterone. *In*; E. Nieschlag and H. M. Behre (eds.), Testosterone-Action, Deficiency, Substitution, pp. 92–114, Springer-Verlag, Berlin, 1990.
49. World Health Organization Task Force on Methods for the Regulation of Male Fertility. Contraceptive efficacy of testosterone-induced azoospermia in normal men. Lancet, *336*: 955—959, 1990.
50. Matsumoto, A. M. Effects of chronic testosterone administration in normal men: Safety and efficacy of high dosage testosterone and parallel dose-dependent suppression of luteinizing hormone, follicle-stimulating hormone, and sperm production. J. Clin. Endocrinol. Metabol., *70*: 282–287, 1990.
51. Yersalis, C. E., Anderson, W. A., Buckley, W. E., and Wright, J. E. Incidence of the non-medical use of anabolic-androgenic steroids. *In*; G. C. Lin and L. Erinoff (eds.), Anabolic Steroid Abuse, National Institute on Drug Abuse Research Monograph 102, US DHHS Publ. No. (ADM) 90-1720, pp. 97–112, NIDA, Rockville, 1990.
52. International Agency for Research On Cancer. Overall Evaluation of Carcinogenicity: An Updating of IARC Monographs Volumes 1 to 42, IARC Monographs on the Evaluation of Carcinogenic Risks to Humans, Suppl. 7, IARC, Lyon, 1987.
53. Sukumar, S., Armstrong, B., Bruyntjes, J. P., Leav, I., and Bosland, M. C. Frequent activation of the Ki-*ras* oncogene at codon 12 in *N*-methyl-*N*-nitrosourea-induced rat prostate adenocarcinomas and neurogenic sarcomas. Mol. Carcinogen., *4*: 362–368, 1991.
54. Sukumar, S., Notario, V., Martin-Zanca, D., and Barbacid, M. Induction of mammary carcinomas in rats by nitroso-methylurea involves malignant activation of H-*ras*-1 locus by single point mutations. Nature, *306*: 658–661, 1983.
55. Sukumar, S. and Barbacid, M. Specific patterns of oncogene activation in transplacentally induced tumors. Proc. Natl. Acad. Sci. U.S.A., *87*: 718–722, 1990.
56. Sukumar, S., Carney, W. P., and Barbacid, M. Independent molecular pathways in initiation and loss of hormone responsiveness in breast carcinomas. Science, *240*: 524–526, 1988.
57. Kumar, R., Sukumar, S., and Barbacid, M. Activation of *ras* oncogenes preceding the onset of neoplasia. Science, *248*: 1101–1104, 1990.
58. Peehl, D. M., Wehner, N., and Stamey, T. A. Activated Ki-*ras* oncogene in human prostatic adenocarcinoma. Prostate, *10*: 281–290, 1987.
59. Carter, B. S., Epstein, J. E., and Isaacs, W. B. *Ras* gene mutations in prostate cancer. Cancer Res., *50*: 6830–6832, 1990.
60. Gumerlock, P. H., Poonamallee, U. R., Meyers, F. J., and deVere White, R. W. Activated *ras* alleles in human carcinoma of the prostate are rare. Cancer Res., *51*: 1632–1637, 1991.
61. Konishi, N., Enomoto, T., Buzard, G., Ohshima, M., Ward, J. M., and Rice, J. M. K-*ras* activation and *ras* p21 expression in latent prostatic carcinomas in Japanese men. Cancer Res., *69*: 2293–2299, 1992.
62. Fearon, E. R. and Vogelstein, B. A genetic model of colorectal tumorigenesis. Cell, *61*: 759–765, 1990.
63. Thompson, T. C., Southgate, J., Kitchener, G., and Land, H. Multistage carcino-

genesis induced by *ras* and *myc* oncogenes in a reconstituted organ. Cell, *56*: 917–930, 1989.
64. Thompson, T. C. Growth factors and oncogenes in prostate cancer. Cancer Cells, *2*: 345–354, 1990.
65. Carter, B. S., Ewing, C. M., Ward, W. S., Treiger, B. F., Aalders, T. W., Schalken, J. A., Epstein, J. I., and Isaacs, W. B. Allelic loss of chromosomes 16q and 10q in human prostate cancer. Proc. Natl. Acad. Sci. U.S.A., *87*: 8751–8755, 1990.
66. Brothman, A. R., Peehl, D. M., Patel, A. M., and McNeal, J.E. Frequency and pattern of karyotypic abnormalities in human prostate cancer. Cancer Res., *50*: 3795–3803, 1990.
67. Brookstein, R., Rio, P., Madreperla, S. A., Hong, F., Allred, C., Grizzle, W. E., and Lee, W.-H. Promoter deletion and loss of retinoblastoma gene expression in human prostate carcinoma. Proc. Natl. Acad. Sci. U.S.A., *87*: 7762–7766, 1990.
68. Brookstein, R., Shew, J.-Y., Chen, P.-L., Scully, P., and Lee, W.-H. Suppression of tumorigenicity of human prostate carcinoma cells by replacing a mutated RB gene. Science, *247*: 712–715, 1990.
69. Leav, I., Ho, S.-M., Ofner, P., Merk, F. B., Kwan, P. W. L., and Damassa, D. Biochemical alterations in sex hormone-induced hyperplasia and dysplasia of the dorsolateral prostates of Noble rats. J. Natl. Cancer Inst., *80*: 1045–1053, 1988.
70. Leav, I., Merk, F. B., Kwan, P. W. L., and Ho, S.-M., Androgen-supported estrogen-enhanced epithelial proliferation in the prostates of intact Noble rats. Prostate, *15*: 23–40, 1989.
71. Ofner, P., Bosland, M. C., and Vena, R. L. Differential effects of diethylstilbestrol and estradiol-17β in combination with testosterone on rat prostate lobes. Toxicol. Appl. Pharmacol., *112*: 300–309, 1992.
72. Drago, J. R. The induction of Nb rat prostatic carcinoma. Anticancer Res., *4*: 255–256, 1984.
73. Yu, M., Cates, J., Leav, I., and Ho, S.-M. Heterogenicity of [^{3}H]estradiol binding sites in the rat prostate: properties and distribution of type I and type II sites. J. Steroid Biochem., *33*: 449–457, 1989.
74. Liehr, J. G., Avitts, T. A., Randerath, E., and Randerath, K. Estrogen-induced endogenous DNA adduction: possible mechanism of hormonal cancer. Proc. Natl. Acad. Sci. U.S.A., *83*: 5301–5305, 1986.
75. Gupta, R. C. Non-random binding of the carcinogen N-hydroxy-2-acetylaminofluorene to the repetitive sequences of rat liver DNA *in vivo*. Proc. Natl. Acad. Sci. U.S.A., *81*: 6943–6947, 1984.
76. Reddy, M. V. and Randerath, K. Nuclease P1-mediated enhancement of sensitivity of ^{32}P-postlabeling test for structurally diverse DNA adducts. Carcinogenesis, *7*: 1543–1551, 1986.

MULTISTAGE CARCINOGENESIS, C. C. HARRIS ET AL. (EDS.),
JAPAN SCI. SOC. PRESS, TOKYO/CRC PRESS, BOCA RATON, PP. 125–133, 1992

Mechanistic Analysis of Multistage Carcinogenesis in the Rat Prostate

Nobuyuki Ito, Tomoyuki Shirai, Tsuneo Masui, Kumiko Ogawa, Toshio Kato, and Satoru Takahashi

First Department of Pathology, Nagoya City University Medical School, Nagoya 467, Japan

Abstract: A new rat model of prostatic carcinomas has been developed using F344 rats and 3,2'-dimethyl-4-aminobiphenyl (DMAB). Immunohistochemical and biochemical investigation using polyclonal antibodies against DMAB-modified DNA showed DMAB-DNA adducts to be formed in all parts of the prostate including the seminal vesicles. DMAB normally induces *in situ* carcinomas limited to the ventral prostate. However, when it is given together with and followed by testosterone propionate (TP), invasive adenocarcinomas, some of which demonstrated metastatic growth in other organs, arose from the dorsolateral and anterior prostate and seminal vesicles, indicating that exogenous testosterone can exert strong enhancing effects on chemically induced carcinogenesis in these lobes of the rat prostate. Sequential observation has indicated that atypical hyperplasias are premalignant lesions and that testosterone plays a key role in the promotion and progression stages of prostate tumor development. By analogy, it is suggested that testosterone may exert equivalent influence on progression of prostate neoplasia in man. In the present studies low incidences of mutations were detected in p53 or K-*ras* genes in noninvasive and invasive rat prostate carcinomas induced by DMAB.

Prostate cancer, which is age-associated, androgen-dependent and of unknown cause, is one of the most common neoplasias in Western countries (*1*, *2*). Because the incidence of prostate cancer is increasing and populations are aging, the death rate is expected to rapidly increase in the next 10 to 15 years (*3*). Epidemiological studies have shown remarkable racial or ethnic variations in the incidences of prostate cancer. However, in spite of striking differences in the prevalence of clinical prostate cancer between Americans and Japanese, little variation has been found with regard to the incidences of latent prostate cancer (*4*). Furthermore, rates of prostate cancer substantially increased in migrants to the United States from Japan and other low-risk countries (*5*). These findings clearly indicate that causal factors responsible for initiation of prostate cancer may be ubiquitous while those endogenous and environmental agents involved in promotion and/or progression may differ with population and country. Detection of factors playing roles in the progression from latent to clinically manifested cancers may be the key to prevention of prostate cancer development. Of the many epidemiological surveys conducted with this aim some have strongly suggested an involvement of high fat and androgens (*6–8*). Investigation using appropriate animal models is therefore necessary to elucidate possible mechanisms underlying the promotion and progression of prostate cancer. In this paper, we review rat prostate cancer models using 3,2′-dimethyl-4-aminobiphenyl (DMAB) and provide recent data on multistep development of prostate cancer in rats.

Induction of Rat Ventral Prostate Carcinomas by DMAB

DMAB, which has been used to induce bladder and colon carcinomas in rats, was also found to induce prostate carcinomas (*9*). We confirmed that the ventral prostate of rats is one of the target organs of DMAB-multiorgan carcinogenicity (10), the incidences of carcinomas with simple protocols being in the range from 3 to 32%. In our first studies, all lesions were located in the ventral lobe and histologically showed cribriform patterns. They were classified as carcinoma *in situ* because most tumors were localized within acini without clear invasive growth.

DMAB is considered to be metabolized to ultimate carcinogenic form(s) through N-oxidation (*11, 12*). Antiserum against DMAB-modified DNA has been developed and applied immunohistochemically to visualize DMAB-DNA adduct formation in the prostate (*13, 14*). It was found that dose-related nuclear staining was present throughout the prostate complex of rats regardless of DMAB-carcinogenic organotropism, suggesting that apparent non-target sites could also give rise to tumors if appropriate additional events occurred. Adduct formation was found to differ among 5 strains of rats tested (F344, ACI/N, Lewis, CD and Wistar), suggesting genetic differences in susceptibility to DMAB prostate carcinogenicity (*15*). Comparative analysis of all data, including the incidences of prostate carcinomas and other types of tumors, demonstrated the F344 rat to be the most appropriate for investigation of DMAB prostate carcinogenesis. Tumors in the ventral prostate in all strains showed a similar morphology.

Effects of Cell Proliferation on the Initiation of DMAB Prostate Carcinogenesis

The enhancing effect of cell proliferation in the target tissue during treatment with carcinogens is a well-known phenomenon in chemical carcinogenesis (*16, 17*). Bosland *et al.* (*18*) also reported enhancement of N-methylnitrosourea (MNU)-induced rat prostate carcinogenesis by application of carcinogen during prostatic cell growth. We induced regenerative cell proliferation in the prostate epithelium 10 times by means of temporary chemical castration by administration of ethinyl estradiol to normal rats or by limited administration of testosterone in orchiectomized rats. Single injections of DMAB were given at each peak of DNA synthesis in the prostate epithelium. Carcinomas of the ventral prostate developed at very high incidence (86%) in the system utilizing chemical castration (*19*) although no such lesions were found in orchiectomized rats (*20*). Assessment of DMAB-DNA adducts, however, revealed levels to be fairly low in the prostate of surgically castrated rats as compared to chemically castrated ones (*14*), probably because of the loss of required activating enzymes for DMAB due to severe atrophy resulting from the orchiectomy. It is concluded that elevation of the carcinogenic response of DMAB by increased cell proliferative activity is only possible under conditions with normal enzymatic activities in the prostate.

Promotion and Progression Effects of Testosterone

Androgens are essential hormones for the development and function of the prostate. The occurrence of prostate cancer in the adult is thought to require the presence of androgens at an early stage of life even though the majority of tumors can grow in the absence of androgen at advanced stages. There is increasing evidence that exogenous testosterone enhances naturally occurring or chemically induced prostate carcinomas in rodents. In 1977, Noble (*21*) induced grossly visible prostate carcinomas by prolonged administration of testosterone propionate (TP) to Noble rats. He also found that a combination of TP and estrone induced tumors in a shorter time period. Pollard *et al.* (*22*) then showed that invasive prostate cancer could be produced in Lobound-Wistar and ACI rats by more than 1 year of treatment with TP. Large prostatic carcinomas also occurred in up to 90% of Lobund-Wistar rats given MNU followed by long-term implantation of TP (*23*). Similar enhancement by TP has been found in other animal systems (*24*).

In our system, when TP was given together and after DMAB administration to F344 rats, invasive adenocarcinomas occurred in the dorso-lateral and anterior prostate and seminal vesicles, some of which metastasized to the abdominal cavity, liver or lung (Table 1) (*25*). DMAB was given sc biweekly at a dose of 50 mg/kg body weight. Animals received 2 cm long Silastic tubes filled with 40 mg TP until the end of the experiment (up to 56 weeks); the tubes were replaced every 6 weeks. The common histological pattern of the induced tumors was of well to poorly differentiated adenocarcinomas accompanied by abundant fibrous stroma, this being compatible with other reports of TP associated prostate tumors. DMAB alone did not induce equivalent tumors and TP alone was not tumorigenic. Development of ventral prostate cancer was rather suppressed. Another experiment in which TP was given after initiation by MNU also resulted in invasive adenocarcinomas arising from the anterior prostate and seminal vesicles (*26*).

Thus, all experimental data clearly show that TP can exert strong enhancing effects (promotion and/or progression) on tumor development in the dorso-lateral and anterior prostate and seminal vesicles. It is not likely that TP-enhancement depends on the carcinogen used as initiator.

Atypical hyperplasias have been suggested to be premalignant proliferative

TABLE 1. Incidences of Invasive Carcinomas of Rat Prostate Induced by DMAB and Testosterone

Treatment	Incidences of carcinomas				
	Prostate			Seminal vesicles	Metastases
	Ventral	Dorso-lateral	Anterior		
1. DMAB+TP	2 (10.5)	9 (47.4)	2 (10.5)	7 (36.8)	5 (26.3)
2. DMAB	7 (35.0)	0 —	0 —	0 —	0 —
3. TP	0 —	0 —	0 —	0 —	0 —

All carcinomas except for those in the ventral prostate were invasive adenocarcinomas.

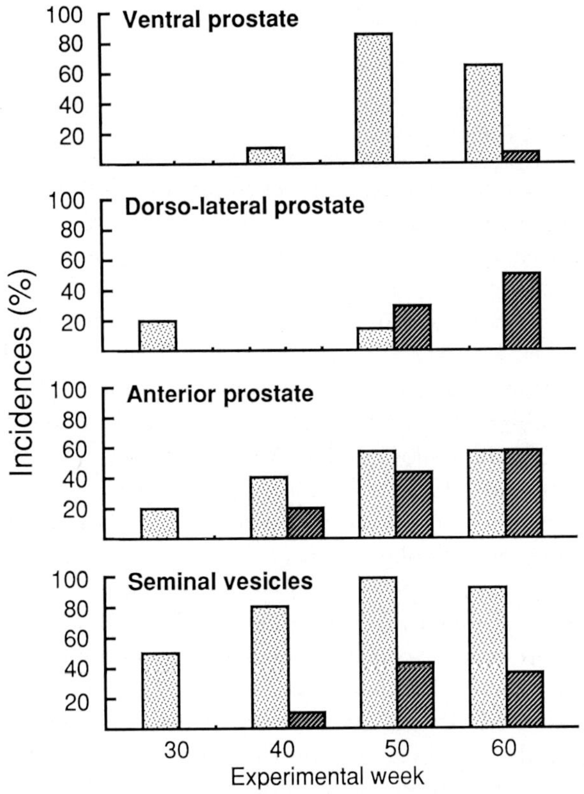

FIG. 1. Sequential changes in the incidences of atypical hyperplasias and carcinomas of the prostate and seminal vesicles. ▒, atypical hyperplasia; ▨, carcinoma.

lesions separate from adenocarcinomas in the ventral prostate (*10, 19, 27*). In order to clarify the process of the development of invasive carcinomas in the dorso-lateral and anterior prostate lobes, animals receiving DMAB and TP were killed sequentially at intervals of 10 weeks. Figure 1 shows sequential changes in incidences of both atypical hyperplasias and carcinomas. Atypical hyperplasias developed from an early stage and increased with time. Carcinomas appeared later and histological observation clearly revealed that most early carcinomas coexisted with atypical hyperplasias in all regions of the accessory sex organs. This finding suggests that atypical hyperplasias are preneoplastic not only in the ventral prostate but also in the other parts of the prostate. Similar findings were reported for Noble rats given TP and estrogen (*28*). In addition, progressive growth from very early carcinomas to invasive advanced carcinomas occurred in the dorso-lateral and anterior prostate and seminal vesicles.

Mechanisms of Testosterone Enhancement

The mechanisms by which TP exerts strong enhancing effects on prostate carcinogenesis in rodents remain unclear. TP administration by tube results in continuous elevation of serum testosterone levels to between 5 and 20 times that

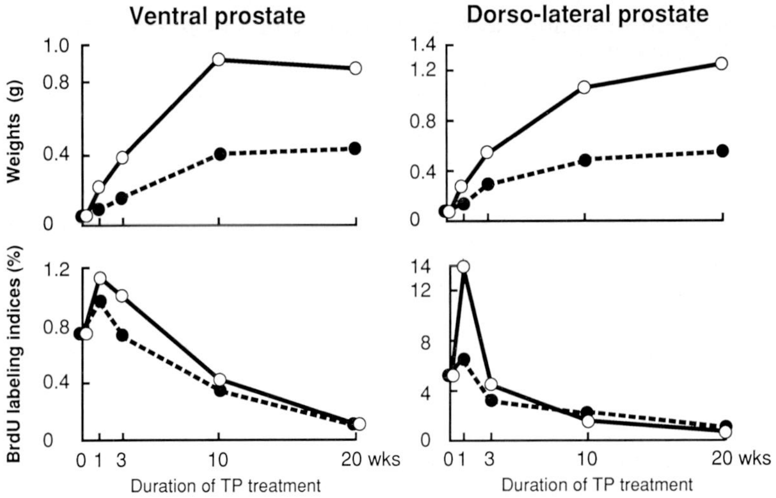

FIG. 2. Effects of continuous treatment of testosterone propionate on the weights and BrdU labeling indices in the epithelial cells of the prostate of rats. ○—○ TP treatment by Silastic tube was implanted in the subcutis, ●---● no-treatment.

of untreated control rats. While steady increase in the weight of the prostate was evident, at least over the first 10 weeks of TP treatment, marked elevation of cell proliferation as assessed by BrdU incorporation was only temporary (Fig. 2). Furthermore, no clear differences in increases in terms of cell proliferation or organ weight between the ventral and dorso-lateral prostates were found (*25*). Thus from a mechanistic viewpoint it is not simply a case of proliferation dependence. A role of estrogen derived from conversion of TP by aromatase has also been suggested (*29*). While Pour *et al.* (*29*) found significant elevation of serum estradiol levels in rats given daily injections of TP for 5 days, this was not evident with continuous administration by tube. In our experiment with animals given TP for up to 20 weeks, similarly, no elevation of serum estradiol was observed. It should be borne in mind that Isaacs (*30*) proposed the ratio of testosterone to estrogen to be one of the factors involved in prostatic carcinogenesis from his studies on ACI/seg rats which spontaneously develop ventral prostate carcinomas. Development of ventral prostate carcinoma, however, was not enhanced by TP in our studies. This is, in fact, in accordance with the result of Isaacs (*30*) that TP treatment failed to facilitate earlier appearance of spontaneous ventral prostate carcinomas in ACI/seg rats. Thus no data are available to explain the differential effects of TP between the ventral lobe and other lobes of the prostate. Clarification of this point should assist in our understanding of prostate cancer development in man.

Oncogene Expression in Tumors Induced by DMAB and TP

Mutation of H-*ras* and K-*ras* oncogenes and of the p53 suppressor gene has been investigated in carcinomas of the ventral and dorso-lateral prostate using the polymerase chain reaction-single strand conformation polymorphism (PCR-SSCP) method (*31*). DNA was obtained from cold acetone-fixed paraffin embedded materials and p53 and K-*ras* gene point mutations were detected in 2 of 13 cases. In contrast, Sukumar *et al.* (*32*) reported a high frequency (70%) of K-*ras* gene G^{35} to A mutations in prostate tumors induced by MNU and TP. This difference in *ras* gene mutation between the two systems may be due to the carcinogen used.

Effects of Other Factors

Diet containing high fat has been applied to many animal systems to clarify the supposed relationship between dietary fat and development of prostate cancer in man (*9*, *33–36*). Corn oil used as a source of high fat has usually been incorporated into the diet at a concentration of 20 to 25% after adjustment for caloric intake. However, none of the experiments, including our recent work with DMAB and MNU (*26*, *37*), showed a positive correlation between high fat and prostate cancer. Although enhancement by high fat was reported by one group when given together with TP (*36*), there was no such influence in the presence of TP in recent work from Pour *et al.* (*29*).

Prolactin, which has been shown to play important roles in regulation of the growth and function of the prostate glands, was also investigated in the DMAB prostate carcinogenesis model to assess whether it exerts a modifying effect (*38*). Hyperprolactinemia was effected by implantation of a prolactin releasing pituitary tumor (MtT/F84), but only results for atypical hyperplasia of the ventral prostate were increased.

Antioxidants (6 naturally occurring species; catechol, resorcinol, hydroquinone, selenium, γ-oryzanol, and α-tocopherol) did not demonstrate any second stage modifying effects on rat prostate carcinogenesis when investigated in our DMAB model (*39*). In another experiment, alteration of cholesterol levels in the serum produced by cholesterol or clofibrate supplementation in the diet, but did not exert any modification of prostate carcinogenesis after the administration of DMAB (*40*). Ohshima *et al.* (*41*) also investigated dietary application of three retinoids to ACI/seg rats without a clear modification of the incidence of spontaneous prostate tumors.

Acknowledgments

The studies performed in the authors' laboratory were supported in part by Grants-in-Aid for Cancer Research from the Ministry of Education, Science and Culture and the Ministry of Health and Welfare of Japan, a Grant-in-Aid from the Ministry of Health and Welfare for a Comprehensive 10 Year Strategy for Cancer Control, Japan and grants from the Society for Promotion of Pathology of Nagoya and the Foundation for Prostate Research, Japan.

REFERENCES

1. Franks, L. M. Etiology, epidemiology, and pathology of prostate cancer. Cancer, *32*: 1092–1095, 1973.
2. Silverberg, E. Statistical and epidemiologic data on urologic cancer. Cancer, (Suppl.) *60*: 692–717, 1987.
3. Chiarodo, A. National Cancer Institute roundtable on prostate cancer: future research directions. Cancer Res., *51*: 2498–2505, 1991.

4. Yatani, R., Chigusa, I., Akazaki, K., Stemmermann, G. N., Welsh, R. A., and Correa, P. Geographic pathology of latent prostate carcinoma. Int. J. Cancer, *29*: 611–616, 1982.
5. Waterhouse, J., Muir, C. S., Correa, P., and Powell, J. (eds.). *In*; "Cancer Incidence in Five Continents," Vol. III, pp. 164, 512, and 513, IARC Scientific Publications No. 15, Lyon, 1976.
6. Ross, R. K., Shimizu, H., Paganini-Hill, A., Honda, G., and Henderson, B. E. Case-control studies of prostate cancer in blacks and whites in southern California. J. Natl. Cancer Inst., *78*: 869–874, 1987.
7. Hill, P., Garbaczewski, L., Helman, P., Walker, A.R.P., Garnes, H., and Wynder, E. L. Environmental factors and breast and prostatic cancer. Cancer Res., *41*: 3817–3818, 1981.
8. Graham, S., Haughey, B., Marshall, J., Priore, R., Byers, T., Mettlin, C., and Pontes, J. E. Diet in the epidemiology of carcinoma of the prostate gland. J. Natl. Cancer Inst., *70*: 687–692, 1983.
9. Katayama, S., Fiala, E., Reddy, B. S., Rivenson, A., Silverman, J., Williams, G., and Weisburger, J. H. Prostate adenocarcinoma in rats: induction by 3,2′-dimethyl-4-aminobiphenyl. J. Natl. Cancer Inst., *68*: 867–873, 1982.
10. Shirai, T., Sakata, T., Fukushima, S., Ikawa, E., and Ito, N. Rat prostate as one of the target organs for 3,2′-dimethyl-4-aminobiphenyl-induced carcinogenesis: effects of dietary ethinyl estradiol and methyltestosterone. Gann, *76*: 803–808, 1985.
11. Flammang, T. J., Westra, J. G., Kadlubar, F. F., and Beland, F. A. DNA adducts formed from the probable proximate carcinogen, N-hydroxy-3,2′-dimethyl-4-aminobiphenyl, by acid catalysis or S-acetyl coenzyme A-dependent enzymatic esterification. Carcinogenesis, *6*: 251–258, 1985.
12. Flammang, T. J. and Kadlubar, F. F. Acetyl coenzyme A-dependent metabolic activation of N-hydroxy-3,2′-dimethyl-4-aminobiphenyl and several carcinogenic N-hydroxy arylamines in relation to tissue and species differences, other acyl donors, and arylhydroxamic acid-dependent acyltransferase. Carcinogenesis, *7*: 919–926, 1986.
13. Tada, M., Aoki, H., Kojima, M., Morita, T., Shirai, T., Yamada, H., and Ito, N. Preparation and characterization of antibodies against 3,2′-dimethyl-4-aminobiphenyl-modified DNA. Carcinogenesis, *10*: 1397–1402, 1989.
14. Shirai, T., Nakamura, A., Fukushima, S., Tada, M., Morita, T., and Ito, N. Immunohistochemical demonstration of carcinogen-DNA adducts in target and non-target tissues of rats given a prostate carcinogen, 3,2′-dimethyl-4-aminobiphenyl. Carcinogenesis, *11*: 653–658, 1990.
15. Shirai, T., Nakamura, A., Fukushima, S., Yamamoto, A., Tada, M., and Ito, N. Different carcinogenic responses in a variety of organs, including the prostate, of five different rat strains given 3,2′-dimethyl-4-aminobiphenyl. Carcinogenesis, *11*: 793–798, 1990.
16. Craddock, V. M. Effects of single treatment with the alkylating carcinogens dimethylnitrosamine, diethylnitrosamine and methanesulphonate, on liver regenerating after partial hepatectomy. II. Alkylation of DNA and inhibition of DNA replication. Chem.-Biol. Interact., *10*: 323–332, 1975.
17. Frei, J. V. Some mechanisms operative in carcinogenesis. A review. Chem.-Biol. Interact., *13*: 1–25, 1976.
18. Bosland, M. C., Prinsen, M. K., and Kroes, R. Adenocarcinomas of the prostate induced by N-nitroso-N-methylurea in rats pretreated with cyproterone acetate and testosterone. Cancer Lett., *18*: 69–78. 1983.
19. Shirai, T., Fukushima, S., Ikawa, E., Tagawa, Y., and Ito, N. Induction of prostate

carcinoma *in situ* at high incidence in F344 rats by a combination of 3,2′-dimethyl-4-aminobiphenyl and ethinyl estradiol. Cancer Res., *46*: 6423–6426, 1986.

20. Shirai, T., Tagawa, Y., Fukushima, S., Asamoto, M., and Ito, N. Lack of tumorigenic response in the prostate gland of castrated F344 rats by 3,2′-dimethyl-4-aminobiphenyl given with methyltestosterone. Cancer Lett., *35*: 1–6, 1987.
21. Noble, R. L. The development of prostatic adenocarcinoma in Nb rats following prolonged sex hormone administration. Cancer Res., *37*: 1929–1933, 1977.
22. Pollard, M., Luckert, P. H., and Schmidt, M. A. Induction of adenocarcinomas in Lobund-Wistar rats by testosterone. Prostate, *3*: 563–568, 1982.
23. Pollard, M., Luckert, P. H., and Snyder, D. L. The promotional effect of testosterone on induction of prostate-cancer in MNU-sensitized L-W rats. Cancer Lett., *45*: 209–212, 1989.
24. Pour, P. M. and Stepan, K. Induction of prostatic carcinomas and lower urinary tract neoplasms by combined treatment of intact and castrated rats with testosterone propionate and N-nitrosobis(2-oxopropyl)amine. Cancer Res., *47*: 5699–5706, 1987.
25. Shirai, T., Tamano, S., Kato, T., Iwasaki, S., Takahashi, S., and Ito, N. Induction of invasive carcinomas in the accessory sex organs other than the ventral prostate of rats given 3,2′-dimethyl-4-aminobiphenyl and testosterone propionate. Cancer Res., *51*: 1264–1269, 1991.
26. Shirai, T., Yamamoto, A., Iwasaki, S., Tamano, S., and Masui, T. Induction of invasive carcinomas of the seminal vesicles and coagulating glands of F344 rats by administration of N-methyl-nitrosourea or N-nitrosobis(2-oxopropyl)amine followed by testosterone propionate with or without high-fat diet. Carcinogenesis, *12*: 2169–2173, 1991.
27. Ward, J. M., Reznik, D.V.M., Stinson, S. F., Lattuada, C. P., Longfellow, D. G., and Cameron, T. P. Histogenesis and morphology of naturally occurring prostatic carcinoma in the ACI/segHapBR rat. Lab. Invest., *43*: 517–522, 1980.
28. Leav, I., Ho, S-M., Ofner, P., Merk, F. B., Kwan, P. W.-L., and Damassa, D. Biochemical alterations in sex hormone-induced hyperplasia and dysplasia of the dorsolateral prostates of Noble rats. J. Natl. Cancer Inst., *80*: 1045–1053, 1988.
29. Pour, P. M., Groot, K., Kazakoff, K., Anderson, K., and Schally, A. V. Effects of high-fat diet on the patterns of prostatic cancer induced in rats by N-nitrosobis(2-oxopropyl)amine and testosterone. Cancer Res., *51*: 4757–4761, 1991.
30. Isaacs, J. T. The aging ACI/Seg versus Copenhagen male rat as a model system for the study of prostatic carcinogenesis. Cancer Res., *44*: 5784–5796, 1984.
31. Orita, M., Suzuki, Y., Sekiya, T., and Hayashi, K. Rapid and sensitive detection of point mutations and DNA polymorphisms using the polymerase chain reaction. Genomics, *5*: 874–879, 1989.
32. Sukumar, S., Armstrong, B., Bruyntjes, J. P., Leav, I., and Bosland, M. C. Frequent activation of the Ki-*ras* oncogene at codon 12 in N-methyl-N-nitrosourea-induced rat prostate adenocarcinomas and neurogenic sarcomas. Mol. Carcinogen., *4*: 362–368, 1991.
33. Katayama, S., Matsumoto, K., and Kitamura, H. Effect of high fat diet and sex steroid on chemically-induced prostate microcancer in rats. Proc. Jpn. Cancer Assoc., *46*: 82, 1987.
34. Bosland, M. C. Rat prostate carcinogenesis: Animal models for the study of mechanisms and risk factors of human prostate cancer development. Fundamental and clinical research in urogenital cancer. Proc. Fourth Int. Sym. Found. Promot. Cancer Res., *4*: 46–47, 1991.
35. Tobisu, K., Kakizoe, T., Tanaka, Y., Takai, K., and Shirai, T. Effect of high fat

diet on spontaneous prostatic adenocarcinoma in ACI/Seg. rat. Proc. Jpn. Cancer Assoc., *49*: 73, 1990.

36. Pollard, M. and Luckert, P. Promotional effects of testosterone and high fat diet on the development of autochthonous prostate cancer in rats. Cancer Lett., *32*: 223–227, 1986.
37. Tagawa, Y., Shirai, T., Fukushima, S., Nakamura, A., Hirose, M., and Ito, N. Lack of modification by dietary unsaturated fat of 3,2′-dimethyl-4-aminobiphenyl-induced rat prostate and colon carcinogenesis. J. Toxicol. Pathol., *2*: 49–53, 1989.
38. Nakamura, A., Shirai, T., Ogawa, K., Wada, S., Fujimoto, N.-A., Ito, A., and Ito, N. Promoting action of prolactin released from a grafted transplantable pituitary tumor (MtT/F84) on rat prostate carcinogenesis. Cancer Lett., *53*: 151–157, 1990.
39. Nakamura, A., Shirai, T., Takahashi, S., Ogawa, K., Hirose, M., and Ito, N. Lack of modification by naturally occurring antioxidants of 3,2′-dimethyl-4-aminobiphenyl-initiated rat prostate carcinogenesis. Cancer Lett., *58*: 241–246, 1991.
40. Tagawa, Y., Ozaki, K., Takahashi, S., Ogawa, K., and Shirai, T. Lack of effects of post-initiation cholesterol on 3,2′-dimethyl-4-aminobiphenyl-induced prostate carcinogenesis. Prostate, *20*: 179–185, 1992.
41. Ohshima, M., Ward, J. M., and Wenk, M. L. Preventive and enhancing effects of retinoids on the development of naturally occurring tumors of skin, prostate gland, and endocrine pancreas in aged male ACI/segHapBR rats. J. Natl. Cancer Inst., *74*: 517–524, 1985.

REGULATION OF CELL GROWTH AND DIFFERENTIATION IN MULTISTAGE CARCINOGENESIS

MULTISTAGE CARCINOGENESIS, C. C. HARRIS ET AL. (EDS.),
JAPAN SCI. SOC. PRESS, TOKYO/CRC PRESS, BOCA RATON, PP. 137–144, 1992

Protein Phosphatases in Cell Division: How Vital Are They?

Mitsuhiro YANAGIDA, Hiroyuki YAMANO, Elisa M. STONE,
Noriyuki KINOSHITA, Tetsuya YOSHIDA, and Kazuhiro SHIOZAKI

Department of Biophysics, Faculty of Science, Kyoto University, Kyoto 606, Japan

Abstract: In contrast to the wealth of information on cellular function of protein kinases, many of which are known to be the products of proto-oncogenes, little is known about how protein dephosphorylation is involved in growth control of normal and malignant cells. In the present study, roles of protein phosphatases in cell division cycle control were examined by molecular genetic approaches using a lower eukaryote, the fission yeast *Schizosaccharomyces pombe*. Nine protein phosphatase genes have been so far identified and characterized in this organism. Each of two (*dis2*$^{+}$, *sds21*$^{+}$, and *ppa1*$^{+}$, *ppa2*$^{+}$) gene products is highly similar to mammalian type 1 and 2A ser/thr phosphatases, respectively. The *ppx1*$^{+}$ product is an intermediate of type 1 and 2A, while the *ppb1*$^{+}$ product is similar to Ca^{2+}-dependent type 2B. At least two protein tyrosine phosphatase genes (*pyp1*$^{+}$ and *pyp2*$^{+}$) exist. The cdc25 protein is now established to be a tyrosine phosphatase that activates cdc2 kinase. Some of these phosphatase genes are interrelated but have distinct, essential functions in cell cycle control. Missense mutations, deletions or high dosage expression of these phosphatase genes affect entry into and exit from mitosis, mitotic chromosome disjunction, cell size and cell shape. They seem to interact with the main regulators of mitosis, cdc2, cdc13/cyclin, cdc25 and wee1, or with mitotic structural components, such as condensed chromosomes or the spindle apparatus. We show that the product of an essential gene, *sds22*$^{+}$, is an important, positive factor in controlling the expression and modulating the activity of dis2 phosphatase.

Protein phosphorylation and dephosphorylation are important post-translational modifications essential for a variety of biological systems. In eukaryotic cell cycle control, the cdc2 protein kinase plays a pivotal role as a component of mitosis promoting factor (*1*), its phosphorylation state changing during the cell cycle and its activity being regulated by tyrosine dephosphorylation (*2*). In contrast to the identification of an ever increasing number of protein kinases (*3*) many of which have been identified as the products of proto-oncogenes, protein dephosphorylation seems to be carried out by a limited number of protein phosphatases (PPase) (*4*); in mammals, there are generally four serine/threonine-specific PPases, that is, type 1 (PP1), 2A (PP2A), 2B (PP2B), and 2C (PP2C). The conservation of amino acid sequences in the catalytic subunits of PP1 and PP2A is very high. Mammalian PP1 and PP2A and fungal counterparts are highly similar and approximately 80% identical in their amino acid sequences (*5, 6*). Protein tyrosine phosphatases (PTPase) have also been found in human and yeast. Their amino acid sequence homology is not as high as in the case of ser/thr phosphatases (*7, 8*). Some receptor proteins contain cytoplasmic domains similar to PTPases and are thought to be a candidate for tumor suppressor genes (*9*).

An apparent paradox is how PPases can counteract the diversity of protein kinases. One possibility is that there may be many more PPases awaiting discovery. Alternatively, the diversity of PPases might be based on the presence of specific modulators, inhibitors and activators.

The importance of protein phosphatases in the cell division cycle was only recently established. Mutations in ser/thr protein phosphatase genes which cause defects in cell division were, in 1989, identified in two lower eukaryotes, namely, *Aspergillus nidulans* (*10*) and the fission yeast *Schizosaccharomyces pombe* (*5*), and a year later in the fruit fly (*11*). A potent phosphatase inhibitor, okadaic acid, was shown in 1988 to be a tumor promoter (*12*). In spite of a wealth of information on the roles of protein kinases in the cell division cycle of normal and malignant cells, the way protein phosphatases are involved in cell division has been little understood. The accumulation of knowledge on protein phosphatases in yeast, however, has been rapid in the past two years, and we are now able to show distinct and essential roles of different protein phosphatases in the fission yeast cell cycle.

Protein Phosphatases Are Essential for Cell Viability

Mutants in the ser/thr phosphatase genes of fission yeast, filamentous fungus and fruit fly were found which cause defects in mitosis (*5, 10, 11*). The fission yeast *dis2*$^+$ gene encodes a polypeptide, ~80% identical to mammalian PP1 (*5*). Another gene *sds21*$^+$ also codes for a PP1-like phosphatase. A cold-sensitive (cs) mutant *dis2-11* displays the phenotypes of chromosome non-disjunction and mitotic defects in the presence of the spindle (*13*). This mutation (alteration from Arg to Gln at the 245th codon) is semi-dominant (Cs$^-$ in haploid and Cs$^+$ in diploid), not only reducing the enzyme activity of the *dis2*$^+$-encoded phosphatase but also that of the other *sds21*$^+$-encoded phosphatase in haploid cells (*6*). The double gene disruption of *dis2*$^+$ and *sds21*$^+$ caused cell lethality, although single gene disruptants were viable (*5*). These findings indicated that these two genes have an overlapping essential function for cell viability.

Fission yeast has two other phosphatase genes (*ppa1*$^+$ and *ppa2*$^+$; ref. *6*) encoding polypeptides ~80% identical to mammalian PP2A. Single gene disruptants are viable but the double gene disruption of *ppa1*$^+$ and *ppa2*$^+$ causes cell lethality so that these two genes share an essential function for cell division. A cs *ppa2* mutant was made by site directed mutagenesis, and causes a dominant-lethal phenotype when overexpressed (*6*).

In addition to these ser/thr phosphatases, the product of the essential gene *cdc25*$^+$ (*1*), which positively controls *cdc2*$^+$ kinase, has been shown to be a protein phosphatase (*14, 15*).

Essential Roles of Different Protein Phosphatases

To understand the roles of protein phosphatases in cell division, it would be highly informative if all of the protein phosphatase genes in one organism were isolated, and the phenotypes of mutants were made and compared. We have been taking this approach for the fission yeast *S. pombe*, and found distinct roles for different phosphatase mutants (*6*, our unpublished result). Nine phosphatase genes so far identified are listed in Table 1.

We have identified six protein ser/thr phosphatase genes (*dis2*$^+$, *sds21*$^+$, *ppa1*$^+$, *ppa2*$^+$, *ppb1*$^+$, and *ppx1*$^+$) in fission yeast (*5*, *6*, *16*, and our unpublished result). As described above, the dis2 and sds21 polypeptides are highly similar to the catalytic subunits of mammalian PP1 phosphatase, while ppa1 and ppa2 resemble PP2A. Their phosphatase activities could be identified in extracts of deletion mutants. Judging from the amounts of protein and from the phosphatase activity, dis2 and ppa2 represent the major PP1 and PP2A-like phosphatases in wild type fission yeast. Their properties of activities are similar to mammalian PP1 and PP2A counterparts (*6*). Amino acid sequence identity between dis2 and sds21 proteins, and between ppa1 and ppa2 proteins are 78–79%, respectively. Identity with their mammalian counterparts is 74–82% (*5*, *6*). Identity between dis2 and ppa2, however, is low (38%, ref. *16*). As stated above, the defective phenotypes of mutants (either cs or double gene disruption) are strikingly different between PP1- and PP2-like mutants; cs *dis2* showed a defective phenotype in chromosome disjunction after entry into mitosis, whereas cs *ppa2* showed a phenotype similar to *wee1*, that is, premature mitosis. One hypothesis is that dis2 and sds21 phosphatases share an essential phosphatase activity in metaphase/anaphase progression and ppa1 and ppa2 phosphatases share another essential activity for the entry into mitosis (see Table 2).

The product of *ppx1*$^+$ gene isolated by hybridization (*6*) has 39, 49 and 71% homology to dis2, ppa2 and the budding yeast SIT4 (*17*) phosphatases, respectively. ppx1 phosphatase is an intermediate form between dis2 and ppa2 and may be a homologue of SIT4, but the disruptants of *ppx1*$^+$ and *SIT4* show different phenotypes.

TABLE 1. Protein Phosphatase Genes Identified in Fission Yeast

Gene	Type	Amino acid specificity	Mutant	Phenotype of gene disruptant	Ref.
dis2	1	ser/thr	cs, del	Viable[a]	(*5*)
sds21	1	ser/thr	del	Viable[a]	(*5*)
ppa1	2A	ser/thr	del	Viable[b]	(*6*)
ppa2	2A	ser/thr	cs, del	Viable[b] (cell size reduction)	(*6*)
ppb1	2B	ser/thr		ND	(upb)
ppx1		ser/thr	del	Viable[c] (cell size and shape)	(*6*, *16*)
cdc25		tyr	ts, del	Lethal[d]	(*1*)
pyx1	PTP	tyr	del	Viable	(*8*)
pyp2	PTP	tyr		ND	(upb)

[a] Lethal when either *sds21*$^+$ or *dis2*$^+$ is also disrupted. [b] Lethal when either *ppa1*$^+$ or *ppa2*$^+$ is also disrupted. [c] Lethal when *ppa2*$^+$ is also disrupted. [d] Viable when *wee1* mutation is introduced. ND: not determined. upb: our unpublished result.

TABLE 2. Phenotype of Different Phosphatase Mutants

Type of mutant	Genes: *dis2*+	Genes: *sds21*+
Arg-245 to Gln	Semi dominant cs Failure to exit mitosis High histone H1 kinase	Normal
Gene disruption	Normal	Normal
Multicopy gene	Normal Reversal of *cdc25-wee1* Failure to rescue *sds22*	Normal Reversal of *cdc25-wee1* Rescue *sds22*
nmt Promoter	Viable, normal	G2 arrest

Type of mutants	*ppa2*+	*ppa1*+	*ppx1*
Arg to Gln	Semi-dominant cs Short cells	ND	ND
Disruption	Viable, short cells Hypersensitive to okadaic acid Rescue cs *dis1*	Normal	Slow growth Short and round
nmt promoter	Normal	ND	ND

Normal: normal growth. ND: not determined.

```
PTP1B    65 DYINASLIKMEEAQRSYILTQGPLPNTCGHFWEMVWE   Charbonneau et al., 1989.
            ****** ** *     **  **        ** ***
pyp1+   323 DYINASFIKTETSN##YIACQGSISRSISDFWHMVWD   Ottilie et al., 1991.
            ** *** *        *****        *** ****
pyp2+       DYMNASHIDVGNKK##YIACQAPKPGTLLDFWNMVWD
```

FIG. 1. Partial amino acid sequence for protein tyrosine phosphatases in fission yeast. The sequence of pyp1 is from reference *8*, while pyp2 is our unpublished result. PTP1B is from human placenta (*7*).

The disruption of *ppx1*+ gene causes slow growth (small colony), displaying significant changes in cell size and shape (our unpublished result). Interestingly, the double disruptant with *ppa2* is lethal, producing the mixed phenotype, but the double disruptant with *dis2* is viable. There may be other intermediate forms in fission yeast; such a phosphatase has been found in *S. cerevisiae* (*18*).

We have isolated a gene (*ppb1*+) encoding a polypeptide similar to type 2B protein phosphatase (PP2B) gene. The gene disruption has not been done. In mammalian cells, the protein product is Ca^{2+}-dependent protein phosphatase (calcineurin). Disruptants of the *S. cerevisiae* PP2B genes are viable (*19*). Therefore, cellular roles of PP2B have not been critically examined. Type 2C protein phosphatase (*4*) was not discovered in fission yeast, although an abundant phosphatase activity similar to mammalian PP2C can be detected in fission yeast cell extracts (*6*).

There are two classes of phosphatase genes, the products of which are capable of removing phosphate from tyrosine in fission yeast. One (*pyp1*+ gene, ref. *8*) is similar to mammalian PTPase. The gene disruptant of *pyp1*+ displayed no phenotype. We found another gene (designated *pyp2*+) encoding a PTP-like polypeptide; the partial sequence is shown in Fig. 1. Determining the phenotype of the double gene disruptant will be of interest. The other class of tyrosine phosphatase is the product of cell cycle regulator *cdc25*$^+$ (*1, 14, 15*). *cdc25* mutant cells are arrested in the G2 phase at the restrictive temperature due to the absence of cdc2 kinase activation by tyr-15 dephosphorylation. If *cdc25*$^+$ is overexpressed, the wee phenotype is observed, due to the premature onset of mitosis.

In short, there are at least four classes of phosphatase activities essential for cell division in fission yeast: 1) the activity shared by dis2 and sds21, 2) ppa1 and ppa2, 3) ppx1 and ppa2, and 4) cdc25. These appear to have different roles in cell division cycle control.

Effect of High Dosage of dis2 and sds21 Phosphatases on the Cell Cycle

In contrast to the disruption phenotype of the *sds21*$^+$ gene (*e.g.*, no effect on cell division), highly expressed *sds21*$^+$ gene was found to display a striking phenotype, that is, the block in G2 phase. Highly elongated cells with a single nucleus and an interphase cytoskeletal structure are produced when the *sds21*$^+$ gene is placed under the control of inducible *nmt1*$^+$ promoter. Interestingly, the G2 block phenotype was not produced and the cells grew normally when the *dis2*$^+$ gene was similarly highly expressed. The amounts of sds21 and dis2 proteins examined by immunoblotting were found to be nearly the same so that the phenotypic difference should not be due to the dosage, but probably due to the differences in protein functions. A finding that supports this notion is that the G2 block phenotype can be produced by modifying the amino acid sequence in the COOH terminus of the dis2 protein (unpublished result).

Another phenotype produced by the high dosage of *dis2*$^+$ and *sds21*$^+$ is again related to the transition from G2 to M phase. If a multicopy plasmid carrying the *dis2*$^+$ or *sds21*$^+$ gene was introduced to the *wee1-cdc25* double mutant, the Ts$^+$ phenotype was reversed to Ts$^-$ (*20*, unpublished result). As the expression level of *sds21*$^+$ from the multicopy plasmid is much less than from the nmtl-inducible promoter, wild type cells carrying the *sds21*$^+$ multicopy plasmid grew at a normal rate (Table 2). Several hypotheses to explain the reversal of the *wee1-cdc25* mutant phenotype are that the high gene dosage of *dis2*$^+$ or *sds21*$^+$ either activates wee1 kinase or inhibits cdc25 phosphatase or inhibits the activation of cdc2/cyclin. All these proteins are known to be phosphorylated. Although full interpretation of this finding needs further investigation, it may be possible to state that the high dosage of dis2 and sds21 phosphatases are implicated in the control of G2/M progression, directly or indirectly by regulating wee1 kinase or cdc25 phosphatase. dis2 phosphatase itself is phosphorylated (unpublished result) so that its activity might also be regulated by phosphorylation and dephosphorylation.

Role of sds22 Protein in Controlling dis2 Phosphatase

The *sds22*$^+$ gene was initially isolated as a high gene dosage suppressor for cs *dis2-11* (*5*). Disruption of the *sds22*$^+$ gene showed that it was essential for division (*21*). Cells of the gene disruptant showed a striking cell cycle phenotype, that is, arrest at metaphase. Consistently, a ts *sds22* mutant recently constructed also showed metaphase arrest at the restrictive temperature (unpublished result). The arrested cells contained a short mitotic spindle and condensed chromosomes arranged to form the metaphase plate-like structure. Therefore, the *sds22*$^{+}$ gene is thought to be required for the metaphase/anaphase progression.

An important property of the *sds22* gene disruptant was that its lethality can be rescued by a multicopy plasmid carrying the *sds21*$^{+}$ gene (*21*). Unexpectedly, a plasmid carrying the *dis2*$^{+}$ gene did not rescue the *sds22* disruptant. A possible explanation for this difference is that dis2 phosphatase acts on chromosome disjunction *via* interaction with *sds22*$^{+}$ whereas *sds21*$^{+}$ will not. A polypeptide similar to sds22 might exist, specifically activated by sds21 phosphatase. The sds22 protein is a relatively small protein, containing eleven tandemly-arranged leucine-rich 22 amino acid repeat units (*21*).

We found that the sds22 and dis2 proteins were co-immunoprecipitated by anti-sds22 antibodies. Immunoprecipitates with anti-sds22 antibodies contained a small amount of dis2 protein (unpublished result). The amount of co-precipitated dis2 protein was increased by the high gene dosage of *dis2*$^{+}$. Thus dis2 and sds22 seem to form a complex. sds21 protein was also present in the immunoprecipitate. This close relationship between dis2 and sds22 was further substantiated by the absence of dis2 protein in disruptant cells of the *sds22*$^{+}$ gene (unpublished result). The loss of sds22 gene function could affect the amount of dis2 protein either *via* transcription, post-transcription or -translation.

These results strongly suggest that a physiological role of sds22 protein is involved in positively regulating dis2 phosphatase. The phenomenon that the loss of sds22 function causes the arrest at mid-mitosis indicates that a particular phosphatase activity dependent on both dis2 and sds22 may be required for the progression from metaphase to anaphase. The substrate of this phosphatase activity is of great interest.

Role of the ppa1^{+} *and ppa2*$^{+}$ *Genes in Mitotic Control*

Antibodies raised against the bacterially-made ppa2 protein were used to identify the products of *ppa1*$^{+}$ and *ppa2*$^{+}$ genes (unpublished result). ppa2 is much more abundant than ppa1, consistent with the assay of protein phosphatase activities in extracts of deletion mutants (*6*). Although viable, gene disruptant cells of *ppa2*$^{+}$ are small in cell size (the semi-wee phenotype). Double disruptant cells of *Δppa1*$^{+}$ *Δppa2* are inviable and produce small, dead cells in a plasmid loss experiment.

A *ppa2*^{cs} mutant constructed by site-directed mutagenesis (from Arg to Gln at the site similar to that of cs *dis2-11*) is again small in cell size and lethal at the restrictive temperature (*6*). Consistently, the potent inhibitor okadaic acid reduces the cell size of wild type (unpublished result). All these results are consistent with the notion that *ppa2*$^{+}$ has a function similar to *wee1*$^{+}$ which inhibits the entry into mitosis, and its loss causes premature mitosis, producing short-sized cells (*1*).

We propose that ppa2 phosphatase is involved in regulating the entry into the M phase. ppa2 phosphatase and wee1 kinase may share an essential function, as the double mutant *Δppa2 wee1-50* was lethal (unpublished result). Consistent with this finding, disruption of *ppa2*$^{+}$ partially suppresses ts *cdc25*. The double mutant *Δppa2 cdc25* supported cell division several times in liquid medium at the restrictive temperature (unpublished result). The progression from G2 to M is inhibited by ppa2 phosphatase which appears to be synergistic with weel and antagonistic to cdc25.

Is ppa2 phosphatase only required in the transition from G2 to M? The finding that *dis1* mutations, which cause a mitotic block and chromosome loss at an extremely high rate (*13*), can be rescued by the deletion of the *ppa2*$^+$ gene (unpublished result) indicates that ppa2 should be involved even after the entry into M phase.

Acknowledgments

The work in the authors' laboratory was supported by grants from the Human Frontier Science Program Organization and the Ministry of Education, Science and Culture of Japan.

REFERENCES

1. Nurse, P. Universal control mechanism regulating onset of M-phase. Nature, *344*: 503–508, 1990.
2. Gould, K.L. and Nurse P. Tyrosine phosphorylation of the fission yeast *cdc2*$^+$ protein kinase regulates entry into mitosis. Nature, *342:* 39–45, 1989.
3. Hunter, T. A thousand and one protein kinases. Cell, *50*: 823–829, 1987.
4. Cohen, P. The structure and regulation of protein phosphatases. Annu. Rev. Biochem., *58*: 453–508, 1989.
5. Ohkura, H., Kinoshita, N., Miyatani, S., Toda, T., and Yanagida, M. The fission yeast *dis2*$^+$ gene required for chromosome disjoining encodes one of two putative type 1 protein phosphatases. Cell, *57*: 997–1007, 1989.
6. Kinoshita, N., Ohkura, H., and Yanagida, M. Distinct, essential roles of type 1 and 2A protein phosphatases in the control of the fission yeast cell division cycle. Cell, *63*: 405–415, 1990.
7. Fischer, E. H., Charbonneau, H., and Tonks, N. K. Protein tyrosine phosphatase: a diverse family of intracellular and transmembrane enzymes. Science, *253*: 401–406, 1991.
8. Ottilie, S., Chernoff, J., Hannig, G., Hoffman, C. S., and Erikson, R. L. A fission-yeast gene encoding a protein with features of protein-tyrosine-phosphatase. Proc. Natl. Acad. Sci. U.S.A., *88*: 3455–3459, 1991.
9. LaForgia, S., Morse, B., Levy, J., Barnea, G., Cannizzaro, L. A., Li, F., Nowell, P. C., Boghosian-Sell, L., Glick, J., Weston, A., Harris, C. C., Drabkin, H., Patterson, D., Croce, C. M., Schlessinger, J., and Huebner, K. Receptor protein-tyrosine phosphatase γ is a candidate tumor suppressor gene at human chromosome region 3p21. Proc. Natl. Acad. Sci. U.S.A., *88*: 5036–5040, 1991.
10. Doonan, J. H. and Morris, N. R. The *bimG* gene of *Aspergillus nidulans*, required for completion of anaphase, encodes a homolog of mammalian phosphoprotein phosphatase 1. Cell, *57*: 987–996, 1989.
11. Axton, J. M., Dombradi, V., Cohen, P. T. W., and Glover, D. M. One of the protein phosphatase 1 isozymes in *Drosophila* is essential for mitosis. Cell, *63*: 33–46, 1990.
12. Suganuma, M., Fujiki, H., Suguri, H., Yoshizawa, S., Hirota, M., Nakayasu, M., Ojika, M., Wakamatsu, K., Yamada, K., and Sugimura, T. Okadaic acid; an additional non-phorbol-12-tetradecanoate-13-acetate-type tumor promoter. Proc. Natl. Acad. Sci. U.S.A., *85*: 1768–1771, 1988.
13. Ohkura, H., Adachi, Y., Kinoshita, N., Niwa, O., Toda, T., and Yanagida, M. Cold-sensitive and caffeine-supersensitive mutants of the *Schizosaccharomyces pombe dis* genes

implicated in sister chromatid separation during mitosis. EMBO J., *7*: 1465–1473, 1988.

14. Dunphy, W. G. and Kumagai, A. The cdc25 protein contains an intrinsic phosphatase activity. Cell, *67*: 189–196, 1991.
15. Gautier, J., Solomon, M. J., Booher, R. N., Bazan, J. F., and Kirschner, M. W. cdc25 is a specific tyrosine phosphatase that directly activates $p34^{cdc2}$. Cell, *67*: 197–211, 1991.
16. Kinoshita, N., Yamano, H., Le Bouffant-Sladechek, F., Kurooka, H., Ohkura, H., Stone, E. M., Takeuchi, M., Toda, T., Yoshida, T., and Yanagida, M. Sister-chromatid separation and protein dephosphorylation in mitosis. Cold Spring Harbor Symp. Quant. Biol., *57*: 621–628, 1991.
17. Arndt, K. T., Styles, C. A., and Fink, G. R. A suppressor of a *HIS4* transcriptional defect encodes a protein with homology to the catalytic subunit of protein phosphatases. Cell, *56*: 527–537, 1989.
18. Da Cruz e Silva, E. F., Hughes, V., McDonald, P., Stark, M. J. R., and Cohen, P. T. W. Protein phosphatase 2Bw and protein phosphatase Z are *Saccharomyces* enzymes. Biochim. Biophys. Acta, *1989*: 269–272, 1991.
19. Liu, Y., Ishii, S., Tokai, M., Tsutumi, H., Ohki, O., Akada, R., Tanaka, K., Tsuchiya, E., Fukui, S., and Miyakawa, T. The *Saccharomyces cerevisiae* genes (CMP1 and CMP2) encoding calmodulin-binding proteins homologous to the catalytic subunit of mammalian protein phosphatase 2B. Mol. Gen. Genet., *227*: 55–59, 1991.
20. Booher, R. and Beach, D. Involvement of a type 1 protein phosphatase encoded by $bws1^+$ in fission yeast mitotic control. Cell, *57*: 1009–1016, 1989.
21. Ohkura, H. and Yanagida, M. Fission yeast $sds22^+$ gene is essential for a mid-mitotic transition and encodes a leucine-rich repeat protein which positively modulates type 1 protein phosphatase. Cell, *64*: 149–157, 1991.

MULTISTAGE CARCINOGENESIS, C. C. HARRIS ET AL. (EDS.),
JAPAN SCI. SOC. PRESS, TOKYO/CRC PRESS, BOCA RATON, PP. 145–152, 1992

Spi1 GTPase Interacts with RCC1 to Maintain Interdependency of Cell Cycle Events

Tomohiro MATSUMOTO and David BEACH

Howard Hughes Medical Institute, Cold Spring Harbor Laboratory, Cold Spring Harbor, NY 11724, U.S.A.

Abstract: A mutant which can enter mitosis at any cell cycle stage has been isolated and characterized in fission yeast. The *pim1* (premature initiation of mitosis) mutant prearrested at G1/S can develop a mitotic spindle and has tightly condensed chromosomes upon shift to the restrictive temperature. *pim1*-induced mitosis requires maturation promoting factor (MPF) activity, but not the essential mitotic inducer, cdc25. The *pim1*$^+$ gene encodes a homolog of regulator of chromosome condensation 1 (RCC1), a regulator of onset of mitosis in mammalian cells.

A multicopy suppressor of *pim1*, *spi1*, was isolated, and found to encode a 25 kDa GTPase. The primary sequence of the spi1 GTPase shows extensive identity (80%) to human TC4, whose function is unknown. The *spi1*/TC4 GTPase defines a novel class in the "*ras*-like" GTPase family, which is distinct from *ras*, *rho*, or *ypt*. Disruption of the *spi1*$^+$ gene causes genomic instability in a heterozygous diploid. These genetic data suggest that *pim1*$^+$ and *spi1*$^+$ interact to coordinate correct entry into mitosis.

Immunological experiments demonstrate that the *pim1*$^+$ and *spi1*$^+$ products are physically associated. Mutation in the *pim1* gene results in lowered affinity of the protein for the *spi1* protein *in vitro*, which may explain why high dosages of the *spi1* protein can rescue the *pim1* mutant *in vivo*. The *pim1*/*spi1* complex dissociates in the presence of Mg^{2+} and GTP. The current data suggests that *pim1*$^+$ acts as a GTP exchanger for the spi1 GTPase.

Understanding how the eukaryote cell cycle is regulated is an essential step toward understanding of the mechanisms which are uncontrolled in cancer growth. We have used the fission yeast, *Schizosaccharomyces pombe*, to study the genes which normally function to couple the processes of DNA replication of mitosis. From a genetic screen designed to target genes on such a pathway, we isolated a temperature sensitive mutant, *pim1*, which initiates mitosis at any cell cycle stage at the restrictive temperature, and isolated two genes by functional complementation. One gene, encoding a homolog of RCC1 (*1*) was shown to be *pim1*$^+$. The other encodes a 25 kDa GTPase (*spi1*$^+$: suppressor of *pim1*). Primary sequence analysis of the *spi1*$^+$ gene showed extensive homology to human TC4 (*2*). The identification of a GTPase having a role in the coupling of cell cycle events is of great interest, given current data from other systems which point to the potential role of GTPases in signal transduction.

The gene encoding the *ras* GTPase was identified as a potential cancer inducing gene (oncogene) in human cells. An extensive effort to search for its homologs or proteins of a similar nature in a variety of organisms has revealed that *ras*-like GTPases define a large superfamily of small molecular weight GTPases. Classified by their primary structure and function, this superfamily has been shown to consist of at least three classes, *ras*, *rho*, and *ypt* (*3*). These GTPases play a role in molecular switchings on signal transduction in the cellular process such as growth control, traffic control during secretion, and vision excitation (*4*). Study of the crystal structure of $p21^{ras}$ and bacterial elongation factor-Tu (EF-Tu) reveals that remarkable common domains (G-1, 2, 3, 4, and 5, Fig. 1a) in both proteins are interacting with guanine nucleotides (*3*). These G-regions are well conserved among all members of the *ras*-like GTPase family, suggesting GTPases are molecular switches built by a common structural design.

Analysis of the amino acid sequences of *spi1*$^{+}$ and TC4 indicated that these GTPases defined a fourth class in the *ras*-like GTPase superfamily. These genetic studies suggested that a novel class of GTPase interacts with RCC1 to maintain interdependency of cell cycle events (*5*).

Immunological experiments have indicated that the *pim1*$^{+}$ and *spi1*$^{+}$ products form a complex, and that this complex dissociates in the presence of Mg^{2+} and GTP. This result suggests that *pim1*$^{+}$ may act as a GTP exchanger for the *spi1* GTPase.

```
                                G-1                         G-2
                1                                                 50
spi1+           MAQPQNVPTFKLVLVGDGGTGKTTFVKRHLTGEFEKKYIATLGVEVHPLH
                 ||      ||||||||||||||||||||||||||||| ||||||||||
TC4            MAAQGEPQVQFKLVLVGDGGTGKTTFVKRHLTGEFEKKYVATLGVEVHPLV
                               | || ||               |  |
RAS-HS                         GAGGVGK               YDPTIEDSY

                           G-3
                51                                                100
spi1+           FHTNFGEICFNVWDTAGQEKLGGLRDGYYIQGQCGIIMFDVTSRITYKNV
                |||| | | ||||||||||| |||||||||| || ||||||||| |||||
TC4             FHTNRGPIKFNVWDTAGQEKFGGLRDGYYIQAQCAIIMFDVTSRVTYKNV
                             ||||||
RAS-Hs                       DTAGQE

                                     G-4                        G-5
                101                                               150
spi1+           PHWWRDLVRVCENIPIVLCGNKVDVKERKVKAKAITFHRKKNLQYYDISA
                | | |||||||||||||||||||| |   ||||| | ||||||||||||||
TC4             PNWHRDLVRVCENIPIVLCGNKVDIKDSKVKAKSIVFHRKKNLQYYDISA
                                    || |                      ||
RAS-Hs                              NKCD                    ETSA

                151                                               200
spi1+           KSNYNFEKPFLWLARKLVGNPNLEFVASPALAPPEVQVDQQLLAQYQQEM
                ||||||||||||||||| | ||||||| ||||||||  |  | |||
TC4             KSNYNFEKPFLWLARKLIGDPNLEFVAMPALAPPEVVMDPALAAQYEHDL
                |
RAS-Hs          K

                201            216
spi1+           NEAAAMPLPDEDDADL
                  |    |||||| ||
TC4             EVAQNPALPDEDD-DL
```

(A)

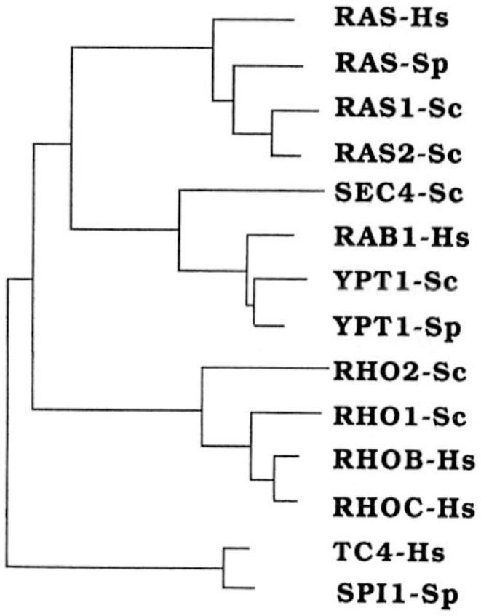

(B)

FIG. 1. A new class in the *ras*-like GTPase superfamily. a: Amino acids in common between the two are shown by a dash. The five conserved regions involved in guanine nucleotide metabolism are underlined and numbered as in ref. *3*. The equivalent G regions of *ras* are indicated. The amino acid sequence of TC4 is taken from ref. *2*, except that at amino acid number 179 of TC4 we found that by altering the frame of the published nucleotide sequence by one base pair, the homology between the two predicted polypeptides was maintained throughout the length of both proteins. Thus, TC4 appears to have a slightly higher molecular weight than first supposed. b: fourteen sequences of *ras* and *ras*-related proteins were analyzed according to ref. *7* by a program called the NJ method (*8*). The length of each horizontal bar represents divergency of each protein. The vertical distance between any two proteins has no significance. References to the sequences are as follows: RAS-Hs: (*9*), RAS-Sp: (*10*), RAS1-Sc and RAS2-Sc: (*11*), SEC4-Sc: (*12*), RAB1-Hs: (*13*), YPT1-Sc: (*14*), YPT1-Sp: (*15*), RHO2-Sc and RHO1-Sc: (*16*), RHOB-Hs and RHOC-HS: (*17*), TC4-Hs: (*2*).

Premature Initiation of Mitosis in the pim1 Mutant

The *pim1* mutant can go into mitosis when cells are shifted to the restrictive temperature even when cells are prearrested at G1/S. The cells show tightly condensed chromosomes and central septa. At a certain time after shift up, the mutants form mitotic spindles. This phenotype suggests that the completion of DNA replication is not necessary for the initiation of mitosis in the *pim1* mutant at the restricitive temperature. We asked whether the mutant could initiate mitosis from "start" of the cell cycle. When the *cdc10 pim1* double mutant is shifted to the restrictive temperature, tightly condensed chromosomes are visible, indicating that *pim1*-induced premature initiation of mitosis occurs in the absence of the normal start signal.

pim1⁺ Encodes a Fission Yeast Homolog of RCC1

Two genes rescuing the temperature sensitivity of the *pim1* mutant were isolated by complementation. Genetic analysis demonstrated that one is the *pim1*$^+$ gene itself. Nucleotide sequence analysis revealed that the gene encodes a homolog of RCC1 (*1*). The loss of function of the RCC1 gene in mammalian cell lines causes premature initiation of mitosis at the G1/S boundary (*6*), suggesting that *pim1*$^+$ and RCC1 are similar to each other not only structurally, but also functionally.

Genetic Interaction between spi1⁺ and pim1⁺

The other gene able to rescue the *pim1* mutation, *spi1*$^+$, was found to encode a 25 kDa GTPase. Sequence analysis showed it to be a homolog of the TC4 gene (Fig. 1a). To test the possibility that *spi1*$^+$ can bypass the function of *pim1*$^+$, the multicopy plasmid carrying the *spi1*$^+$ gene was introduced into a null mutant of *pim1* in which no *pim1*$^+$ gene product is thought to be expressed. High dosages of *spi1*$^+$ gene could not rescue the null mutant of *pim1*, whereas the *pim1*$^+$ gene could. Therefore, the *spi1*$^+$ gene can rescue the *pim1* mutant only in the presence of the *pim1* gene product. The *spi1*$^+$ gene was disrupted by the *ura4* gene and a heterozygous diploid was constructed. Following sporulation the diploid yielded two viable and two lethal progenys, indicating that the *spi1*$^+$ gene is essential. Interestingly, the diploid showed an abnormal nuclear structure as revealed by DAPI staining. Some cells showed tightly condensed chromosomes beside interphase nuclei, or several small satellite nuclei. This phenotype seems somewhat similar to that of the *pim1* mutant.

spi1/TC4 GTPase Defines a Novel Class in the ras-like GTPase Superfamily

Phylogenetic analysis based on the primary structure of the proteins can be used to reveal evolutionary relationships between proteins, and to define some particular families. Such an analysis of the *ras*-like GTPase family, from which over 50 genes have been isolated from a wide range of species, showed that the *spi1*/TC4 genes do not fit any known classes, but are a novel class (Fig. 1b). In contrast to the other classes in the family, the *spi1*/TC4 genes lack the characteristic carboxy-terminal domain (CAAX) which is essential for association to the cytosolic membrane.

Physical Interaction between pim1⁺ and spi1⁺

Immunological experiments using anti-pim1 and anti-spi1 antibodies showed that both proteins are abundant in fission yeast. *pim1*$^+$ was estimated at 0.15% of the total protein and *spi1*$^+$ at 0.65%. Indirect immunofluorescent staining revealed that *pim1*$^+$ localized in the nucleus, and *spi1*$^+$ predominantly on the nuclear envelope. Assuming that all *pim1*$^+$ protein is present in the nucleus, we calculated that 4 or 5 molecules of *pim1*$^+$ protein exist per 1 kb DNA (data not shown).

To test the possibility that the gene products interact physically, immunoprecipitations were done using the anti-pim1 antibody. In the immunoprecipitate, *pim1*$^+$ and *spi1*$^+$ were found to form a complex. This *pim1*$^+$/*spi1*$^+$ complex was resistant to high salt washes (420 mM NaCl), but we found that the presence of Mg^{2+} and GTP dissociated this complex. As shown in Fig. 2, after incubation of the complex in the presence of Mg^{2+} and GTP, 95% of the *spi1*$^+$ protein was found dissociated from *pim1*$^+$ protein. We did not detect any GTPase activity in the complex (data not shown).

The nature of the *pim1* mutant protein was tested. The immunoprecipitation was done using extracts from wild-type and *pim1-46* strains. The amount of the *pim1* product brought down by the antibody was similar in both extracts at 0 time (top

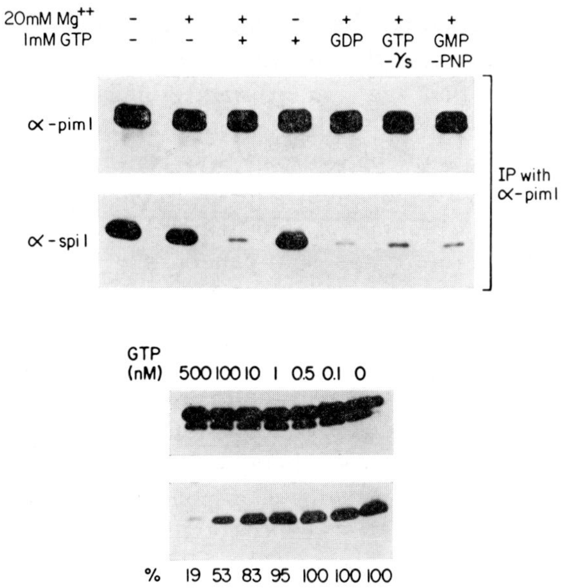

FIG. 2. The effect of Mg^{2+} and GTP on the *pim1*+/*spi1*+ complex. Top panel: immunoprecipitations were carried out in the wild type cell extract using anti-pim1 antibody. The immunocomplex was incubated for 40 min at room temperature in the presence or absence of Mg^{2+}, GTP, or a GTP analog. The samples were run on SDS-PAGE, and transferred to nylon membrane. The upper and lower portions of the membrane were Western blotted using either anti-*pim1* antibody or anti-*spi1* antibody, respectively. Bottom panel: GTP was added to the immunocomplex to the final concentration shown for each lane. Each sample was Western blotted as in the top panel. The amount of *spi1*+ protein remaining in the complex is shown as a % at the bottom of each lane.

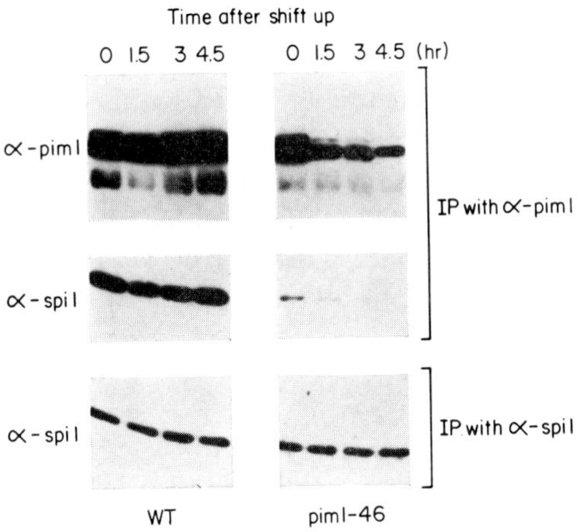

FIG. 3. *pim1* mutant protein. Immunoprecipitations were done using wild-type (left panels) or *pim1-46* extracts (right panels). Samples were taken at 90-min intervals following temperature shift up. Top and middle panels: immunoprecipitations with anti-pim1 antibody were Western blotted using anti-pim1 antibody (top panels) or anti-spi1 antibody (middle panels). Bottom panels: immunoprecipitations were Western blotted using anti-spi1 antibody. WT: wild type.

panels in Fig. 3). However, the amount of the *spi1*$^+$ product bound to the *pim1* product was much less in the *pim1-46* strain than that in wild-type even at time 0 (middle panels in Fig. 3). This indicates that the mutant *pim1* protein has less binding affinity to the *spi1*$^+$ product under these conditions (note that the total amount of *spi1*$^+$ is not altered in the *pim1-46* strain: bottom panels in Fig. 3). It is very likely that the high dosage of *spi1*$^+$ product could compensate for the lower affinity of *pim1* mutant protein *in vivo*. In addition, the mutant *pim1* protein was found to be degraded following a shift to restrictive temperature (top right panel in Fig. 3).

Function of pim1$^+$*/RCC1*

We took advantage of yeast genetics to study the interdependency of cell cycle events, and showed that the fission yeast RCC1 homolog interacts with a novel class of *ras*-like GTPases (*5*). The identification of a GTPase interacting with RCC1 leads to the idea that a GTPase signal cascade is acting as a molecular switch to turn on mitotic events upon the completion of DNA replication. Study of other GTPase signal cascades has suggested that the regulation of the GTPase activity involves at least two factors, a guanine nucleotide release protein (GNRP) and a GTPase activating protein (GAP) (*3*). The effect of GTP on the *pim1*$^+$/*spi1*$^+$ complex suggests the most probable role of *pim1*$^+$ is as a GNRP for this system. Loss of function of *pim1*$^+$ locks the spi1 GTPase cycle in an inactive state, resulting in the premature initiation of mitosis.

Similar genetic approaches have been utilized in organisms such as *Saccharomyces cerevisiae* and *Aspergillus nidulans*. RAD9 from *S. cerevisiae* and *bim*E7 from *A. nidulans* have been characterized as genes involved in cell cycle dependency (*18*, *19*); however the primary structure of these genes do not show any common identity with either RCC1 (*pim1*$^+$) or *spi1*$^+$. It may be possible that they function as a GAP or other interacting protein for the *spi1* GTPase. The nucleotide sequence of *bim*E7 suggests that the gene product has a nuclear targeting signal and transmembrane region (*21*).

Homologs of RCC1 from various organisms have been identified and shown to be abundant in nucleus (*20*, *22*, *23*) as in fission yeast. We have estimated that the *pim1*$^+$ product exists in nucleus at a ratio of 4 or 5 molecules to 1 kb DNA (roughly one molecule per nucleosome unit). This ratio may hint at how the *pim1*$^+$ gene product is regulating the *spi1* GTPase cycle; possibly, the *pim1*$^+$ product senses the state of chromatin (or DNA) with respect to its replication state, and activates the spi1 GTPase cycle to inhibit mitosis until completion of DNA replication.

REFERENCES

1. Ohtsubo, M., Kai, R., Furuno, N., Sekiguchi, T., Sekiguchi, M., Hayashida, H., Kuma, K., Miyata, T., Fukushige, S., Murotsu, T., Matsubara, K., and Nishimoto, T. Isolation and characterization of the active cDNA of the human cell cycle gene (RCC1) involved in the regulation of onset of chromosome condensation. Genes Dev., *1*: 585–593, 1987.
2. Drivas, G. T., Shih, A., Coutavas, E., Rush, M. G., and D'Eustachio, P. Charac-

terization of four novel *ras*-like genes expressed in a human teratocarcinoma cell line. Mol. Cell. Biol., *10*: 1793–1798, 1990.

3. Bourne, H. R., Sanders, D. A., and McCormick, F. The GTPase superfamily: conserved structure and molecular mechanism. Nature, *349*: 117–127, 1991.
4. Stryer, L. G. Proteins: a family of signal transduction. Annu. Rev. Cell Biol., *2*: 391–419, 1986.
5. Matsumoto, T. and Beach, D. Premature initiation of mitosis in yeast lacking RCC1 homolog or an interacting GTPase. Cell, *66*: 347–360, 1991.
6. Nishimoto, T., Eilen, E , and Basilico, C. Premature chromosome condensation in a tsDNA-mutant of BHK cells. Cell, *15*: 475–483, 1978.
7. Xiong, Y. and Eickbush, T. H. Origin and evolution of retroelements based upon their reverse transcriptase sequences. EMBO J., *9*: 3353–3362, 1990.
8. Saitou, N. and Nei, M. The neighbor-joining method: a new method for reconstructing phylogenetic trees. Mol. Biol. Evol., *4*: 406–425, 1987.
9. Capon, D. J., Chen, E. Y., Levinson, A. D., Seeburg, P. H., and Goeddel D. V. Complete nucleotide sequences of the T24 human bladder carcinoma oncogene and its normal homologue. Nature, *302*: 33–37, 1983.
10. Fukui, Y. and Kaziro, Y. Molecular cloning and sequence analysis of a *ras* gene from *Schizosaccharomyces pombe*. EMBO J., *4*: 687–691, 1985.
11. Powers, S., Katooka, T., Fasano, O., Goldfarb, M., Strathern, J., Broach, J., and Wigler, M. Gene in *S. cerevsiae* encoding proteins with domains homologous to mammalian *ras* proteins. Cell, *36*: 607–612, 1984.
12. Salminen, A. and Novick, P. J. A *ras*-like protein is required for a post-Golgi event in yeast secretion. Cell, *49*: 527–538, 1987.
13. Zahraoui, A., Touchot, N., Chardin, P., and Tavitian, A. The human *Rab* genes encode a family of GTP-binding proteins related to yeast YPT1 and SEC4 products involved in secretion. J. Biol. Chem., *264*: 12394–12401, 1989.
14. Gallwitz, D., Donath, C., and Sander, C. A yeast gene encoding a protein homologous to the human c-*has*/*bas* proto-oncogene product. Nature, *306*: 704–707, 1983.
15. Miyake, S. and Yamamoto, M. Identification of *ras*-related, YPT family genes in *Schizosaccharomyces pombe*. EMBO J., *9*: 1417–1422, 1990.
16. Madaule, P , Axel, R., and Myers, A. M. Characterization of two members of the *rho* gene family from the yeast *Saccharomyces cerevisiae*. Proc. Natl. Acad. Sci. U.S.A., *84*: 779–783, 1987.
17. Chardin, P., Madaule, P., and Tavitian, A. Coding sequence of human *rho* cDNAs clone 6 and clone 9. Nucl. Acids Res., *16*: 2717, 1988.
18. Weinert, T. A. and Hartwell, L. H. The RAD9 gene controls the cell cycle response to DNA damage in *Saccharomyces cerevisiae*. Science, *241*: 317–322, 1988.
19. Osmani, S. A., Engle, D. B., Doonan, J. H., and Morris, N. R. Spindle formation and chromatin condensation in cells blocked at interphase by mutation of a negative cell cycle control gene. Cell, *52*: 241–251, 1988.
20. Bischoff, F. R., Maier, G., Tilz, G., and Ponstingl, H. A 47-kDa human nuclear protein recognized by antikinetochore autoimmune sera is homologous with the protein encoded by RCC1, a gene implicated in onset of chromosome condensation. Proc. Natl. Acad. Sci. U.S.A., *87*: 8617–8621, 1990.
21. Engle, D. B., Osmani, S. A., Osmani, A. H., Rosborough, S., Xiang, X., and Morris, N. R. A negative regulator of mitosis in *Aspergillus* is a putative membrane-spanning protein. J. Biol. Chem., *265*: 16132–16137, 1990.
22. Frasch, M. The maternally expressed *Drosophila* gene encoding the chromatin-binding protein BJ1 is a homolog of the vertebrate gene regulator of chromatin condensation,

RCC1. EMBO J., *5*: 1225–1236, 1991.

23. Clark, K. L., Ohtsubo, M., Nishimoto, T., Goebl, M., and Sprague, G. F., Jr. The yeast SRM1 protein and human RCC1 protein share analogous functions. Cell Regul., *2*: 781–792, 1991.

MULTISTAGE CARCINOGENESIS, C. C. HARRIS ET AL. (EDS.),
JAPAN SCI. SOC. PRESS, TOKYO/CRC PRESS, BOCA RATON, PP. 153–170, 1992

The *trk* Family of Oncogenes and Neurotrophin Receptors

Fabienne LAMBALLE, Rüdiger KLEIN, and Mariano BARBACID

Department of Molecular Biology, Bristol-Myers Squibb Pharmaceutical Research Institute, Princeton, New Jersey 08543-4000, U.S.A.

Abstract: To date more than twenty five different oncogenes have been identified in human neoplasias. One of these oncogenes is *trk*, a transforming gene originally isolated from a colon carcinoma biopsy by using gene transfer assays. This oncogene encodes a chimeric molecule that contains the 221 amino terminal residues of a non-muscle tropomyosin followed by the transmembrane and cytoplasmic domains of the *trk* proto-oncogene product, a tyrosine protein kinase receptor. *trk* oncogenes have also been identified in a significant fraction of thyroid papillary carcinomas. Some of these *trk* oncogenes contain sequences derived from genes other than tropomyosin. One such gene is *tpr*, a gene first identified as a component of the human *met* oncogene. The *trk* proto-oncogene, non-muscle tropomyosin and *tpr* map in the long arm of chromosome 1. Therefore, *trk* oncogenes are likely to result from internal rearrangements or from unequal cross-overs between two chromosome 1s. Recent studies have demonstrated that the product of the *trk* proto-oncogene, gp140^{trk}, is the functional receptor for nerve growth factor (NGF). NGF elicits the rapid phosphorylation of gp140^{trk} on tyrosine residues. Moreover, addition of NGF to NIH3T3 cells expressing gp140^{trk} induces the transient expression of c-Fos, DNA synthesis and morphologic transformation. Finally, transfection of the *trk* proto-oncogene into NGF non-responsive PC12 mutant cells restores NGF responsiveness. Two additional genes designated *trk*B and *trk*C have recently been isolated in our laboratory. These genes are highly related to the *trk* proto-oncogene and encode tyrosine protein kinases which serve as functional receptors for the NGF-related neurotrophins brain-derived neurotrophic factor (BDNF) and neurotrophic-3 (NT-3), respectively. Whether mutations in these novel members of the *trk* family of receptor genes are also implicated in human cancer remains to be determined.

Since their discovery a decade ago, human oncogenes (both growth promoting and growth suppressing oncogenes) have been identified in more than one-third of all human malignancies. In most cases, these oncogenes have been extensively characterized at the molecular level and their mechanism of activation has been elucidated. The development of polymerase chain reaction (PCR) and related technologies have made it possible to utilize these oncogenes as probes for a variety of clinical applications including cancer diagnosis, prognosis and quantitation of

TABLE 1. Proto-oncogenes of Known Function

Oncogene	Proto-oncogene		Function
	Gene	Protein	
v-*sis*	c-*sis*	c-Sis	PDGF
v-*erb*B	c-*erb*B	c-ErbB	EGF receptor
v-*fms*	c-*fms*	c-Fms	CSF-1 (M-CSF) receptor
v-*kit*	c-*kit*	c-Kit	Steel factor receptor
met	proto-*met*	Met	Hepatocyte growth factor receptor
trk	proto-*trk*	Trk	NGF receptor
v-*mos*	c-*mos*	c-Mos	Oocyte cytostatic factor
v-*fos*	c-*fos*	c-Fos	Component of AP-1 transcription factor
v-*jun*	c-*jun*	c-Jun	Component of AP-1 transcription factor
v-*rel*	c-*rel*	c-Rel	Component of NF-κB transcription factor
v-*erb*A	c-*erb*A	TRα-1	Thyroid hormone receptor

residual disease in patients in remission. However, the ultimate goal of molecular oncology is to utilize oncogenes as targets for cancer therapy. In a not too distant future, we should be able to generate inhibitors of oncogene function that will not interfere with the physiological function of their normal alleles, the cellular proto-oncogenes. However, the development of such specific inhibitors will require a more profound knowledge of the mechanisms by which oncogenes contribute to neoplasia and even more importantly, a precise understanding of the role that proto-oncogenes play in normal cells.

During the last few years, the physiological role of various proto-oncogene products has been elucidated (Table 1). First, the v-*sis* oncogene was found to be allelic to the B chain of platelet-derived growth factor (PDGF) (*1, 2*). Subsequently, the v-*erb*B and v-*fms* retroviral oncogenes were found to be derived from cellular proto-oncogenes encoding the epidermal growth factor (EGF) and colony-stimulating factor (CSF)-1 receptors, respectively (*3, 4*). More recently the c-Kit proto-oncogene product has been identified as the receptor for steel factor (SF) (*5, 6*) and the Met protein as the receptor for the hepatocyte growth factor (HGF) (also known as the scatter factor) (*7, 8*). Other examples of recent assignments of defined biological functions to the products of proto-oncogenes include the identification of the c-Mos protein as the cytostatic factor responsible for preventing oocytes to enter the mitotic cycle (*9*), and the identification of the c-Fos, c-Jun, and c-Rel proteins as members of the AP-1 (c-Fos and c-Jun) (*10*) and NF-κB (c-Rel) (*11*, 12) transcription factors (Table 1).

These findings have had a highly significant impact on our efforts to establish the molecular basis of neoplastic transformation. Unfortunately, these observations may not have an immediate impact on human cancer since most of the above proto-oncogenes have not been directly implicated in the development of human tumors.

Our laboratory has concentrated its research efforts on the molecular characterization of the *trk* oncogene, a transforming gene originally identified in a colon carcinoma biopsy by means of gene transfer assays (*13*). Subsequent studies have indicated that the involvement of the *trk* oncogene in colon cancer is sporadic. However, *trk* oncogenes have been identified in about 25–30% of human papillary carcinomas (*14*). In this report, we summarize our current knowledge on the structure and mechanisms of activation of human *trk* oncogenes as well as recent findings that have led to the demonstration that its normal allele, the *trk* proto-oncogene (*15*), is the functional receptor for nerve growth factor (NGF) (*16–22*). In addition, we describe the isolation of two *trk*-related genes (*trk*B and *trk*C) recently identified in our laboratory (*23–26*) whose products also serve as receptors for other NGF-related neurotrophins such as brain-derived neurotrophic factor (BDNF) and neurotrophin-3 (NT-3) (*21, 26–30*).

The trk Oncogene

Molecular characterization of the *trk* oncogene present in a colon carcinoma biopsy revealed a hybrid molecule consisting of seven of the eight exons of a non-muscle tropomyosin gene followed by sequences coding for the putative transmembrane and cytoplasmic domains of a novel member of the supergene family of tyrosine kinase receptors, now known as the *trk* proto-oncogene (*13, 15*) (Fig. 1). Comparison of the deduced amino acid sequences of the *trk* oncogene and proto-oncogene products indicated that the transforming protein lacks the signal peptide and most of the putative extracellular ligand-binding domain (360 out of a total of 375 residues) of the normal *trk* gene product (*13, 15*). No differences were observed within the *trk*-derived sequences. These observations indicate that the fusion of tropomyosin sequences is sufficient to confer transforming properties to the *trk* tyrosine kinase (*13, 15*) (Fig. 1).

The *trk* proto-oncogene and the non-muscle tropomyosin gene involved in its malignant activation map in the long arm of chromosome 1 (*31, 32*). Therefore, this

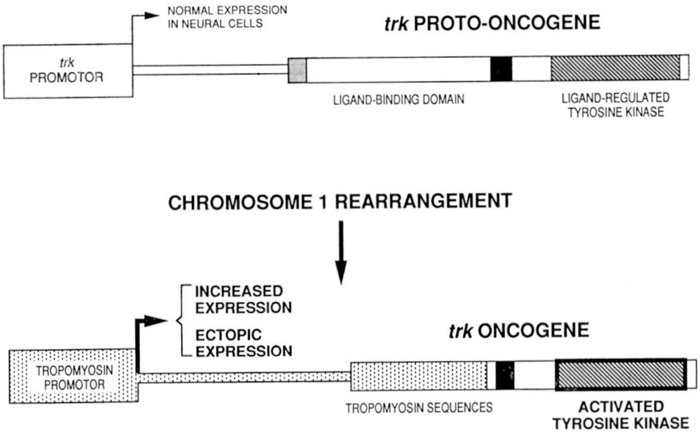

FIG. 1. Schematic representation of the mechanism of activation of a human *trk* oncogene isolated from a colon carcinoma biopsy (*13*). Thick boxes represent putative promoter sequences. Medium size boxes represent coding sequences. They include: signal peptide (shaded box), ligand binding domain (indicated open box), transmembrane region (black box), tyrosine kinase catalytic domain (stapled box) and tropomyosin sequences (dotted box). Thin boxes represent non-coding sequences derived from the *trk* locus (open box) or the non-muscle tropomyosin gene (dotted box). Structural as well as non-structural alterations likely to contribute to the transforming properties of the *trk* oncogene are highlighted.

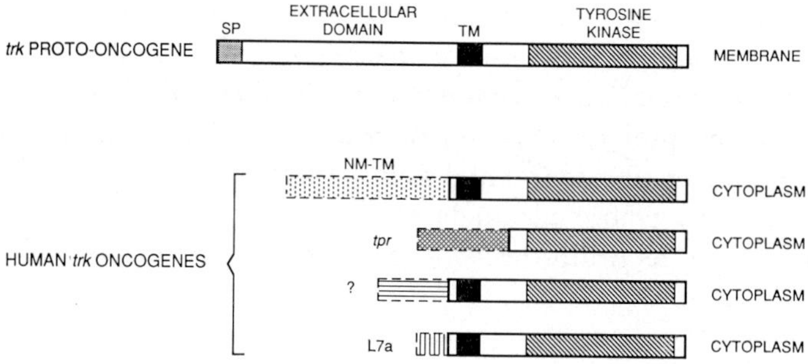

FIG. 2. Comparison of the structure of the products of various human *trk* oncogenes with that of the normal *trk* proto-oncogene product. The indicated domains correspond to: signal peptide (SP, shaded box), extracellular domain (indicated open box), transmembrane region (TM, black box), tyrosine kinase catalytic domain (stapled box), non-muscle tropomyosin (NM-TM, dotted box), *tpr* gene (hatched box), ribosomal protein L7a (vertical bars) and unknown (horizontal bars) sequences. The right column indicates the respective subcellular location of these proteins.

trk oncogene was presumably generated by a chromosome 1 rearrangement involving either an unequal cross-over or an internal deletion/inversion. Figure 1 summarizes the various structural as well as non-structural alterations that this chromosomal rearrangement caused in the *trk* locus. Some, if not all, of these changes are likely to contribute to the oncogenic properties of the *trk* oncogene. First of all, expression of the *trk* oncogene in the tumor cells is likely to be regulated by the tropomyosin promoter. This alteration results in the ectopic and increased expression of the *trk* kinase. In addition, replacement of the extracellular domain of the *trk* proto-oncogene by tropomyosin sequences also results in major structural changes. These structural alterations deregulate the kinase activity of the *trk* gene by a mechanism likely to involve dimerization of the *trk* catalytic domain (see below).

It is also interesting to notice that the product of the *trk* oncogene is no longer associated with membranes since the amino-terminal tropomyosin moiety does not have a signal peptide (Fig. 2). However, removal of the amino-terminal moiety of the *trk* proto-oncogene product including the signal peptide and the extracellular domain is not sufficient to activate its transforming potential (*33*). Similarly, replacement of these sequences by those derived from β-actin or β-globin genes does not result in the generation of *trk* oncogenes (*33*). Moreover, addition of a signal peptide to the colon carcinoma *trk* oncogene had no deleterious effect on its transforming activity in spite of the fact that more than 98% of its gene product is associated with cellular membranes (*33*). These results support the concept that the subcellular localization of *trk* oncogene product may not be a major factor in determining its transforming properties.

The molecular structure of some of the *trk* oncogenes identified in thyroid tumors has been recently unveiled (*34*). These *trk* oncogenes exhibit an overall structure similar to the original colon carcinoma isolate, coding for hybrid molecules with a similar subset of *trk* proto-oncogene-derived sequences. However, these oncogenes differ in the nature of the foreign sequences that replace the putative ligand-binding domain of the *trk* gene (Fig. 2). In one case, the activating sequences were contributed by the same non-muscle tropomyosin locus that participated in the generation of the colon carcinoma oncogene. Two additional *trk* oncogene isolates contain sequences derived from the *tpr* locus (*34*). This gene was first identified as part of the *met* oncogene, the transforming allele of the HGF receptor (*35*). Sequences present in the fourth thyroid *trk* oncogene isolate remain to be identified. Finally, a *trk* oncogene in which the extracellular sequences were replaced by a fragment of the L7a ribosomal protein has been recently isolated from a human breast carcinoma cell line, apparently activated during gene transfer (*36*) (Fig. 2).

Comparison of the various amino-terminal sequences of these *trk* oncogenes has failed to reveal any common structural motif(s) that might be considered directly responsible for their transforming properties. *In vitro* analysis of various *trk* oncoproteins did not reveal increased levels of tyrosine phosphorylating activity. However, these *trk* proteins exhibit higher levels of tyrosine phosphorylation *in vivo* than their normal counterpart, the *trk* proto-oncogene product (unpublished observations). Physiological activation of tyrosine protein kinase receptors by their cognate ligands is mediated by an oligomerization step which results in transphosphorylation of specific tyrosine residues (*37*). Thus, the *trk* oncoproteins may owe their transforming properties to the formation of stable dimeric structures that result in their constitutive activation. Dimerization may take place in the products of the tropomyosin-containing *trk* oncogenes, since tropomyosins are known to exist as dimeric α-helical coiled-coil structures (*38*). In support of this hypothesis, replacement of the non-muscle tropomyosin sequences present in certain *trk* oncogenes by those encoding the smooth and skeletal muscle tropomyosin isoforms results in novel *trk* chimeric genes with efficient transforming activity (*33*, *39*). Unfortunately, examination of the *tpr*- and L7a-derived sequences present in other *trk* oncogenes did not reveal any structural motifs that may predict the formation of dimers. Therefore, it is possible that constitutive activation of *trk* oncoproteins might be accomplished by alternative mechanisms that do not involve dimerization.

The trk Proto-oncogene

The human *trk* proto-oncogene codes for a protein of 790 amino acid residues that displays the basic characteristic features of tyrosine protein kinase cell surface receptors (*15*) (Fig. 3). They include a 32 amino acid-long signal peptide, a putative ligand-binding domain rich in consensus N-glycosylation sites, a single transmembrane domain, a catalytic règion highly related to that of known tyrosine protein kinases, and a short carboxy-terminal tail of fifteen amino acid residues. Analysis of the deduced amino acid sequence of the *trk* proto-oncogene product indicates that this gene does not belong to any of the well characterized subfamilies of tyrosine kinase cell surface receptors. Its extracellular domain shows no homology with those of other growth factor receptors. Indeed, the *trk* proto-oncogene product, as well as those encoded by the other members of the *trk* family of receptors (see below), have an unique array of structural motifs in their extracellular domains that include a leucine-rich (LR) region with significant homology to that of the LRM gene family followed by two immunoglobulin-like domains (Fig. 3), that may be responsible for their interaction with their respective ligands (unpublished observations).

Biochemical analysis of NIH3T3 cells expressing *trk* proto-oncogene cDNA

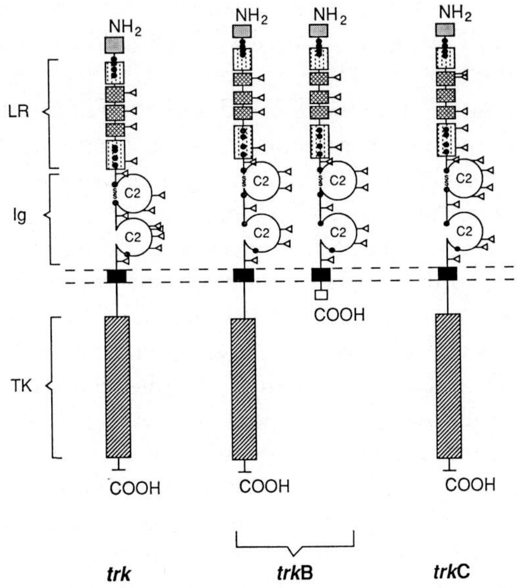

FIG. 3. Schematic representation of the structural domains of the known members of the *trk* family of tyrosine protein kinases. From top (amino-terminus) to bottom (carboxy-terminus): Signal peptide (shaded boxes); amino-terminal (dotted boxes), central (cross-hatched boxes) and carboxy-terminal (dotted boxes) domains of an LR region homologous to the extracellular domain of the LRM glycoprotein family; Ig-like domains (C2); transmembrane region (black boxes); and tyrosine kinase catalytic domain (TK) (hatched boxes). The open box represents the carboxy-terminal domain of the non-catalytic isoform encoded by the *trk*B locus. Symbols within the extra-cellular domains indicate cysteine residues (solid circles) and consensus N-glycosylation sites (triangles).

clones indicated that the primary translational product of this gene is a 110 kDa glycoprotein with a polypeptidic backbone of 80 kDa (*15*). This 110 kDa glycoprotein becomes further glycosylated, presumably during its transport to the plasma membrane, to yield a 140 kDa glycoprotein (*15*). Both gp110^{trk} and gp140^{trk} proteins exhibit *in vitro* kinase activity specific tyrosine residues. ^{125}I-surface labelling of NIH3T3 cells expressing a complete cDNA clone of the *trk* proto-oncogene indicated that only the heavily glycosylated 140 kDa isoform is located on the cell surface (*15*). These observations indicate that gp140^{trk} is the mature human *trk* proto-oncogene product.

*trk*B

The *trk* proto-oncogene is a prototype of a small subfamily of tyrosine protein kinase genes (Fig. 3). Screening of mammalian cDNA libraries with *trk*-derived probes has revealed at least two related loci designated *trk*B (*23–25*) and *trk*C (*26*). *trk*B appears to be a large and complex locus (≥100 kbp) with an intricate transcription pattern (*23–25*). At least six different transcripts ranging in size from 2.0 kb to 9.0 kb have been identified in mouse tissues. These transcripts code for at least two different classes of cell surface receptors (*24*).

One of the products of the *trk*B gene is gp145^{trkB}, a heavily glycosylated molecule with tyrosine protein kinase activity (*23–25*) (Fig. 3). gp145^{trkB} is synthesized from two transcripts (9.0 kb and 5.5 kb) likely to differ in their polyadenylation signals. The deduced amino acid sequence of this glycoprotein indicates a polypeptidic backbone of 821 amino acid residues which exhibits all the characteristic features of tyrosine kinase cell surface receptors. Comparison of the amino acid sequence of the *trk*B gp145^{trkB} and *trk* gp140^{trk} proteins indicates a high degree of homology in both their extracellular domains (57% homology, 38% identity) and kinase catalytic regions (88% homology, 73% identity). In addition, both molecules exhibit a short carboxy-terminal tail (15 amino acid residues) characteristic of this gene family.

The mouse *trk*B locus also codes for a second class of molecules that lack a kinase catalytic domain (*24, 25*) (Fig. 3). One of these proteins is gp95^{trkB}, a glycoprotein identical to gp145^{trkB} from amino acid residues 1 to 465 which encompass the signal peptide, extracellular domain and transmembrane region. However, gp95^{trkB} has a very short cytoplasmic domain of 23 residues of which the last eleven bare no resemblance with any of the sequences present in gp145^{trkB} (*24, 25*). Northern blot analysis of *trk*B transcripts using probes derived from cDNA clones coding for gp95^{trkB} indicate that the synthesis of this putative non-catalytic receptor is directed by transcripts of 8.2 kb and 2.5 kb. Both of these mRNA species may be derived from the same transcriptional unit. The presence of a consensus polyadenylation site 400 bp downstream from the end of the coding sequences is likely to be responsible for the generation of the 2.5 kb mRNA species.

*trk*C

Recent studies in our laboratory have revealed the existence of *trk*C, a third member of the mammalian *trk* gene family of receptors (*26*) (Fig. 3). Nucleotide sequence analysis of *trk*C cDNA clones of porcine origin revealed a 825 amino acid-long putative tyrosine kinase with all the structural features characteristic of cell surface receptors. The extracellular domain of the *trk*C gene product is 53% homologous (35% identical) to that of the *trk* proto-oncogene and 52% homologous (39% identical) to the corresponding domain of the catalytic *trk*B protein including ten of the twelve cysteine residues present in this *trk*C domain are conserved in the *trk* and *trk*B gene products (*26*). Moreover, the extracellular domain of the *trk*C protein also possesses the LR and Ig motifs present in the *trk* and *trk*B gene products (Fig. 3). Even higher homologies were observed when we compared the respective catalytic domains of these three genes (86% homology with the human *trk* gene and 90% homology with the mouse *trk*B). Thus, it appears that the *trk*C gene is equally related to *trk* and *trk*B (*26*). The *trk*C protein also exhibits the short carboxy-terminal tail (15 residues) characteristic of the other members of the *trk* gene family.

Expression of the trk Gene Family in Neural Tissues

Expression studies involving Northern blot analysis, *in situ* hybridization and immunocytochemical techniques indicate that the members of the *trk* gene family are preferentially, if not exclusively expressed in the nervous system (*23, 24, 40, 41*)

TABLE 2. Pattern of Expression of the *trk* Gene Family in Neural Tissues

Structure	*trk* Gene expression		
	trk	*trk*B[a]	*trk*C
Central nervous system			
Cerebral cortex	—	+++[b]	+++
Corpus callosum	—	—[b]	ND
Thalamus	—	+++[b]	ND
Hippocampus	—	+++[b]	+++
Fimbria hippocampus	—	—	ND
Choroid plexus	—	+++[c]	—
Ependymal layer of ventricles	—	+++[c]	—
Cerebellum: Purkinje cells	—	+++	—
Cerebellum: granular cell layer	—	—	+++
Brainstem	—	+	ND
Spinal cord	—	+++	ND
Peripheral nervous system			
Cranial Ganglia: V	+++	+	ND
VII	—	+++	ND
VIII	—	+++	ND
IX/X superior	+++	+++	ND
IX/X inferior	—	+++	ND
Dorsal root ganglia	+++	+	ND
Autonomic nervous system	—	+++	ND
Cranio-facial structures			
Eye: retina, ophthalmic nerve	—	+++	ND
Vestibular system: inner ear	—	+	ND
Nasal chamber	—	+	ND
Snout	—	+	ND
Submaxillary gland	—	+	ND
Palate, tongue, tooth Buds	—	+	ND

a) Unless otherwise indicated, *trk*B expression was determined with a probe that recognizes all *trk*B transcripts.
b) Transcripts encoding gp145^{trkB}. c) Transcripts encoding gp95^{trkB}. ND, not done.

(Table 2). *In situ* hybridization analysis of mouse embryos revealed that the *trk* proto-oncogene is expressed in dorsal root ganglia, as well as in visceral sensory ganglia such as the fifth (trigeminal), superior ninth (superior) and tenth (jugular) cranial ganglia (*40*). This pattern of expression is highly specific, since other neighboring cranial ganglia such as the eighth (acoustic), inferior ninth (petrosal) and tenth (nodose) ganglia do not exhibit detectable *trk* gene transcripts (*40*). *trk* proto-oncogene transcripts are also absent in other related structures of the brain such as the trigeminal nerve that arrives into the *trk*-expressing trigeminal ganglion from the base of the myelencephalon.

Analysis of late (17.5-day old) embryos and adult mouse brain indicates that *trk* gene expression continues to be limited to visceral sensory ganglia of neural crest origin (dorsal root, trigeminal and superior ninth and tenth ganglia). No *trk* expression could be detected in other sensory ganglia of non-neural crest origin (acoustic ganglion) or in other cranial ganglia that are not strictly sensory (*40*). Detailed analysis of adult sensory ganglia indicates that *trk* gene expression occurs in neurons but not in the surrounding glia. However, only about half of the neurons present within a particular ganglion appear to contain *trk* gene transcripts. Since sensory ganglia contain functionally distinct neurons, it might be possible to assign *trk* gene expression to a particular subtype of neurons.

Expression of the *trk*B locus during mouse embryonic development can be first detected in 9.5-day old embryos (*23, 41*). At this time, *trk*B is expressed in a wide variety of rudimental structures of the developing central nervous system (CNS) and peripheral nervous system (PNS) including the forebrain, caudal midbrain, hindbrain, spinal cord, the trigeminal ganglion and differentiating neural crest cells, which will form the dorsal root ganglia. In 13.5-day old embryos, the pattern of *trk*B expression appears to reflect the entire network of the developing CNS and PNS. *trk*B expression is maintained throughout this network during late fetal development, once the scaffolding for the entire nervous system is fully constructed (*23, 41*). Unlike the *trk* proto-oncogene whose expression is confined to sensory neurons of neural crest origin, *trk*B transcripts are found in cells derived from both the neuroepithelium and the neural crest (Table 2).

In the adult mouse, most *trk*B expression is found in the brain and the spinal cord (*23, 24, 41*). However, low levels of *trk*B transcripts could also be observed in lung and muscle (8.2 kb, 2.5 kb, and 2.0 kb transcripts) as well as in ovaries (8.2 kb and 2.5 kb transcripts). Traces of two distinct mRNA species (2.8 kb and 2.5 kb) were found in testis. Whether these mRNAs correspond to *trk*B transcripts that use different polyadenylation signals (a phenomenon quite common in testis) or correspond to transcripts of a related locus, remains to be determined. *In situ* hybridization analysis of mouse brain tissue revealed that *trk*B transcripts can be identified in most structures of the cerebrum including the cortical layers, thalamus, hippocampus and choroid plexus (*23, 24, 41*) (Table 2). Either low levels or absence of *trk*B transcripts occur in the corpus callosum, the parafasicular and reticular thalamic nuclei and in the fimbria hippocampus. In the cerebellum, *trk*B expression appears to be more restricted, with high levels in the Purkinje cell layer and the caudal peduncle, but low levels or no expression in other cells such as those of the granular layer (Table 2).

Not all *trk*B transcripts are equally distributed throughout mouse neural tissues. Indeed, *in situ* hybridization studies using probes specific for transcripts encoding the catalytic ($gp145^{trkB}$) and non-catalytic ($gp95^{trkB}$) *trk*B gene products revealed a highly specialized pattern of expression (*24*). Transcripts coding for $gp145^{trkB}$ are present in the cerebral cortex and the pyramidal cell layer of the hippocampus, but not in the choroid plexus or the ependymal lining of the cerebral ventricles. In contrast, transcripts encoding the non-catalytic receptor-like $gp95^{trkB}$ protein were found in the choroid plexus and the ependymal lining of the ventricles but not in the cerebral cortex or the hippocampus (Table 2). In summary, transcripts encoding structurally distinct *trk*B proteins are expressed in functionally distinct structures of the adult mouse brain (*24*).

This pattern of expression has provided some insights regarding the possible function of the non-catalytic *trk*B gene product(s) (*24*). The ependyma is a ciliated epithelial cell layer that participates in the circulation of the cerebrospinal fluid from the ventricles into the interstitial space between neurons and neuroglia. The choroid plexus is known to serve as an active barrier between the blood supply and the cerebrospinal fluid. Therefore, it is possible that gp95^{trkB} may have a role in the active transport of its ligands within the brain as well as across the blood-brain barrier. gp95^{trkB} may also serve as a clearance receptor. Interestingly, the receptor implicated in clearance of the atrial natriuretic peptide lacks the cytoplasmic guanyl cyclase domain present in a related atrial natriuretic peptide receptor involved in signal transduction (*42*). Further studies involving probes specific for other *trk*B transcripts and additional CNS and PNS structures are needed to unveil the functional complexity of the mammalian *trk*B locus.

Northern blot analysis of a series of adult mouse tissues indicates that *trk*C is preferentially expressed in the brain (*26*). No detectable expression could be observed in RNAs isolated from lung, heart, intestine, kidney, spleen, liver, testes, and muscle. Low levels of *trk*C expression may occur in the ovaries. *In situ* hybridization studies revealed *trk*C transcripts in various brain structures, most notably in the hippocampus, cerebral cortex and the cerebellum (Table 2). In the hippocampus, expression was highest in the pyramidal cell layer and in the dentate gyrus (*26*). In the cerebral cortex, we identified high levels of *trk*C expression in clusters of cells located in the external layers. Finally, specific *trk*C hybridization in the cerebellum was localized in the granular layer, but not in the white matter or in the Purkinje cell layer or the molecular layer (*26*). These preliminary studies suggest that *trk*C may have an expression pattern somewhat complementary to that of the related *trk*B gene (Table 2).

The trk Proto-oncogene Encodes the Functional Receptor for NGF

The specific pattern of expression of the members of the *trk* gene family is consistent with a potential role as receptors for neurotrophic factors. To date, five neurotrophic factors have been characterized at the molecular level. They include the four members of the NGF gene family, NGF (*43*), BDNF (*44, 45*), NT-3 (*46–50*), and NT-4 (*51*), as well as the ciliary neurotrophic factor (CNTF) (*52, 53*). Each of these factors have been implicated in the development and survival of specific subsets of neurons. NGF recognizes two types of receptors which display different

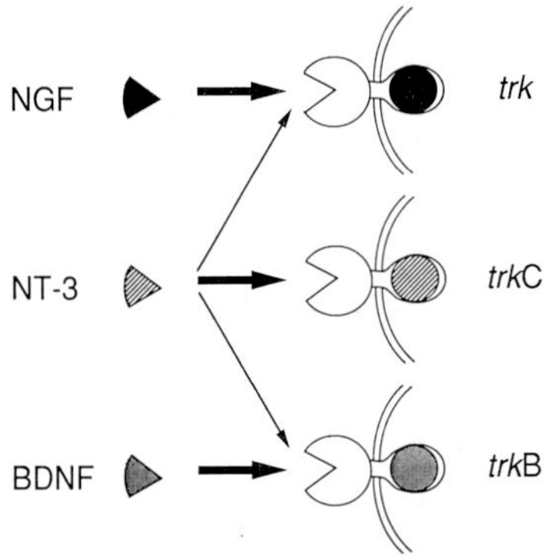

FIG. 4. Schematic representation of the known interactions between the NGF family of neurotrophins and the *trk* family of tyrosine protein kinase receptors.

affinities and biological properties. The high affinity receptors ($K_d \simeq 10^{-10}$ to 10^{-11} M) appear to be responsible for the major biological responses to NGF (*54*). The low affinity receptors ($K_d \simeq 10^{-8}$ to 10^{-9} M) are cysteine-rich glycoproteins encoded by the well characterized LNGFR gene (*55, 56*). The high affinity receptors have been identified as molecular species of 130,000 to 150,000 daltons (*54*), structurally distinct from the low affinity receptors (*57, 58*).

Recent evidence indicates that NGF may utilize signal transduction pathways involving the phosphorylation of tyrosine residues (*59*). More recently, Meakin and Shooter reported that the high affinity receptors could be immunoprecipitated by anti-phosphotyrosine antibodies (*57*). These observations suggested to us that the high affinity NGF receptor might be a member of the tyrosine protein kinase family. We have recently obtained experimental evidence that conclusively demonstrate that the *trk* receptor, gp140^{trk} is the functional, high affinity receptor for NGF (*16, 21*) (Fig. 4). This claim is supported by various independent lines of evidence, including: (i) NGF efficiently binds to non-neural NIH3T3 mouse fibroblasts and Sf9 insect cells only when they express the *trk* proto-oncogene product; (ii) NGF can be chemically cross-linked to the product of the *trk* proto-oncogene independently of whether it is ectopically expressed in NIH3T3 cells or is present in PC12 cells; (iii) cells expressing the *trk* proto-oncogene depict high affinity NGF receptors regardless of their species of origin or their developmental lineage; (iv) the product of the *trk* proto-oncogene becomes rapidly phosphorylated on tyrosine residues upon incubation of PC12 cells with NGF; and (v) the tyrosine kinase activity of the *trk* proto-oncogene product can be stimulated by NGF (*16, 21*).

Similar results have been independently obtained by other investigators (*17–20, 22*). Kaplan *et al.* first demonstrated the induction of tyrosine phosphorylation in gp140^{trk} upon NGF treatment of PC12 cells (*17*). Subsequently, Hempstead, Kaplan and co-workers demonstrated direct binding of NGF to gp140^{trk} receptors (*18, 20*). However, these authors have proposed that the high affinity NGF receptor is a heterodimeric molecule composed of gp140^{trk} and gp75^{LNGFR}, the product of the previously described LNGFR gene (*18*). This model is in conflict with our results showing high affinity binding of NGF to gp140^{trk} expressed in NIH3T3 cells which do not contain gp75^{LNGFR} (*16, 21*) and with the demonstration by Glass *et al.* that BDNF supports the survival of *trk*B expressing cells (see below) in the absence of the low affinity gp75^{LNGFR} NGF receptor (*30*). Moreover, our results (*21*), along with those of Nebreda *et al.*, using *Xenopus* oocytes (*20*) have indicated that the interaction of NGF with gp140^{trk} receptors triggers a pleiotropic cascade of signal transduction events even in the absence of gp75^{LNGFR}.

Addition of NGF to quiescent NIH3T3 cells expressing gp140^{trk} receptors (E25-48 cell line) resulted in the induction of DNA synthesis in essentially each of the cells that expressed gp140^{trk} receptors (*21*). As indicated above, such a response does not require the presence of additional factors nor the expression of the low affinity NGF receptor. The most dramatic illustration of the mitogenic properties of NGF resides in its ability to induce E25-48 cells to grow in semi-solid agar and to induce the morphologic transformation of NIH3T3 cells transfected with the *trk* proto-oncogene (Table 3). These observations indicate that NGF has a mitogenic activity comparable to that of growth factors with oncogenic potential such as v-*sis*/PDGF,

TABLE 3. NGF Confers Transforming Activity to the Product of the *trk* Proto-oncogene

trk allele	Plasmid		Transforming activity (foci/10^5 NIH3T3 cells)	
			−NGF	+NGF
trk proto-oncogene	pDM69	1 μg	0	>300
		100 ng	0	>300
		10 ng	0	292
		1 ng	0	23
trk oncogene	pDM16	100 ng	>300	>300
		1 ng	120	113

TABLE 4. Transformation of NIH3T3 Cells by Co-expression of the *trk* Proto-oncogene with NGF and NT-3, but Not with BDNF

Transfected DNA[a]	Number of foci
None	0
trk 1 μg	0
NGF 1 μg	0
BDNF 1 μg	0
NT-3 1 μg	0
trk 1 μg+NGF 1 μg	<500
trk 1 μg+NGF 0.1 μg	350
trk 1 μg+BDNF 1 μg	0
trk 1 μg+BDNF 0.1 μg	0
trk 1 μg+NT-3 1 μg	190
trk 1 μg+NT-3 0.1 μg	39

[a] Transfected DNAs included pMEX-derived expression plasmids pDM69 (*trk* proto-oncogene) (*15*), pLTRS-NGF (NGF) (*19*), pLL42 (BDNF) (*28*), and pLL43 (NT-3) (*28*).

EGF/transforming growth factor α (TGFα) and some of the members of the FGF family. Removal of NGF from morphologically transformed cultures of NIH3T3 cells expressing the normal *trk* proto-oncogene causes the rapid reversion of their transformed phenotype. These results indicate that cellular transformation is a direct response to the mitogenic stimulus of NGF on gp140^{trk} receptors (*21*).

gp140^{trk} Is Also a Receptor for NT-3

The product of the *trk* proto-oncogene may also serve as a receptor for neurotrophic factors other than NGF (*19*) (Fig. 4). Competition experiments indicated that NT-3, but not BDNF, partially displaced [^{125}I]-NGF from binding to gp140^{trk} (*21*). Since saturating amounts of NT-3 only displaced about 60% of the bound NGF, it is likely that this factor competes for overlapping but not identical binding sites. The interaction of NT-3 with gp140^{trk} receptors elicits a limited functional response. Co-transfection of NIH3T3 cells with plasmids encoding the *trk* proto-oncogene product and each of the three neurotrophins NGF, BDNF, and NT-3 led to the efficient transformation of cells co-expressing gp140^{trk} and NGF and to a lesser extent of those co-expressing gp140^{trk} and NT-3 (Table 4). Moreover, addition to gp140^{trk} expressing NIH3T3 cells of partially purified NT-3 protein produced in a baculovirus expression system induced tyrosine phosphorylation of gp140^{trk} and stimulated thymidine incorporation (*21*).

The trkB Tyrosine Protein Kinase gp145^{trkB} Is a Receptor for BDNF and NT-3

Co-transfection of NIH3T3 cells with expression plasmids encoding gp145^{trkB} and BDNF also elicits the morphologic transformation of the recipient cells with an efficiency of at least 10^4 ffu per μg of DNA (Table 5). These findings raised the possibility that the *trk*B kinase gp145^{trkB} might be the functional receptor of BDNF (*29*). Additional experimental evidence supporting this concept includes (i) induction of DNA synthesis by BDNF in quiescent NIH3T3 cells expressing gp145^{trkB} receptors but not in their parental NIH3T3 cells; (ii) the rapid phosphorylation in tyrosine residues of gp145^{trkB} molecules in cells exposed to BDNF; (iii) the constitutive tyrosine phosphorylation of gp145^{trkB} in cells constitutively expressing BDNF and (iv) the efficient displacement of [^{125}I]-labeled NT-3 from binding to cells expressing gp145^{trkB} receptors. These results, taken together, firmly establish gp145^{trkB} as a functional receptor for BDNF (*27–30*) (Fig. 4).

gp145^{trkB} also serves as a functional receptor for NT-3 since this tyrosine protein kinase efficiently binds [^{125}I]-labeled NT-3 (*27–30*) (Fig. 4). Moreover, addition of NT-3 to cells expressing gp145^{trkB} induces its rapid phosphorylation on tyrosine residues and allows quiescent cells to enter the S phase. However, the mitogenic activity of NT-3 on these cells appears to be more limited than that of BDNF (*29*, *30*). Co-transfection of expression plasmids encoding gp145^{trkB} and NT-3 led to the morphologic transformation of NIH3T3 cells with an efficiency 100 to 200-fold lower than that observed when the *trk*B gene was co-expressed with BDNF (Table 5). Whether the interaction of NT-3 with gp145^{trkB} has physiological relevance remains to be determined.

trkC Is the Primary Receptor for NT-3

*trk*C is the third known member of the *trk* family of tyrosine protein kinase

TABLE 5. The *trk*B Receptor Is Activated by BDNF and to a Lesser Extent by NT-3, but Not by NGF

Transfected DNA[a]	Number of foci
None	0
*trk*B 1 μg	0
NGF 1 μg	0
BDNF 1 μg	0
NT-3 1 μg	0
*trk*B 1 μg+NGF 1 μg	0
*trk*B 1 μg+NGF 0.1 μg	0
*trk*B 1 μg+BDNF 1 μg	>500
*trk*B 1 μg+BDNF 0.1 μg	>500
*trk*B 1 μg+NT-3 1 μg	100
*trk*B 1 μg+NT-3 0.1 μg	22

[a] Transfected DNAs included pMEX-derived expression plasmids pFRK44 (*trk*B) (*23*), pLTRSNGF (NGF) (*19*), pLL42 (BDNF) (*28*), and pLL43 (NT-3) (*28*).

TABLE 6. The *trk*C Receptor Is Specifically Activated by NT-3

Transfected DNA[a]	Number of foci
None	0
*trk*C 1 μg	0
NGF 1 μg	0
BDNF 1 μg	0
NT-3 1 μg	0
*trk*C 1 μg+NGF 1 μg	0
*trk*C 1 μg+NGF 0.1 μg	0
*trk*C 1 μg+BDNF 1 μg	0
*trk*C 1 μg+BDNF 0.1 μg	0
*trk*C 1 μg+NT-3 1 μg	>500
*trk*C 1 μg+NT-3 0.1 μg	>500

[a] Transfected DNAs included pMEX-derived expression plasmids pFL20 (*trk*C) (*26*), pLTRSNGF (NGF) (*19*), pLL42 (BDNF) (*28*), and pLL43 (NT-3) (*28*).

genes (*26*). The product of the *trk*C gene, gp145^{trkC}, is also a neurotrophin receptor as demonstrated by its ability to bind with high affinity (K_d=26 pM) and to be cross-linked to [^{125}I]-labeled NT-3. As indicated above, this neurotrophin also interacts with gp140^{trk}, gp145^{trkB} and gp75^{LNGFR}. However, gp145^{trkC} appears to be specific for NT-3 since this receptor does not bind either NGF or BDNF (*26*) (Fig. 4). Whether gp145^{trkC} may bind other neurotrophins remains to be determined.

NT-3 can activate mitogenic signalling in NIH3T3 cells through gp145^{trkC} receptors (*26*). NT-3 elicits the rapid phosphorylation of gp145^{trkC} in tyrosine residues and induces resting NIH3T3 cells expressing gp145^{trkC} receptors to enter the S phase. Moreover, co-expression of gp145^{trkC} and NT-3 results in the morphologic transformation of NIH3T3 cells (Table 6). Quantitative studies indicate that co-expression of gp145^{trkC} and NT-3 is about two orders of magnitude more efficient in transforming NIH3T3 cells than when NT-3 is co-expressed with either gp140^{trk} or gp145^{trkB} (*21, 29*). Moreover, NT-3 exhibits more limited biological activity than BDNF on either NIH3T3 (*29*) or PC12 (*30*) cells expressing gp145^{trkB} receptors. Based on these observations, we would like to propose that gp145^{trkC} is a primary receptor for NT-3. However, confirmation of this hypothesis must await the outcome of similar studies in neuronal cells.

The present studies demonstrate that the *trk* family of tyrosine protein kinases are functional receptors for the NGF family of neurotrophins (Fig. 4). These findings provide an important framework of ligand/receptor relationships to study the molecular mechanisms that govern the differentiation, growth and survival of neurons. The recent isolation of additional neurotrophins (*51*) and neuronal tyrosine protein kinase receptors (*60*) indicate that tyrosine phosphorylation is likely to play a very significant role in controlling signalling pathways in neurons.

REFERENCES

1. Doolittle, R. F., Hunkapiller, M. W., Hood, L. E., Devare, S. G., Robbins, K. C., Aaronson, S. A., and Antoniades, H. N. Simian sarcoma virus oncogene, v-*sis*, is derived from the gene (or genes) encoding a platelet-derived growth factor. Science, *221*:

275–277, 1983.

2. Deuel, T. F., Huang, J. S., Huang, S. S., Stroobant, P., and Waterfield, M. D. Expression of a platelet-derived growth factor-like protein in simian sarcoma virus transformed cells. Science, *221*: 1348–1350, 1983.
3. Downward, J., Yarden, Y., Mayes, E., Scrace, G., Totty, N., Stockwell, P., Ullrich, A., Schlessinger, J., and Waterfield, M. D. Close similarity of epidermal growth factor receptor and v-*erb*-B oncogene protein sequences. Nature, *307*: 521-527, 1984.
4. Sherr, C. J., Rettenmier, C. W., Sacca, R., Roussel, M. F., Look, A. T., and Stanley, E. R. The c-*fms* proto-oncogene product is related to the receptor for the mononuclear phagocyte growth factor, CSF-1. Cell, *41*: 665–676, 1985.
5. Zsebo, K. M., Williams, D. A., Geissler, E. N., Broudy, V. C., Martin, F. H., Atkins, H. L., Hsu, R. Y., Birkett, N. C., Okino, K. H., Murdock, D. C., Jacobsen, F. W., Langley, K. E., Smith, K. A., Takeishi, T., Cattanach, B. M., Galli, S. J., and Suggs, S. V. Stem cell factor is encoded at the Sl locus of the mouse and is the ligand for the c-*kit* tyrosine kinase recepor. Cell, *63:* 213–224, 1990.
6. Huang, E., Nocka, K., Beier, D. R., Chu, T. Y., Buck, J., Lahm, H. W., Wellner, D., Leder, P., and Besmer, P. The hematopoietic growth factor KL is encoded by the Sl locus and is the ligand of the c-*kit* receptor, the gene product of the W locus. Cell, *63*: 225–233, 1990.
7. Bottaro, D. P., Rubin, J. S., Faletto, D. L., Chan, A. M., Kmiecik, T. E., Vande Woude, G. F., and Aaronson, S. A. Identification of the hepatocyte growth factor receptor as the c-*met* proto-oncogene product. Science, *251*: 802–804, 1991.
8. Naldini, L., Vigna, E., Narsimhan, R. P., Gaudino, G., Zarnegar, R., Michalopoulos, G. K., and Comoglio, P. M. Hepatocyte growth factor (HGF) stimulates the tyrosine kinase activity of the receptor encoded by the proto-oncogene c-MET. Oncogene, *6*: 501–504, 1991.
9. Sagata, N., Watanabe, N., Vande Woude, G. F., and Ikawa, Y. The c-*mos* proto-oncogene product is a cytostatic factor responsible for meiotic arrest in vertebrate eggs. Nature, *342*: 512–518, 1989.
10. Curran, T. and Franza, B. R., Jr. Fos and Jun: the AP-1 connection. Cell, *55*: 395–397, 1988.
11. Ghosh, S., Gifford, A. M., Riviere, L. R., Tempst, P., Nolan, G. P., and Baltimore, D. Cloning of the p50 DNA binding subunit of NF-kappa B: homology to rel and dorsal. Cell, *62*: 1019–1029, 1990.
12. Kieran, M., Blank, V., Logeat, F., Vandekerckhove, J., Lottspeich, F., Le Bail, O., Urban, M. B., Kourilsky, P., Baeuerle, P. A., and Israel, A. The DNA binding subunit of NF-kappa B is identical to factor KBF1 and homologous to the rel oncogene product. Cell, *62*: 1007–1018, 1990.
13. Martin-Zanca, D., Hughes, S. H., and Barbacid, M. A human oncogene formed by the fusion of truncated tropomyosin and protein tyrosine kinase sequences. Nature, *319*: 743–748, 1986.
14. Bongarzone, I., Pierotti, M. A., Monzini, N., Mondellini, P., Manenti, G., Donghi, R., Pilotti, S., Grieco, M., Santoro, M., Fusco, A., Vecchio, G., and Della Porta, G. High frequency of activation of tyrosine kinase oncogenes in human papillary thyroid carcinoma. Oncogene, *4*: 1457–1462, 1989.
15. Martin-Zanca, D., Oskam, R., Mitra, G., Copeland, T., and Barbacid, M. Molecular and biochemical characterization of the human *trk* proto-oncogene. Mol. Cell. Biol., *9*: 24–33, 1989.
16. Klein, R., Jing, S. Q., Nanduri, V., O'Rourke, E., and Barbacid, M. The *trk* proto-oncogene encodes a receptor for nerve growth factor. Cell, *65*: 189–197, 1991.

17. Kaplan, D. R., Martin-Zanca, D., and Parada, L. F. Tyrosine phosphorylation and tyrosine kinase activity of the *trk* proto-oncogene product induced by NGF. Nature, *350*: 158–160, 1991.
18. Hempstead, B. L., Martin-Zanca, D., Kaplan, D. R., Parada, L. F., and Chao, M. V. High-affinity NGF binding requires coexpression of the *trk* proto-oncogene and the low-affinity NGF receptor. Nature, *350*: 678–683, 1991.
19. Kaplan, D. R., Hempstead, B. L., Martin-Zanca, D., Chao, M. V., and Parada, L. F. The *trk* proto-oncogene product: a signal transducing receptor for nerve growth factor. Science, *252*: 554–558, 1991.
20. Nebreda, A. R., Martin-Zanca, D., Kaplan, D. R., Parada, L. F., and Santos, E. Induction by NGF of meiotic maturation of Xenopus oocytes expressing the *trk* proto-oncogene product. Science, *252*: 558–561, 1991.
21. Cordon-Cardo, C., Tapley, P., Jing, S. Q., Nanduri, V., O'Rourke, E., Lamballe, F., Kovary, K., Klein, R., Jones, K. R., Reichardt, L. F., and Barbacid, M. The *trk* tyrosine protein kinase mediates the mitogenic properties of nerve growth factor and neurotrophin-3. Cell, *66*: 173–183, 1991.
22. Loeb, D. M., Maragos, J., Martin-Zanca, D., Chao, M. V., Parada, L. F., and Greene, L. A. The *trk* proto-oncogene rescues NGF responsiveness in mutant NGF-nonresponsive PC12 cell lines. Cell, *66*: 961–966, 1991.
23. Klein, R., Parada, L. F., Coulier, F., and Barbacid, M. *trk*B, a novel tyrosine protein kinase receptor expressed during mouse neural development. EMBO J., *8*: 3701–3709, 1989.
24. Klein, R., Conway, D., Parada, L. F., and Barbacid, M. The *trk*B tyrosine protein kinase gene codes for a second neurogenic receptor that lacks the catalytic kinase domain. Cell, *61*: 647–656, 1990.
25. Middlemas, D. S., Lindberg, R. A., and Hunter, T. *trk*B, a neural receptor protein-tyrosine kinase: evidence for a full-length and two truncated receptors. Mol. Cell. Biol., *11*: 143–153, 1991.
26. Lamballe, F., Klein, R., and Barbacid, M. *trk*C, a new member of the *trk* family of tyrosine protein kinases, is a receptor for neurotrophin-3. Cell, *66*: 967–979, 1991.
27. Squinto, S. P., Stitt, T. N., Aldrich, T. H., Davis, S., Bianco, S. M., Radziejewski, C., Glass, D. J., Masiakowksi, P., Furth, M. E., Valenzuela, D. M., DiStefano, P. S., and Yancopoulos, G. D. *trk*B encodes a functional receptor for brain-derived neurotrophic factor and neurotrophin-3 but not nerve growth factor. Cell, *65*: 885–893, 1991.
28. Soppet, D., Escandon, E., Maragos, J., Middlemas, D. S., Reid, S. W., Blair, J., Burton, L. E., Stanton, B. R., Kaplan, D. R., Hunter, T., Nikolics, K., and Parada, L. F. The neurotrophic factors brain-derived neurotrophic factor and neurotrophin-3 are ligands for the *trk*B tyrosine kinase receptor. Cell, *65*: 895–903, 1991.
29. Klein, R., Nanduri, V., Jing, S. A., Lamballe, F., Tapley, P., Bryant, S., Cordon-Cardo, C., Jones, K. R., Reichardt, L. F., and Barbacid, M. The *trk*B tyrosine protein kinase is a receptor for brain-derived neurotrophic factor and neurotrophin-3. Cell, *66*: 395–403, 1991.
30. Glass, D. J., Nye, S. H., Hantzopoulos, P., Macchi, M. J., Squinto, S. P., Goldfarb, M., and Yancopoulos, G. D. TrkB mediates BDNF/NT-3-dependent survival and proliferation in fibroblasts lacking the low affinity NGF receptor. Cell, *66*: 405–413, 1991.
31. Miozzo, M., Pierotti, M. A., Sozzi, G., Radice, P., Bongarzone, I., Spurr, N. K., and Della Porta, G. Human TRK proto-oncogene maps to chromosome 1q32-q41. Oncogene, *5*: 1411–1414, 1990.

32. Morris, C. M., Hao, Q. L., Heisterkamp, N., Fitzgerald, P. H., and Groffen, J. Localization of the TRK proto-oncogene to human chromosome bands 1q23-1q24. Oncogene, *6*: 1093–1095, 1991.
33. Coulier, F., Martin-Zanca, D., Ernst, M., and Barbacid, M. Mechanism of activation of the human *trk* oncogene. Mol. Cell. Biol., *9*: 15–23, 1989.
34. Greco, A. and Pierotti, M. Isolation and characterization of an oncogene generated by a somatic rearrangement between *trp* and *trk* genes in human papillary thyroid carcinomas. Submitted for publication.
35. Park, M., Dean, M., Cooper, C. S., Schmidt, M., O'Brien, S. J., Blair, D. G., and Vande Woude, G. F. Mechanism of *met* oncogene activation. Cell, *45*: 895–904, 1986.
36. Ziemiecki, A., Muller, R. G., Fu, X. C., Hynes, N. E., and Kozma, S. Oncogenic activation of the human *trk* proto-oncogene by recombination with the ribosomal large subunit protein L7a. EMBO J., *9*: 191–196, 1990.
37. Ullrich, A. and Schlessinger, J. Signal transduction by receptors with tyrosine kinase activity. Cell, *61*: 203–212, 1990.
38. Zot, A. S. and Potter, J. D. Structural aspects of troponin-tropomyosin regulation of skeletal muscle contraction. Annu. Rev. Biophys. Chem. *16*: 535–559, 1987.
39. Barnes, D., Clayton, L., Chumbley, G., and MacLeod, A. R. Activation of the *trk* oncogene by alternatively spliced muscle and non-muscle tropomyosin sequences. Oncogene, *4*: 259–262, 1989.
40. Martin-Zanca, D., Barbacid, M., and Parada, L. F. Expression of the *trk* proto-oncogene is restricted to the sensory cranial and spinal ganglia of neural crest origin in mouse development. Genes Dev., *4*: 683–694, 1990.
41. Klein, R., Martin-Zanca, D., Barbacid, M., and Parada, L. F. Expression of the tyrosine kinase receptor gene *trk*B is confined to the murine embryonic and adult nervous system. Development, *109*: 845–850, 1990.
42. Fuller, F., Porter, J. G., Arfsten, A. E., Miller, J., Schilling, J. W., Scarborough, R. M., Lewicki, J. A., and Schenk, D. B. Atrial natriuretic peptide clearance receptor. Complete sequence and functional expression of cDNA clones. J. Biol. Chem., *263*: 9395–9401, 1988.
43. Levi-Montalcini, R. The nerve growth factor: thirty-five years later. EMBO J., *6*: 1145–1154, 1987.
44. Barde, Y. A., Edgar, D., and Thoenen, H. Purification of a new neurotrophic factor from mammalian brain. EMBO J., *1*: 549–553, 1982.
45. Leibrock, J., Lottspeich, F., Hohn, A., Hofer, M., Hengerer, B., Masiakowksi, P., Thoenen, H., and Barde, Y. A. Molecular cloning and expression of brain-derived neurotrophic factor. Nature, *341*: 149–152, 1989.
46. Maisonpierre, P. C., Belluscio, L., Squinto, S., Ip, N. Y., Furth, M. E., Lindsay, R. M., and Yancopoulos, G. D. Neurotrophin-3: a neurotrophic factor related to NGF and BDNF. Science, *247*: 1446–1451, 1990.
47. Hohn, A., Leibrock, J., Bailey, K., and Barde, Y. A. Identification and characterization of a novel member of the nerve growth factor/brain-derived neurotrophic factor family. Nature, *344*: 339–341, 1990.
48. Ernfors, P., Ibanez, C. F., Ebendal, T., Olson, L., and Persson, H. Molecular cloning and neurotrophic activities of a protein with structural similarities to nerve growth factor: developmental and topographical expression in the brain. Proc. Natl. Acad. Sci. U.S.A., *87*: 5454–5458, 1990.
49. Jones, K. R. and Reichardt, L. F. Molecular cloning of a human gene that is a member of the nerve growth factor family. Proc. Natl. Acad. Sci. U.S.A., *87*: 8060–8064, 1990.
50. Rosenthal, A., Goeddel, D. V., Nguyen, T., Lewis, M., Shih, A., Laramee, G. R.,

Nikolics, K., and Winslow, J. W. Primary structure and biological activity of a novel human neurotrophic factor. Neuron, *4*: 767–773, 1990.
51. Hallbook, F., Ibanez, C. F., and Persson, H. Evolutionary studies of the nerve growth factor family reveal a novel member abundantly expressed in Xenopus ovary. Neuron, *6*: 845–858, 1991.
52. Stockli, K. A., Lottspeich, F., Sendtner, M., Masiakowski, P., Carroll, P., Gotz, R., Lindholm, D., and Thoenen, H. Molecular cloning, expression and regional distribution of rat ciliary neurotrophic factor. Nature, *342*: 920–923, 1989.
53. Lin, L. F., Mismer, D., Lile, J. D., Armes, L. G., Butler, E. T., 3d, Vannice, J. L., and Collins, F. Purification, cloning, and expression of ciliary neurotrophic factor (CNTF). Science, *246*: 1023–1025, 1989.
54. Hosang, M. and Shooter, E. M. Molecular characteristics of nerve growth factor receptors on PC12 cells. J. Biol. Chem., *260*: 655–662, 1985.
55. Chao, M. V., Bothwell, M. A., Ross, A. H., Koprowski, H., Lanahan, A. A., Buck, C. R., and Sehgal, A. Gene transfer and molecular cloning of the human NGF receptor. Science, *232*: 518–521, 1986.
56. Radeke, M. J., Misko, T. P., Hsu, C., Herzenberg, L. A., and Shooter, E. M. Gene transfer and molecular cloning of the rat nerve growth factor receptor. Nature, *325*: 593–597, 1987.
57. Meakin, S. O. and Shooter, E. M. Molecular investigations on the high-affinity nerve growth factor receptor. Neuron, *6*: 153–163, 1991.
58. Weskamp, G., and Reichardt, L. F. Evidence that biological activity of NGF is mediated through a novel subclass of high affinity receptors. Neuron, *6*: 649–663, 1991.
59. Maher, P. A. Nerve growth factor induces protein-tyrosine phosphorylation. Proc. Natl. Acad. Sci. U. S.A., *85*: 6788–6791, 1988.
60. Lai, C. and Lemke, G. An extended family of protein-tyrosine kinase genes differentially expressed in the vertebrate nervous system. Neuron, *6*: 691–704, 1991.

MULTISTAGE CARCINOGENESIS, C. C. HARRIS ET AL. (EDS.),
JAPAN SCI. SOC. PRESS, TOKYO/CRC PRESS, BOCA RATON, PP. 171–181, 1992

Abnormalities of Growth Factor Systems in Transformed Airway Epithelial Cells

Paul NETTESHEIM, Patrice C. FERRIOLA, Alice T. ROBERTSON,
Tomohisa IWANAGA, Ronald STEIGERWALT, and Joyce E. RUNDHAUG

Laboratory of Pulmonary Pathobiology, National Institute of Environmental Health Sciences, Research Triangle Park, North Carolina 27709, U.S.A.

Abstract: The role of the peptide growth factors transforming growth factor α (TGFα) and transforming growth factor β (TGFβ) in the regulation of proliferation of normal and transformed airway epithelial cells was studied. Normal as well as transformed rat tracheal epithelial (RTE) cell cultures secrete similar amounts of TGFα during logarithmic growth. Once normal RTE cell cultures reach the plateau phase of growth, they down-regulate TGFα expression at the RNA and protein level; in contrast, transformed cells do not down-regulate TGFα. Using neutralizing TGFα antiserum and a tyrphostin TGFα/EGF receptor tyrosine kinase inhibitor, we show that the secreted TGFα is utilized by both normal and transformed cells as an autocrine mitogenic factor.

Normal RTE cells are highly sensitive to the growth inhibitory effects of TGFβ, particularly during early phases of logarithmic growth. At late logarithmic and plateau phases of proliferation, cultures of normal RTE cells secrete large amounts of TGFβ. That the endogenous TGFβ is exerting growth inhibitory effects can be demonstrated by adding TGFβ antisera to the cultures which causes a burst of proliferation. Many transformed RTE cell lines exhibit a markedly reduced sensitivity to the growth inhibitory effects of TGFβ. However, the cells remain responsive to regulation of ECM genes by TGFβ. The transformed cell lines examined secrete less than one tenth the amount of TGFβ of normal cells. Our studies show that the autocrine TGFβ growth restraining mechanism is inoperative in many of the RTE cell transformants.

We conclude, therefore, that alterations in TGFα and TGFβ regulation of cell proliferation are important factors contributing to the abnormal growth behavior of transformed RTE cells.

Over the last 20 years a great number of regulatory peptides have been isolated and shown to be important in the control of cell growth and differentiation. Many neoplasms exhibit abnormalities in the expression of these growth factors or their receptors (*1, 2*). The autocrine hypothesis of cancer postulates that disturbances of growth factor systems are responsible for the autonomous growth behavior of neoplasms. For the last several years we have tested the autocrine hypothesis and it's relevance in respiratory carcinogenesis, focusing our attention on two peptide growth

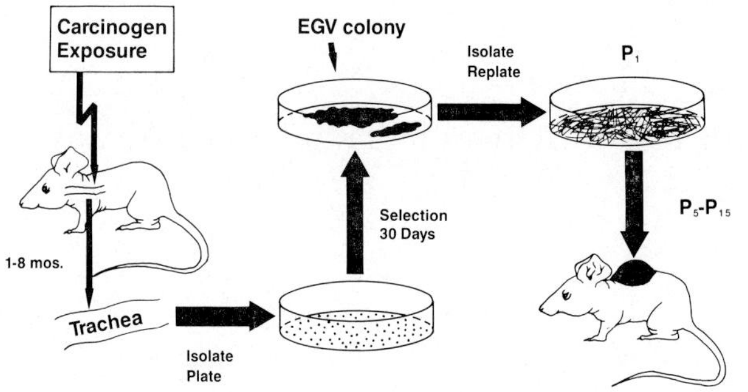

FIG. 1. *In vitro* assay for detection of preneoplastic stem cell variants formed *in vivo*, following exposure of tracheas to carcinogens. Rats are exposed to a tracheal carcinogen. At different times after carcinogen exposure tracheas are removed, the epithelium is dissociated and the cells are cultured. Four days after plating, selection for transformed stem cells is begun, which form large colonies within 3 to 5 weeks. The EGV-colonies are isolated, replated and subcultured repeatedly. Different passages (P5–P15) are inoculated into compatible hosts to test for neoplastic potential (from ref. *6*).

factors, namely transforming growth factor α (TGFα) and transforming growth factor β (TGFβ), one a mitogen, the other a growth inhibitor of epithelial tissues (*3, 4*). For these studies we have used the rat tracheal epithelial (RTE) transformation system (Fig. 1), which has proven to be a useful experimental model for the study of multistage carcinogenesis (*5, 6*). During the course of these studies we have obtained new insights regarding not only growth regulation of neoplastic airway epithelium but also regarding the role of autocrine factors in controlling proliferation of normal cells. In this presentation we will summarize evidence indicating that neoplastically transformed airway cells concomitantly exhibit several defects in TGFα and TGFβ pathways, which explains at least in part, their abnormal proliferative activity. We will also discuss findings which indicate that the growth of normal cells is controlled by the same regulatory systems, and that the major distinction between normal and neoplastic cells may not be whether or not they produce growth factors, but rather, whether the secretion of autocrine factors and the responses to them are appropriately regulated.

Characteristics of Growth Behavior of Normal and Transformed Rat Tracheal Epithelial Cells

Two major features of *in vitro* growth behavior distinguish normal tracheal cells from transformed cells. Normal cells have a limited growth capacity and are dependent on a number of different peptide growth factors. In contrast, transformed RTE cells, so-called immortal growth variants, have an unlimited growth capacity and most of them are independent of exogenous growth factors. The transition from normal to transformed growth behavior is perhaps best illustrated by the experiment shown in Fig. 2. The growth pattern of control and carcinogen exposed cells is virtually indistinguishable during the early phases of culture. However, soon after selection for transformed cell variants is begun, growth in the control cultures ceases, while the carcinogen exposed cultures continue to proliferate. During this time Enhanced Growth Variant Colonies (EGV-colonies) arise. Many of these EGV-

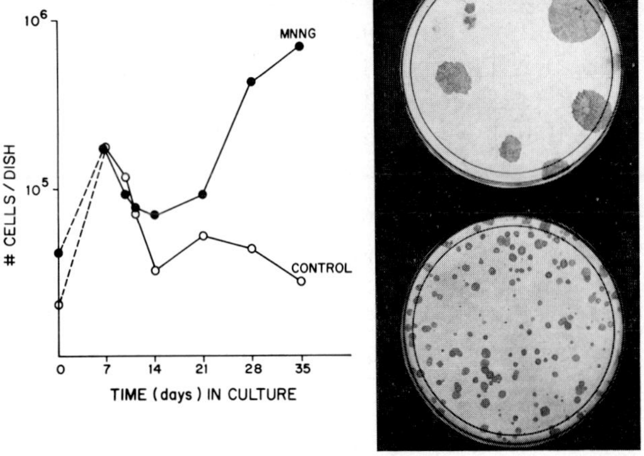

FIG. 2. Left: growth of normal and transformed primary rat tracheal epithelial cells. (○) Normal cells; (●) cells exposed to N-methyl-N′-nitro-N-nitrosoguanidine, MNNG. Cells are seeded on an x-irradiated fibroblast feeder layer in serum containing media and are exposed to MNNG; 4 days later the feeder cells are removed by mild trypsinization to select for transformed colonies (*5*). Right, Bottom: day-7 colonies of normal cells. Right, top: transformed colonies after 5 weeks of selection (from ref. *6*).

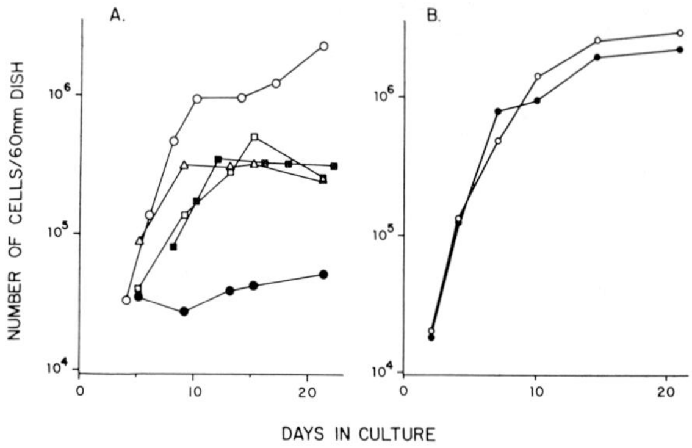

FIG. 3. Changes in growth factor dependence of normal and transformed RTE cells. A) Growth of primary RTE cells in the presence or absence of epidermal growth factor (E) and bovine pituitary extract (B). Cells were plated in complete serum-free medium (CSFM; ○) or in SFM-E/-B (●). Cells were plated in CSFM and media was changed to SFM-E/-B on day 1 (□), day 3 (△) or day 6 (■) after plating. B) Growth of a neoplastically transformed cell line in CSFM (○) or in SFM-E/-B (●) (Modified from ref. *9*).

colonies can be subcultured, become immortal cell lines and ultimately become neoplastic (*5–7*).

The second major distinction between normal and transformed RTE cells lies in the difference in growth factor dependence (*8*). In order to examine growth factor dependence and the role of autocrine growth factors, we have used serum-free media which contain among other peptide growth factors, epidermal growth factor (EGF) and bovine pituitary extract (BPE) (*9*, 10). Primary RTE cell cultures require these factors for maximum proliferation and cells plated without EGF/BPE undergo very little proliferation (Fig. 3a). The growth factors can be removed once proliferation has been initiated, and the cultures can undergo several rounds of cell replication, but plateau phase of growth is reached at a lower cell density than in cultures propagated in the continued presence of EGF and BPE. In contrast, many of the neoplastically transformed cell lines are independent of EGF and BPE for proliferation (Fig. 3B).

Autocrine TGFα Growth Regulation in Transformed RTE Cells

Why are transformed RTE cells EGF independent? The simplest hypothesis, but by no means the only conceivable one, is that transformed cells produce their

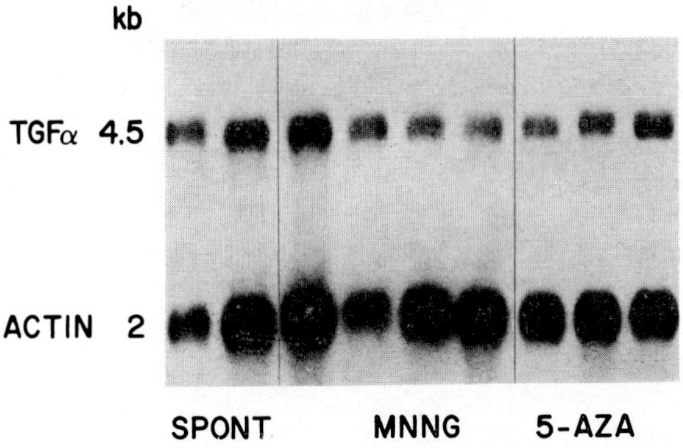

FIG. 4. Northern analysis of TGFα mRNA from immortalized RTE cell lines generated by diverse carcinogens. SPONT, spontaneously immortalized cell lines; MNNG, 5-AZA, cells immortalized following exposure of primary RTE cells to the alkylating agent MNNG and the hypo-methylating agent 5-azacytidine. Lanes 2, 5, 6, 8, and 9 represent cell lines isolated from tumors following injection of immortalized cell lines into nude mice while lanes 1, 3, 4, and 7 are cells lines with neoplastic potential (from ref. *10*).

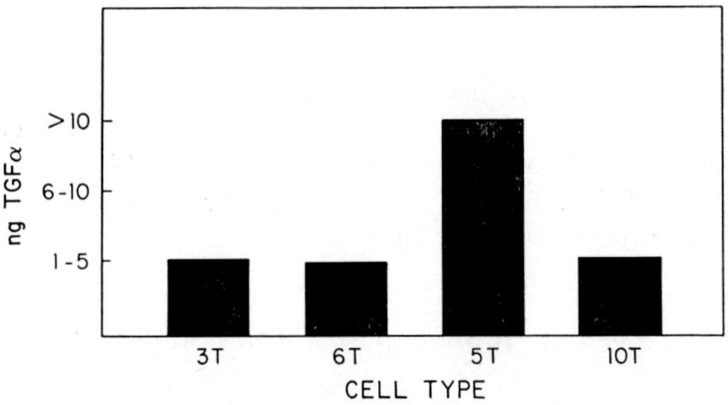

FIG. 5. TGFα secretion by neoplastic RTE cell lines. Data are presented as approximate amounts of TGFα collected from 25 ml of media conditioned by subconfluent neoplastic cell lines for 24 hr. TGFα was quantitated by both a radioreceptor assay which used conditioned media to compete with ^{125}I-EGF binding to 5637 bladder carcinoma cells, and by a radioimmunoassay which used conditioned media to compete with TGFα for binding of a specific antiserum. Results were similar with both assays (from ref. *8*).

own EGF-like factor, namely TGFα. TGFα is a 50 amino acid peptide which is structurally and functionally homologous with EGF. Both growth factors bind to and activate the same cellular receptor, an integral membrane protein with intrinsic tyrosine kinase activity. Ligand activation of the TGFα/EGF receptor leads to phosphorylation of protein substrates and initiation of a signal transduction cascade which induces cell division (*3*).

We examined TGFα expression in preneoplastic and neoplastic cell lines transformed from primary RTE cells either spontaneously or following exposure to chemical carcinogens. All of the cell lines studied express TGFα transcript (Fig. 4) and 4/4 cell lines examined secrete TGFα into the media as determined by radioimmune assay (Fig. 5) and Western blotting using TGFα specific antiserum. The cell line EGV-5T, which we studied in some detail, secretes at least two forms of TGFα, the seemingly fully processed form of 6.0 kD and a larger, presumptive pro-

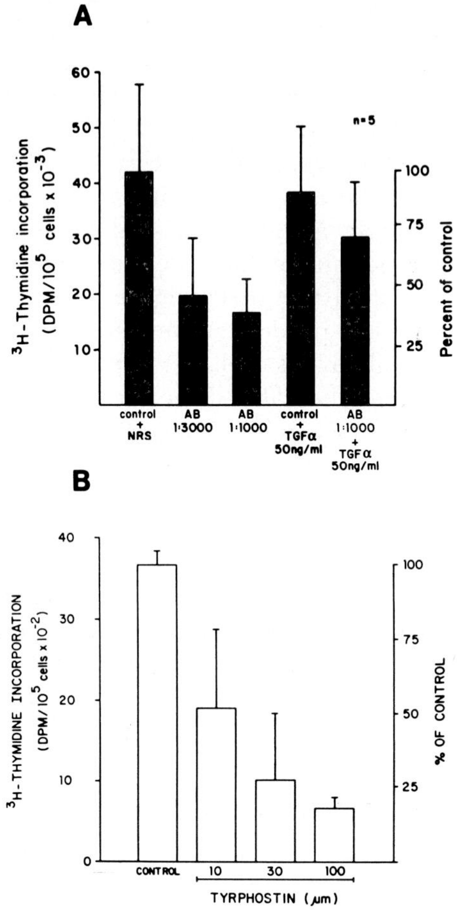

FIG. 6. A) Effect of TGFα antiserum on DNA synthesis of neoplastic, EGV5T cells. ^{3}H-thymidine incorporation by mid log phase EGV5T cultures propagated in the absence of EGF was measured following a 24 hr exposure to rat TGFα antibody. NRS=normal rabbit serum. B) Effect of tyrphostin on DNA synthesis of EGV5T cells, ^{3}H-thymidine incorporation was measured 24 hr after tyrphostin exposure (modified from ref. *10*).

TGFα, which is approximately 14.3 kD in size. That the endogenous growth factor is indeed acting as an autocrine mitogen can be demonstrated in two ways. Addition of TGFα-specific, neutralizing antiserum to the media results in significant reduction of DNA synthesis (Fig. 6). The other approach is to inhibit TGFα/EGF-receptor tyrosine kinase activity with a tyrphostin compound. Since activation of the kinase is a necessary step in transduction of the signal generated by binding of the ligand to the receptor, inhibiting the receptor kinase activity is expected to decrease TGFα dependent proliferation. As shown in Fig. 6B, addition of the tyrphostin Tyr8 to the cultures inhibits DNA synthesis (and growth, not shown, *10*). Together, these data indicate that at least a significant portion of the proliferative activity in cultures of transformed RTE cells is dependent on autocrine TGFα.

TGFα Autocrine Growth Regulation of Normal RTE Cells

TGFα expression is low in most normal, adult tissues, so low, that originally, it was thought to be expressed only in embryonic and neoplastic tissues (*2*). However, in recent years, in situ hybridization studies as well as immunocytochemical studies have shown that TGFα is expressed at low levels in many adult epithelial tissues (for review see *3*). Our first Northern blot analysis of RNA from primary RTE cell cultures also suggested that TGFα expression is very low (*9*). Close examination of primary RTE cell cultures shows that normal cells not only express TGFα message but also secrete measurable quantities of TGFα into the media. Using the same methods described for examining the autocrine role of TGFα in transformed cells, (see Fig. 6) we have found that a significant portion of the proliferative activity in primary RTE cultures is dependent on endogenous TGFα (*11*). In EGF/BPE deprived cultures, TGFα antibody as well as tyrphostin significantly inhibit DNA synthesis. However, these studies also demonstrate very important differences between normal and transformed cells in the regulation of TGFα expression. They show that primary cultures of RTE cells markedly down regulate expression of TGFα message shortly after reaching plateau of growth and drastically reduce TGFα secretion (Table 1). In contrast, transformed cells show very little evidence for such regulation. The amounts of TGFα produced per unit cell number in late primary cultures are less than 1/10 that in plateau cultures of transformed cells. As a result the concentrations of TGFα reached in media conditioned by transformed RTE cultures are 5 times higher (and some times more) than in primary cultures.

In conclusion, we showed that secretion of TGFα is not a unique feature of

TABLE 1. TGFα Secretion Primary *vs*. Transformed RTE (CSFM-48 hr)

	ng/10^6c	ng/dish	pM
RTE			
Log	0.92	0.40	17.5
Plateau	0.11	0.35	15.5
EGV10			
Log	2.84	0.76	33.0
Plateau	2.47	1.84	80.5

transformed cells. Proliferation of both cell types is at least in part dependent on an autocrine TGFα pathway. However transformed RTE cells constitutively express high levels of TGFα regardless of growth state, while normal cells down regulate TGFα when reaching plateau of growth. These differences in regulation of TGFα expression may be crucial for the differences in growth behavior of normal and transformed cells.

The Alternative Hypothesis: Growth Restraining Mechanisms Are Abnormal in Transformed RTE Cells

The abnormalities in the TGFα system just described may be important, but do they fully explain the enhanced growth capacity of transformed RTE cells?

A growth restraining mechanism which seems to be operating in almost all epithelial tissues that have been studied is mediated by TGFβ and it's cognate receptors (for review see *4*). TGFβ belongs to a large superfamily of multifunctional regulatory peptides. Three different isoforms of TGFβ are expressed in mammalian cells and their expression is differentially regulated in various tissues. All TGFβ isoforms are secreted in latent form and are cleaved from a latency complex by mechanisms not yet fully understood, in order to become biologically active. Two specific membrane receptors that are essential in transducing signals generated by TGFβ binding have been identified on nearly all cell types. The TGFβs not only regulate growth but control many other cell functions including extracellular matrix production and degradation.

Like many other epithelial cells, primary RTE cells are exquisitely sensitive to the growth inhibitory effects of TGFβ1 (Fig. 7) and TGFβ2, not shown. Thus, even very small amounts secreted into the cellular environment may have profound effects. Normal RTE cell cultures express TGFβ1 but TGFβ2 RNA transcripts are not detectable (*12*). Three TGFβ1 transcripts are seen on Northern blots of RNA

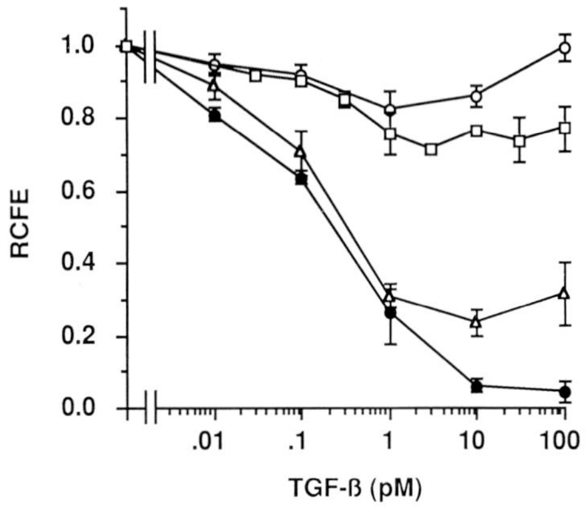

Fig. 7. Effect of TGFβ1 on colony formation of normal and transformed rat tracheal epithelial cells. Normal primary RTE cells (●) and transformed cell lines EGV6 (○); EGV9 (△); EGV5 (□) were treated with different concentrations of TGFβ1 for 7 days. RCFE=relative colony forming efficiency=number of colonies in treated cultures/number of colonies in control cultures (from ref. *12*).

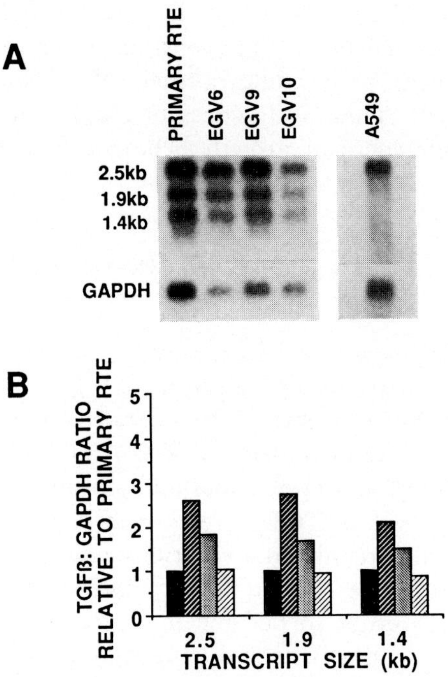

FIG. 8. TGFβ1 mRNA expression in primary RTE cultures and transformed cell lines. Northern analysis was performed with poly A$^+$ enriched RNA from late logarithmic growth phase cultures of primary RTE cells, and of EGV6, EGV9, and EGV10 cell lines. A549 RNA is shown for comparison. A) Autoradiograms of Northern blots probed for TGFβ1 and glyceraldehyde-3-phosphate dehydrogenase (GAPDH). B) Plot of ratio of densitometry determinations of TGFβ1/GAPDH signals for each of the three TGFβ1 transcripts (■) Primary RTE, (▨) EGV6, (▤) EGV9, (▩) EGV10 (from ref. *12*).

from both primary and transformed RTE cells (Fig. 8). The 2.5 kb message is commonly expressed in many tissues and cell lines. The 1.9 kb message is usually a less prominent RNA species but was recently shown by Qian *et al.* to be highly expressed in infarcted myocardial tissue (*13*). The 1.4 kb transcript which we regularly see expressed in cultured RTE cells has not been previously characterized and it's significance is currently uncertain. TGFβ is produced and secreted by normal RTE cells as can be shown by radio-receptor competition assay (Fig. 9). Most of the secreted TGFβ is in latent form. However, small amounts are activated and retard the growth of primary RTE cultures. This becomes apparent when TGFβ neutralizing antibodies are added to the cultures and induce an increase in DNA synthesis (not shown). Thus, an autocrine TGFβ growth restraining mechanism is operative in normal RTE cell cultures.

Reports in the literature indicate that TGFβ is often overexpressed in neoplastic cells and that the excess TGFβ secretion may have a paracrine effect on the tumor associated mesenchymal tissues, stimulating tumor growth indirectly by stimulating angiogenesis and stromal development (*14*, *15*). We are addressing the question of how transformed RTE cells manage to escape the growth inhibitory effects of TGFβ. As described above, normal RTE cells are highly sensitive to growth inhibition by TGFβ. Therefore, it was important to determine whether transformed cells differ

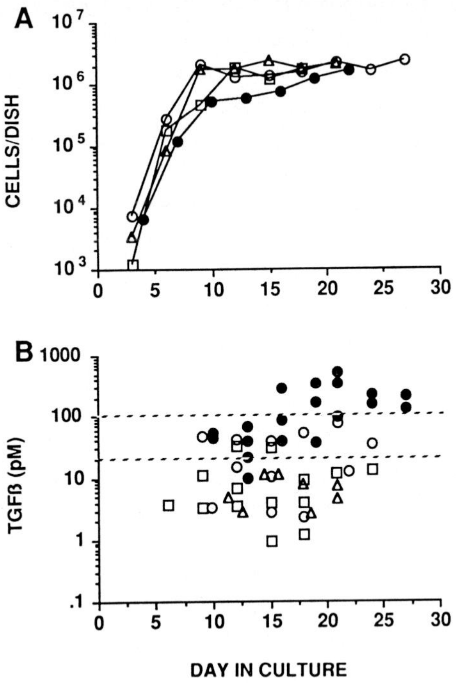

FIG. 9. Secretion of TGFβ by primary RTE cells and three transformed RTE cell lines. A) Representative growth curves for primary (●) and EGV cell line cultures (○, EGV6; △, EGV9; □, EGV10). B) Concentration of total TGFβ in media conditioned for 72 hr periods. Media were collected beginning 24 hr after start of cultures. Symbols are the same as in (A). Concentrations of total TGFβ in conditioned media were determined by radioreceptor assay (from ref. *12*).

from normal cells in their response to TGFβ. Using a colony forming assay to quantitate TGFβ responsiveness it can be shown that many of the transformed cell lines have significantly reduced responses to TGFβ (Fig. 7). The degree of TGFβ sensitivity varies widely: some cell lines are strongly growth inhibited like normal cells while others barely respond at all. The changes in TGFβ sensitivity do not seem to be due to a loss of TGFβ membrane receptors (*12*). Radioligand binding assays show no relationship between the number of binding sites and TGFβ responsiveness and receptor crosslinking studies also fail to show any correlation between expression of the three cellular binding proteins and responsiveness to TGFβ growth inhibition. Thus we conclude that the loss of TGFβ responsiveness must either result from defects in receptor function or from defective signal transduction pathways downstream of the receptor.

We also examined mRNA expression and TGFβ secretion by the transformed cell lines (see Fig. 8). Expression of TGFβ1 mRNA by transformed cells is similar to or slightly higher than expression in normal RTE cells and does not change significantly as a function of the cultures' growth state. In contrast, TGFβ secretion is markedly reduced in cultures of transformed cells (see Fig. 9).

These data show that transformed RTE cells are defective in at least two aspects of the TGFβ system: a) many (but not all) transformed RTE cell lines have a substantially reduced capacity to respond to the growth inhibitory effects of TGFβ and b) transformed RTE cell cultures secrete significantly lower levels of TGFβ than normal RTE cell cultures. Together, these two abnormalities render the TGFβ system non-operational as a growth restraining mechanism in many RTE cell transformants. The mechanisms underlying both of these defects are under investigation.

Conclusions

Our studies strongly suggest that the transforming growth factors alpha and beta are two important autocrine factors regulating proliferation of normal rat tracheal epithelial cell cultures. They also raise a number of intriguing questions. TGFα appears to be most important as a mitogen during early stages of logarithmic growth of normal RTE cell cultures. Whether the down-regulation of TGFα expression in late primary cultures causes the reduction in proliferation rates or whether it is the result of other events occurring in steady state cultures, such as the action of autocrine TGFβ and/or terminal cell differentiation (*16*, *17*), is an unresolved question.

TGFβ is secreted by primary RTE cells in large amounts in late logarithmic growth and plateau phase cultures and is growth inhibitory. To what extent the two growth factors regulate each other's expression or function is not known and is currently under investigation. Also uncertain is whether endogenous TGFβ is the main factor inducing terminal differentiation of primary RTE cells or whether TGFβ production is a byproduct of the process of terminal differentiation.

In transformed RTE cells both growth factor pathways are abnormal. Transformed RTE cells fail to down regulate TGFα expression, as normal cells do, when the cultures reach the plateau phase of growth. Also, many transformed RTE cell lines are hypo-responsive to TGFβ and secrete significantly less TGFβ than normal RTE cells. These abnormalities of TGFβ and TGFβ pathways are believed to play a critical role in the transformed growth behavior of immortalized, neoplastic RTE cells.

REFERENCES

1. Sporn, M. B. and Roberts, A. B. Autocrine growth factors and cancer. Nature, *313*: 745–747, 1985.
2. Derynck, R., Goeddel, D.V., Ullrich, A., Gutterman, J. U., Williams, R. D., Bringman, T. S., and Berger, W. H. Synthesis of messenger RNAs for transforming growth factors alpha and beta and the epidermal growth factor receptor by human tumors. Cancer Res., *47*: 707–712, 1987.
3. Carpenter, G. and Wahl, M. L. The epidermal growth factor family. *In*; M. B. Sporn and A. B. Roberts (eds.), Handbook of Pharmacology and Experimental Therapeutic, pp. 69–171, Springer-Verlag, Heidelberg, 1990.
4. Roberts, A. B. and Sporn, M. B. (eds.). The transforming growth factor-betas. *In*; Peptide Growth Factors and their Receptors: Handbook of Experimental Pharmacology, pp. 419–472, Springer-Verlag, Heidelberg, 1990.
5. Nettesheim, P. and Barrett, J. C., Tracheal epithelial cell transformation: a model system for studies on neoplastic progression. *In*; L. Goldgerg (ed.), Critical Review of

Toxicology, Vol. 12, pp. 215–239, CRC Press, Boca Raton, 1984.
6. Nettesheim, P., Fitzgerald, D. J., Kitamura, K., Walker, C. L., Gilmer, T. M., Barrett, J. C., and Gray, T. E. *In vitro* analysis of multistage carcinogenesis. Environ. Health Perspec., *75*: 71–79, 1987.
7. Walker, C. L. and Nettesheim, P. *In vitro* neoplastic progression of transformants generated by diverse carcinogens. Cancer Res., *49*: 4427–4430, 1989.
8. Ferriola, P. C., Steigerwalt, R., Robertson, A. T., and Nettesheim, P. Abnormalities in growth regulation of transformed rat tracheal epithelial cells. Pathobiology, *58*: 28–36, 1990.
9. Ferriola, P. C., Walker, C. L., Robertson, A. T., Earp, H. S., Rusnak, D. W., and Nettesheim, P. Altered growth factor dependence and transforming growth factor gene expression in transformed rat tracheal epithelial cells. Mol. Carcinogen., *2*: 1–9, 1990.
10. Ferriola, P. C., Earp, H. S., DiAugustine, R., and Nettesheim, P. Role of TGFα and its receptor in proliferation of immortalized rat tracheal epithelial cells: studies with tyrphostin and TGFα antisera. J. Cell Physiol., *147*: 166–175, 1991.
11. Ferriola, P. C., Robertson, A. T., Rusnak, D. W., DiAugustine, R., and Nettesheim, P. EGF dependence and TGFα autocrine growth regulation in primary RTE cells. J. Cell. Physiol., *152*: 302–309, 1992.
12. Steigerwalt, R. W., Rundhaug, J. E., and Nettesheim, P. Transformed rat tracheal epithelial cells exhibit alterations in TGFβ secretion and TGFβ responsiveness. Mol. Carcinogen., in press.
13. Qian, S. W., Kondaiah, P., Casscells, W., Roberts, A. B., and Sporn, M. B. A second messenger RNA species of transforming growth factor β1 in infarcted rat heart. Cell Regulation, *2*: 241–249, 1991.
14. Coffey, R. J., Goustin, A. S., Soderquist, A. M., Shipley, G. D., Wolfshol, J., Carpenter, G., and Moses, H. L. Transforming growth factor α and β expression in human colon cancer lines: implication for an autocrine model. Cancer Res., *47*: 4590–4594, 1987.
15. Schwarz, L. C., Wright, J. A., Gingras, M.-C., Kondaiah, P., Danielpour, D., Pimentel, M., Sporn, M. B., and Greenberg, A. H. Aberrant TGFβ production and regulation in metastatic malignancy. Growth Factors, *3*: 115–127, 1990.
16. Nettesheim, P., Smits, H. L., George, M. A., Gray, T., and Jetten, A. M. Squamous differentiation in normal and transformed rat tracheal epithelial cells. Carcinogenesis, *10*: 743–748, 1989.
17. Gray, T., Rundhaug, J., and Nettesheim, P. Critical variables controlling cell proliferation in primary cultures of rat tracheal epithelial cells. *In vitro* Cell. Dev. Biol., in press.

MULTISTAGE CARCINOGENESIS, C. C. HARRIS ET AL. (EDS.),
JAPAN SCI. SOC. PRESS, TOKYO/CRC PRESS, BOCA RATON, PP. 183–195, 1992

TGFβ Regulation of Epithelial Cell Proliferation: Role of Tumor Suppressor Genes

Harold L. Moses,*[1] Jennifer A. Pietenpol,*[1] Karl Münger,*[2] Catherine S. Murphy,*[1] and Edmund Y. Yang*[1]

Department of Cell Biology, Vanderbilt University School of Medicine, Nashville, Tennessee 37232, U.S.A.[1] *and Laboratory of Tumor Virus Biology, National Cancer Institute, Bethesda, Maryland 20892, U.S.A.*[2]

Abstract: Transforming growth factor β1 (TGFβ1) is the prototype of a large family of polypeptides involved in growth control, extracellular matrix production, and development. The TGFβs have marked stimulatory effects on connective tissue formation. They are chemotactic for fibroblasts, indirect mitogens for certain mesenchymal cells and stimulators of extracellular matrix deposition. The TGFβs are also potent inhibitors of proliferation of most cell types in culture, and *in vivo* studies have indicated that the predominant effect of TGFβ1 on cell proliferation is inhibition. We have investigated the mechanism of TGFβ1 inhibition of skin keratinocyte growth. Earlier studies demonstrated that TGFβ1 inhibition of keratinocyte proliferation involves suppression of c-*myc* transcription, and indirect evidence suggested that the product of the retinoblastoma tumor susceptibility gene, pRB, may be involved in this process. More recently, we have shown that transient expression of pRB in skin keratinocytes can repress human c-*myc* promoter/CAT transcription as effectively as TGFβ1. The same c-*myc* promoter region, termed the TGFβ control element (TCE), was required for regulation by both TGFβ1 and pRB. Oligonucleotides containing the TCE bound to several nuclear factors in mobility shift assays and a cellular protein of approximately 106 kD in Southwestern assays. Binding of these factors could be demonstrated in cells with or without normal pRB, and the binding of some factors was rapidly inhibited by TGFβ1 treatment of TGFβ-sensitive but not TGFβ-insensitive cells. These data indicate that pRB can function to inhibit c-*myc* transcription and suggest the involvement of cellular factor(s) in addition to pRB in the TGFβ1 pathway for suppression of c-*myc* transcription. Studies with other cell types have shown that another tumor suppressor gene, p53, can also regulate transcription of c-*myc* in transient assays. Whereas wild type p53 markedly suppressed transcription, four different mutant p53 clones caused transactivation. The data support the hypothesis that pRB and p53 can both cause growth inhibition by blocking the expression of the protooncogene, c-*myc*, and indicate that tumor suppressor genes may function in the response pathway for diffusible negative growth regulators such as TGFβ.

Over the past decade there have been remarkable advances in our understanding of the diffusible factors that regulate cell proliferation and the molecular mechanisms involved in this regulation. Much of the work has centered around the growth stimulatory peptides and their relationship to cellular protooncogenes. It is now widely recognized that protooncogenes code for growth factors, growth factor receptors, molecules involved in growth factor signal transduction, and transcription factors that are necessary for the growth factor response (reviewed in *1*). Work with oncogenes has been particularly important in identifying genes involved in the growth factor-receptor-response pathway and in pinpointing important regulatory steps in this growth stimulatory response.

While negative regulators of cell proliferation have been hypothesized to be important for a number of decades, this field did not gain respectability until the demonstration that transforming growth factor β1 (TGFβ1) is a potent inhibitor of proliferation of many cell types (*2*). TGFβ1 remains as the prototypic diffusible negative regulator of cell proliferation and is known to have an extraordinary diversity of biological effects in addition to the inhibition of cell proliferation (reviewed in *3*). TGFβ1 is now known to belong to a very large family of related molecules with a wide range of regulatory activities during embryologic development and in the adult state. Of the numerous TGFβ-like molecules, the mammalian TGFβ1, TGFβ2, and TGFβ3 proteins have been shown to be potent inhibitors of cell proliferation (*4*). Recent studies (*5–8*) have indicated that antioncogenes, or tumor suppressor genes, are probably involved in the response pathway for the negative regulation of cell proliferation by TGFβ1. The growth inhibitory effects of TGFβ1 in one *in vivo* model system and evidence for oncogene and tumor suppressor gene involvement in the growth inhibitory pathway for TGFβ1 will be reviewed.

TGFβ Regulation of Cell Proliferation In Vitro

Although originally described as a factor that stimulated soft agar growth of rodent fibroblasts (*9*, *10*), it is unlikely that TGFβ1, or any of the TGFβs, are direct mitogens for any cell type. They are probably indirect mitogens for certain mesenchymal cells through induction of autocrine stimulation by endogenous growth factors (*11*, *12*). TGFβ1 was first demonstrated to be a growth inhibitor in studies comparing the biological activities of the growth inhibitor from African green monkey (BSC-1) cells originally described by Holley *et al.* (*13*) and human platelet derived TGFβ1 (*2*). It is now known that the BSC-1 growth inhibitor is identical to TGFβ2 (*14*). Subsequent studies have demonstrated that TGFβ1 and TGFβ2 are the most potent growth inhibitory polypeptides known for a wide variety of cell types in culture including most epithelial cells, endothelial cells, most lymphoid cells, and many myeloid cells (for review, see *3*). TGFβ3 has also been shown to be growth inhibitory for epithelial cell types in culture (*4*). In general, the inhibitory effects of the TGFβs are reversible, and where studied, the TGFβs cause growth arrest in the G1 phase of the cell cycle (*15*).

TGFβ Regulation of Cell Proliferation In Vivo

TGFβ1 and TGFβ2 have also been demonstrated to be inhibitory for cell proliferation *in vivo*. Silberstein and Daniel (*16*) reported that TGFβ1 administered in semi-solid pellets reversibly inhibits mammary epithelial cell proliferation *in vivo*. Russell *et al.* (*17*) found that TGFβ1 and TGFβ2, administered intravenously, inhibited the early phase of liver regeneration following partial hepatectomy. Inhibition of hematopoietic cell proliferation has been demonstrated by Goey *et al.* (*18*) following intraarterial administration of TGFβ1. Evidence has been presented for TGFβ1 suppression of the immune response to immunogenic tumors and of cytotoxic T lymphocyte production *in vivo* (*19*, *20*).

Additional *in vivo* studies have demonstrated that TGFβ1 has remarkable effects on the chicken chorioallantoic membrane (CAM) (*21*). When TGFβ1 was focally applied to the CAM, gross angiogenesis was induced. Furthermore, a central hypercellular lesion was observed characterized by increases in fibroblast, epithelial, and endothelial cell densities. The formation of this lesion was quite rapid, and in fact, within 4 hr of TGFβ1 treatment both fibroblasts and epithelial cells accumulated to increased densities at the point of treatment, where the concentrations of TGFβ1 would be highest. However, the density changes induced by TGFβ1 were not mediated by increases in proliferation. Fibroblasts, endothelial cells, and epithelial cells were markedly growth inhibited in the central area of TGFβ1 application. Since fibroblasts and epithelial cells rapidly increased in density in the face of proliferative inhibition, their accumulation must have been due to stimulated cell

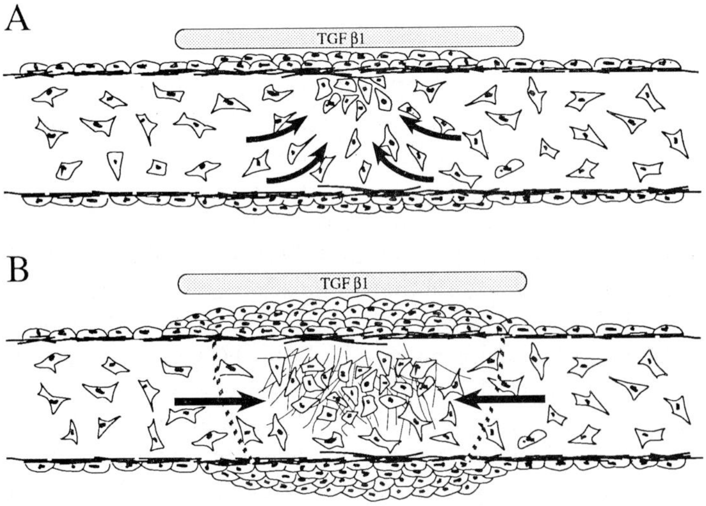

FIG. 1. *In vivo* effects of TGFβ1 on the chicken CAM. When TGFβ1 is locally applied to the CAM in the form of a methylcellulose disk (stippled ovals), TGFβ1 diffuses into the CAM and forms a concentration gradient. (A) Within 4 hr, fibroblasts and epithelial cells accumulate centrally through chemotaxis (arrows). (B) Beyond 8 hr, when more TGFβ1 has diffused into the CAM, centrally accumulated cells form a zone of growth inhibition (demarcated by dashed lines), and chemotaxis probably occurs from more peripheral regions (arrows). Angiogenesis then occurs by 16 hr (*21*).

migration from regions peripheral to the site of TGFβ1 treatment (*21*).

These studies are reminiscent of *in vitro* studies in which it has been demonstrated that the chemotactic effects of TGFβ1 occur at a much lower (sub-picomolar) concentration than that required for other TGFβ1 effects (*22*). At higher concentrations (picomolar levels) TGFβ1 is no longer chemotactic and other biologic effects are induced, including growth inhibition and simulation of extracellular matrix production. The observations of TGFβ1 effect in the CAM suggest that similar concentration-dependent mechanisms may specify different zones of cellular function *in vivo* (Fig. 1). With initial TGFβ1 administration, rapid inward chemotaxis of cells is observed (Fig. 1A). But, with continued administration, and increased diffusion of TGFβ1 into the CAM, the region of chemotactic stimulation moves outward peripherally (Fig. 1B). As cells migrate centrally and accumulate, where TGFβ1 concentrations are higher, their proliferation is inhibited and they devote their energies to performing differentiated functions, which in the case of the fibroblasts is deposition of extracellular matrix and in the case of the endothelial cells is formation of capillary tubes and secretion of basement membrane materials. Thus, TGFβ1-induced growth inhibition is an integral, and perhaps necessary, component of the mesenchymal reorganization stimulated in the CAM. Similar functions may be stimulated by TGFβ1 in the physiological contexts of wound healing and embryogenesis as well as in the pathological process of neoplasia. Many cancer cells have lost the growth inhibitory response to TGFβ (*15, 23, 24*) and produce increase quantities of TGFβ1 (*25*) which could play a role in tumor stroma formation and angiogenesis as illustrated by the CAM studies (*21*). TGFβ produced by tumors could also enhance tumor growth by suppression of immune surveillance (*19*).

TGFβ Effects on Early Growth Factor Induced Events

In studying the mechanisms of TGFβ growth inhibition, we have utilized secondary cultures of human skin keratinocytes grown in low-calcium, serum-free medium (*15, 24*) and a continuous line of mouse keratinocytes cultured in low-calcium, serum-containing medium (*26, 27*). Both cell types require epidermal growth factor (EGF) TGFα for proliferation and retain the ability to differentiate under high calcium conditions. TGFβ1, TGFβ2, and TGFβ3 are potent inhibitors for the keratinocytes (*4, 27*). The cells were found to be reversibly inhibited in their growth by the TGFβs with the majority of the cells blocked in the G1 phase of the cell cycle (*15, 27*). In considering the mechanisms by which the TGFβs inhibit cell proliferation, cytotoxicity can be excluded; the inhibition is reversible (*15, 27*). Induction of terminal differentiation, although reported for bronchial epithelial cells (*23*), does not appear to be a general phenomenon and does not occur in either the human foreskin keratinocytes or in the mouse keratinocyte cell line (*15, 27*). It is possible that prior growth inhibition of keratinocytes by the TGFβs may render them more susceptible to induction of differentiation by physiologically inducers such as calcium. TGFβ1 does not appear to interfere with growth factor-receptor interactions or with many of the early events induced by growth stimulatory factors including some signal transduction events (*27, 28*). For example, EGF induction of c-*fos* in mouse keratinocytes is not inhibited by TGFβ1 even though EGF stimulation of DNA synthesis is inhibited (*26*).

Perhaps the best evidence that TGFβ does not interfere with early growth factor induced events is the data demonstrating that TGFβ1 can prevent EGF-stimulated DNA synthesis in epithelial cells even when added late in G1, long after early events induced by EGF have occurred (*6, 29, 30*). Following EGF addition to the mouse keratinocytes that have been growth arrested by depletion of EGF, there is a 12 hr lag phase prior to entry of the cells into the S phase of the cell cycle (*27*). TGFβ1 was shown to inhibit subsequent entry into S phase if added at any time up to the G1/S boundary (*6*). Thus, in considering mechanisms of TGFβ growth inhibition, events other than those induced early by growth factors must be examined.

The Role of c-myc in Growth Inhibition by TGFβ

The protooncogene, c-*myc*, has been shown to be necessary for proliferation of a number of cell types (for review, see *8*). The addition of TGFβ1 to rapidly growing human and mouse keratinocytes resulted in a rapid reduction of c-*myc* mRNA and protein (*26*). Half-maximal reduction in c-*myc* mRNA following TGFβ addition occurred in approximately 30 min. Since the half-life of c-*myc* mRNA following addition of actinomycin D is approximately 20 min, the effects of TGFβ on suppression of c-*myc* must occur quite rapidly, yet protein synthesis is probably required for TGFβ suppression of c-*myc* (*26*). Since TGFβ rapidly reduces c-*myc*, we have investigated whether c-*myc* is necessary for cell proliferation in the mouse keratinocytes. The addition of antisense c-*myc* oligonucleotides was demonstrated to rapidly reduce c-*myc* protein and to inhibit cell proliferation as effectively as TGFβ1 (*31*).

Like other immediate-early genes, c-*myc* is induced rapidly by the addition of EGF to quiescent cells of many types, including skin keratinocytes (*26*). However, unlike other immediate-early genes, c-*myc* expression remains elevated throughout G1 and S phases (*26, 32*). Thus, c-*myc* expression could be a target of TGFβ1 effects even in late G1. Expression of c-*myc* mRNA and protein were shown to be rapidly inhibited by TGFβ1 addition throughout G1 and S phases of the cell cycle (*26, 32*). Use of antisense c-*myc* oligonucleotides that inhibit *myc* protein synthesis inhibited progression through the cell cycle in a pattern very similar to that observed with TGFβ1 (*32*). The oligonucleotides inhibited progression into S phase when added at any point in G1 but had no inhibitory effect when added during S phase. This indicates that in keratinocytes the c-*myc* protein may be important for the initiation of S phase but is not absolutely required for progression in S phase and that the cell cycle state specific effects of TGFβ1 may be related to the stage of the cell cycle at which c-*myc* is needed. In addition, the data are compatible with TGFβ suppression of c-*myc* being a critical component in the pathway for TGFβ1-induced growth inhibition.

The mechanism of TGFβ suppression of c-*myc* was investigated. Nuclear run-on assays utilizing single-stranded, exon- and intron-specific probes demonstrated that the block in c-*myc* expression by TGFβ1 occurred at the level of transcriptional initiation (*31*). Studies with the series of 5′ deletion c-*myc*/chloramphenicol acetyltransferase constructs indicated that a *cis* regulatory element which resides between positions −100 and +71 relative to P1 transcription start site, is responsible for the TGFβ1 suppression. Based on this data, it was proposed that the mechanism of TGFβ1 growth inhibition involves synthesis or modification of a protein that may interact with a specific *cis* element in the 5′ regulatory region of c-*myc* gene resulting in inhibition of transcriptional initiation of this gene (*31*).

Requirement for pRB in TGFβ1 Suppression of c-myc Transcription

In considering other proteins that may be involved in TGFβ1 regulation of c-*myc* transcription, evidence indicated that the protein product of the retinoblastoma gene, pRB, was a likely candidate. pRB has properties of a cell cycle regulatory factor (*33*). It is a differentially phosphorylated 105 kD nuclear protein that has been postulated to contribute to growth suppression, directly or indirectly (*34*). Evidence of tumor suppressor activity by pRB is provided by the observations that loss or inactivation of the Rb gene has been found in a variety of malignant cell types including retinoblastomas, osteosarcomas, small cell carcinoma of the lung, and carcinomas of the breast, bladder and prostate (see *6* for review). Furthermore, introduction of a cloned Rb gene into cells results in marked changes in morphology, decreased growth rates, and reduced tumorigenic potential in neoplastic cells (*35, 36*).

Additional evidence for a role of pRB in growth regulation has come from studies with DNA tumor virus transforming gene products. It has been demonstrated that pRB associates with the transforming proteins of SV40 (*37*), adenovirus (*38*), and HPV-16 (*39*). The specific transforming proteins are large T antigen (TAg), E1A, and E7, respectively. Furthermore, mutant forms of these virus proteins that do not bind pRB are transformation defective. It has been hypothesized that binding of pRB by DNA viral transforming proteins may block the growth suppressive activity of pRB resulting in some of the aberrations of growth control associated with transformation by these viruses (*37–39*).

Keratinocytes transformed by the DNA tumor viruses SV40 and HPV-16 or HPV-18 have been shown to be resistant to the growth inhibitory effects of TGFβ1 (*6*). Further, TGFβ1 was unable to suppress c-*myc* mRNA levels in these DNA tumor virus-transformed cells. Subsequent studies tested whether blocking of TGFβ1 suppression of c-*myc* expression is mediated through the pRB binding domain of the DNA tumor virus transforming proteins. Transient expression in non-transformed keratinocytes of the DNA tumor virus proteins that bind pRB including HPV-16 E7, adenovirus E1A and SV40 TAg, prevented TGFβ1 suppression of c-*myc* expression. Mutants of E1A and TAg that impaired association with pRB failed to block the TGFβ1 suppression of c-*myc* (*6*).

Thus, the data indicate that a cellular protein interacting with the conserved domain of the DNA viral oncoproteins is necessary for TGFβ1 suppression of c-*myc* transcription. However, proteins other than pRB bind to the pRB binding domain of the DNA viral transforming proteins (*38, 40–42*), and their involvement in this cannot be excluded. To further examine the possible involvement of pRB in the TGFβ1 pathway for suppression of c-*myc* transcription, the effect of expression of pRB on c-*myc* expression was determined (*5*). Transient expression of pRB in skin

TIE in transin/stromelysin	-709	G A G T T G G T G A -700
TCE in c-*myc*	-86	G C A G A G G G C G T G G G G G A A A A G A A -63
RCE in c-*fos*	-71	G G G C G C G C G G T G G G G A G A C C G C G G T G G C A C -102

FIG. 2. Sequence of TCE in comparison to TIE and RCE. See text for discussion.

keratinocytes was shown to repress transcription of the human c-*myc* promoter as effectively as TGF-β1. The same c-*myc* promoter region was required for regulation by both TGF-β1 and pRB. These sequences, termed the TGF-β control element (TCE), lie between −86 and −63 relative to the P1 transcription start site. The demonstration that transient expression of pRB inhibits *myc* transcription like TGF-β1 and requires the same promoter element as TGFβ1 provides additional evidence in favor of pRB being that component in this TGF-β1 pathway targeted by the DNA tumor virus oncoproteins.

Kerr *et al.* (*43*) have presented results indicating that TGFβ1 suppression of transin/stromelysin gene transcription is mediated through binding of a *fos* containing protein complex to a promoter sequence, termed the TGFβ1 inhibitory element (TIE). TIE also shows a region of sequence similarity to a region of the TCE (Fig. 2). A second region of sequence similarity to TCE within the human c-*myc* promoter is outside the 5′ region shown to be necessary for TGFβ1 suppression of c-*myc* transcription. Robbins *et al.* (*44*) have reported that expression of pRB in mouse fibroblasts suppresses transcription of c-*fos* and have identified an element, termed the retinoblastoma control element (RCE), in the c-*fos* promoter necessary for this suppression. More recently, sequences homologous to the RCE have been identified in the TGFβ1, β2, and β3 promoters by Kim *et al.* (*45*). Cotransfection with an RB expression plasmid was shown to regulate expression from TGFβ1 promoter/CAT constructs positively or negatively depending of the cell type. This group also reported that sequences similar to the RCE are present in the human c-*myc* promoter and that RB over-expression enhances c-*myc* expression in mink lung (Mv1Lu) cells which are very sensitive to the growth inhibitory effect of TGFβ (*45*). One of the sequences in the c-*myc* promoter they reported to be similar to the RCE is in the same region as TCE, but is on the noncoding strand (Fig. 2).

We have examined the effect of TGFβ1 treatment or over-expression of pRB on c-*myc* expression in the Mv1Lu cells. TGFβ1 suppressed transcription while RB had little or no effect (C. S. Murphy, J. A. Pietenpol, and H. L. Moses, unpublished observations). Since pRB did not suppress transcription of c-*myc* in the Mv1Lu cells, it was suspected that another tumor suppressor gene such as p53 that encodes a DNA-binding protein might be involved. Expression of wild-type p53 was found to regulate transcription of c-*myc* in transient assays in these cells. Whereas wild type p53 markedly suppressed transcription, four different mutant p53 clones caused transactivation. Preliminary data indicate that the TCE is not required for wild type p53 suppression or mutant p53 transactivation of c-*myc*. This indicates that cell type differences may exist in the tumor suppressor genes involved in the response pathway for suppression of c-*myc* expression and growth inhibition. The possibility that p53 may be involved in the response pathway for growth inhibition by TGFβ1 in the Mv1Lu cells in a manner analogous to pRB in the keratinocytes is currently being investigated.

TCE Binding to Cellular Proteins

Evidence for keratinocyte protein binding to the TCE was obtained in both gel mobility shift (*5*) and Southwestern assays (*8*). By gel shift, TCE formed three retarded complexes (TCE-I, TCE-II, and TCE-III), whereas Southewestern blots showed TCE binding predominantly to one major protein of approximately 106 kD, termed p106. Which, if any, of the bands in the gel shift assay corresponds to the protein detected in the Southwestern assay is not known. However, the binding to p106 was rapidly decreased by TGFβ1 treatment. In the gel shift assay binding to the TCE-II complex and not TCE-I or TCE-II was rapidly diminished by TGFβ1 treatment. This suggests that TCE binding to TCE-II and p106 may be due to related phenomena. The observation that binding in both assays is down regulated by TGFβ1 treatment argues in favor of both binding assays reflecting biologically relevant protein-DNA interactions.

Because pRB is a nuclear phosphoprotein of 105–110 kD that is capable of binding DNA (*46*) and because pRB appears to be involved in the suppression of c-*myc* transcription in response to TGF-β1 treatment, the possibility of TCE binding directly to pRB was examined. No binding of the TCE oligonucleotide was obtained with cellular proteins co-precipitated with antibodies to DNA tumor viral oncoproteins (*5, 8*). Additional evidence that TCE is not binding to pRB in the Southwestern analysis is provided by experiments on extracts from retinoblastoma cell lines (WERI and Y-79) lacking the RB gene and a human prostatic adenocarcinoma cell line (DU-145) that has an exon 21 deleted RB gene and produces a smaller functionally defective RB protein (*5, 8*). TCE binding to the shifted complexes and to p106 was observed in extracts from these cell lines similar to that observed with normal human foreskin keratinocytes.

Unlike the TGF-β1 regulation of protein binding seen in the TGFβ1-sensitive keratinocytes, there was no repression of TCE-protein binding in protein extracts from TGF-β1-treated SV40-transformed human foreskin keratinocytes (HFK/SV40) or DU-145 cells that are insensitive to the growth inhibitory effect of TGF-β1 (*6, 8*). While the Southwestern data indicate that pRB does not bind to the TCE, pRB could be part of a multi-protein complex involved in regulation of c-*myc* transcription through the TCE. In addition, the data suggest that the TCE binding protein (p106) detected by Southwestern analysis and TCE-II detected by gel shift analysis may be a positive transcriptional factor for c-*myc*, since TGFβ1 down-regulates binding. The observations: 1) that binding is decreased rapidly following TGF-β1 treatment of keratinocytes with kinetics similar to the decrease in c-*myc* mRNA abundance and 2) that binding is not decreased following TGFβ1 treament of SV40/HFK cells that are resistant to the c-*myc* suppressive and growth inhibitory effect of TGFβ1 (*6*) are consistent with this hypothesis.

The studies discussed here indicate that p106 may play a role in TGFβ1 suppression of c-*myc* and of keratinocyte cell growth. We have proposed a model to describe the mode of action of p106 (Fig. 3). The p106 protein may be a positive transcription factor for c-*myc*, inducing transcription of the gene and increasing cell growth. It is possible that TGFβ1, in concert with proteins like pRB, inhibits the action of p106 decreasing its binding to the TCE and thereby inhibiting c-*myc*

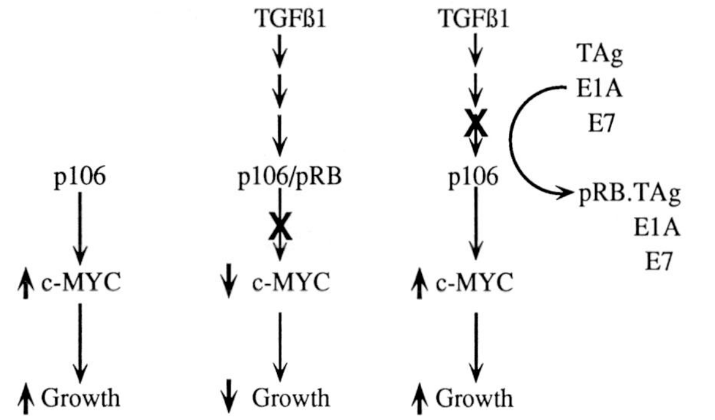

FIG. 3. Schematic model of TGFβ1 inhibitory action on keratinocyte cell growth. This model represents possible modes of action for TGFβ1 inhibition of c-*myc* expression and, subsequently, cell growth (see text).

transcription and cell growth. Various pRB-binding oncoproteins may remove pRB from this pathway, thereby causing the cells to become insensitive to TGFβ1 inhibition. Obviously, other models are possible and further delineation of the exact sequence of events in this important pathway will require cloning of the p106 gene and expression in appropriate systems to examine potential p106 binding to pRB and to show a direct effect of p106 on c-*myc* gene transcription.

Effect of TGFβ1 Treatment on pRB Phosphorylation State

Following growth factor stimulation of quiescent keratinocytes, TGFβ1 can inhibit progression into S phase at any point prior to the G1/S transition but does not inhibit progression through the S phase of the cell cycle (*6*). Since pRB is underphosphorylated during G1 and hyperphosphorylated during S and G2 (*33*), the G1/S specific phosphorylation of pRB becomes an attractive target for the growth inhibitory activities of TGFβ1 (*30*). However, in TGFβ1 treated primary human keratinocytes and a series of human papilloma virus and SV40 transformed human keratinocyte cell lines, the phosphorylation status of pRB strictly correlated with cell growth (*32*). Treatment of rapidly growing nontransformed keratinocytes with TGFβ1 caused a decrease in pRB phosphorylation over a period of several hours that correlated with growth arrest of the cells. In addition, placement of keratinocytes in amino acid-deficient or growth factor-depleted medium, growth conditions that cause a G1 arrest similar to TGFβ1 treatment also caused a slow decrease in the phosphorylation state of pRB. In the transformed keratinocytes that are resistant to the growth inhibitory effect of TGFβ, treatment with TGFβ1 had no effect on pRB phosphorylation. Thus, no evidence was found for a direct effect of TGFβ1 on the phosphorylation status of these cells indicating that the pRB dependent suppression of c-*myc* transcription by TGFβ1 in keratinocytes is not mediated through an alteration in the phosphorylation state of pRB.

Conclusions

Control of keratinocyte proliferation as with other cell types involves both

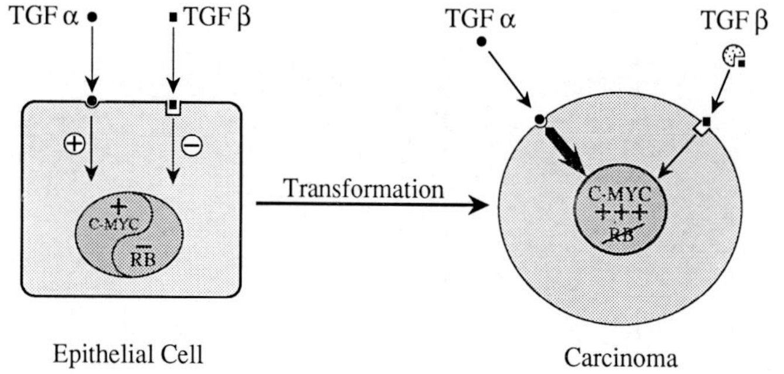

FIG. 4. Model for positive and negative growth factor regulation of keratinocyte proliferation. TGFβ1 suppresses transcription of c-*myc*, a protooncogene required for cell proliferation utilizing a pathway that requires the protein product of the retinoblastoma susceptibility gene (pRB) (see text). This predicts that one mechanism for loss of the growth inhibitory response in carcinoma cells is mutational inactivation of the Rb gene.

positive and negative polypeptide regulators that bind to cell surface membrane receptors. The keratinocytes produce the same peptides that stimulate or inhibit their proliferation. For example, keratinocytes produce TGFα and TGFα stimulates keratinocyte (*47*) (Fig. 4). Keratinocytes also secrete TGFβ which can reversibly inhibit their proliferation (Fig. 4). TGFβ is secreted in a latent form that could be activated in the medium or at the cell membrane by proteolytic action resulting in a negative effect on cell proliferation. It is likely that autocrine regulation by both stimulators and inhibitors of proliferation is an important physiological mechanism of regulation of keratinocyte proliferation. The presence of opposing regulatory pathways should allow for a more precise control of cell proliferation than would an on/off stimulatory pathway provided by the growth factors. The growth inhibitory polypeptides probably play as important a role in the control of cell proliferation as the growth stimulatory factors. Data summarized here indicate that the mechanism of TGFβ1 growth inhibition in skin keratinocytes involves suppression of transcription of the protooncogene, c-*myc*, the expression of which is required for cell proliferation. The data further indicate that the tumor suppressor gene product, pRB, is a critical component in this pathway. This would predict that one mechanism for loss of the growth inhibitory response to TGFβ1 in carcinoma cells could be mutational inactivation of the Rb gene (Fig. 4).

REFERENCES

1. Goustin, A. S., Leof, E. B., Shipley, G. D., and Moses, H. L. Perspectives in cancer research: growth factors and cancer. Cancer Res., *46*: 1015–1029, 1986.
2. Tucker, R. F., Shipley, G. D., Moses, H. L., and Holley, R. W. Growth inhibitor from BSC-1 cells closely related to the platelet type β transforming growth factor. Science, *226*: 705–707, 1984.
3. Moses, H. L. The biological actions of transforming growth factor β. *In*; V. Sara, K. Hall, and H. Low (eds.), Growth Factors From Genes to Clinical Application, pp. 141–155, Raven Press, New York, 1990.
4. Graycar, J. L., Miller, D. A., Arrick, B. A., Lyons, R. M., Moses, H. L., and Derynck,

R. Human transforming growth factor-β3: recombinant expression, purification, and biological activities in comparison with transforming growth factors-β1 and -β2. Mol. Endocrinol., *3*: 1977–1986, 1989.

5. Pietenpol, J. A., Münger, K., Howley, P. M., Stein, R. W., and Moses, H. L. Factor-binding element in the human c-*myc* promoter involved in transcriptional regulation by transforming growth factor β1 and by the retinoblastoma gene product. Proc. Natl. Acad. Sci. U.S.A., *88*: 10227–10231, 1991.
6. Pietenpol, J. A., Stein, R. W., Moran, E., Yaciuk, P., Schlegel, R., Lyons, R. M., Pittelkow, M. R., Münger, K., Howley, P. M., and Moses, H. L. TGF-β1 inhibition of c-*myc* transcription and growth in keratinocytes is abrogated by viral transforming proteins with pRB binding domains. Cell, *61*: 777–785, 1990.
7. Moses, H. L., Yang, E. Y., and Pietenpol, J. A. TGF-β stimulation and inhibition of cell proliferation: new mechanistic insights. Cell, *63*: 245–247, 1990.
8. Murphy, C. S., Pietenpol, J. A., Münger, K., Howley, P. M., and Moses, H. L. c-*myc* and pRB: role in TGFβ1 inhibition of keratinocyte proliferation. Cold Spring Harbor Symp., in press.
9. Roberts, A. B., Anzano, M. A., Lamb, L. C., Smith, J. M., and Sporn, M. B. New class of transforming growth factors potentiated by epidermal growth factor: isolation from non-neoplastic tissues. Proc. Natl. Acad.. Sci. U.S.A., *78*: 5339–5343, 1981.
10. Moses, H. L., Branum, E. B., Proper, J. A., and Robinson, R. A. Transforming growth factor production by chemically transformed cells. Cancer Res., *41*: 2842–2848, 1981.
11. Leof, E. B., Proper, J. A., Goustin, A. S., Shipley, G. D., DiCorleto, P. E., and Moses, H. L. Induction of c-*sis* mRNA and activity similar to platelet-derived growth factor by transforming growth factor-β: a proposed model for indirect mitogenesis involving autocrine activity. Proc. Natl. Acad. Sci. U.S.A., *83*: 2453–2457, 1986.
12. Battegay, E. J., Raines, E. W., Seifert, R. A., Bowen-Pope, D. F., and Ross, R. TGF-β induces bimodal proliferation of connective tissue cells *via* complex control of an autocrine PDGF loop. Cell, *63*: 515–524, 1990.
13. Holley, R. W., Armour, R., and Baldwin, J. H. Density-dependent regulation of growth of BSC-1 cells in cell culture: growth inhibitors formed by the cells. Proc. Natl. Acad. Sci. U.S.A., *75*: 1864–1866, 1978.
14. Hanks, S. K., Armour, R., Baldwin, J. H., Maldonado, F., Spiess, J., and Holley, R. W. Amino acid sequence of the BSC-1 cell growth inhibitor (polyergin) deduced from the nucleotide sequence of the cDNA. Proc. Natl. Acad. Sci. U.S.A., *85*: 79–82, 1988.
15. Shipley, G. D., Pittelkow, M. R., Wille, J. J., Jr., Scott, R. E., and Moses, H. L. Reversible inhibition of normal human prokeratinocyte proliferation by type β transforming growth factor-growth inhibitor in serum-free medium. Cancer Res., *46*: 2068–2071, 1986.
16. Silberstein, G. B. and Daniel, C. W. Reversible inhibition of mammary gland growth by transforming growth factor-β. Science, *237*: 291–293, 1987.
17. Russell, W. E., Coffey, R. J., Jr., Ouellette, A. J., and Moses, H. L. Type β transforming growth factor reversibly inhibits the early proliferative response to partial hepatectomy in the rat. Proc. Natl. Acad. Sci. U.S.A., *85*: 5126–5130, 1988.
18. Goey, H., Keller, J. R., Back, T., Longo, D. L., Ruscetti, F. W., and Wiltrout, R. H. Inhibition of early murine hemopoietic progenitor cell proliferation after *in vivo* locoregional administration of transforming growth factor-β 1. J. Immunol., *143*: 877–880, 1989.
19. Torre-Amione, G., Beauchamp, R. D., Koeppen, H., Park, B. H., Schreiber, H., Moses, H. L., and Rowley, D. A. A highly immunogenic transfected with a murine

transforming growth factor type β1 cDNA escapes immune surveillance. Proc. Natl. Acad. Sci. U.S.A., *87*: 1486–1490, 1990.
20. Fontana, A., Frei, K., Bodmer, S., Hofer, E., Schreier, M. H., Palladino, M. A., Jr., and Zinkernagel, R. M. Transforming growth factor-b inhibits the generation of cytotoxic T cells in virus-infected mice. J. Immunol., *143*: 3230–3234, 1989.
21. Yang, E. Y. and Moses, H. L. Transforming growth factor β1-induced changes in cell migration, proliferation, and angiogenesis in the chicken chorioallantic membrane. J. Cell Biol., *111*: 731–741, 1990.
22. Postlethwaite, A. E., Keski-Oja, J., Moses, H. L., and Kang, A. H. Stimulation of the chemitactic migration of human fibroblasts by transforming growth factor β. J. Exp. Med., *165*: 251–256, 1987.
23. Masui, T., Wakefield, L. M., Lechner, J. F., LaVeck, M. A., Sporn, M. B., and Harris, C. C. Type β transforming growth factor is the primary differentiation-inducing serum factor for normal human bronchial epithelial cells. Proc. Natl. Acad. Sci. U.S.A., *83*: 2438–2442, 1986.
24. Moses, H. L., Tucker, R. F., Leof, E. B., Coffey, R. J., Jr., Halper, J., and Shipley, G. D. Type β transforming growth factor is a growth stimulator and a growth inhibitor. *In*; J. Feramisco, B. Ozanne and C. Stiles (eds.), Growth Factors and Transformation. Cancer Cells 3, pp. 65–71, Cold Spring Harbor Press, New York, 1985.
25. Derynck, R., Jarrett, J. A., Chen, E. Y., Eaton, D. H., Bell, J. R., Assoian, R. K., Roberts, A. B., Sporn, M. B., and Goeddel, D. V. Human transforming growth factor-β complementary DNA sequence and expression in normal and transformed cells. Nature, *316*: 701–705, 1985.
26. Coffey, R. J., Jr., Bascom, C. C., Sipes, N. J., Graves-Deal, R., Weissman, B. E., and Moses, H. L. Selective inhibition of growth-related gene expression in murine keratinocytes by transforming growth factor β. Mol. Cell. Biol., *8*: 3088–3096, 1988.
27. Coffey, R. J., Jr., Sipes, N. J., Bascom, C. C., Graves-Deal, R., Pennington, C. Y., Weissman, B. E., and Moses, H. L. Growth modulation of mouse keratinocytes by transforming growth factors. Cancer Res., *48*: 1596–1602, 1988.
28. Chambard, J.-C. and Pouyssegur, J. TGF-β inhibits growth factor-induced DNA synthesis in hamster fibroblasts without affecting the early mitogenic events. J. Cell. Physiol., *135*: 101–107, 1988.
29. Howe, P. H., Draetta, G., and Leof, E. B. Transforming growth factor β1 inhibition of p34cdc2 phosphorylation and histone H1 kinase activity is associated with G1S-phase growth arrest. Mol. Cell. Biol., *11*: 1185–1194, 1991.
30. Laiho, M., DeCaprio, J. A., Ludlow, J. W., Livingston, D. M., and Massague, J. Growth inhibition by TGF-β linked to suppression of retinoblastoma protein phosphorylation. Cell, *62*: 175–185, 1990.
31. Pietenpol, J. A., Holt, J. T., Stein, R. W., and Moses, H. L. Transforming growth factor β-1 suppression of c-*myc* gene transcription: role in inhibition of keratinocyte proliferation. Proc. Natl. Acad. Sci. U.S.A., *87*: 3758–3762, 1990.
32. Münger, K., Pietenpol, J. A., Pittelkow, M. R., Holt, J. T., and Moses, H. L. TGFβ regulation of c-*myc* expression, pRB phosphorylation, and cell cycle progression in keratinocytes. Cell Growth Diff., *3*: 291–298, 1992.
33. DeCaprio, J. A., Ludlow, J. W., Lynch, D., Furukawa, Y., Griffin, J., Piwnica-Worms, H., Huang, C.-M., and Livingston, D. M. The product of the retinoblastoma susceptibility gene has properties of a cell cycle regulatory element. Cell, *58*: 1085–1095, 1989.
34. Friend, S. H., Bernards, R., Rogelj, S., Weinberg, R. A., Rapaport, J. M., Albert, D. M., and Dryja, T. P. A human DNA segment with properties of the gene that

predisposes to retinoblastoma and osteosarcoma. Nature, *323*: 643–646, 1986.

35. Huang, H.-J. S., Yee, J.-K., Shew, J.-Y., Chen, P.-L., Bookstein, R., Friedmann, T., Lee, E. Y.-H. P., and Lee, W-H. Suppression of the neoplastic phenotype by replacement of the RB gene in human cancer cells. Science, *242*: 1563–1566, 1988.
36. Takahashi, R., Hashimoto, T., Xu, H.-J., Hu, S.-X., Matsui, T., Miki, T., Bigo-Marshall, H., Aaronson, S. A., and Benedict, W. F. The retinoblastoma gene functions as a growth and tumor suppressor in human bladder carcinoma cells. Proc. Natl. Acad. Sci. U.S.A., *88*: 5257–5261, 1991.
37. DeCaprio, J. A., Ludlow, J. W., Figge, J., Shew, J.-Y., Huang, C.-M., Lee, W.-H., Marsilio, E., Paucha, E., and Livingston, D. M. SV40 large tumor antigen forms a specific complex with the product of the retinoblastoma susceptibility gene. Cell, *54*: 275–283, 1988.
38. Whyte, P., Buchkovich, K. J., Horowitz, J. M., Friend, S. H., Raybuck, M., Weinberg, R. A., and Harlow, E. Association between an oncogene and an anti-oncogene: the adenovirus E1A proteins bind to the retinoblastoma gene product. Nature, *334*: 124–129, 1988.
39. Dyson, N., Howley, P. M., Münger, K., and Harlow, E. The human papilloma virus-16 E7 oncoprotein is able to bind to the retinoblastoma gene product. Science, *243*: 934–937, 1989.
40. Dyson, N., Buchkovich, K., Whyte, P., and Harlow, E. The cellular 107K protein that binds to adenovirus E1A also associates with the large T antigens of SV40 and JC virus. Cell, *58*: 249–255, 1989.
41. McCormick, F., Clark, R., Harlow, E., and Tjian, R. SV40 T antigen binds specifically to a cellular 53 K protein *in vitro*. Nature, *292*: 63–65, 1981.
42. Whyte, P., Williamson, N. M., and Harlow, E. Cellular targets for transformation by the adenovirus E1A proteins. Cell, *56*: 67–75, 1989.
43. Kerr, L. D., Miller, D. B., and Matrisian, L. M. TGF-β1 inhibition of transin-stromelysin gene expression is mediated through a *fos* binding sequence. Cell, *61*: 267–278, 1990.
44. Robbins, P. D., Horowitz, J. M., and Mulligan, R. C. Negative regulation of human c-*fos* expression by the retinoblastoma gene product. Nature, *346*: 668–671, 1990.
45. Kim, S. J., Lee, H. D., Robbins, P. D., Busam, K., Sporn, M. B., and Roberts, A. B. Regulation of transforming growth factor β1 gene expression by the product of the retinoblastoma-susceptibility gene. Proc. Natl. Acad. Sci. U.S.A., *88*: 3052–3056, 1991.
46. Lee, W.-H., Shew, J. Y., Hong, F. D., Sery, T. W., Donosco, L. A., Young, L.-J., Bookstein, R., and Lee, E. Y.-H. P. The retinoblastoma susceptibility gene encodes a nuclear phosphoprotein associated with DNA binding activity. Nature, *329*: 642–644, 1987.
47. Coffey, R. J., Jr., Derynck, R., Wilcox, J. N., Bringman, T. S., Goustin, A. S., Moses, H. L., and Pittelkow, M. R. Production and auto-induction of transforming growth factor-alpha in human keratinocytes. Nature, *328*: 817–820, 1987.

MULTISTAGE CARCINOGENESIS, C. C. HARRIS ET AL. (EDS.),
JAPAN SCI. SOC. PRESS, TOKYO/CRC PRESS, BOCA RATON, PP. 197–204, 1992

Transforming and c-*fos* Promoter/enhancer-stimulating Activities of a GDP/GTP Exchange Protein for Small GTP-binding Proteins

Yoshimi TAKAI, Kozo KAIBUCHI, Akira KIKUCHI, Masahito KAWATA, Takuya SASAKI, and Takeshi YAMAMOTO

Department of Biochemistry, Kobe University School of Medicine, Kobe 650, Japan

Abstract: There is a superfamily of *ras* p21/*ras* p21-like small GTP-binding proteins (G proteins). Small G proteins have GDP-bound inactive and GTP-bound active forms which are interconvertible by GDP/GTP exchange and GTPase reactions. The former and latter reactions are regulated by GDP/GTP exchange proteins (GEPs) and GTPase activating proteins (GAPs), respectively. We have isolated two types of GEP: one is a stimulatory type called GDP dissociation stimulator (GDS) and the other is an inhibitory type called GDP dissociation inhibitor (GDI). Among the GEPs thus far isolated, only *smg* GDS is active on Ki-*ras* p21. This GEP is also active on *smg* p21 and *rho* p21, but is inactive on Ha-*ras* p21. For the action of *smg* GDS, the post-translational processing of the C-terminal region of its substrate small G proteins is essential. Point-mutated Ki-*ras* p21 strongly transforms NIH/3T3 cells and markedly stimulates the c-*fos* promoter/enhancer in this cell line, whereas normal Ki-*ras* p21 is almost inactive in these activities. *smg* GDS induces the Ki-*ras* p21 activation which eventually leads to the transformation of NIH/3T3 cells and to the stimulation of the c-*fos* promoter/enhancer in this cell line. Thus, *smg* GDS plays an important role in regulating the activity of Ki-*ras* p21 as well as of other small G proteins.

There is a *ras* p21-related small G protein superfamily which consists of more than forty members (Table 1). Each of these members is composed of a single polypeptide with Mr values between 20,000 and 36,000 that has a consensus amino acid sequence responsible for GDP/GTP-binding and GTPase activities (*1*, *2*). Among these small G proteins, we have found *smg* p25A, -B, and -C, and *smg* p21A and -B. Small G proteins can be classified into at least four groups according to their primary structures and possible functions. As shown in Fig. 1, small G proteins have GDP-bound inactive and GTP-bound active forms which are interconvertible by GDP/GTP exchange and GTPase reactions (*2*). The former and latter reactions are regulated by GDP/GTP exchange proteins (GEPs) and GTPase activating proteins (GAPs), respectively (*2*, *3*). There are two types of GEP: one is a stimulatory type called GDP dissociation stimulator (GDS) and the other is an inhibitory type called GDP dissociation inhibitor (GDI) (*2*, *4*). GDS stimulates the dissociation of GDP

TABLE 1. The Small G Protein Superfamily

	ras	*rho*	*rab*	Others
Mammal	Ha-*ras*	*rho*A	*rab*1	*arf*1
	Ki-*ras*	*rho*B	*rab*2	*arf*2
	N-*ras*	*rho*C	*rab*3A/*smg*-25A	*arf*3
	R-*ras*	*rac*1	*rab*3B/*smg*-25B	*TC*4/*ran*
	ral	*rac*2	*smg*-25C	
	*rap*1A/*smg*-21A/K*rev*-1	G25K	*rab*4	
	*rap*1B/*smg*-21B	*TC*10	*rab*5	
	*rap*2		*rab*6	
	*TC*21		*rab*7	
			*rab*8	
			*rab*9	
			*rab*10	
			*rab*11	
			ram	
Yeast	*RAS*1	*RHO*1	*YPT*1	*ARF*1
	*RAS*2	*RHO*2	*YPT*2	*ARF*2
	*RSR*1	*CDC*42	*YPT*3	*SAR*1
			*SEC*4	*SPI*1
			*SAS*1	
			*SAS*2	
			*ryh*1	

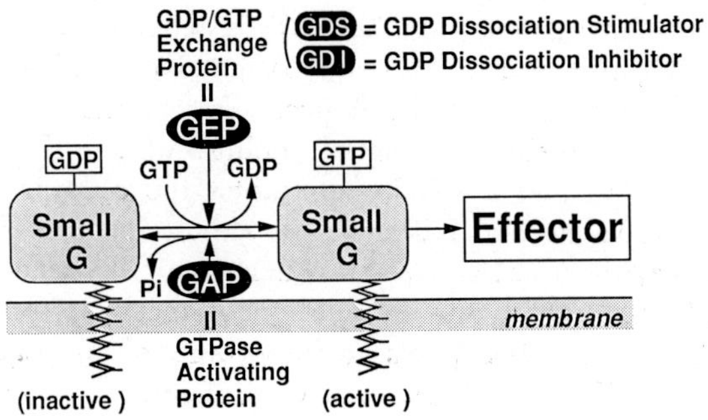

FIG. 1. Mode of activation of small G proteins.

from and thereby the subsequent binding of GTP to small G proteins, whereas GDI inhibits both reactions. The GTP-bound active form of small G proteins interacts with their specific effector proteins and thus exert their functions.

Among the proteins directly interacting with small G proteins, *ras* p21 GAP was first identified and has been well characterized (*3*). Point-mutated *ras* p21 is frequently found in human carcinomas such as colorectal carcinomas, lung carcinomas, and pancreas carcinomas. Point-mutated *ras* p21 is reduced in intrinsic GTPase activity and becomes insensitive to the GAP action (*3*). In this way, the GTP-bound active form of *ras* p21 is continuously produced in the cells expressing point-mutated *ras* p21, thereby inducing transformation of the cells. Moreover, the neurofibromatosis type 1 (NF1) gene has been shown to encode a protein having *ras* p21 GAP activity (*5*). It is likely that reduction of the activity of this NF1 protein

TABLE 2. Specificity of GEPs for Small G Proteins

	Ki-*ras* p21	Ha-*ras* p21	*smg* p21	*rho* p21	*rac* p21	*smg* p25A	*SEC4* p24	*rab*11 p24
smg GDS	+	−	+	+	+	−	−	−
smg p25 GDI	−	−	−	−	−	+	+	+
rho GDI	−	−	−	+	+	−	−	−

causes the continuous activation of *ras* p21. Following the discovery of *ras* p21 GAP, *rho* p21 GAP, and *smg* p21 GAPs were discovered (*2*).

In contrast to GAP, there are several reports suggesting the presence of GDS for *ras* p21, but in none of these cases has the protein been well characterized (2). In our laboratory, we have purified one GDS and two GDIs, cloned their cDNAs, and determined their primary structures: they are *smg* GDS, *smg* p25 GDI, and *rho* GDI (*2*). We first thought that these GEPs were specific for each small G protein: *smg* GDS for *smg* p21, *smg* p25 GDI for *smg* p25A, and *rho* GDI for *rho* p21, but have recently clarified that they are active on a group of small G proteins as shown in Table 2 (*2, 6*). Particularly, we found that *smg* GDS is active on Ki-*ras* p21 as well as on *smg* p21 and *rho* p21 (*6*). *smg* GDS is a single polypeptide with 558 amino acids and a calculated Mr value of about 61,000. We further found that *smg* GDS exhibits cell transforming and c-*fos* promoter/enhancer-stimulating activities in cooperation with Ki-*ras* p21 in NIH/3T3 cells (*7*). In this review article, we describe the function and mode of action of this *smg* GDS.

Two Actions of smg GDS

smg GDS is active on at least Ki-*ras* p21, *smg* p21, and *rho* p21 among many small G proteins (*6*). *smg* GDS forms a complex with both the GDP-bound and GTP-bound forms of each substrate small G protein at a molar ratio of 1: 1, and thereby stimulates the dissociation of GDP and GTP from and the subsequent association of both nucleotides with each substrate small G protein to the same degree in a cell-free system (*2, 6*). However, since the intracellular concentration of GTP is much higher than that of GDP, *smg* GDS may stimulate the GDP/GTP exchange reaction in intact cells. In the case of *smg* p25 GDI and *rho* GDI, interaction is only with the GDP-bound form of their substrate small G proteins (*2*). Ki-*ras* p21, *smg* p21, and *rho* p21 bind to membranes through a hydrophobic and polybasic C-terminal region as described below (*2*). *smg* GDS forms a complex with both the GDP-bound and GTP-bound forms of small G proteins, and thereby inhibits their binding to membranes and induces their dissociation from the membranes (*2*). Thus, *smg* GDS has two actions: one is to regulate GDP/GTP exchange reaction and the other is to regulate the translocation of small G proteins between the cytosol and membranes.

Post-translational Processing of Small G Proteins and smg GDS Actions

Small G proteins have unique cDNA-predicted C-terminal structures and undergo post-translational processing as shown in Fig. 2. Ki-*ras* p21, *smg* p21, and

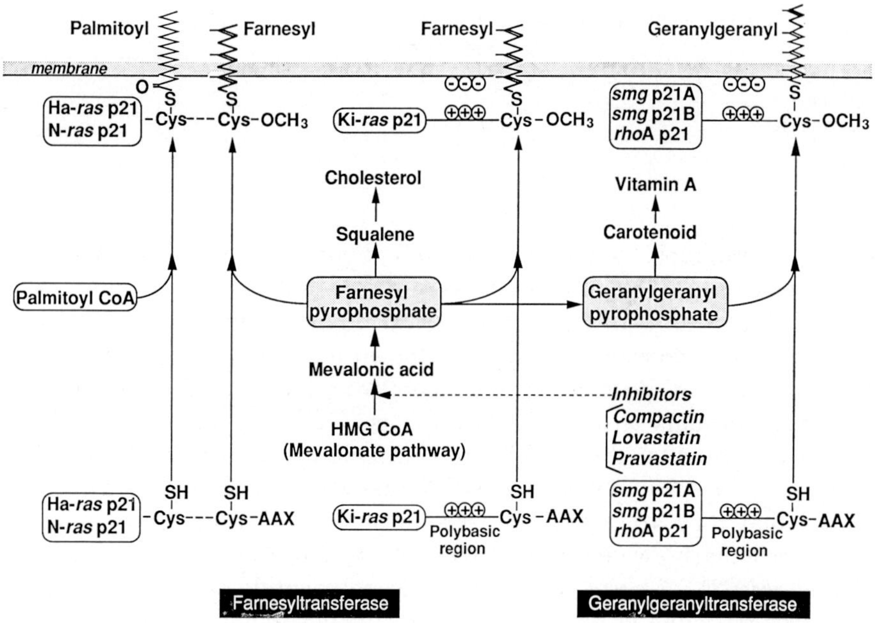

FIG. 2. Post-translational processing of the C-terminal region of small G proteins.

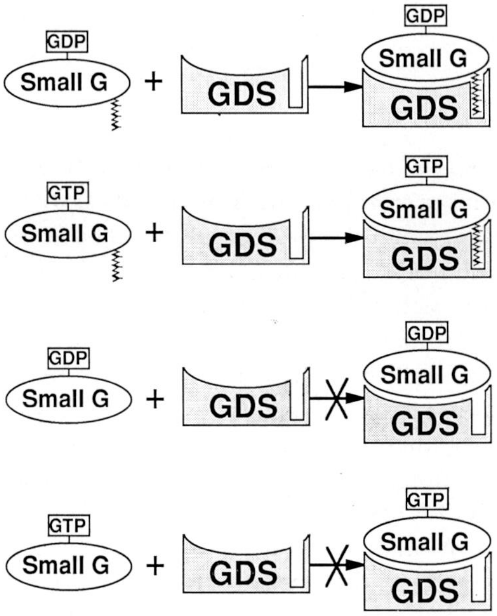

FIG. 3. Necessity of the post-translational processing of small G proteins for their interaction with *smg* GDS.

rho p21 have a CAAX C-terminal structure (A: an aliphatic amino acid; X: any amino acid). They are post-translationally modified: they are first farnesylated for Ki-*ras* p21 or first geranylgeranylated for *smg* p21 and *rho* p21 at the cysteine residue, the AAX portion is then removed by proteolysis, and, finally, the exposed cysteine residue is carboxyl methylated (*2*, *8*). All of these small G proteins have a polybasic region upstream of the prenylated cysteine residue (*1*, *2*). Ha- and N-*ras* p21s also have a CAAX C-terminal structure but lack the polybasic region and have a second cysteine residue which is palmitoylated (*2*). Among these steps of the post-translational processing, that of prenylation is the rate-limiting step. Phenyltransferases specific for *ras* p21, *smg* p21, and *rho* p21 have been identified and well characterized (*2*). *smg* GDS is active on the post-translationally modified form of its substrate small G proteins, whereas *smg* GDS is inactive on the post-translationally unmodified form as shown in Fig. 3. *smg* p25 GDI and *rho* GDI are also active only on the post-translationally processed form of their substrate small G proteins. In contrast, all the GAPs thus far reported including *ras* p21 GAP, *rho* p21 GAP, and *smg* p21 GAPs are active on both the post-translationally modified and unmodified forms of their substrate small G proteins.

Transforming Activity of smg GDS

Point-mutated Ki-*ras* p21 strongly transforms NIH/3T3 cells, whereas normal Ki-*ras* p21 is slightly active in this function (*1*). Overexpression of both *smg* GDS and Ki-*ras* p21 strongly transforms NIH/3T3 cells, whereas overexpression of either *smg* GDS or Ki-*ras* p21 alone transforms the cells only to a small extent (*7*). In the cells in which both *smg* GDS and Ki-*ras* p21 are overexpressed, the ratio of GTP to GDP attached to Ki-*ras* p21 increases in comparison with that in the cells in which only Ki-*ras* p21 is overproduced (*7*). These results indicate that *smg* GDS induces the Ki-*ras* p21 activation which eventually leads to the transformation of NIH/3T3 cells.

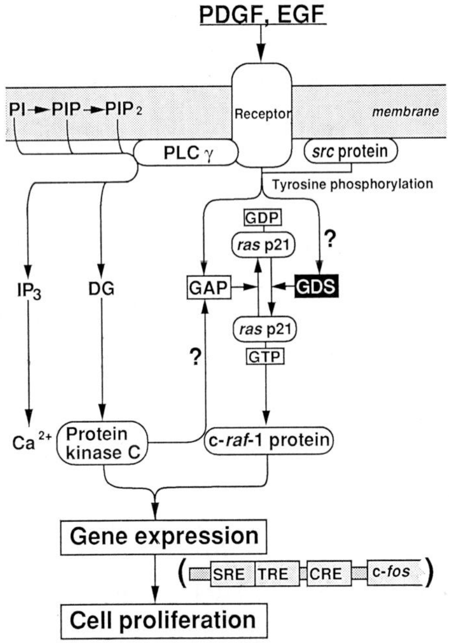

FIG. 4. Possible modes of activation and action of *ras* p21.

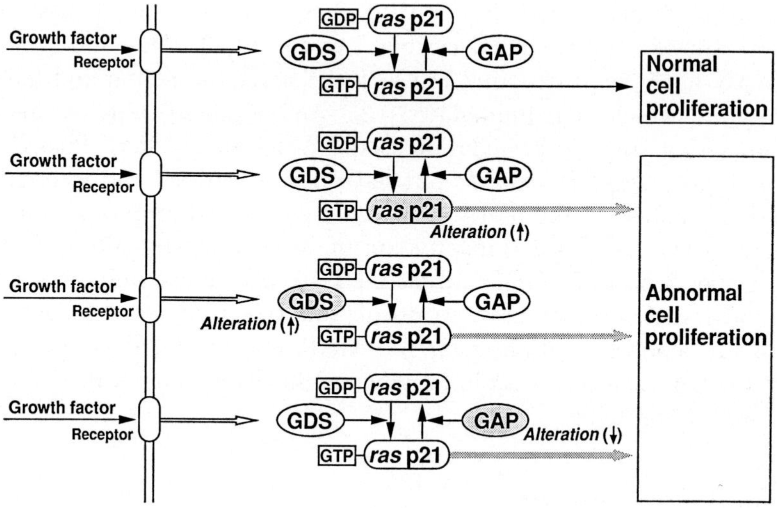

FIG. 5. Possible mechanisms of carcinogenesis through *ras* p21 and its regulatory proteins.

The *ras* p21 activity is regulated by the tyrosine kinase-type growth factor receptors, such as the PDGF and EGF receptors, and the non-receptor type tyrosine kinases, such as the *src* protein (Fig. 4) (*2*). In lymphocytes, protein kinase C also activates *ras* p21. There is increasing evidence that *ras* p21 is the down-stream of these intracellular signaling pathways. On the other hand, point-mutated *ras* p21 has been detected in 30–50% of various cancers including colorectal carcinomas and lung carcinomas. It is theoretically possible that either decrease in the *ras* p21 GAP activity or increase in the *smg* GDS activity causes the continuous activation of *ras* p21 as shown in Fig. 5. Consistently, the NF-1 protein has been shown to exhibit *ras* p21 GAP activity (*5*). Therefore, it is tempting to speculate that some abnormality may be present in *smg* GDS, which is always active on Ki-*ras* p21 even without a growth factor signal, in cancers whose *ras* p21 is not mutated.

c-fos Promoter/enhancer-stimulating Activity of smg GDS

We and others have previously reported that point-mutated *ras* p21 stimulates the c-*fos* promoter/enhancer in NIH/3T3 cells (*2*). Overexpression of both *smg* GDS and Ki-*ras* p21 markedly stimulates the c-*fos* promoter/enhancer in NIH/3T3 cells, whereas overexpression of either *smg* GDS or Ki-*ras* p21 alone only weakly stimulates it (*7*). This result, together with the fact that *smg* GDS activates Ki-*ras* p21 in both cell-free and intact cell systems, indicates that *smg* GDS induces the Ki-*ras* p21 activation which eventually leads to the activation of the c-*fos* promoter/enhancer (Fig. 4).

The c-*fos* promoter/enhancer element consists of at least a serum response element (SRE), TPA-response element (TRE), and cAMP-response element (CRE) (*9*). *ras* p21 stimulates both SRE and TRE but not CRE (*2*). Moreover, this *ras* p21 action is not mediated by protein kinase C or A (*2*). Protein kinase C stimulates both SRE and TRE, and protein kinase A stimulates CRE. The N-terminal truncated activated form of the c-*raf*-1 protein also stimulates the c-*fos* promoter/enhancer in NIH/3T3 cells (*2*). In this case again, this c-*raf*-1 protein stimulates both SRE and TRE but not CRE in a manner independent of protein kinases C and A (*2*). Increasing evidence indicates that the c-*raf*-1 protein may be the downstream of *ras* p21 and may mediate at least a part of the actions of *ras* p21 (*2*) (Fig. 4), but it remains to be clarified how *ras* p21 regulates the activity of the c-*raf*-1 protein.

Mode of Activation of Small G Proteins by smg GDS

It is not yet known how *smg* GDS activates Ki-*ras* p21 and *rho* p21, but *smg* p21 is phosphorylated by protein kinase A and activation of this phosphorylation is initiated by *smg* GDS (*2, 10*). *smg* p21B is phosphorylated by protein kinase A at Ser^{179} in the C-terminal region (*10*). This site is between the polybasic region and the prenylated cysteine residue. *smg* p21A also has a potential phosphorylation site in a similar region (*2*). The protein kinase A-catalyzed phosphorylation of *smg* p21 makes it sensitive to the two actions of *smg* GDS: stimulating the GDP/GTP exchange reaction of *smg* p21 and translocating it between the cytosol and membranes (*2, 10*). Thus, the protein kinase A-catalyzed phosphorylation of *smg* p21 initiates its activation by *smg* GDS. It should be emphasized that the signal from protein kinase A is not transduced to the regulatory protein of *smg* p21 but to *smg* p21 itself.

It is very interesting that both Ki-*ras* p21 and *rho* p21 have a potential phosphorylation site between the polybasic region and the prenylated cysteine residue in the C-terminal region. There are several reports that Ki-*ras* p21 is phosphorylated by protein kinases C and A (*2*). However, we were unable to confirm these earlier observations, and it is still not known whether these small G proteins are phosphorylated by protein kinase C or A or by an unidentified protein kinase.

ras p21 GAP has been shown to be phosphorylated at its tyrosine residue and to interact with the phosphotyrosine of the PDGF and EGF receptors through the *src* homology region 2 (SH2) domain of *ras* p21 GAP (*3*). However, it remains to be clarified whether this modification of *ras* p21 GAP affects its activity. At this time, it appears possible that the signal is transduced not only to *ras* p21 GAP but also to *smg* GDS. Further studies are necessary to establish how *ras* p21 is regulated by various growth factors.

REFERENCES

1. Barbacid, M. *ras* genes. Annu. Rev. Biochem., *56*: 779–827, 1987.
2. Takai, Y., Kaibuchi, K., Kikuchi, A., and Kawata, M. Small GTP-binding proteins. Int. Rev. Cytol., *133*: 187–222, 1992.
3. McCormick, F. *ras* GTPase activating protein: Signal transmitter and signal terminator. Cell, *56*: 5–8, 1989.
4. Kaibuchi, K., Mizuno, T., Fujioka, H., Yamamoto, T., Kishi, K., Fukumoto, Y., Hori, Y., and Takai, Y. Molecular cloning of the cDNA for a stimulatory GDP/GTP exchange protein for *smg* p21s, *ras* p21-like small GTP-binding proteins, and its characterization. Mol. Cell. Biol., *11*: 2873–2880, 1991.
5. Xu, G., Lin, B., Tanaka, K., Dunn, D., Wood, D., Gesteland, R., White, R., Weiss, R., and Tamanoi, F. The catalytic domain of the neurofibromatosis type 1 gene product stimulates *ras* GTPase and complements *ira* mutants of *S. cerevisiae*. Cell, *63*:

835–841, 1990.
6. Mizuno, T., Kaibuchi, K., Yamamoto, T., Kawamura, M., Sakoda, T., Fujioka, H., Matsuura, Y., and Takai, Y. A stimulatory GDP/GTP exchange protein for *smg* p21 is active on the post-translationally processed form of c-Ki-*ras* p21 and *rho*A p21. Proc. Natl. Acad. Sci. U.S.A., *88*: 6442–6446, 1991.
7. Fujioka, H., Kaibuchi, K., Kishi, K., Yamamoto, T., Kawamura, M., Sakoda, T., Mizuno, T., and Takai, Y. Transforming and c-*fos* promoter/enhancer-stimulating activities of a stimulatory GDP/GTP exchange protein for small GTP-binding proteins. J. Biol. Chem., *267*: 926–930, 1992.
8. Katayama, M., Kawata, M., Yoshida, Y., Horiuchi, H., Yamamoto, T., Matsuura, Y., and Takai, Y. The posttranslationally modified C-terminal structure of bovine aortic smooth muscle *rho*A p21. J. Biol. Chem., *266*: 12639–12645, 1991.
9. Verma, I. M. and Sassone-Corsi, P. Proto-oncogene *fos*: complex but versatile regulation. Cell, *51*: 513–514, 1987.
10. Hata, Y., Kaibuchi, K., Kawamura, S., Hiroyoshi, M., Shirataki, H., and Takai, Y. Enhancement of the actions of *smg* p21 GDP/GTP exchange protein by the protein kinase A-catalyzed phosphorylation of *smg* p21. J. Biol. Chem., *266*: 6571–6577, 1991.

GENETIC INSTABILITY AND MULTISTAGE CARCINOGENESIS

MULTISTAGE CARCINOGENESIS, C. C. HARRIS ET AL. (EDS.),
JAPAN SCI. SOC. PRESS, TOKYO/CRC PRESS, BOCA RATON, PP. 207–219, 1992

5-Methylcytosine as an Endogenous Mutagen in the p53 Tumor Suppressor Gene

William M. Rideout III,*[1] Gerhard A. Coetzee,*[2] Aria F. Olumi,*[1] Charles H. Spruck,*[1] and Peter A. Jones*[1]

USC/Kenneth Norris Jr. Comprehensive Cancer Center, Los Angeles, California 90033, U.S.A.[1] and *UCT/MRC Research Unit for the Cell Biology of Atherosclerosis, Department of Medical Biochemistry, University of Cape Town Medical School, Observatory 7925, South Africa*[2]

Abstract: Approximately 4% of cytosine residues in human DNA are modified post-synthetically into 5-methylcytosine (5mC) which is the only modified base present in vertebrate DNA. The function of 5mC is not fully understood, but methylation of promoter regions is often associated with transcriptional inactivity and may be part of a gene silencing mechanism. While undermethylation of promoter regions is correlated with expression, the same does not seem to be true for the remainder of genes since many genes are expressed while containing 5mC in their coding regions. This is significant because 5mC is known to be inherently mutagenic and it has been suggested that it is responsible for 30–40% of all human germline point mutations.

We have used direct genomic sequencing to examine the methylation status of CpG sequences which serve as potential methylation sites in the human p53 gene. These sites, which are known to be hotspots for mutations in several human cancers, were found to be methylated in the target human tissues examined. The results suggest that 5mC may play a substantial role as an endogenous mutagen in the p53 gene and that the generation of these mutations does not require the direct interaction of a carcinogen with DNA.

We have also compared the spectrum of p53 mutations reported in the literature for various human tumors. The patterns of mutations seen in different tumor types vary considerably and 5mC contributes to 63% of point mutations in colorectal cancer but only 13% in lung cancer. Mutations in lung cancer are therefore caused by a different mechanism than colorectal cancer and this presumably requires the direct interaction of carcinogens with DNA. Assessment of the proportion of 5mC induced mutations in the p53 gene therefore allows for an estimate of the relative importance of endogenous and exogenous mechanisms of carcinogenesis.

5-Methylcytosine, a Fifth Base in Vertebrate DNA

5-Methylcytosine (5mC) comprises on average about 1% of the base composition of vertebrate genomes. This modified base is found almost exclusively in the doublet

CpG (*1*) and nearest-neighbor studies show a strong suppression of this dinucleotide to one-fifth the level expected from simple base composition, and a corresponding elevation of TpG and CpA dinucleotides. These shifts in dinucleotide frequencies have been hypothesized to be due to an increased rate of mutation of 5mC to T due to spontaneous deamination (*2, 3*). However, it is quite likely that current CpG levels in vertebrate genomes represent an equilibrium state between their erasure by methylation driven mutation and the generation of new CpGs by other mutational events (*4*).

Regions of DNA within mammalian genomes that are not suppressed for CpG content are called CpG islands and are frequently associated with genes and gene promoters (*5, 6*). CpG islands are thought to escape methylation and subsequent mutation, thereby maintaining their existence (*5*).

5-Methylcytosine is synthesized after DNA replication by DNA methyltransferase, which transfers the methyl group from S-adenosylmethionine to the 5 position carbon in the pyrimidine ring of incorporated cytosines (*7*). Eukaryotic methyltransferases achieve site-specificity by methylating cytosines at the hemimethylated CpG dinucleotides generated during replication of methylated CpGs (*7*). This results in the propagation of specific methylation patterns from one cell generation to the next (*8*). However, the control and regulation of *de novo* methylation and demethylation are not known.

Potential Functions of 5-Methylcytosine

The best-known and well-characterized example of gene repression associated with extensive methylation occurs on the X-chromosome in the somatic cells of mammalian females (*9*). Cells achieve dosage compensation by inactivating almost all of one copy of the X-chromosome. Transfection of DNA from cell lines with the hypoxanthine phosphoribosyltransferase (HPRT) gene on an inactivated X-chromosome into HPRT deficient cells cannot confer resistance to HAT medium; therefore, the heavily methylated X-chromosome is transcriptionally silent (*10*). This transcriptional dormancy may be reliably maintained by cytosine methylation throughout the usually unmethylated CpG islands in the promoters of genes like PGK1 (*11*). Reactivation of the inactive PGK1 gene by 5-azacytidine, which is a powerful inhibitor of DNA methyltransferase (*12*), is accompanied by the demethylation of many CpGs within the promoter (*13*). This silencing of promoters by methylation provides normally irreversible regulation of the gene for the life of the animal.

Transcriptional repression by methylation has also been postulated in other systems. The addition of 5-azacytidine to immortalized embryonic fibroblast cell lines such as 10T1/2, induces the formation of several differentiated cell types including myocytes, adipocytes, and chondrocytes (*14–16*). The differentiation events correlate with the expression of previously silent determination genes, like MyoD (*17*), as well as cell type specific markers like acetylcholine receptors (*15*), in myocytes. These experiments imply that demethylation induced by the drug is causing the changes in phenotype, but this remains to be proven.

Transient transfection assays of various *in vitro* methylated or unmethylated genes have also demonstrated an irrefutable connection between methylation status and gene expression (*18–22*). This transcriptional silencing appears to be accomplished through direct or indirect mechanisms. The binding of some transcription factors to their target DNA sequences such as cyclic-AMP responsive element binding protein (CREB) (*23*) and c-*myc* (*24*) are inhibited by CpG methylation. On the other hand, the ubiquitous Sp1 transcription factor is not methylation sensitive and binds equally well to methylated and unmethylated target sequences (*25*). Indirect inhibition apparently occurs when the methyl-CpG binding protein (MeCP-1) binds to methylated sequences in or near gene promoters and blocks the access of transcription factors to the promoter (*26*).

5-Methylcytosine, an Endogenous Mutagen

The presence of 5mC in vertebrate genomes correlates with many possible beneficial functions, but it is becoming increasingly clear that 5mC bestows a significant mutational burden on vertebrates. The rates of spontaneous deamination of 5mC to T and C to U have been studied primarily *in vitro* by inducing deamination with heat and high pH. The extrapolated rates for 5mC and C deamination in ssDNA at the physiological conditions of 37°C and pH 7.4 have been estimated as 9.5×10^{-10} sec^{-1} and 2.1×10^{-10} sec^{-1}, respectively (*27, 28*). Methylation enhances the rate of deamination in single-stranded DNA by approximately 4.5-fold. The rates of C deamination, observed under the mild physiological conditions of a sensitive bacterial genetic assay, are 1×10^{-10} sec^{-1} and 7×10^{-13} sec^{-1} for ssDNA and dsDNA, respectively (*29*). Since the human haploid genome (6×10^9 bases) contains 1% 5mC and the rate of deamination of 5mC in dsDNA can be estimated as 3.15×10^{-12} sec^{-1} (4.5 times the deamination rate of C in dsDNA), this would yield about 16 5 mC deamination events per day per haploid genome. This frequency may be insufficient to account for the number of mutations observed at CpGs, however, it might be further enhanced by periods of single-strandedness occurring during replication and transcription.

Deamination of 5mC and C results in T-G and U-G mismatches, respectively. The later are efficiently repaired by uracil glycosylases that excise the aberrant base (*30, 31*). Mismatches of T-G are hypothetically more problematic to repair in the correct direction, since T is normally found in DNA. However, specific mismatch repair systems exist in both prokaryotes and eukaryotes that preferentially remove the T and restore the C: G base-pair.

Prokaryotes and eukaryotes have apparently evolved efficient repair mechanisms to cope with the increased mutational load created by 5mC. The very short patch repair mechanism (VSP), described for *Escherichia coli* requires the *vsr* gene (*32*). This mechanism recognizes T-G mismatches only in specific nucleotide sequences, which are associated with DNA cytosine methylase (Dcm) recognition sites. In bacteria deficient for the *vsr* gene and competent for *dcm* methylation, reintroduction of the *vsr* gene is able to reduce the rate of mutation at Dcm methylase sites by 4-fold (*32*). This demonstrates the value of having a mechanism to counteract the deleterious effects of 5mC. A thymine DNA glycosylase specific for G-T mismatches is found in HeLa nuclear extracts which depyrimidates the T followed by DNA polymerase β, filling in the apyrimidic excision gap (*33*). Previous studies

TABLE 1. Contribution of CpG to Human Germline Point Mutations

Gene	Disease	Transitions at CpG/ total point mutations	Reference
Factor IX	Hemophilia	70/194 (36%)	(*73*)
Low density lipoprotein receptor	Familial hypercholesterolemia	8/18 (44%)	(*74*)
Glucose-6-phosphate dehydrogenase	G6PD deficiency	4/9 (44%)	(*36*)

in vitro indicated that this repair mechanism in HeLa cells approached 95% fidelity for removing the T from a T: G mismatch (*34*). Despite specific mismatch-excision repair mechanisms a large number of mutations still occur at potentially methylated CpGs.

Germline Mutations

The enhanced mutability of CpG dinucleotides in vertebrates was first noticed by the fact that a preponderance of human restriction fragment length polymorphisms (RFLPs) are revealed by enzymes that contain CpG in their recognition sequences (*e.g.*, Mspl-CCGG, Taql-TCGA) (*35*). Their prevalence in detecting RFLPs supports the idea that CpGs and 5mC create mutational hotspots.

The hypothesis that methylated CpGs constitute mutation hotspots has been supported by the analysis of germline point mutations resulting in human genetic diseases. Table 1 lists a few of the many germline mutations in human genes which have been sequenced. The prominent role of CpG participation in more than 30% of point mutations is clearly evident and in a comprehensive review of 139 disease-causing mutations, 52 (37.4%) were in CpG sequences and 44 (31.7%) were of the type predicted by deamination of 5mC (*36*). These mutation frequencies indicate that approximately one-third of all genetic disease-causing mutations could be caused by 1% of the DNA bases acting as an endogenous mutagen. For this hypothesis to be correct, methylation must be present at the CpG sites in question. We showed that the CpG at codon 408 in the low density lipoprotein receptor (LDLR) gene, a position known to have undergone a germline mutation, is methylated *in vivo* (*37*). The high mutability observed throughout the LDLR locus is most likely in part due to the presence of methylated CpG residues.

Tumor Suppressor Genes

Carcinogenesis results from multiple genetic changes with chromosomal rearrangements and deletions, gene amplification, and point mutations all potentially contributing to tumorigenesis. Events which activate oncogenes such as the *myc* and *ras* gene families in a dominant fashion and promote cell growth and transformation have been well characterized (*38*). Recently genetic alterations that promote malignancy by the inactivation of genes necessary for maintaining cell normality have also been identified. These negative regulators of cell growth have been termed tumor suppressor genes. Several genes have been isolated as candidate

TABLE 2. CpG as a Hotspot for Germline Point Mutations in Tumor Suppressor Genes

Gene	Tumor	Transitions at CpG/ point mutations	Reference
Rb	Retinoblastoma	3/8	(*75*)
p53	Li-Fraumeni syndrome	2/6	(*76, 77*)
p53	Ependymoma	0/1	(*78*)
APC/DP2.5	Familial adenomatous polyposis	4/8	(*45, 79*)

tumor suppressor genes including the retinoblastoma (Rb) (*39–41*), Wilms' tumor (WT1) (*42, 43*), deleted in colorectal carcinoma (DCC) (*44*), DP2.5 adenomatous polyposis coli (APC) (*45–47*), neurofibromatosis type-1 (NF-1) (*48*), and p53 genes (*49*).

Germline Mutations in Tumor Suppressor Genes

Germline mutations have recently been found in several tumor suppressor genes which are thought to predispose patients for the development of certain cancers such as retinoblastoma and Li-Fraumeni Syndrome (LFS). Analysis of the few point mutations which have been published, once again underscores the prominent role of CpG in spontaneous mutation (Table 2). It is remarkable that of the total of 17 mutations so far reported 6 or 35% have occurred at CpG. The data in Table 2 are clearly too preliminary for detailed analysis but the role of CpG seems very similar to that for other human germline mutations (Table 1).

Somatic Mutations in a Tumor Suppressor Gene

The p53 gene is the most frequently mutated gene associated with adult tumors and chromosome 17p which harbors the gene is often reduced to homozygosity in tumors. Loss of heterozygosity detected by RFLP studies suggests that the p53 gene plays a prominent role in the tumorigenesis and progression of many of the most common types of adult tumors including lung, colorectum, bladder, brain, gastric, liver, ovary, endometrium, leukemia, and esophageal carcinomas (*50*). In bladder and colorectal carcinomas the loss of heterozygosity at 17p and the prior mutation of the remaining p53 allele are late stage events during tumor progression (*51–53*).

The 53-kD nuclear phosphoprotein, p53, appears to negatively regulate the cell cycle (*54*), but several of the characterized mutations that alter protein function also encourage cellular proliferation and led to the initial classification of p53 as an oncogene (for review see *49*). Mutations in p53 are not all equally effective in generating malignancy (*55*). Several mutations appear doubly injurious to normal cell growth because these mutant forms of p53 confer growth advantages in addition to destroying the normal growth suppressive function of p53 (*56*). Introduction of the wild-type p53 gene into colorectal carcinoma cells that have mutant p53 alleles suppresses their growth, providing direct evidence for the negative regulatory role for p53 (*57*).

The p53 gene has 5 highly conserved domains among fish, birds, amphibians, and mammals (*58*) and 98% of the mutations identified in tumors and tumor cell

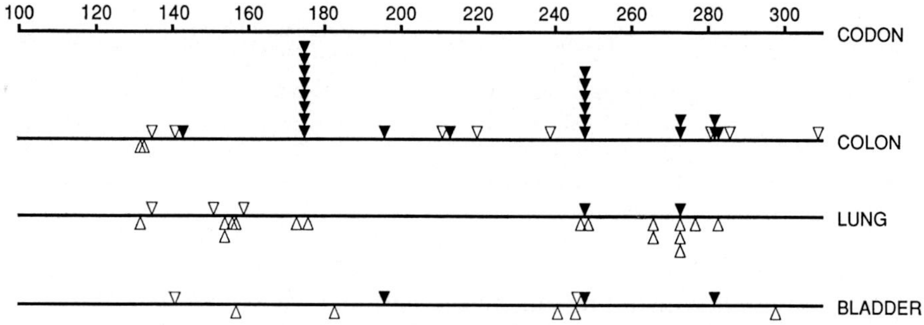

FIG. 1. Mutation patterns of p53 in common adult tumors. The pattern of point mutations in the p53 gene from colon (*53*), lung (*80*), and bladder (*51*) tumors is shown. Each arrow represents a single mutation at the codon indicated. Transitions are symbolized by downward pointing triangles, with the filled triangles marking transitions at CpGs. Transversions are symbolized by upward pointing triangles. The coding region of p53 from codons 100 to 310 is depicted which includes the four conserved domains where 98% of the p53 point mutations occur (*50*). We demonstrated that two of the three most frequently mutated codons or hotspots, 175 and 273, are methylated in genomic DNAs (*37*). (Reprinted with permission from Bioessays (*81*)).

lines are scattered throughout the four domains contained between codons 110 to 307 in exons 5 through 8 (*50*). This region of p53 is amenable to mutational screening by polymerase chain reaction-single stranded conformational polymorphism (PCR-SSCP) analysis which has become the preferred method for rapid detection of point mutations in tumor DNA samples (*59*). These inactivating mutations encompass transitions, transversions, and deletions, illustrating the ease of destroying gene function through several kinds of mutation. This contrasts with the limited number of point mutations that activate proto-oncogenes such as codons 12, 13, or 61 in H-*ras*. The domains of highly-conserved amino acids are crucial for the proper function of the p53 phosphoprotein and are also involved in the binding and inactivation of the protein by growth-altering viral proteins like SV40 large T antigen, adenovirus 5 E1b protein, and the E6 proteins of the human papilloma viruses 16 and 18 (*60–63*).

Somatic mutations in p53 have been studied in a wide variety of cancer types and the spectra of mutation varies strikingly among the different tumor types (Fig. 1). The percentage of transitions that concur with the model of 5mC-induced deamination events varies drastically from 67% in colon cancer to a low of 9.5% in lung cancer, whereas the percentage of transversions is 6.5% in colon cancer and as much as 76% in lung cancer. There are 22 CpGs in the 544 bases of exons 5 through 8, therefore, approximately 8% of the bases accounts for an average of 40% of the mutations in all three cancers and up to 67% of the p53 mutations detected in colorectal carcinoma. This specificity of p53 mutation with respect to tumor type is probably indicative of the etiology of carcinogenic insults the tissues experience. Comparing these mutations to the pattern of genetic disease causing point mutations (Tables 1 and 2) indicates that 5mC probably acts as an endogenous mutagen in both germline and somatic tissues.

Methylation at CpGs in p53 in normal tissues may account for the frequency of transitions at those sites prevalent in many diverse human tumors. On the other hand, transcriptionally active genes might be expected to be unmethylated because of the often observed inverse relationship of methylation and gene expression (*18, 19, 22*). However, many genes (such as HPRT and PGK) are expressed with 5mC in their coding sequences despite the often-seen relationship between gene inactivation and methylation (*64, 65*). The variability of methylation necessitates direct examination of the methylation status for CpG sequences observed to be hotspots for mutation. We directly examined the *in vivo* methylation status at several of the most commonly mutated CpGs in p53 by ligation-mediated polymerase chain reaction (LM-PCR) genomic sequencing (*11, 66*). Cytosine methylation was present at codons 175, 273, and 282 as well as all of the neighboring CpGs observed in white blood cell, sperm, and urothelial cell DNAs (*37*). These codons are mutational hotspots (*i.e.*, mutated in more than one tumor) in colon cancer and have also been shown to be mutated in several other tumor types (Fig. 1). The fact that these sites are indeed methylated *in vivo* supports the hypothesis that 5mC is an endogenous mutagen contributing to multiple recurrences of identical somatic mutations.

Molecular Epidemiology

The broad spectrum of mutation and tumor specific pattern of mutation in p53 makes it an attractive candidate for studies in molecular epidemiology (*67*). Many carcinogens function through direct interaction with DNA which result in definitive and characteristic mutations. For example, alkylating agents attack the O^6 position of guanine and result in transitions from G to A (*68*), benzo(a)pyrene, on the other hand, causes transversions of G to T (*69*), and melphalan predominantly generates A to T transversions (*70*). Tobacco-induced lung cancer frequently contains G to T transitions in the p53 gene which could be due to benzo(a)pyrene in cigarette smoke or to another of the many carcinogenic agents in tobacco. In hepatocellular carcinomas from areas with endemic hepatitis B and high exposures to aflatoxin B1 a specific transversion at codon 249, G to T, has been observed. This is consistent with the type of mutation aflatoxin B1 induces in experimental systems (*71, 72*). For cancers where there are no well-recognized experimentally-demonstrated carcinogens (*e.g.*, colon cancer, leukemias, and sarcomas), 5mC may be a predominant mutagen. The frequencies and types of point mutations in p53 found in these tumor types could then be compared to mutations occurring in tumors from populations with a higher than normal incidence of cancer (*67*). These comparisons could indicate the involvement of an exogenous mutagen participating in carcinogenesis for those at risk. For example, lung cancers from cigarette smokers may have a higher percentage of G to C transversions in the p53 gene, indicative of carcinogens that attack guanines, than lung cancers from nonsmokers or from those exposed to asbestos. The utility of the p53 gene for molecular epidemiology is due to several factors, (i) the ease of p53 inactivation by a multitude of possible mutations, (ii) the significant percentage of involvement in nearly every type of human adult cancer, (iii) the simplicity of screening for mutations in the highly conserved domains in exons 5–8 by PCR-SSCP, and (iv) the unique patterns of mutations seen in different tumor types.

Conclusion and Perspectives

The functions of 5mC remain debatable, but the magnitude of its role in both germline and somatic mutations is impressive. For both categories an average of nearly one-third of all point mutations that have been described are consistent with the model of spontaneous deamination-induced transitions at 5mC. We have shown the presence of methylation in the LDLR and the p53 tumor suppressor genes at hotspots for CpG transitions which provides supportive evidence for the model. The rate of mutation at CpGs in the germline in tumor suppressor genes and other genes is probably not easily perturbed because it is dependent on the endogenous mutagen, 5mC. This results in the consistent value of approximately 35% of all point mutations in the germline occurring at CpGs. In comparison, the overall contribution of presumably methylated CpGs to somatic mutations in the p53 gene in cancer is similar. These values reflect the predictable nature of deamination events at 5mCs. In contrast, the contribution of CpG to mutagenesis in a particular tissue or cancer can vary dramatically as seen in both lung and colon cancers (Fig. 1). This departure from the consistent nature of 5mC-induced mutations could indicate the involvement of exogenous carcinogens in a particular tumor type. In the case of colon cancer, alterations and instability in methylation patterns could enhance the rate of 5mC to T mutations. Exogenous agents that affect the rate of G: T mismatch repair in somatic tissues may also participate in carcinogenesis. Perhaps early-stage events that increase the rate of the cell division will result in more rapid accumulation of deamination-induced mutations. Faster cell division would provide less time for mismatch repair as well as an increased frequency of DNA in the single stranded form during replication, which would also enhance the deamination rate. For lung cancer, the slow accumulation of 5mC to T mutations is most likely overshadowed by the numerous exogenous mutagens present in cigarette smoke. Departure from the predicted background of 5mC-induced mutations in the p53 gene would provide clues about the prevalence of mutagens that act directly on DNA and clues about the nature of those interactions.

Acknowledgment

This work was supported by the United Cancer Research Society and by the National Cancer Institute (grant R35 CA49758).

REFERENCES

1. Doskocil, J. and Sorm, F. Distribution of 5-methylcytosine in pyrimidine sequences of deoxyribonucleic acids. Biochim. Biophys. Acta, *55*: 933–959, 1962.
2. Coulondre, C., Miller, J. H., Farabaugh, P. J., and Gilbert, W. Molecular basis of base substitution hotspots in *Escherichia coli*. Nature, *274*: 775–780, 1978.
3. Lindahl, T. and Nyberg, B. Heat induced deamination of cytosine residues in deoxyribonucleic acids. Biochemistry, *13*: 3405–3410, 1974.
4. Sved, J. and Bird, A. The expected equilibrium of the CpG dinucleotide in vertebrate genomes under a mutation model. Proc. Natl. Acad. Sci. U.S.A., *87*: 4692–4696, 1990.
5. Bird, A. P. CpG-rich islands and the function of DNA methylation. Nature, *321*: 15–21, 1986.

6. Gardiner-Garden, M. and Frommer, M. CpG islands in vertebrate genomes. J. Mol. Biol., *196*: 261–282, 1987.
7. Adams, R. L., Gardiner, K., Rinaldi, A., Bryans, M., McGarvey, M., and Burdon, R. H. Mouse ascites DNA methylase: characterization of size, proteolytic breakdown and nucleotide recognition. Biochim. Biophys. Acta, *868*: 9–16, 1986.
8. Wigler, M., Levy, D., and Perucho, M. The somatic replication of DNA methylation. Cell, *24*: 33–40, 1981.
9. Grant, S. G. and Chapman, V. M. Mechanisms of X-chromosome regulation. Annu. Rev. Genet., *22*: 199–233, 1988.
10. Liskay, R. M. and Evans, R. J. Inactive X chromosome DNA does not function in DNA-mediated cell transformation for the hypoxanthine phosphoribosyl-transferase gene. Proc. Natl. Acad. Sci. U.S.A., *77*: 4895–4898, 1980.
11. Pfeifer, G. P., Steigerwald, S. D., Mueller, P. R., Wold, B., and Riggs, A. D. Genomic sequencing and methylation analysis by ligation mediated PCR. Science, *246*: 810–813, 1989.
12. Jones, P. A. and Taylor, S. M. Cellular differentiation, cytidine analogs and DNA methylation. Cell, *20*: 85–93, 1980.
13. Hansen, R. S. and Gartler, S. M. 5-Azacytidine-induced reactivation of the human X chromosome-linked PGK1 gene is associated with a large region of cytosine demethylation in the 5′ CpG island. Proc. Natl. Acad. Sci. U.S.A., *87*: 4174–4178, 1990.
14. Constantinides, P. G., Jones, P. A., and Gevers, W. Functional striated muscle cells from non-myoblast precursors following 5-azacytidine treatment. Nature, *267*: 364–366, 1977.
15. Constantinides, P. G., Taylor, S. M., and Jones, P. A. Phenotypic conversion of cultured mouse embryo cells by Aza pyrimidine nucleosides. Dev. Biol., *66*: 57–71, 1978.
16. Taylor, S. M. and Jones, P. A. Multiple new phenotypes induced in 10T 1/2 and 3T3 cells treated with 5-azacytidine. Cell, *17*: 771–779, 1979.
17. Davis, R. L., Weintraub, H., and Lassar, A. B. Expression of a single transfected cDNA converts fibroblasts to myoblasts. Cell, *51*: 987–1000, 1987.
18. Vardimon, L., Kressmann, A., Cedar, H., Maechler, M., and Doerfler, W. Expression of a cloned adenovirus gene is inhibited by *in vitro* methylation. Proc. Natl. Acad. Sci. U.S.A., *79*: 1073–1077, 1982.
19. Stein, R., Razin, A., and Cedar, H. *In vitro* methylation of the hamster adenine phosphoribosyltransferase gene inhibits its expression in mouse L cells. Proc. Natl. Acad. Sci. U.S.A., *79*: 3418–3422, 1982.
20. Busslinger, M., Hurst, J., and Flavell, R. A. DNA methylation and the regulation of globin gene expression. Cell, *34*: 197–206, 1983.
21. Keshet, I., Yisraeli, J., and Cedar, H. Effect of regional DNA methylation on gene expression. Proc. Natl. Acad. Sci. U.S.A., *82*: 2560–2564, 1985.
22. Yisraeli, J., Frank, D., Razin, A., and Cedar, H. Effect of *in vitro* DNA methylation on beta-globin gene expression. Proc. Natl. Acad. Sci. U.S.A., *85*: 4638–4642, 1988.
23. Iguchi-Ariga, S. M. and Schaffner, W. CpG methylation of the cAMP-responsive enhancer/promoter sequence TGACGTCA abolishes specific factor binding as well as transcriptional activation. Genes Dev., *3*: 612–619, 1989.
24. Prendergast, G. C. and Ziff, E. B. Methylation-sensitive sequence-specific DNA binding by the c-Myc basic region. Science, *251*: 186–189, 1991.
25. Harrington, M. A., Jones, P. A., Imagawa, M., and Karin, M. Cytosine methylation does not affect binding of transcription factor Sp1. Proc. Natl. Acad. Sci. U.S.A., *85*: 2066–2070, 1988.

26. Boyes, J. and Bird, A. DNA methylation inhibits transcription indirectly *via* a methyl-CpG binding protein. Cell, *64*: 1123–1134, 1991.
27. Wang, R. Y., Kuo, K. C., Gehrke, C. W., Huang, L. H., and Ehrlich, M. Heat- and alkali-induced deamination of 5-methylcytosine and cytosine residues in DNA. Biochim. Biophys. Acta, *697*: 371–377, 1982.
28. Ehrlich, M., Norris, K. F., Wang, R. Y., Kuo, K. C., and Gehrke, C. W. DNA cytosine methylation and heat-induced deamination. Biosci. Rep., *6*: 387–393, 1986.
29. Frederico, L. A., Kunkel, T. A., and Shaw, B. R. A sensitive genetic assay for the detection of cytosine deamination: determination of rate constants and the activation energy. Biochemistry, *29*: 2532–2537, 1990.
30. Shenoy, S., Ehrlich, K. C., and Ehrlich, M. Repair of thymine•guanine and uracil•guanine mismatched base-pairs in bacteriophage M13mp18 DNA heteroduplexes. J. Mol. Biol., *197*: 617–626, 1987.
31. Ehrlich, M., Zhang, X. Y., and Inamdar, N. M. Spontaneous deamination of cytosine and 5-methylcytosine residues in DNA and replacement of 5-methylcytosine residues with cytosine residues. Mutat. Res., *238*: 277–286, 1990.
32. Lieb, M. Spontaneous mutation at a 5-methylcytosine hotspot is prevented by very short patch (VSP) mismatch repair. Genetics, *128*: 23–27, 1991.
33. Wiebauer, K. and Jiricny, J. Mismatch-specific thymine DNA glycosylase and DNA polymerase beta mediate the correction of G.T mispairs in nuclear extracts from human cells. Proc. Natl. Acad. Sci. U.S.A., *87*: 5842–5845, 1990.
34. Brown, T. C. and Jiricny, J. Different base/base mispairs are corrected with different efficiencies and specificities in monkey kidney cells. Cell, *54*: 705–711, 1988.
35. Barker, D., Schafer, M., and White, R. Restriction sites containing CpG show a higher frequency of polymorphism in human DNA. Cell, *36*: 131–138, 1984.
36. Cooper, D. N. and Krawczak, M. The mutational spectrum of single base-pair substitutions causing human genetic disease: patterns and predictions. Hum. Genet., *85*: 55–74, 1990.
37. Rideout, W. M. III, Coetzee, G. A., Olumi, A. F., and Jones, P. A. 5-Methylcytosine as an endogenous mutagen in the human LDL receptor and p53 genes. Science, *249*: 1288–1290, 1990.
38. Suarez, H. G. Activated oncogenes in human tumors. Anticancer Res., *9*: 1331–1343, 1989.
39. Friend, S. H., Bernards, R., Rogelj, S., Weinberg, R. A., Rapaport, J. M., Albert, D. M., and Dryja, T. P. A human DNA segment with properties of the gene that predisposes to retinoblastoma and osteosarcoma. Nature, *323*: 16–22, 1986.
40. Lee, W. H., Bookstein, R., Hong, F., Young, L. J., Shew, J. Y., and Lee, E. Y. Human retinoblastoma susceptibility gene: cloning, identification, and sequence. Science, 1394–1399, 1987.
41. Fung, Y. K., Murphree, A. L., T'ang, A., Qian, J., Hinrichs, S. H., and Benedict, W. F. Structural evidence for the authenticity of the human retinoblastoma gene. Science, *236*: 1657–1661, 1987.
42. Gessler, M., Poustka, A., Cavenee, W., Neve, R. L., Orkin, S. H., aud Bruns, G. A. Homozygous deletion in Wilms tumours of a zinc-finger gene identified by chromosome jumping. Nature, *343*: 774–778, 1990.
43. Call, K. M., Glaser, T., Ito, C. Y., Buckler, A. J., Pelletier, J., Haber, D. A., Rose, E. A., Kral, A., Yeger, H., Lewis, W. H., Jones, C., and Housman, D. E. Isolation and characterization of a zinc finger polypeptide gene at the human chromosome 11 Wilms' tumor locus. Cell, *60*: 509–520, 1990.
44. Fearon, E. R., Cho, K. R., Nigro, J. M., Kern, S. E., Simons, J. W., Ruppert, J. M.,

Hamilton, S. R., Preisinger, A. C., Thomas, G., Kinzler, K. W., and Vogelstein, B. Identification of a chromosome 18q gene that is altered in colorectal cancers. Science, *247*: 49–56, 1990.

45. Groden, J., Thliveris, A., Samowitz, W., Carlson, M., Gelbert, L., Albertsen, H., Joslyn, G., Stevens, J., Spirio, L., Robertson, M., Sargeant, L., Krapcho, K., Wolff, E., Burt, R., Hughes, J. P., Warrington, J., McPherson, J., Wasmuth, J., Le Paslier, D., Abderrahim, H., Cohen, D., Leppert, M., and White, R. Identification and characterization of the familial adenomatous polyposis coli gene. Cell, *66*: 589–600, 1991.
46. Joslyn, G., Carlson, M., Thliveris, A., Albertsen, H., Gelbert, L., Samowitz, W., Groden, J., Stevens, J., Spirio, L., Robertson, M., Sargeant, L., Krapcho, K., Wolff, E., Burt, R., Hughes, J. P., Warrington, J., McPherson, J., Wasmuth, J., Le Paslier, D., Abderrahim, H., Cohen, D., Leppert, M., and White, R. Identification of deletion mutations and three new genes at the familial polyposis locus. Cell, *66*: 601–613, 1991.
47. Kinzler, K. W., Nilbert, M. C., Li-Kuo, S., Vogelstein, B., Bryan, T. M., Levy, D. B., Smith, K. J., Preisinger, A. C., Hedge, P., McKechnie, D., Finniear, R., Markham, A., Groffen, J., Boguski, M. S., Altschul, S. F., Horii, A., Ando, H., Miyoshi, Y., Miki, Y., Nishisho, I., and Nakamura, Y. Identification of FAP locus genes from chromosome 5q21. Science, *253*: 661–665, 1991.
48. Xu, G. F., O'Connell, P., Viskochil, D., Cawthon, R., Robertson, M., Culver, M., Dunn, D., Stevens, J., Gesteland, R., White, R., and Weiss, R. The neurofibromatosis type 1 gene encodes a protein related to GAP. Cell, *62*: 599–608, 1990.
49. Lane, D. P. and Benchimol, S. p53: oncogene or anti-oncogene? Genes Dev., *4*: 1–8, 1990.
50. Hollstein, M., Sidransky, D., Vogelstein, B., and Harris, C. C. p53 mutations in human cancers. Science, *253*: 49–53, 1991.
51. Sidransky, D., Von, E. A., Tsai, Y. C., Jones, P. A., Summerhayes, I., Marshall, F., Paul, M., Green, P., Hamilton, S. R., Frost, P., and Vogelstein, B. Identification of p53 gene mutations in bladder cancers and urine samples. Science, *252*: 706–709, 1991.
52. Olumi, A. F., Tsai, Y. C., Nichols, P. W., Skinner, D. G., Cain, D. R., Bender, L. I., and Jones, P. A. Allelic loss of chromosome 17p distinguishes high grade from low grade transitional cell carcinomas of the bladder. Cancer Res., *50*: 7081–7083, 1990.
53. Baker, S. J., Preisinger, A. C., Jessup, J. M., Paraskeva, C., Markowitz, S., Willson, J. K., Hamilton, S., and Vogelstein, B. p53 gene mutations occur in combination with 17p allelic deletions as late events in colorectal tumorigenesis. Cancer Res., *50*: 7717–7722, 1990.
54. Martinez, J., Georgoff, I., Martinez, J., and Levine, A. J. Cellular localization and cell cycle regulation by a temperature-sensitive p53 protein. Genes Dev., *5*: 151–159, 1991.
55. Finlay, C. A., Hinds, P. W., Tan, T. H., Eliyahu, D., Oren, M., and Levine, A. J. Activating mutations for transformation by p53 produce a gene product that forms an hsc70-p53 complex with an altered half-life. Mol. Cell. Biol., *8*: 531–539, 1988.
56. Hinds, P., Finlay, C., and Levine, A. J. Mutation is required to activate the p53 gene for cooperation with the ras oncogene and transformation. J. Virol., *63*: 739–746, 1989.
57. Baker, S. J., Markowitz, S., Fearon, E. R., Willson, J. K., and Vogelstein, B. Suppression of human colorectal carcinoma cell growth by wild-type p53. Science, *249*: 912–915, 1990.
58. Soussi, T., Caronde, F. C., and May, P. Structural aspects of the p53 protein in relation

to gene evolution. Oncogene, *5*: 945–952, 1990.

59. Hensel, C. H., Xiang, R. H., Sakaguchi, A. Y., and Naylor, S. L. Use of the single strand conformation polymorphism technique and PCR to detect p53 gene mutations in small cell lung cancer. Oncogene, *6*: 1067–1071, 1991.
60. Lane, D. P. and Crawford, L. V. T-antigen is bound to host protein in SV40-transformed cells. Nature, *278*: 261–263, 1979.
61. Linzer, D. I. H. and Levine, A. J. Characterization of a 54K dalton cellular SV40 tumor antigen present in SV40 transformed cells and uninfected embryonal carcinoma cells. Cell, *17*: 43–52, 1979.
62. Sarnow, P., Ho, Y. S., Williams, J., and Levine, A. J. Adenovirus E1b-58 kd tumor antigen and SV40 large tumor antigen are physically associated with the same 54 kd cellular protein in transformed cells. Cell, *28*: 387–394, 1982.
63. Werness, B. A., Levine, A. J., and Howley, P. M. Association of human papillomavirus types 16 and 18 E6 proteins with p53. Science, *248*: 76–79, 1990.
64. Wolf, S. F., Jolly, D. J., Lunnen, K. D., Friedmann, T., and Migeon, B. R. Methylation of the hypoxanthine phosphoribosyltransferase locus on the human X chromosome: implications for X-chromosome inactivation. Proc. Natl. Acad. Sci. U.S.A., *81*: 2806–2810, 1984.
65. Keith, D. H., Singer, S. J., and Riggs, A. D. Active X chromosome DNA is unmethylated at eight CCGG sites clustered in a guanine-plus-cytosine-rich island at the 5′ end of the gene for phosphoglycerate kinase. Mol. Cell. Biol., *6*: 4122–4125, 1986.
66. Mueller, P. R. and Wold, B. *In vivo* footprinting of a muscle specific enhancer by ligation mediated PCR. Science, *246*: 780–786, 1989.
67. Jones, P. A., Buckley, J. D., Henderson, B. E., Ross, R. K., and Pike, M. C. From gene to carcinogen: a rapidly evolving field in molecular epidemiology. Cancer Res., *51*: 3617–3620, 1991.
68. Loechler, E., Green, C., and Essigmon, J. *In vivo* mutagenesis by O^6-methylguanine built into a unique site in a viral genome. Proc. Natl. Acad. Sci. U.S.A., *81*: 6271–6275, 1984.
69. Mazur, M. and Glickman, B. Sequence specificity of mutations induced by benzo[a]pyrene-7,8-diol-9,10-epoxide at endogenous APRT gene in CHO cells. Somat. Cell Mol. Genet., *14*: 393–400, 1988.
70. Wang, P., Bennet, R. A. O., and Porvirk, L. F. Melphalan-induced mutagenesis in an SV40 based shuttle vector: predominance of A.T to T.A transversions. Cancer Res., *50*: 7527–7531, 1990.
71. Hsu, I. C., Metcalf, R. A., Sun, T., Welsh, J. A., Wang, N. J., and Harris, C. C. Mutational hotspot in the p53 gene in human hepatocellular carcinomas [see comments]. Nature, *350*: 427–428, 1991.
72. Bressac, B., Kew, M., Wands, J., and Ozturk, M. Selective G to T mutations of p53 gene in hepatocellular carcinoma from southern Africa. Nature, *350*: 429–431, 1991.
73. Giannelli, F., Green, P. M., High, K. A., Lzier, J. N., Lillicrap, D. P., Ludwig, M., Olak, K., Reitsma, P. M., Goossens, M., Yoshioka, A., Sommer, S., and Brownlee, G. G. Haemophilia B: database of point mutations and short additions and deletions. Nucl. Acids Res., *18*: 4053–4059, 1990.
74. Hobbs, H. H., Russell, D. W., Brown, M. S., and Goldstein, J. L. The LDL receptor locus in familial hypercholesterolemia: mutational analysis of a membrane protein. Annu. Rev. Genet., *24*: 133–170, 1990.
75. Yandell, D. W., Campbell, T. A., Dayton, S. H., Petersen, R., Walton, D., Little, J. B., McConkie, R. A., Buckley, E. G., and Dryja, T. P. Oncogenic point mutations in the human retinoblastoma gene: their application to genetic counseling. N. Engl.

J. Med., *321*: 1689–1695, 1989.
76. Srivastava, S., Zou, Z. Q., Pirollo, K., Blattner, W., and Chang, E. H. Germ-line transmission of a mutated p53 gene in a cancer-prone family with Li-Fraumeni syndrome. Nature, *348*: 20–27, 1990.
77. Malkin, D., Li, F. P., Strong, L. C., Fraumeni, J. F. J., Nelson, C. E., Kim, D. H., Kassel, J., Gryka, M. A., Bischoff, F. Z., Tainsky, M. A., and Friend, S. H. Germ line p53 mutations in a familial syndrome of breast cancer, sarcomas, and other neoplasms. Science, *250*: 1233–1238, 1990.
78. Metzger, A. K., Sheffield, V. C., Duyk, G., Daneshvar, L., Edwards, M. S. B., and Cogen, P. H. Identification of a germ-line mutation in the p53 gene in a patient with an intracranial ependymoma. Proc. Natl. Acad. Sci. U.S.A., *88*: 7825–7829, 1991.
79. Nishisho, I., Nakamura, Y., Miyoshi, Y., Miki, Y., Ando, H., Horii, A., Koyama, K., Utsunomiya, J., Baba, S., Hedge, P., Markham, A., Krush, A. J., Petersen, G., Hamilton, S. R., Nilbert, M. C., Levy, D. B., Bryan, T. M., Preisinger, A. C., Smith, K. J., Su, L., Kinzler, K. W., and Vogelstein, B. Mutations of chromosome 5q21 genes in FAP and colorectal cancer patients. Science, *253*: 665–669, 1991.
80. Chiba, I., Takahashi, T., Nau, M. M., D'Amico, D., Curiel, D. T., Mitsudomi, T., Buchhagen, D. L., Carbone, D., Piantadosi, S., Koga, H., Reissman, P. T., Slamon, D. J., Holmes, E. C., and Minna, J. D. Mutations in the p53 gene are frequent in primary, resected non-small cell lung cancer. Lung Cancer Study Group. Oncogene, *5*: 1603–1610, 1990.
81. Jones, P. A., Rideout, W. M. III, Shen, J., Spruck, C. H., and Tsai, Y. C. Methylation, mutation and cancer. Bioessays, *14*: 33–36, 1992.

MULTISTAGE CARCINOGENESIS, C. C. HARRIS ET AL. (EDS.),
JAPAN SCI. SOC. PRESS, TOKYO/CRC PRESS, BOCA RATON, PP. 221–229, 1992

Endogenous Mutations and Cancer

Thomas M. Reid, Michael Fry, and Lawrence A. Loeb

The Joseph Gottstein Memorial Cancer Research Laboratory, Department of Pathology SM-30, University of Washington, Seattle, Washington 98195, U.S.A.

Abstract: We have analyzed two aspects concerning the relationship between mutations and cancer. Firstly, we consider the possibility that spontaneous mutations result from normal cellular processes. Errors in DNA replication, depurination of DNA, and damage to DNA by oxygen free radicals are important potential sources of endogenous mutations. Mutations produced by DNA polymerases *in vitro* are clustered, and consist predominantly of single-base substitutions. Analysis of termination sites during copying by DNA polymerase-α indicates that certain pause sites are associated with misincorporation of single non-complementary nucleotides, and thus pause sites could be associated with mutagenic hotspots. Depurination results predominantly in transversion mutations resultant from the incorporation of deoxyadenosine opposite abasic sites. Mutations resulting from oxygen free radical damage to DNA are predominantly single-base substitutions: C->T, G->C, and G->T being the most frequent. In addition, there is an unusual mutation that results from oxygen free radical damage to DNA, two adjacent cytidines being substituted by two thymidines.

The frequency of mutations observed in tumors appears to be much greater than that predicted from the known rates for spontaneous mutagenesis. Recent observations suggest that many human tumors contain four or more independent mutations. If these multiple mutations are each required for tumor development, then the occurrence of malignancies based on normal mutation rates would be exceedingly rare, and it may be necessary to postulate that tumors result from an increase in the rate of endogenous mutagenesis. Genes that are likely targets for inducing such a mutator phenotype include: DNA primase, DNA polymerases, enzymes involved in nucleotide metabolism, and genes that code for other processes that guarantee the partitioning of chromosomes during cell division.

Cytological observations indicate that the pathogenesis of cancer proceeds by sequential steps, from normal cells to pre-malignant foci to localized tumors, to invasive tumors, and finally to metastatic lesions (*1*). There is increasing evidence that these processes are associated with mutations. Firstly, we will consider possible sources for spontaneous mutations; we have investigated three mutagenic processes that occur at unusually high frequency, and thus have the potential to contribute to the spectrum of spontaneous mutation (*2*). Secondly, we will explore the possibility that tumor progression results from genetic instability (*3*). A progression of phenotypic changes have been described in many human tumors. These include somatic chromosomal abnormalities, as well as point mutations. The problem is the multiplicity of mutations may be greater than that which would be predicted from normal spontaneous mutation rates. We have postulated that the large number of mutations observed in many human tumors could be the result of the induction of a mutator phenotype in cancer cells (*4*).

Spontaneous Mutagenesis

While damage to cellular DNA by environmental chemicals is a key causal event in the etiology of certain human cancers, there are also endogenous cellular processes that produce the same types of damage. These endogenous processes could contribute to spontaneous mutagenesis and might also be a causal factor in carcinogenesis (*2*). Several processes that damage DNA and therefore could logically contribute to background or so called "spontaneous mutagenesis" have already been identified. As in the case of DNA damage by exogenous chemical agents, spontaneous damage would need to occur at a high enough frequency to exceed the cell's capacity for DNA repair. Only unrepaired DNA damage could be responsible for spontaneous mutations and, following the same logic, spontaneous cancers. In addition, mutations could be the direct result of misincorporations during DNA replication that were not corrected by post-synthetic mismatch correction mechanisms.

A model linking DNA damage to mutagenesis and carcinogenesis is presented in Fig. 1. In this model, random mutations result from misincorporations by DNA polymerases opposite unrepaired DNA damage. DNA damage occurring in cells that do not divide, such as neurons, cannot be propagated to successive generations and thus is not associated with malignancy. Also, mutations would not result from error-free DNA repair processes, nor from damaged DNA that is replicated without causing a change in the nucleotide sequence of the newly made DNA product. A major factor linking DNA damage to mutagenesis is the copying of damaged

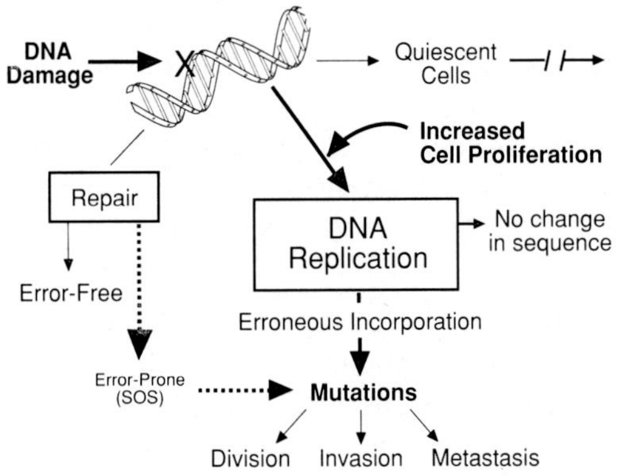

FIG. 1. A model that depicts the relationship of unrepaired DNA damage to mutagenesis and carcinogenesis. Factors that increase cell proliferation increase the frequency of copying past unrepaired DNA lesions during cell replication.

DNA by DNA polymerases during each cell division cycle; DNA polymerases copy past the damaged DNA and can insert non-complementary nucleotides opposite the site of damage. In procaryotes, SOS error-prone DNA repair synthesis (*5*) can be induced by DNA damage, possibly by facilitating replication past DNA lesions, but it is uncertain whether such a response exists in human cells. Mutation would be predominantly random, however some of these randomly distributed mutations would occur in key genes that alter the growth properties of cells, allowing them to escape homeostatic mechanisms that regulate cell division and in genes that might promote metastasis. In this scheme, any process that increases the likelihood of division in cells containing DNA damage would also increase the likelihood of mutations and malignancy. Stimuli for cell division could include increases in autocrine and paracrine growth factors, virus induced transformation, as well as regenerative stimuli brought about simply by the death of adjacent cells and tissues.

Oxygen Free Radicals

Among endogenous reactive species generated in cells with a high potential for damaging DNA are oxygen free radicals. Cellular processes that yield oxygen free radicals include: respiration, phagocytosis, cell injury and drug metabolism (*6*). Even though these radicals are short-lived, they react with diverse macromolecules in their environment. Damage to DNA by oxygen free radicals appears to be continuous and very extensive. Based on urinary excretion of two major products of DNA damage by oxygen free radicals, thymine glycol and 8-hydroxyguanosine, it has been estimated that reactive oxygen species introduce twenty thousand lesions in DNA in each somatic cell per day (*7, 8*). It seems probable that not every one of these 20,000 DNA alterations per cell is repaired prior to the onset of DNA replication.

Considering the postulated involvement of oxygen free radicals in major human disease (*6*), it is surprising that little is known about the mechanism of mutagenesis by oxygen free radicals. Studies on DNA damage and mutagenesis by oxygen free radicals have been hampered by a vast array of interactions. On the basis of alterations resulting from exposure of nucleosides to oxygen free radicals *in vitro*, it has been estimated that over 100 different types of modifications in DNA are produced by oxygen free radicals (*9*). As a result of this complexity, it has been difficult to assign a particular type of oxygen free radical or a specific modification in DNA as the causative factor that produces a specific type of mutation. To surmount this complexity, we have taken a different approach. We first established the types of mutations produced by exposure of biologically active DNA to oxygen free radicals *in vitro* (*10*), and then we have started to investigate the chemical lesions that are responsible for the specific mutation (*11*).

Studies on mutagenesis *in vitro* by agents that generate oxygen free radicals have used both reversion assays (*12*) and forward mutation assays (*13*). Reversion assays measure the frequency and types of mutations at a defined mutant locus on a DNA molecule. Forward mutation assays are inherently less sensitive, but provide a wide spectrum of mutations and sequence contexts produced as a result of DNA damage by oxygen free radicals. So far, our analysis indicates that many agents that

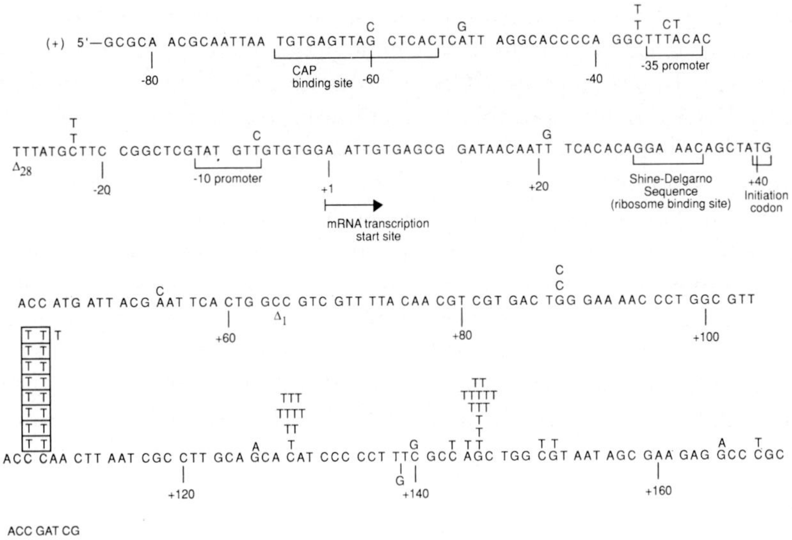

FIG. 2. Spectrum of mutations induced by copper. The DNA sequence of the viral strand of M13mp2 starting at the first nucleotide after the *lac*I termination codon and through the coding sequence of amino acid 47 of the *lac*Z gene is shown. Single-base substitutions are displayed above the wild type sequence and indicate the nucleotide found in the viral (+) strand. Deletions are shown below the viral sequence. Reproduced with permission (*15*).

TABLE 1. Frequent Mutations Produced by Agents that Generate Oxygen Free Radicals

Mutation	Percent of mutations			
	Cu (15)	Fe (10)	HL-60 (14)	Methylene blue (17)
C->T	34	20	9	1
G->C	4	39	21	60
G->T	26	18	21	25
T->C	4	6	11	8
CC->TT	15	0	6	0

All of the above spectra were obtained using the *lac*Zα gene. The numbers in parentheses refer to the original references.

generate oxygen free radicals cause mutations *in vitro*. This list includes transition metals (Cu^{+}, Fe^{2+}, and Ni^{2+}), myeloperoxidase and stimulated polymorphonuclear leukocytes (*14*). Using this forward mutation assay (*15*), one can detect a wide variety of nucleotide sequence alterations produced within a portion of the *lac*Z gene and its regulatory region. The mutagenic spectrum produced by exposure of DNA to copper *in vitro* is shown in Fig. 2. Of the mutations induced by Cu, 90% are single-base substitutions. Mutations are not random. There are hot spots at positions +107, +108, +129, and +145. Nucleotide sequence alterations at positions +107 and +108 were found to be tandem single-based substitutions. The presence of tandem single-based substitutions at adjacent cytidine residues may be diagnostic for mutagenesis by oxygen free radicals (*15*) and/or UV irradiation.

A tabulation of the types of mutations produced by different lesions that generate oxygen free radicals is given in Table 1. The C->T substitutions presumably are caused by damage to template cytidine residue, resulting in base pairing with dATP at high frequency. The G->C substitutions are presumably mediated by G: G base-pairs. The G->T transversions could be mediated by the formation of 8-hydroxy-guanosine which preferentially base-pairs with thymidine (*11, 18, 19*), or could be the result of a labile adduct that depurinates (*vide infra*). Tandem C->T substitutions have been detected frequently with copper (*15*) and with DNA exposed to oxygen bursts by differentiated HL-60 cells (*14*).

Abasic Sites

The chemical bonds within DNA are not entirely stable in aqueous solution. Depurination is the most frequent change, resulting in cleavage of the N-glycosylic bond leaving the phosphodiester backbone intact (*20, 21*). It has been calculated that each cell undergoes 10,000 depurinations per day (*21*). When DNA polymerases encounter abasic sites, they most frequently incorporate deoxyadenosine as a single-base substitution (*22*). Accordingly, if depurination is a major source of spontaneous mutations, then the spectrum of spontaneous mutations should be heavily biased towards substitutions by deoxyadenosine opposite template purines.

Errors in DNA Replication

In order for DNA replication not to be a key factor in spontaneous mutagenesis, DNA synthesis must be an exceptionally accurate process. During each cell division, some three billion nucleotides are copied in each human cell. The frequencies of misincorporation by purified DNA polymerases have been investigated extensively using both reversion and forward mutation assays (*23, 24*). The combined data indicates that DNA polymerases are highly error prone when compared to the low frequency of spontaneous mutations. The error rates of purified DNA polymerases vary from 1 in 5,000 to less than 1 in 1 million (*25*). The most frequent errors are single-base substitutions and, of these, transitions are more frequent than transversions. In addition to misincorporation during the course of DNA synthesis, we have recently demonstrated that pause sites by DNA polymerase-α, a major DNA replication and repair enzyme of mammalian cells (*23*), are associated with misincorporation at the 3′-terminal nucleotide of the growing DNA chain (*26*). This observation carries the possibility that *in vivo* mutational "hot spots" may, in some cases, be generated as a result of pausing by a replicating DNA polymerase. Such a possibility is testable, since genes with well defined highly mutable nucleotide clusters such as *ras* (*27*) or p53 (*28*) can be copied *in vitro* and the locations of sites for pausing and misinsertion can be evaluated.

Spontaneous Mutation in Eucaryotic Cells

Comparison of the frequency of the types of mutations produced by singular pathways *in vitro* with actual spontaneous mutations in cancer cells may yield important clues to the contribution of an individual pathway to mutagenesis and/or carcinogenesis. Studies on the spectrum of spontaneous mutations have mainly involved the insertion of recombinant shuttle vectors into eucaryotic cells, or the polymerase chain reaction (PCR) amplifications of specific endogenous chromosomal genes. Even though an analysis of endogenous genes with respect to malignancy is most pertinent, the spectrum of mutations recovered may be determined by phenotypic selection in culture. Nevertheless, studies on the non-essential gene, hypoxanthine phosphoribosyltransferase, indicate that the majority of spontaneous mutations in mammalian cells are G: C->A: T transitions (*29*). Studies on the *ras* genes in human cancers are restricted to a few loci (*27*). In the case of colon cancer, mutations occur predominantly at codon 12, and are predominantly single-base transitions, favoring replication errors or oxygen damage as a potential source. On the other hand, studies with the K-*ras* gene in human pancreatic adenocarcinoma yield a different result; the predominant changes are G->T transversions, suggesting depurination as a possible cause. The most extensive studies have been on the p53 gene. In hepatocarcinoma, the predominant substitution is G: C->T: A (*30*), and is compatible with aflatoxin-induced DNA damage (possibly *via* depurination), or damage by oxygen free radicals with the production of 8-hydroxyguanosine. Recent studies on squamous cell carcinoma reveal a high frequency of dinucleotide changes involving two adjacent cytidines mutated to two thymines. These unique mutations are compatible with mutagenesis *via* UV radiation or *via* DNA damage by oxygen free radicals. Conversely, it is interesting to speculate that the lack of this marker mutation among the p53 mutations that have been sequenced in internally located tumors argues against a significant contribution of oxygen free radicals to mutagenesis during tumor progression.

Mutations during Multi-stage Carcinogenesis

Current evidence indicates that multiple mutations are associated with the malignant phenotype. Sequential chromosome abnormalities have been reported in a variety of human cancers. Of human colon cancer, 25–50% have been shown to contain more than nine mutations (*30, 31*). It is conceivable that we are observing only a small fraction of mutations found in tumors, since most of our observations have relied on cytological changes that include genomic rearrangements, large deletions, and chromosomal loss.

A reasonable estimate for the overall frequency of mutations in human somatic cells is 1.4×10^{-10} mutations per nucleotide per cell generation. This estimate is based on reported frequencies of mutations in single copy genes, and on the frequency of electrophoretic mutational variant proteins at unselected loci (*4*). Moreover, the somatic mutation rate is similar to the human germinal mutation rate. If one assumes that any mutation can cause a tumor (the worst case scenario) and that human tumors asise in one or a few cells, then the potential target for oncogenic mutations is very large. If only one dominant mutation is required, then billions of tumors might arise spontaneously during a normal life span. A two mutational hypothesis yields a more realistic number. However, recent observations suggest that many human tumors contain four or more independent mutations (*4, 31*). If these mutations are required for tumor development, then the occurrence of malignancies based on normal mutation rates would be exceedingly rare. It may, therefore, be necessary to postulate that many tumors exhibit a mutator phenotype.

A number of explanations can be advanced to account for the multiple mutations leading to tumor progression. Firstly, cancer causing genes could contain sequences that mutate at exceptionally high frequencies. These "hot spots" could be due to the nucleotide sequence of DNA or due to pause sites during DNA replication. However, based on estimates of enhanced mutagenesis at known "hot spots", the contribution of "hot spots" would be at most 10^4 times greater than the average mutation frequency per nucleotide per genome (*4*), and thus is unlikely to be a major factor in multiple mutations that appear in human cancers. Secondly, a single mutagenic event could cause multiple locus deletions that inactivate a series of adjacent genes, including tumor suppressor genes, and there is evidence to support the hypothesis that deletions are important in the inactivation of tumor suppressor genes (*32*); however, a preponderance of deletions in the spontaneous mutation spectrum of human tumor cells remains to be demonstrated. On the other hand, the presence of large numbers of deletions specifically in cancer cells might be mediated by the activation of a unique mechanism in these cells. Thirdly, continued DNA damage by exogenous chemicals may be constantly occurring in cancer cells, and these cells may be defective in the repair of this damage. However, there is no reason to hypothesize that DNA in tumor cells is particularly susceptible to damage by chemical carcinogens. In fact, human cancer cells are frequently more resistant to the lethal effects of many chemical carcinogens. Fourthly, each mutation could confer a selective advantage. After each mutation, there could be an expansion of the mutant population to provide a large clonal population of target cells for the next mutagenic event. Considering the clonal origin of cancer (*33*), such a selective mechanism is likely to be important in tumor progression. Selective clonal expansion is likely to account for some of the multiplicity of mutations that are observed in tumors. However, there are difficulties in interpretation. In the case of tumor suppressor genes, one would have to postulate that a single mutation at a recessive locus imparts to these hemizygous mutant cells a major selective growth advantage.

The alternate attractive hypothesis to account for the high frequency of mutations observed in cancer cells is the involvement of a mutator phenotype. Evidence to support a higher frequency of mutagenesis in cancer cells compared to normal cells is controversial (*34*, *35*). If a mutagenic phenotype underlies these mutations, then important targets for tumor progression would be genes required to maintain the normal sequence of DNA, as well as the stringent location of genes within each chromosome, and the accurate segregation of chromosomes during cell division. Putative genes that could be damaged during tumor progression include those that encode DNA polymerases, enzymes involved in the metabolism of deoxynucleotides, proteins involved in the correction of errors during DNA replication, proteins involved in DNA repair, and as yet unidentified genes that guarantee the proper partitioning of chromosomes during the cell cycle. In total, there may be some 50–100 target genes that could affect the accumulation of mutations during tumor progression.

Acknowledgments

This work was supported by an OIG grant, CA39903, to LAL and a postdoctoral fellowship to TMR, CA08855, from the National Cancer Institute, and grants from the United States—Israel Binational Fund, the Fund for Basic Research administered by the Israel Academy of Science and Humanities and the Israel Cancer Association to MF.

MF is currently at the Rappaport Institute for Research in the Medical Sciences, Technion —Israel Institute of Technology, Haifa, Israel.

REFERENCES

1. Foulds, L. The experimental study of tumor progression: A review. Cancer Res., *14*: 327–339, 1954.
2. Loeb, L. A. Endogenous carcinogenesis: Molecular oncology into the Twenty-first century—Presidential Address. Cancer Res., *49*: 5489–5496, 1989.
3. Nowell, P. C. The clonal evolution of tumor cell populations. Science, *194*: 23–28, 1976.
4. Loeb, L. A. Mutator phenotype may be required for multistage carcinogenesis. Cancer Res., *51*: 3075–3079.
5. Walker, G. C. Mutagenesis and inducible response to deoxyribonucleic acid damage in *Escherichia coli*. Microbiol. Rev., *48*: 60–93, 1984.
6. Klebanoff, S. J. Phagocytic cells: Products of oxygen metabolism. *In*; J. I. Gallin, I. M. Goldstein, and R. Snyderman (eds.), Inflammation: Basic Principles and Clinical Correlates, pp. 391–444, Raven Press, New York, 1988.
7. Cathcart, R., Scheiers, E., Saul, R. L., and Ames, B. N. Thymine glycol and thymidine glycol in human and rat urine: A possible assay for oxidative DNA damage. Proc. Natl. Acad. Sci. U.S.A., *81*: 5633–5637, 1984.
8. Shigenaga, M. K., Cimeno, C. J., and Ames, B. N. Urinary 8-hydroxy-2′deoxy-guanosine as a biological marker of *in vivo* oxidative DNA damage. Proc. Natl. Acad. Sci. U.S.A., *86*: 9697–9701, 1989.
9. Hutchinson, F. Chemical changes induced in DNA by ionizing radiation. Prog. Nucl. Acid Res. Mol. Biol., *32*: 115–154, 1985.
10. McBride, T. J., Preston, B. D., and Loeb, L. A. Mutagenic spectrum resulting from DNA damage by oxygen radicals. Biochemistry, *30*: 207–213, 1991.
11. Cheng, K. C., Cahill, D. S., Kasai, H., Nishimura, S., and Loeb, L. A. 8-hydroxy-guanine, an abundant form of oxidative DNA damage, causes G—>T and A—>C substitutions. J. Biol. Chem., *267*: 166–172, 1992.
12. Loeb, L. A., James, E. A., Waltersdorph, A. M., and Klebanoff, S. J. Mutagenesis by the autoxidation of iron using isolated DNA. Proc. Natl. Acad. Sci. U.S.A., *85*: 3918–3922, 1988.
13. Kunkel, T. A. Mutational specificity of depurination. Proc. Natl. Acad. Sci. U.S.A., *81*: 1494–1498, 1984.
14. Reid, T. M. and Loeb, L. A. Mutagenic specificity of oxygen radicals produced by human leukemia cells. Cancer Res., *52*: 1082–1086, 1992.
15. Tkeshelashvili, T. K., McBride, T. J., Spence, K., and Loeb, L. A. Mutation spectrum of copper-induced DNA damage. J. Biol. Chem., *266*: 6401–6406, 1991.
16. Schaaper, R. M., Danforth, B. N., and Glickman, B. W. Mechanisms of spontaneous mutagenesis: An analysis of the spectrum of spontaneous mutation in the *E. coli lac*I gene. J. Mol. Biol., *189*: 273–284, 1986.
17. McBride, T. J., Schneider, J. E., Floyd, R. E., and Loeb, L. A. Unpublished results.
18. Wood, M. L., Dizdaroglu, M., Gajewski, E., and Essigmann, J. M. Mechanistic studies of ionizing radiation and oxidative mutagenesis: genetic effects of a single 8-hydroxy-guanine (7-hydro-8-oxoguanine) residue inserted at a unique site in a viral genome. Biochemistry, *29*: 7024–7032, 1990.
19. Shibutani, S., Takeshita, M., and Grollman, A. O. Insertion of specific bases during

DNA synthesis past the oxidation-damaged base 8-oxo-dG. Nature, *349*: 431–434, 1991.
20. Lindahl, T. and Andersson, A. Rate of chain breakage at apurinic sites in double-stranded deoxyribonucleic acid. Biochemistry, *11*: 3618–3623, 1972.
21. Loeb, L. A. and Preston, B. D. Mutagenesis by apurinic/apyrimidinic sites. Annu. Rev. Genet., *20*: 201–230, 1986.
22. Schaaper, R. M., Kunkel, T. A., and Loeb, L. A. Infidelity of DNA synthesis associated with bypass of apurinic sites. Proc. Natl. Acad. Sci. U.S.A., *80*: 487–491, 1983.
23. Fry, M. and Loeb, L. A. Mammalian DNA Polymerases, CRC Press, Boca Raton, 1986.
24. Reyland, M. and Loeb, L. A. On the fidelity of DNA replication: XX. Isolation of high fidelity DNA polymerase-primase complexes by immunoaffinity chromatography. J. Biol. Chem., *262*: 10824–10830, 1987.
25. Kunkel, T. A. Exonucleolytic proofreading. Cell, *53*: 837–840, 1988.
26. Fry, M. and Loeb, L. A. A DNA polymerase-α pause site is a hot spot for nucleotide misinsertion. Proc. Natl. Acad. Sci. U.S.A., *89*: 763–767, 1992.
27. Bos, J. The *ras* gene family and human carcinogenesis. Mutat. Res., *195*: 255–271, 1988.
28. Levine, A. L., Momand, J., and Finlay, C. A. The p53 tumor suppressor gene. Nature, *351*: 453–456, 1991.
29. Albertini, R. J., Nicklas, J. A., O'Neill, J. P., and Robison, S. H. *In vivo* somatic mutations in humans: measurement and analysis. Annu. Rev. Genet., *24*: 305–326, 1990.
30. Hollstein, M., Sidransky, D., Vogelstein, B., and Harris, C. C. p53 mutations in human cancers. Science, *253*: 49–53, 1991.
31. Fearon, E. R. and Vogelstein, B. A genetic model for colorectal tumorigenesis. Cell, *61*: 759–767, 1990.
32. Kaden, D., Gadi, I. K., Bardwell, L., Gelman, R., and Sager, R. Spontaneous mutation rates of tumorigenic and nontumorigenic Chinese hamster embryo fibroblast cell lines. Cancer Res., *49*: 3374–3379, 1989.
33. Fialkow, P. J. The origin and development of human tumors studied with cell markers. N. Engl. J. Med., *291*: 26–35, 1974.
34. Elmore, E., Kakunaga, T., and Barrett, J. C. Comparison of spontaneous mutation rates of normal and chemically transformed human skin fibroblasts. Cancer Res., *43*: 1650–1655, 1983.
35. Seshadri, R., Kutlaca, R. J., Trainor, K., Matthews, C., and Morley, A. A. Mutation rate of normal and malignant human lymphocytes. Cancer Res., *47*: 407–409, 1987.

MULTISTAGE CARCINOGENESIS, C. C. HARRIS ET AL. (EDS.),
JAPAN SCI. SOC. PRESS, TOKYO/CRC PRESS, BOCA RATON, PP. 231–238, 1992

Mammalian G2 Regulatory Genes and Their Possible Involvement in Genetic Instability in Cancer Cells

Hiroto OKAYAMA,[*1,*2] Akihisa NAGATA,[*1] Makoto IGARASHI,[*2]
Kimihiko SUTO,[*1] and Shigeki JINNO[*1]

Department of Molecular Genetics, Research Institute for Microbial Diseases, Osaka University, Osaka 565, Japan [*1] *and The Okayama Cell Switching Project, ERATO, Kyoto 606, Japan*[*2]

Abstract: In the fission yeast *Schizosaccharomyces pombe*, mitosis is initiated following the activation of the *cdc2*$^+$/cyclin B kinase. The *cdc2*$^+$/cyclin B kinase is positively regulated by *cdc25*$^+$ tyrosine phosphatase and negatively regulated by *wee1*$^+$/*mik1*$^+$ tyrosine kinases.

This regulatory system is evolutionarily conserved throughout higher eukaryotes. *Drosophila* and humans contain a *cdc25*$^+$ gene homolog called String and CDC25Hs (hereafter referred to as CDC25Hu1), respectively. We recently cloned a *wee1*$^+$ homolog (WEE1Hu) and two additional *cdc25*$^+$ homologs (CDC25Hu2 and CDC25Hu3) from human cells. Consequently, human cells contain at least one *wee1*$^+$ and three *cdc25*$^+$ homologs. Both CDC25Hu1 and CDC25Hu2 resemble the *cdc25*$^+$ gene not only in structure and function but also in the mode of expression. They are expressed mostly in G2. On the other hand, CDC25Hu3 is expressed mostly in early S, indicating that it has some novel function in the early phase of the cell cycle. In all the cell lines examined, CDC25Hu2 is expressed to a greater extent than CDC25Hu1 or CDC25Hu3. The expression of CDC25Hu2 is particularly high in various cancer cells including those transformed by SV40 or human papilloma virus type 16 E6, E7, both of which are well known for their ability to induce genomic instability. In addition, there is a noticeable correlation between the extent of aneuploidy and the level of CDC25Hu2 expression in the cancer cells examined.

In view of the fact that overexpression of *cdc25*$^+$ under certain conditions induces genomic instability in the fission yeast, overexpression of CDC25Hu2 associated with many cancer cells might play at least a role in the induction of their chromosomal abnormalities.

The G2 phase of the cell cycle is the period when the timing of entry into mitosis is regulated through a complex biochemical process. This commitment process is controlled by at least two physiological conditions: 1) the completion of DNA replication and 2) nutrient availability (*1*). The first manifestation of cell commitment to enter mitosis is the activation of the *cdc2*$^+$/cyclin B kinase (*2–4*). The activity of *cdc2*$^+$ kinase is regulated by post-translational modifications and by association with cyclin B protein. *cdc2*$^+$ kinase becomes phosphorylated at threonine 167 early in the cell cycle followed by binding to cyclin B protein (*5*, *6*). The cyclin-bound, phosphorylated *cdc2*$^+$ kinase is further phosphorylated at the tyrosine 15 residue (and threonine 14 in mammalian cells) to become an inactive form (*5*, *6*). The inactive *cdc2*$^+$ kinase is activated by dephosphorylation at tyrosine 15 (and also at threonine 14 in mammalian cells) (*7*, *8*). In *Schizosaccharomyces pombe*, a set of genes that includes *cdc25*$^+$, *wee1*$^+$, *mik1*$^+$, and *nim1*$^+$ participates in this regulatory process (Fig. 1). *wee1*$^+$, a mitotic inhibitor encoding a specific tyrosine kinase, mediates a signal for nutrient availability/cell size, and inhibits *cdc2*$^+$/cyclin B kinase by presumably phosphorylating the tyrosine 15 residue (*9*). *wee1*$^+$ has a functionally redundancy to another kinase *mik1*$^+$ (*10*) and is, in turn, negatively regulated by *nim1*$^+$ kinase (*11*). *cdc25*$^+$, a mitotic inducer encoding a specific tyrosine phosphatase, mediates a signal for the completion of DNA synthesis and activates *cdc2*$^+$ kinase by dephosphorylating the tyrosine 15 residue (*12*, *13*).

This regulatory system is evolutionarily conserved throughout higher eukaryotes. All the eukaryotes so far investigated have *cdc2*$^+$ kinase and cyclins. Homologs of *cdc25*$^+$ have been found in *Saccharomyces cerevisiae*, *Drosophila* and humans (*14*–18) and a homolog of *wee1*$^+$ in humans (*19*). All these homologs are structurally and functionally similar to the *S. pombe* genes.

Structure and Biological Activity of a Human Homolog of wee1$^+$

The human *wee1*$^+$ homolog cDNA (WEE1Hu) we cloned is 2.8 kb long and encodes a 49 kDa protein with a typical serine/threonine kinase domain in the middle of the coding region. The kinase domain is essential for its function: any deletion or insertion that influences the kinase domain resulted in complete inactivation of complementation activity. Among protein kinases, WEE1Hu has the highest amino acid homology with *wee1*$^+$ (29%) and *mik1*$^+$ (24%). Whereas the *mos* and *raf* oncogenes also have significant homology with WEE1Hu, they cannot complement a *wee1* mutation.

WEE1Hu shares remarkable similarity in function with the *wee1*$^+$ gene. WEE1Hu

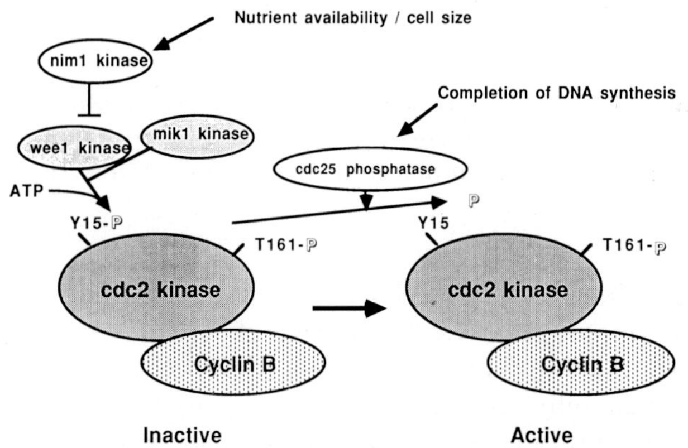

FIG. 1. Regulation of the *cdc2*$^+$/cyclin B protein kinase in *S. pombe*.

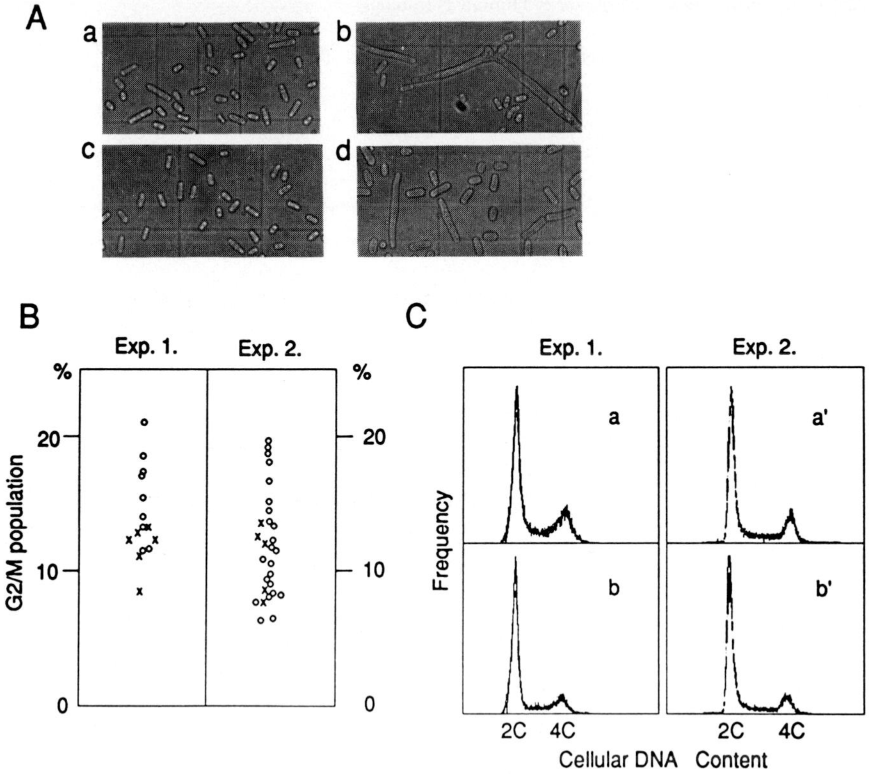

FIG. 2. Effects of WEE1Hu overexpression on yeast and rat cells. A. Effect of WEE1Hu overexpression on wild type *S. pombe*. a, b, c, and d: cells transfected with pcL-WEE1Hu (SV40 promoter) (a), pcMVL-WEE1Hu (human cytomegalovirus promoter) (b), pcMVL-WEE1Hu with a frameshift at the EcoT22I site (c), or the *S. pombe wee1*$^+$ gene inserted in the pAL-SK vector (d). B and C. Effect of WEE1Hu overexpression on the G2/M population of rat cells. Circles and crosses represent independent colonies stably transfected, respectively, with either pcD2-WEE1Hu or pcD2-fsEcoT22I (a frameshift mutant of WEE1Hu, see Fig. 3) (or pcDneo in Exp. 1) as a negative control. Colonies with the highest G2/M population were chosen from those transfected with WEE1Hu and from the control cells obtained in the two separate experiments, and their actual analysis patterns are shown in C. 2C and 4C represent the G1 and G2/M phases, respectively.

very effectively complements an *S. pombe* strain with a temperature-sensitive *wee1* mutation which either overproduces *cdc25*$^+$ or contains the *cdc2*-3w mutation. Overexpression of the *wee1*$^+$ gene in wild-type *S. pombe* strongly inhibits G2 to M progression, and, as a result, highly elongated cells are formed (Fig. 2) (*19*). Overexpression of WEE1Hu in *S. pombe* led to the formation of similarly elongated cells. WEE1Hu has a similar effect on mammalian cells. Expression of WEE1Hu in NRK cells resulted in a 50–70% increase over the control in 30% of stably transfected cells in G2. This suggests an inhibition of G2 progression by WEE1Hu, and thus, WEE1Hu has a strikingly similar function to *S. pombe wee1*$^+$.

Recently Parker and Piwanica-Worms found that the WEE1Hu protein produced in *Escherichia coli* had a tyrosine, but not threonine kinase activity (*20*). It can phosphorylate only the tyrosine 15 residue of *cdc2*$^+$ kinase. These results indicate

TABLE 1. Properties of Three *cdc25* Human Homologs

Name	mRNA size	Protein MW	Expression	Cell Cycle Dependency	Complementation of *S. pombe*
CDC25Hu1	2.2 kb	53 kDa	Low	G2	+
CDC25Hu2	3.2 kb	63 kDa	High	G2	++
CDC25Hu3	3.4 kb	58 kDa	Medium	late G1–early S	+++

```
CDC25Hu2    MEVPQPEPAPGSALSPAGVCGGAQRPGHLPGLLLGSHGLLGSPVRAAASSPVTTLTQTMHDLAG

CDC25Hu2 LGSRSRLTHLSLSRRASESSLSSESSESSDAGLCMDSPSPMDPHMAEQTFEQAIQAASRIIRNEQFA
CDC25Hu1                                 MSTELFSSTREEGSSGSGPSFRSNQRKMLNLLLERDTSFTVC

CDC25Hu3 MRRIHSLPQKLLGCSPALKRSHSDSLD-------HDIFQLIDPDENKENEAFEF----KKPVRPVSR
CDC25Hu2 IRRFQSMPVRLLGHSPVLRNITNSQAPDGRRKSEAGSGAASSSGEDKENDGFVF----KMPWKPTHP
CDC25Hu1 PDVPRTPVGKFLGDSANLSILSGGTPKCCLDLSNLSSGEITATQLTTSADLDETGHLDSSGLQEVHL

CDC25Hu3 GCLHS-HGLQEGKDLFTQRQNSAPARM-LSSNERDSSEPGNFIPLFTPQSPV--TATLSD--EDDGF
CDC25Hu2 SSTHALAEWASRREAFAQRPSSAPDLMCLSPDR--KMEVEELSPLALGRFSL--TPAEGDTEEDDGF
CDC25Hu1 AGMNHDQHLM--KCSPAQLLCSTPNGLDRGHRKRDAMCSSSANKENDNGNLVDSEMKYLG--SPITT

CDC25Hu3 VDLLDGENLKNEEETPSCMASLWTAPLVMRTTNLDNR--------CKLFDSPSLCSSSTRSVLKRPE
CDC25Hu2 VDILESD-LKDDDAVPPGMESLISAPLVKTLEKEEEKDLVMYSKCQRLFRSPSMPCSVIRPILKRLE
CDC25Hu1 VPKLDKNPNLGEDQAEEISDELMEFSLKDQEAKVSRSG---------LYRSPSMPENLNRPRLKQVE

CDC25Hu3 RSQEESPPGSTKRRKSMSGASPKESTNPEKAHETLHQSLSLASSPKGTIENILDNDPRD--LIGDFS
CDC25Hu2 RPQDRDTPVQNKRRRSVTPPEEQQEAEEPKARVLRSKSL-----CHDEIENLLDSDHRE--LIGDYS
CDC25Hu1 KFKDNTIPDKVK-KKYFSGQGKLRKGLCLKKTV----SL-----CDITITQMLEEDSNQGHLIGDFS

CDC25Hu3 KGYLFHTVAGKHQDLKYISPEIMASVLNGKFANLIKEFVIIDCRYPYEYEGGHIKGAVNLHMEEEVE
CDC25Hu2 KAFLLQTVDGKHQDLKYISPETMVALLTGKFSNIVDKFVIVDCRYPYEYEGGHIKTAVNLPLERDAE
CDC25Hu1 KVCALPTVSGKHQDLKYVNPETVAALLSGKFQGLIEKFYVIDCRYPYEYLGGHIQGALNLYSQEELF

CDC25Hu3 DFLLKKPIVPTDG-KRVIVVFHCEFSSERGPRMCRYVRERDRLGNEYPKLHYPELYVLKGGYKEFFM
CDC25Hu2 SFLLKSPIAPCSLDKRVILIFHCEFSSERGPRMCRFIRERDRAVNDYPSLYYPEMYILKGGYKEFFP
CDC25Hu1 NFFLKKPIVPLDTQKRIIIVFHCEFSSERGPRMCRCLREEDRSLNQYPALYYPELYILKGGYRDFFP

CDC25Hu3 KCQSYCEPPSYRPMHHEDFK-EDLKKFRTKSRTWAGEKSKREMYSRLKKL*
CDC25Hu2 QHPNFCEPQDYRPMNHEAFKDE-LKTFRLKTRSWAGERSRRELCDRLQDQ*
CDC25Hu1 EYMELCEPQSYCPMHHQDHKTE-LLRCRSQSKVQEGERQLREQIALLVKDMSP*
```

FIG. 3. Amino acid comparison among the three *cdc25*$^+$ human homologs. Identical amino acids are shaded.

that WEE1Hu is a true counterpart of *wee1*$^+$ and, moreover, that phosphorylation at the threonine 14 residue of the *cdc2*$^+$ kinase found in mammalian cells is catalyzed by some other enzyme.

Structure and Expression of Three cdc25 Human Homologs

One such homolog cDNA was isolated first by Sadhu *et al.* (*15*) using the polymerase chain reaction method with primers corresponding to the regions highly

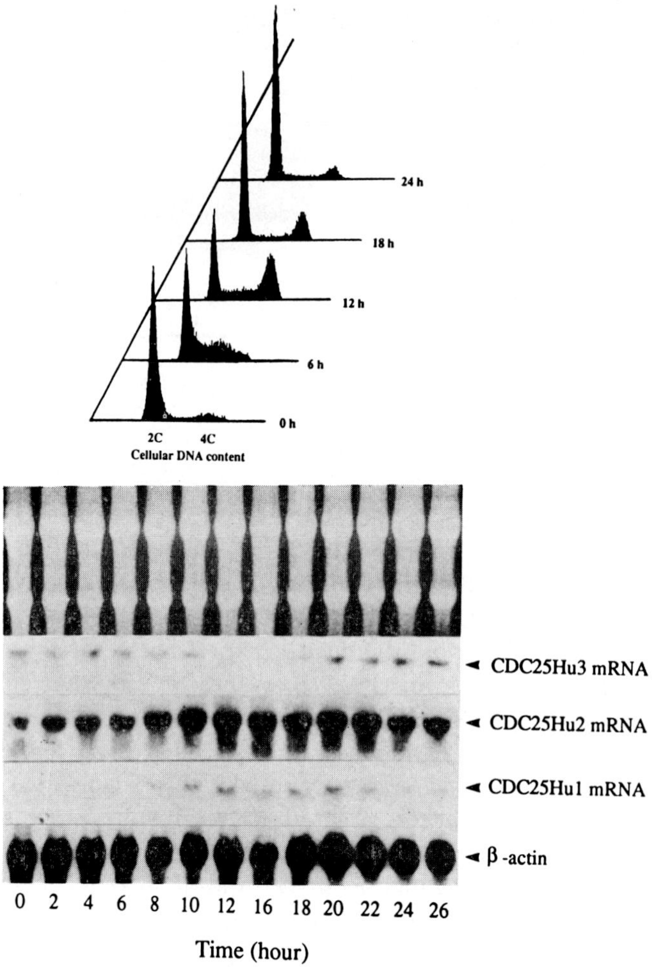

FIG. 4. Cell cycle dependency of CDC25Hu3 expression. a, b, and c: RNA blot analysis of the expression of CDC25Hu3 (a), CDC25Hu2 (b) and CDC25 (c) in HeLa cells. HeLa cells were doubly blocked with thymidine at early S and then released to proceed through the cell cycle. The cell cycle progression was monitored with a fluorescence-activated cell analyzer that measured the DNA content in each cell (upper figure). Fraction of the cells was harvested every 2 hr, total RNA was prepared, and Northern blot analysis was carried out.

conserved between the *S. pombe cdc25*$^+$ gene and its *S. cerevisiae* counterpart MIH1 (*16*). Subsequently, we and others isolated two additional homologs from human cells (*17, 18*), and thus humans contain at least three *cdc25*$^+$ homologs; homology properties are summarized in Table 1. They differ in the size and the sequence of mRNA and encoded proteins, the level and cell cycle dependency of expression, and the ability to complement a *cdc25* mutant. The three homologs share significant sequence similarity with one another (Fig. 3), and this similarity is particularly evident in the C-terminal 150 amino acids, where the functional domain resides (*15*). Among the three, CDC25Hu2 and CDC25Hu3 are more closely related in structure. Perhaps as a reflection of this, CDC25Hu2 and Hu3 complement a *cdc25* mutation much more efficiently than Hu1.

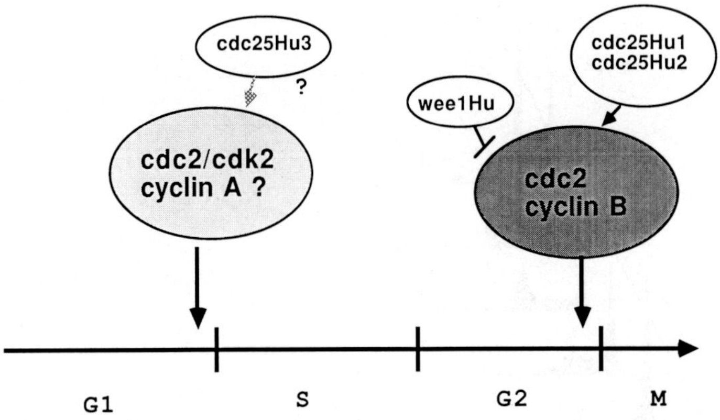

FIG. 5. Proposed model for the regulation of the cell cycle in mammalian cells.

One striking difference among the three is the cell cycle dependency of their expression. HeLa cells were arrested in early S by double thymidine block and released to proceed through the cell cycle. Every 2 hr, cells were harvested and their cell cycle patterns were analyzed by flow cytometry. Simultaneously, RNA was prepared and analyzed by Northern blotting for the expression of the three homologs along with β-actin as an internal control (Fig. 4). As indicated by the cell cycle pattern, HeLa cells entered the G2/M phases 12 hr after release. The messages for CDC25Hu1 and Hu2 peaked in G2/M phases. Thus, CDC25Hu1 and Hu2 share remarkable similarity with the *S. pombe cdc25*$^{+}$ gene, and this is consistent with their function as mitotic inducers. On the other hand, CDC25Hu3 was expressed in S phase, its expression decreased G2/M phase and increased in G1, suggesting that this homolog may have some novel function in G1 and/or S.

In summary, a mammalian system controlling the G2 to M transition shares striking similarity with the fission yeast system, but is more complex (Fig. 5). CDC25Hu1 and CDC25Hu2 are likely to be counterparts of *cdc25*$^{+}$, but the reason humans contain two counterparts is unclear. Humans also have WEE1Hu, a true counterpart of *wee1*$^{+}$, which has not been found in any other organisms than *S. pombe*. CDC25Hu3, in contrast, may have some function early in the cell cycle.

Overexpression of cdc25 Human Homologs in Cancer Cells

In *S. pombe*, dysregulated expression of G2 control genes results in abnormal cell division. Typical consequences are formation of anucleate or aneuploid cells or cells with fragmented chromosomes (*1, 10*). Many malignant cancer cells contain varying extents of chromosome abnormalities: aneuploidy, translocations and deletions (*21, 22*). We found that many cancers contain various degrees of disarray in the expressions of CDC25Hu1, Hu2, Hu3, cdc2, and WEE1Hu. Particularly interesting is highly elevated constitutive expression of the CDC25Hu2 gene in SV40-transformed cells (*17*), since SV40 is well known for its ability to induce genetic instability as well as immortalization (*23, 24*). Overexpression of CDC25Hu2 is a primary event and occurs immediately after SV40 transformation (*17*). Moreover, over-

TABLE 2. Expression Levels of *cdc25* Homologs *vs.* Aneuploidy

Cell line	Origin	Expression level			
		Aneuploidy	CDC25Hu1	CDC25Hu2	CDC25Hu3
Miz-1	Embryonic fibroblast (limb)	—	ND	+	ND
AH	Skin fibroblast	—	ND	+	ND
OR-4	Adult skin fibroblast	—	ND	+	ND
HH4	Spherocytosis patient (B lymphoblast)	—	ND	+	ND
Hut11	Fibrosarcoma (skin)	+	ND	+	+
Hut14	Fibrosarcoma (skin)	+	+	+++	+
Ht1080	Fibrosarcoma (acetabulum)	+	ND	+	+
CaLu-3	Adenocarcinoma (lung)	++	+	++	+
PC-3	Adenocarcinoma (prostate)	++	++	+++	++
HT29	Adenocarcinoma (colon)	++	++	+++	++
HeLa	Epitheloid carcinoma (cervix)	++	++	+++	+++
KB	Epidermoid carcinoma (oral)	++	+	++++	+++
ME180	Epidermoid carcinoma (cervix)	++	++	++++	+
T24	Transitional-cell carcinoma (bladder)	++	+	++++	+
Malme-3M	Malignant melanoma (skin)	++	ND	++++	+
SW480	Adenocarcinoma (colon)	++	+++	+++++	+++++
A204	Rhabdomyosarcoma	++	ND	+++++	+
GM637	SV40-transformed lung fibroblast	++	++	+++++	+++
XPSV40	SV40-transformed skin fibroblast	++	+++	+++++	++
VMRC-MELG	Malignant melanoma (skin)		ND	+++	+
MeWo	Malignant melanoma (skin)		+	+++	+
C32TG	Amelanotic melanoma (skin)		+	+++	+
PA-1	Teratocarcinoma (ovary)		++	+++	++++

ND: not detectable.

expression of CDC25Hu2 was also found in the E6, E7 gene of malignant human papilloma virus type 16 (*17*), which is another well-known transforming gene that induces genomic instability. Furthermore, we found a significant correlation between overexpression of CDC25Hu2 and aneuploidy in 13 human tumor cell lines examined (Table 2).

REFERENCES

1. Enoch, T. and Nurse, P. Mutation of yeast cell cycle control genes abolishes dependence of mitosis on DNA replication. Cell, *60*: 665–673, 1990.
2. Lee, M. G., Norbury, C. J., Spurr, N. K., and Nurse, P. Regulated expression and phosphorylation of a possible mammalian cell-cycle control protein. Nature, *333*: 676–679, 1988.
3. Dunphy, W. G. and Newport, J. W. Unveiling of mitotic control mechanisms. Cell, *58*: 1013–1016, 1988.
4. Norbury, C. J. and Nurse, P. Control of the eukaryote cell cycle by $p34^{cdc2}$ homologues. Biochim. Biophys. Acta, *989*: 85–95, 1989.
5. Ducommun, B., Brambilla, P., Felix, M.-A., Franza, B. R. Jr., Karsenti, E., and Draetta, G. cdc2 phosphorylation is required for its interaction with cyclin. EMBO J., *10*: 3311–3319, 1991.

6. Gould, K. L., Moreno, S., Owen, D. J., Sazer, S., and Nurse, P. Phosphorylation at Thr 167 is required for *Schizosaccharomyces pombe* $p34^{cdc2}$ function. EMBO J., *10*: 3297–3309, 1991.
7. Norbury, C., Blow, J., and Nurse, P. Regulatory phosphorylation of the $p34^{cdc2}$ protein kinase in vertebrates. EMBO J., *10*: 3321–3329, 1991.
8. Krek, W. and Nigg, E. A. Mutations of $p34^{cdc2}$ phosphorylation sites induce premature mitotic events in HeLa cells: evidence for a double block to $p34^{cdc2}$ kinase activation in vertebrates. EMBO J., *10*: 3331–3341, 1991.
9. Russell, P. and Nurse, P. Negative regulation of mitosis by *wee1*$^+$, a gene encoding a protein kinase homologue. Cell, *49*: 559–567, 1987.
10. Lundgren, K., Walworth, N., Booher, R., Dembsiki, M., Kirschner, M., and Beach, D. *mik1* and *wee1* cooperate in the inhibitory tyrosine phosphorylation of cdc2. Cell, *64*: 1111–1122, 1991.
11. Russell, P. and Nurse, P. The mitotic inducer *nim1*$^+$ functions in a regulatory network of protein kinase homologs controlling the initiation of mitosis. Cell, *49*: 569–576, 1987.
12. Russell, P. and Nurse, P. *cdc25*$^+$ functions as a mitotic inducer in the mitotic control of fission yeast. Cell, *45*: 145–153, 1986.
13. Kumagai, A. and Dunphy, W. G. The cdc25 protein controls tyrosine dephosphorylation of the cdc2 protein in a cell-free system. Cell, *64*: 903–914, 1991.
14. Edgar, B. A. and O'Farrell, P. H. Genetic control of cell division patterns in the Drosophila embryo. Cell, *57*: 177–187, 1989.
15. Sadhu, K., Reed, S. T., Richardson, H., and Russell, P. Human homolog of fission yeast *cdc25* mitotic inducer is predominantly expressed in G2. Proc. Natl. Acad. Sci. U.S.A., *87*: 5139–5143, 1990.
16. Russell, P., Moreno, S., and Reed, S. I. Conservation of mitotic controls in fission and budding yeasts. Cell, *57*: 295–303, 1989.
17. Nagata, A., Igarashi, M., Jinno, S., Suto, K., and Okayama, H. An additional homolog of the fission yeast *cdc25*$^+$ gene occurs in humans and is highly expressed in some cancer cells. New Biologist, *3*: 959–968, 1991.
18. Glaktionov, K. and Beach, D. Specific activation of cdc25 tyrosine phosphatases by B-type cyclins: evidence for multiple roles of mitotic cyclins. Cell, *67*: 1181–1194, 1991.
19. Igarashi, M., Nagata, A., Jinno, S., Suto, K., and Okayama, H. *Wee1*$^+$-like gene in human cells. Nature, *353*: 80–83, 1991.
20. Parker, L. and Piwanica-Worms, H. WEE1Hu encodes a tyrosine kinase that inhibits $p34^{cdc2}$/cyclin B kinase activity by phosphorylation of $p34^{cdc2}$ on tyr 15. Cold Spring Harbor Meeting (Abstr.), 1992.
21. Mertens, F., Heim, S., Mandahl, N., Johansson, B., Rydholm, A., Biorklund, A., Wennerberg, J., Jonsson, N., and Mitelman, F. Clonal chromosome aberrations in a keratocanthoma and a basal cell papilloma. Cancer Genet. Cytogenet., *39*: 227–232, 1989.
22. Stambridge, E. J. Human tumor suppressor genes. Annu. Rev. Genet., *24*: 615–657, 1990.
23. Nichols, W. W., Girardi, A. J., Bradt, C. I., Hill, R., Cody, C. Cytogenetic changes induced in human diploid fibroblasts by tsA58 SV40 at permissive and restrictive temperatures. Mutat. Res., *150*: 327–332, 1985.
24. Ray, F. A., Peabody, D. S., Cooper, J. L., Cram, S., and Kraemer, P. M. SV40 T antigen alone drives karyotype instability that precedes neoplastic transformation of human diploid fibroblasts. J. Cell. Biochem., *42*: 13–31, 1990.

MULTISTAGE CARCINOGENESIS, C. C. HARRIS ET AL. (EDS.),
JAPAN SCI. SOC. PRESS, TOKYO/CRC PRESS, BOCA RATON, PP. 239–248, 1992

Cellular Targets of the Oncoproteins Encoded by the Cancer Associated Human Papillomaviruses

Peter M. HOWLEY, Karl MÜNGER, Helen ROMANCZUK,
Martin SCHEFFNER, and Jon M. HUIBREGTSE

Laboratory of Tumor Virus Biology, National Cancer Institute, Bethesda, Maryland 20892, U.S.A.

Abstract: Insight into the mechanisms by which DNA tumor viruses transform cells has come from the recognition that the virus-encoded oncoproteins interact specifically with important cell regulatory proteins. The "high risk" human papillomaviruses such as HPV-16 and HPV-18 which are associated with human anogenital carcinomas encode two transforming genes (E6 and E7) which are expressed in HPV positive cancers and derived cell lines. E7 shares functional and structural features with the adenovirus E1A proteins. Like Ad E1A and the large T proteins of the polyomaviruses, E7 can complex pRB. The E7 proteins of the "high risk" HPVs associate with pRB with approximately a 10-fold higher affinity than do the E7 proteins of the "low risk" HPVs, and important biological differences between the E7 proteins of these two groups of HPVs are determined by amino-terminal sequences which include the pRB binding domain.

Like SV40 large T and Ad 5 E1B, the E6 oncoprotein encoded by the "high risk" HPVs can form a complex with p53. *In vitro*, E6 promotes the degradation of p53 and this degradation involves the ubiquitin-dependent protease system. The selective degradation of cellular proteins such as p53 with negative regulatory functions provides a novel mechanism of action for dominant acting oncoproteins.

The relevance of the inactivation of the normal functions of pRB and p53 in human cervical carcinogenesis has recently been demonstrated by the analysis of these two genes and their products in a series of HPV-positive and HPV-negative cell lines. Each of five HPV-positive cervical cancer cell lines expressed normal pRB and low levels of wild type p53 proteins, which are presumed to be altered in function as a consequence of association with the HPV oncoproteins. In contrast, mutations were identified in the p53 and RB genes expressed in the HPV-negative cervical carcinoma cell lines, C33-A and HT-3. These results support the hypothesis that the inactivation of the normal functions of the tumor suppressor proteins pRB and p53 are important steps in human cervical carcinogenesis, either by mutation or through complex formation with HPV E6 and E7 oncoproteins.

The evidence now associating specific human papillomaviruses (HPVs) with certain human anogenital cancers, including human cervical cancer, is quite strong. Epidemiology implicates a venereally transmitted agent in human cervical carcinoma and indicates a prolonged latency of perhaps twenty to twenty-five years (*1, 2*). Investigators evaluated a number of genital pathogenic organisms as potential etiologic factors over the years. Herpes simplex virus (HSV) type 2 was considered a potential etiologic agent, in the late 1960's (*3, 4*). No convincing molecular biology evidence for the presence of HSV nucleic acids in cervical cancers was found, however (*5*). A role for HSV as a potential cofactor perhaps working in concert with the HPVs has not been ruled out and remains a possibility that merits further study.

The initial evidence suggesting a role of HPV infection with cervical cancer was provided by cytologists who recognized that the morphologic abnormalities that constitute cervical dysplasia (also referred to as cervical intraepithelial neoplasia or CIN) were a consequence of a papillomavirus infection (*6–8*). A papillomavirus etiology for cervical dysplasia was further established by the demonstration of papillomavirus capsid antigens in the nuclei of some cells in about 50% of cervical dysplasia lesions (*9, 10*). The link of a papillomavirus infection of the cervix, to cervical dysplasia, recognized as a pre-neoplastic lesion with the potential to progress to cervical cancer, inspired an evaluation of cervical cancer tissues for the evidence of HPV DNA.

There are over 65 different types of HPVs (*11*). About 20 of these HPVs are found in anogenital lesions, and these HPVs can be further classified as either "high risk" or low risk" on the basis of the lesions with which they are associated. The "low risk" viruses (HPV-6 and HPV-11) are associated with venereal warts, also known as condyloma acuminata, which rarely progress to cancer. In contrast, the "high risk" viruses (including HPV-16 and -18) are associated with CIN and cancer. HPV-16 and HPV-18 DNAs were initially cloned from cervical carcinoma tissues (*12, 13*). Using these two DNAs as hybridization probes, approximately 70% of the human cervical carcinomas can be shown to contain DNA of these HPV types (*14*). Additional HPVs have been subsequently cloned and also shown to be associated with invasive cervical carcinomas (*15*). The "high risk" genital tract HPVs include types 16, 18, 31, 33, 35, 39, 45, 51, 52, and 56, which are found in cases of moderate and severe dysplasia and in invasive cervical carcinomas.

Approximately 85% of cervical carcinomas contain a "high risk" HPV DNA (*16*). Studies of cervical cancers and of HPV positive cervical cancer cell lines have shown that the DNA is usually integrated (*14*). In those cases where the DNA is integrated, the pattern of integration is clonal indicating that the association of the HPV precedes the clonal outgrowth of the tumor. The integrated state of the HPV DNA in cervical cancers contrasts with the extrachromosomal state of the viral DNA in the benign precursor lesions (*17*). Integration of the genome is apparently a random event with regard to the site of integration in the host chromosome since the HPV DNA is found in different locations in different cancers and derived cell lines. Of note, however, is that integration has occurred sometimes in the vicinity of known oncogenes. In the HeLa cell line (an HPV-18 positive human cervical carcinoma cell line), integration of the viral genome occurred within 50 kilobases of c-myc on chromosome 8 (*18*). It is not yet known whether integration in the vicinity of an oncogene provides a selective advantage to the cell and, as such, contributes to the progression of a pre-neoplastic lesion to a cancer.

The integration pattern of the viral genome, however, reveals specificity with respect to where the double-stranded circular viral genome is opened and disrupted as a consequence of the integration. It often occurs in the E1/E2 region of the viral genome (*19, 20*) disrupting the E2 viral transcriptional regulatory circuit. The E2 open reading frame encodes a DNA binding regulatory protein which effects transcription and DNA replication. E2 has been most extensively studied in the bovine papillomavirus where its products have been shown to act both positively and negatively in transcriptional regulation (*21*). For HPV-16 and HPV-18, E2 acts chiefly to repress activity of the promoter from which the E6 and E7 genes are transcribed (*22–24*). HPV is transcriptionally active in cervical cancer and the patterns of viral RNA reveal specific expression of the E6 and E7 genes (*19, 25, 26*). Thus, it has been proposed that integration of the viral genome in cervical cancers, with the disruption of the E1 and E2 regulatory genes, might provide a selective advantage due to the deregulated expression of the E6 and E7 oncoproteins. We have have recently carried out a genetic analysis of whether indeed E1 and/or E2 negatively regulate the viral immortalization functions. Mutation of either the E1 gene or the E2 gene in the background of a "wild type" HPV genome resulted in a marked increase in immortalization capacity. Mutations were also generated in the E2 binding sites located upstream of the viral promoter which directs the synthesis of the viral E6 and E7 transforming genes. E2 negatively regulates the expression of this promoter through binding at adjacent sites. Surprisingly, the mutation of these sites only partially relieves the negative effect of E2 on viral immortalization, implicating additional mechanisms in the E2 repression of viral immortalization functions (*27*). This study supports the hypothesis that a selective growth advantage is provided by the integration of the viral genome in a manner which results in the loss of expression of either E1 or E2.

Continued expression of E6 and E7 are necessary for the proliferation of cervical carcinoma cells. Antisense RNA experiments suggest a requirement for the expression of E6 and E7 for the proliferation of C4-I cells, an HPV-18 positive cervical carcinoma cell line (*28*). The expression of BPV-1 E2 in HeLa cells (another HPV-18 positive cervical cancer cell line) prevents their continued cell proliferation, and it has been proposed that this occurs through the transcriptional repression of the E6 and E7 genes (22). This finding is in agreement with the genetic study described above that E1 and E2 negatively regulate the immortalization functions of the "high risk" HPVs (*27*).

The E6 and E7 genes of the "high risk" papillomaviruses, such as HPV-16 and 18, have transforming properties. These genes contrast with the E6 and E7 genes of the "low risk" HPVs, such as HPV-6 and 11, which are either non-transforming or are only very weakly transforming. The E6 and E7 genes of the "high risk" HPVs together are capable of efficiently immortalizing primary human keratinocytes (*29, 30*) whereas these same gene products from the "low risk" viruses are incapable of efficiently immortalizing primary human keratinocytes (*31*).

The E7 gene product of HPV-16 has been well studied and is 98 amino acids in size. It has an aberrant slow mobility in polyacrylamide gels, binds zinc, and is phosphorylated on serines by casein kinase II (*32–34*). E7 is expressed in benign lesions as well as cancers (*26*). E7 has adenovirus E1A-like transcriptional modulatory and transformation properties (*35*). Like adenovirus E1A, it is capable of transactivating the adenovirus E2 promoter (*35*). This transactivation property is similar to that of the 12S E1A product, rather than to that of the 13S E1A product, in that E7 is not capable of transactivating the adenovirus E3 promoter or the adenovirus E4 promoter (*36*).

As a viral transforming protein, E7 can transform established rodent cells such as NIH 3T3 cells (*35, 37–40*). It can cooperate with an activated ras oncogene to fully transform baby rat kidney cells or rat embryo fibroblasts (*35, 41*). E7 can also cooperate with the E6 gene of the "high risk" HPVs to efficiently immortalize primary human keratinocytes (*29, 30*) and primary human diploid fibroblasts (*42*). Striking similarities in the sequence exist between the amino terminal 37 amino acids and the conserved regions 1 and 2 of adenovirus E1A (*35*), which are involved in transformation.

The viral encoded oncoproteins of the DNA tumor viruses (including the HPVs) interact specifically with critical cellular regulatory proteins. The oncogenic properties of these viruses are in part a consequence of these specific interactions. The E7 proteins encoded by the oncogenic genital tract HPVs, the adenovirus E1A protein, and the SV40 large T antigen are all nuclear proteins and share certain characteristics. Each can extend the lifespan of primary cells, cooperate with other cytoplasmic oncoproteins such as ras to fully transform primary rat cells, induce DNA synthesis in growth-arrested cells, transform established rodent cells, and modulate transcription from certain promoters (reviewed in *43*). The regions of amino acid sequence similarity between E7 and adenovirus E1A noted above are also shared with the T antigens encoded by the polyomaviruses. These conserved regions have been shown to participate in the binding of a number of important cellular regulatory proteins, including the product of the retinoblastoma tumor suppressor gene, pRB (*43–46*), and a recently cloned 107K protein (*34*). The similar biologic properties of the transforming oncoproteins of these different viruses probably derive from their ability to target a similar set of cell regulatory proteins. The amino terminal domain of the E7 proteins is highly conserved among the "high risk" HPVs and the "low risk" HPVs. The E7 proteins of all of these genital tract HPVs can complex pRB, although there is a significant difference in the affinity of these complexes (*46*). The E7 proteins from the "low risk" HPVs types 6 and 11 associate with pRB with about a ten-fold lower affinity than do the E7 proteins of the "high risk" HPV types 16 and 18. Complex formation between the E7 proteins and pRB requires the integrity of the region similar to conserved region 2 of adenovirus E1A (*34, 46, 47*).

We have recently carried out a structural and functional comparison of the E7 proteins encoded by the low-risk and high risk human papillomaviruses. In this study we have demonstrated that the major determinant which distinguished the transformation potential of the E7 proteins of the oncogenic and non-oncogenic genital tract HPVs correlated with affinity for binding the retinoblastoma protein (*48*). A series of chimeric proteins consisting of domains of the oncogenic and non-oncogenic proteins was constructed to determine the domains of E7 responsible for the difference in transformation potential and to define the regions of E7 responsible for the different biochemical properties. We have previously mapped the differences in biological and biochemical properties to the amino terminal half of E7 (*49*). This region of E7 contains the domains similar to conserved regions 1 and 2 of the

TABLE 1. The Status of pP53 and pRB in Human Cervical Cancer Cell Lines[a)]

Cell line	HPV	pRB	p53	Codon	Mutation	Amino acid
HeLa	HPV-18	WT	WT	—	—	—
C4-II	HPV-18	WT	WT	—	—	—
SiHa	HPV-16	WT	WT	—	—	—
CASKI	HPV-16	WT	WT	—	—	—
ME180	HPV-39[b)]	WT	WT	—	—	—
C33-A	Negative	Mutated	Mutated	273	CGT to TGT	Arg to Cys
HT-3	Negative	Mutated	Mutated	245	GGC to GTC	Gly to Val

[a)] The specific details of the studies providing the data for this summary have been published by Scheffner *et al.*, 1991 (*55*). [b)] The ME180 cell line contains and expresses HPV DNA sequences closely related to HPV-39 (*56*).

adenovirus E1A oncoprotein. The region of E7 similar to conserved region 2 consists of a binding domain for pRB and a casein kinase II phosphorylation site. The transformation potential of the chimeric E7 proteins segregated with the pRB binding domain of the high risk E7 protein. This domain was itself responsible for the more avid binding of pRB by the E7 proteins of the oncogenic *versus* non-oncogenic HPV types. A comparison of the pRB binding domains of the E7 proteins of the genital tract HPVs revealed a consistent amino acid difference between the "high risk" and "low risk" viruses. A single amino acid substitution (Asp 21 to Gly) in the high risk virus was shown to be the principal determinant responsible for the difference in pRB binding and transformation capacity (*48*).

The transforming properties of the E6 protein were unveiled by studies using primary human squamous epithelial cells which are the normal host cells for HPVs (*29, 30*). Efficient immortalization of primary human keratinocytes requires both E6 and E7 (*29, 30*). The transformation property of the E6 proteins of the "high risk" viruses prompted the investigation of whether E6, like the SV40 large T antigen and the E1B protein encoded by adenovirus 5, targeted p53. Association of the E6 proteins of the "high risk" HPV types, but not of the "low risk" HPV types with p53, could be demonstrated using E6 and human p53 synthesized *in vitro* using rabbit reticulocyte lysates (*50*). In SV40 and adenovirus 5 trnasformed cells, the levels of p53 are increased and the half life of the protein extended (*51, 52*). In contrast, HPV containing cervical carcinomas and HPV transformed cells generally contain very low levels of p53 (*55*). Thus, although the E6 oncoproteins, like the transforming proteins of these different DNA tumor viruses, target p53, the consequence of the protein-protein interaction is different. Experiments examining the consequence of the interaction of the E6 oncoprotein of the "high risk" HPVs with p53 demonstrated that the E6 oncoproteins that are encoded by the oncogenic HPVs and bind p53 stimulate the degradation of p53 in rabbit reticulocyte lysates (*53*). The E6 promoted degradation of p53 is ATP-dependent and involves the ubiquitin protease system (*53*). The selective degradation of a cellular protein by a viral gene product is a novel mechanism of action for dominant-acting viral or cellular oncoproteins.

The establishment of the transforming functions of the E6 and E7 oncoproteins of the "high risk" HPVs in their normal host cell supports a role for these viruses in carcinogenic progression. It seems quite clear that the oncogenic HPVs exert some of their proliferative and cancer promoting effects through the interactions of the E6 and E7 oncoproteins with key cellular regulatory proteins. In a benign HPV infection, the interaction of E6 and E7 with the pRB and p53 tumor suppressor gene products must provide some advantage to the virus, possibly by expanding the pool of cells which will make viral particles by inducing cellular proliferation, or by providing the necessary intra-cellular environment for vegetative viral DNA replication. In the HPV-positive cancers, expression of E6 and E7 appears to be deregulated as a consequence of the integration of the viral genome. As with SV40 and adenovirus, expression of the HPV oncoproteins may contribute to chromosome instability and aneuploidy, leading to other cellular mutations necessary for progression to invasive cancer. Other cytogentic studies have implicated genetic changes in the short arm of human chromosome 3P in carcinogenic progression in human cervical cancers (*54*).

We have recently studied the state of the pRB and p53 genes in cervical carcinoma cell lines which either do or do not contain HPV. As already mentioned, approximately 15% of human cervical cancers are negative for HPV DNA sequences (*16*). In the study summarized in Table 1, the RB and p53 genes were found to be wild type in each of the HPV-positive cell lines examined (*55*). Normal forms of the pRB protein were found in each of five HPV-positive cell lines. An abnormally fast migrating pRB protein was detected in the two HPV-negative lines and mutations were documented in each of the pRB genes in each of these cell lines. In addition, there had been a loss of the normal pRB allele. Sequence analysis of the RNA revealed deletions, which could be accounted for by specific mutations at splice junctions in the DNA (*55*). Low levels of the p53 protein were found in each of the five HPV-positive cell lines consistent with the hypothesis that E6 targets the degradation of the cellular p53 protein. Sequence analysis of the cDNA corresponding to the conserved region of the p53 gene revealed that indeed the p53 genes were wild type for each of the five HPV-positive cell lines. In contrast, mutations were found in each of the p53 genes in the two HPV-negative cell lines (Table 1). The point mutations resulted in amino acid substitutions in the genes in the C33-A and HT-3 cell lines affecting the p53 codons 273 and 245, respectively. These data suggest that p53 and pRB are central targets in cervical carcinogenesis. The inactivation of the cellular proteins can occur either through the complex formation with the viral E6 and E7 oncoproteins, as is the case in HPV-positive cervical cancers, or by specific mutations of the genes, as appears to be the case in the HPV-negative cervical cancers.

Acknowledgment

We are grateful to Carol Comlish for her excellent editorial assistance in the preparation of this manuscript.

REFERENCES

1. Kessler, I. I. Human cervical cancer as a venereal disease. Cancer Res., *36*: 783–791, 1976.
2. zur Hausen, H. Human papillomaviruses and their possible role in squamous cell carcinomas. Curr. Top. Microbiol. Immunol., *78*: 1–30, 1977.

3. Rawls, W. E., Tompkins, W. A. F., Figueroa, M. E., and Melnick, J. L. Herpes simplex virus type 2: association with carcinoma of the cervix. Science, *161*: 1255–1256, 1968.
4. Nahmias, A. J., Josey, W. E., Naib, Z. M., Luce, C. F., and Guest, B. A. Antibodies to herpes virus hominus types 1 and 2 in humans. II. Women with cervical cancer. Am. J. Epidemiol., *91*: 547–552, 1970.
5. zur Hausen, H. Herpes simplex virus in human genital cancer. Int. Rev. Exp. Pathol., *25*: 307–326, 1983.
6. Meisels, A. and Fortin, R. Condylomatous lesions of the cervix and vagina. I. Cytologic patterns. Acta Cytol., *20*: 505–509, 1976.
7. Purola, E. and Savia, E. Cytology of gynecologic condyloma acuminatum. Acta Cytol., *21*: 26–31, 1977.
8. Laverty, C. R., Russell, P., Hills, E., and Booth, N. The significance of noncondylomatous wart virus infection of the cervical transformation zone. Acta Cytol., *22*: 195–201, 1978.
9. Kurman, R. J., Shah, K. H., Lancaster, W. D., and Jenson, A. B. Immunoperoxidase localization of papillomavirus antigens in cervical dysplasia and vulvar condylomas. Am. J. Obstet. Gynecol., *140*: 931-935, 1981.
10. Walker, P. G., Singer, A., Dyson, J. L., Shah, K. V., To, A., and Coleman, D. V. The prevalence of human papillomavirus antigen in patients with cervical intraepithelial neoplasia. Br. J. Cancer, *48*: 99–101, 1983.
11. DeVilliers, E.-M. Heterogeneity of the human papillomavirus group. J. Virol., *63*: 4898–4903, 1989.
12. Durst, M., Gissmann, L., Idenburg, H., and zur Hausen, H. A papillomavirus DNA from a cervical carcinoma and its prevalence in cancer biopsy samples from different geographic regions. Proc. Natl. Acad. Sci. U.S.A., *80*: 3812–3815, 1983.
13. Boshart, M., Gissmann, L., Ikenberg, H., Kleinheinz, A., Scheurlen, W., and zur Hausen, H. A new type of papillomavirus DNA, its presence in genital cancer biopsies and in cell lines derived from cervical cancer. EMBO J., *3*: 1151–1157, 1984.
14. zur Hausen, H. and Schneider, A. The role of papillomaviruses in human anogenital cancer. *In*; N. P. Salzman and P. M. Howley (eds.), Papillomaviruses, pp. 245–263, New York, Plenum, 1987.
15. Beaudenon, S., Kremsdorf, D., Croissant, O., Jablonska, S., Wain-Hobson, S., and Orth, G. A novel type of human papillomavirus associated with genital neoplasias. Nature, *321*: 246–249, 1986.
16. Riou, G., Favre, M., Jeannel, D., Bourhis, J., Le Doussal, V., and Orth, G. Association between poor prognosis in early-stage invasive cervical carcinomas and non-detection of HPV DNA. Lancet, *335*: 1171–1174, 1990.
17. Durst, M., Kleinheinz, A., Hotz, M., and Gissmann, L. The physical state of human papillomavirus type 16 DNA in benign and malignant genital tumours. J. Gen. Virol., *66*: 1515–1525, 1985.
18. Durst, M., Croce, C., Gissmann, L., Schwarz, E., and Huebner, K. Papillomavirus sequences integrate near cellular oncogenes in some cervical carcinomas. Proc. Natl. Acad. Sci. U.S.A., *84*: 1070–1074, 1987.
19. Baker, C. C., Phelps, W. C., Lindgren, V., Braun, M. J., Gonda, M. A., and Howley, P. M. Structural and transcriptional analysis of human papillomavirus type 16 sequences in cervical carcinoma cell lines. J. Virol., *61*: 962–971, 1987.
20. Schwarz, E., Freese, U. K., Gissmann, L., Mayer, W., Roggenbuck, B., Stremlau, A., and zur Hausen, H. Structure and transcription of human papillomavirus sequences in cervical carcinoma cells. Nature, *314*: 111–114, 1985.
21. McBride, A. A., Romanczuk, H., and Howley, P. M. The papillomavirus E2 regu-

latory proteins. J. Biol. Chem., *266*: 18411–18414, 1991.
22. Thierry, F. and Yaniv, M. The BPV1-E5 trans-acting protein can be either an activator or a repressor of the HPV18 regulatory region. EMBO J., *6*: 3391–3397, 1987.
23. Bernard, B. A., Bailly, C., Lenoir, M,-C., Darmon, M., Thierry, F., and Yaniv, M. The human papillomavirus type 18 (HPV18) E2 gene product is a repressor of the HPV18 regulatory region in human keratinocytes. J. Virol., *63*: 4317–4324, 1989.
24. Romanczuk, H., Thierry, F., and Howley, P. M. Mutational analysis of *cis* elements involved in E2 modulation of human papillomavirus type 16 P_{97} and type 18 P_{105} promoters. J. Virol., *64*: 2849–2859, 1990.
25. Schneider-Gadicke, A. and Schwarz, E. Different human cervical carcinoma cell lines show similar transcription patterns of human papillomavirus type 18 early genes. EMBO J., *5*: 2285–2292, 1986.
26. Smotkin, D. and Wettstein, F. O. Transcription of human papillomavirus type 16 early genes in a cervical cancer and a cancer-derived cell line and identification of the E7 protein. Proc. Natl. Acad. Sci. U.S.A., *83*: 4680–4684, 1986.
27. Romanczuk, H. and Howley, P. M. Disruption of either the E1 or the E2 regulatory gene of HPV-16 increases viral immortalization capacity. Proc. Natl. Acad. Sci. U.S.A., *89*: 3159–3163, 1992.
28. von Knebel-Doeberitz, M., Oltersdorf, T., Schwarz, E., and Gissmann, L. Correlation to modified human papillomavirus early gene expression with altered growth properties in C4-I cervical carcinoma cells. Cancer Res., *48*: 3780–3786, 1988.
29. Munger, K., Phelps, W. C., Bubb, V., Howley, P. M., and Schlegel, R. The E6 and E7 genes of the human papillomavirus type 16 together are necessary and sufficient for transformation of primary human keratinocytes. J. Virol., *63*: 4417–4421, 1989.
30. Hawley-Nelson, P., Vousden, K. H., Hubbert, N. L., Lowy, D. R., and Schiller, J. T. HPV16 E6 and E7 protein cooperate to immortalize human foreskin keratinocytes. EMBO J., *8*: 3905–3910, 1989.
31. Barbosa, M. S., Vass, W. C., Lowy, D. R., and Schiller, J. T. *In vitro* biological activities of the E6 and E7 genes vary among HPVs of different oncogenic potential. J. Virol., *65*: 292–298, 1991.
32. Barbosa, M. S., Lowy, D. R., and Schiller, J. T. Papillomavirus polypeptides E6 and E7 are zinc-binding proteins. J. Virol., *63*: 1404–1407, 1989,
33. Firzlaff, J. M., Galloway, D. A., Eisenman, R. N., and Luscher, B. The E7 protein of human papillomavirus type 16 is phosphorylated by casein kinase II. New Biologist, *1*: 44–53, 1989.
34. Barbosa, M. S., Edmonds, C., Fisher, C., Schiller, J. T., Lowy, D. R., and Vousden, K. H. The region of the HPV E7 oncoprotein homologous to adenovirus E1a and SV40 large T antigen contains separate domains for Rb binding and casein kinase II phosphorylation. EMBO J., *9*: 153–160, 1990.
35. Phelps, W. C., Yee, C. L., Münger, K., and Howley, P. M. The human papillomavirus type 16 E7 gene encodes transactivation and transformation functions similar to those of adenovirus E1A. Cell, *53*: 539–547, 1988.
36. Phelps, W. C., Bagchi, S., Barnes, J. A., Raychaudhuri, P., Krause, V., Munger, K., Howley, P. M., and Nevins, J. R. Analysis of trans-activation by HPV-16 E7 and adenovirus 12S E1A suggests a common mechanism. J. Virol., *65*: 6922–6930, 1991.
37. Kanda, T., Watanabe, S., and Yoshiike, K. Immortalization of primary rat cells by human papillomavirus type 16 subgenomic DNA fragments controlled by the SV40 promoter. Virology, *165*: 321–325, 1988.
38. Vousden, K. H., Doniger, J., DiPaolo, J. A., and Lowy, D. R. The E7 open reading frame of human papillomavirus type 16 encodes a transforming gene. Oncogene

Res., *3*: 167–175, 1988.

39. Bedell, M. A., Jones, K. H., Grossman, S. R., and Laimins, L. A. Identification of human papillomavirus type 18 transforming genes in immortalized and primary cells. J. Virol., *63*: 1247–1255, 1989.
40. Tanaka, A., Noda, T., Yajima, H., Hatanaka, M., and Ito, Y. Identification of a transforming gene of human papillomavirus type 16. J. Virol., *63*: 1465–1469, 1989.
41. Matlashewski, G., Schneider, J., Banks, L., Jones, N., Murray, A., and Crawford, L. Human papillomavirus type 16 DNA cooperates with activated ras in transforming primary cells. EMBO J., *6*: 1741–1746, 1987.
42. Watanabe, S., Kanda, T., and Yoshiike, K. Human papillomavirus type 16 transformation of primary human embryonic fibroblasts requires expression of open reading frames E6 and E7. J. Virol., *63*: 965–969, 1989.
43. Whyte, P., Williamson, N. M., and Harlow, E. Cellular targets for transformation by the adenovirus E1A proteins. Cell, *56*: 67–75, 1989.
44. DeCaprio, J. A., Ludlow, J. W., Figge, J., Shew, J.-Y., Huang, C.-M., Lee, W.-H., Marsillo, E., Paucha, E., and Livingston, D. M. SV40 large tumor antigen forms a specific complex with the product of the retinoblastoma susceptibility gene. Cell, *54*: 275–283, 1988.
45. Ewen, M. B., Ludlow, J. W., Marsilio, E., DeCaprio, J. A., Millikan, R. C., Cheng, S. H., Pauch, E., and Livingston, D. M. An N-terminal transformation-governing sequence of SV40 large T antigen contributes to the binding of both p110 Rb and a second cellular protein, p120. Cell, *58*: 257–267, 1989.
46. Munger, K., Werness, B. A., Dyson, N., Phelps, W. C., and Howley, P. M. Complex formation of human papillomavirus E7 proteins with the retinoblastoma tumor suppressor gene product. EMBO J., *8*: 4099–4105, 1989.
47. Edmonds, C. and Vousden, K. H. A point mutational analysis of human papillomavirus type 16 E7 protein. J. Virol., *63*: 2650–2656, 1989.
48. Heck, D. V., Yee, C. L., Howley, P. M., and Munger, K. Efficiency of binding the retinoblastoma protein correlates with the transforming capacity of the E7 oncoproteins of the human papillomaviruses. Proc. Natl. Acad. Sci. U.S.A., *89*: 4442–4446, 1992.
49. Munger, K., Yee, C. L., Phelps, W. C., Pietenpol, J. A., Moses, H. L., and Howley, P. M. Biochemical and biological differences between E7 oncoproteins of the high- and low-risk human papillomavirus types are determined by amino-terminal sequences. J. Virol., *65*: 3943–3948, 1991.
50. Werness, B. A., Levine, A. J., and Howley, P. M. Association of human papillomavirus types 16 and 18 E6 proteins with p53. Science, *248*: 76–79, 1990.
51. Oren, M., Maltzman, W., and Levine, A. J. Post-translational regulation of the 54K cellular tumor antigen in normal and transformed cells. Mol. Cell. Biol., *1*: 101–110, 1981.
52. Reich, N. C., Oren, M., and Levine, A. J. Two distinct mechanisms regulate the levels of a cellular tumor antigen. Mol. Cell. Biol., *3*: 2143–2150, 1983.
53. Scheffner, M., Werness, B. A., Huibregtse, J. M., Levine, A. J., and Howley, P. M. The E6 oncoprotein encoded by human papillomavirus types 16 and 18 promotes the degradation of p53. Cell, *63*: 1129–1136, 1990.
54. Yokota, J., Tsukada, Y., Nakajima, T., Gotoh, M., Shimosato, Y., Mori, N., Tsunokawa, Y., Sugimura, T., and Terada, M. Loss of heterozygosity on the short arm of chromosome 3 in carcinoma of the uterine cervix. Cancer Res., *49*: 3598–3601, 1989.
55. Scheffner, M., Munger, K., Byrne, J. C., and Howley, P. M. The state of the p53 and retinoblastoma genes in human cervical carcinoma cell lines. Proc. Natl. Acad. Sci. U.S.A., *88*: 5523–5527, 1991.

56. Reuter, S., Delius, H., Kahn, T., Hofmann, B., zur Hausen, H., and Schwarz, E. Characterization of a novel human papillomavirus DNA in the cervical carcinoma cell line ME 180. J. Virol., *65*: 5564–5568, 1991.

MULTISTAGE CARCINOGENESIS, C. C. HARRIS ET AL. (EDS.),
JAPAN SCI. SOC. PRESS, TOKYO/CRC PRESS, BOCA RATON, PP. 249–257, 1992

Chemically Induced Tumors in Transgenic Mice Carrying Prototype Human c-Ha-*ras* Genes

Motoya KATSUKI,*[1] Kiyoshi ANDO,*[1] Atsuhiko SAITOH,*[1] Satoru DOI,*[1] Minoru KIMURA,*[1] Ri-ichi TAKAHASHI,*[2] Takanori HASEGAWA,*[2] Minesuke YOKOYAMA,*[2] Tatsuji NOMURA,*[2] Mitsuo IZAWA,*[3] and Susumu NISHIMURA*[3]

Department of DNA Biology, School of Medicine, Tokai University, Isehara, Kanagawa 259-11, Japan[1] *Central Institute for Experimental Animals, Kawasaki, Kanagawa 216, Japan*[2], *and Biology Division, National Cancer Center Research Institute, Tokyo 104, Japan*[3]

Abstract: Three independent transgenic mouse lines carrying human prototype c-Ha-*ras* genes were established. Approximately 50% of the transgenic offspring of these lines developed spontaneous tumors within 18 months. Types of tumors were restricted to angiosarcomas, skin papillomas and lung or Harderian adenocarcinomas. Interestingly, all angiosarcomas (16/16) had point mutations at the 61st codon of the transgenes. Furthermore, they were also very susceptible to the chemical carcinogens, N-methyl-N′-nitrosourea (MNU) and dimethylbenzanthracene (DMBA). Within 12 weeks after administration of MNU, the transgenic mice developed forestomach papillomas and then carcinomas very frequently, at the rate of almost 100% and almost all of the tumors had point mutations in their transgenes at the 12th codon from GGC (Gly) to GAC (Asp). All the carcinomas of the forestomach, lung and spleen induced by DMBA had point mutations at the 61st codon from CAG (Gln) to CTG (Leu). Because no somatic point mutations in the transgenes have ever been detected in normal tissues of the affected mice, these mutations seemingly activated the human prototype c-Ha-*ras* transgene. From these results, it is suggested that the somatic mutation of the human c-Ha-*ras* transgene plays a causative role in the occurrence of natural tumors and those induced by MNU or DMBA administration in transgenic mice. This transgenic mouse provides a unique screening system for chemicals that induce or suppress the tumorigenesis.

ras family genes (Ha-, Ki-, and N-*ras*) are assumed to play a crucial role in signal transduction involved in the regulation of cell proliferation and differentiation in normal eukaryotic cells (*1*). Activated types of *ras* oncogenes are frequently found in human cancers and appear to be implicated in their development (*2*). A somatic point mutation in the 12th or 61st codon and less frequently in the 13th or 59th codon of the *ras* gene seems to acquire transforming activity in *in vitro* cell culture systems such as the NIH3T3 cell line (*1*). However, the *in vivo* effects of these mutational changes of the *ras* oncogenes in the development of animal and human cancers remain to be elucidated.

Many animal tumors in which *ras* oncogenes have been reproducibly found to be activated were induced by a variety of chemical carcinogens (*1, 3–5*). For example, in rat mammary carcinomas induced by a single dose of methylnitrosourea (MNU) during puberty, the c-Ha-*ras* oncogene was activated in 82% of the treated rats (*6*). MNU is known to cause GC to AT transition in DNA *via* the formation of O^6-methylguanine (*7*). The skin papillomas and carcinomas induced by the initiator dimethylbenzanthracene (DMBA) followed by multiple applications of the promoter 12-O-tetradecanoyl-phorbol-13-acetate (TPA) showed a very high frequency (90%) of activation of the c-Ha-*ras* oncogene in the mouse (*8*).

Transgenic animal models carrying an activated *ras* gene under the control of a certain type of promoter and accomplishing their targeted expression in the expected tissues were also generated (*9–12*). For example, transgenic mice expressing an activated c-Ha-*ras* oncogene from a suprabasal keratin promoter developed skin hyperkeratosis and papillomas (*12*).

We have generated unique transgenic mouse models carrying the prototype human c-Ha-*ras* gene with its own promoter (*13*). We report here that these transgenic mouse lines were extraordinarily tumorigenic and also susceptible to carcinogens.

Transgenic Mice

The structure of the human prototype c-Ha-*ras* DNA injected into mouse zygotes is shown in Fig. 1. It was constructed by ligation of each normal part of a human activated c-Ha-*ras* gene with single point mutation at the 12th codon (BB in, Fig. 1) or the 61st codon (MM in Fig. 1). This gene was incapable of transforming NIH3T3 cells (*14*).

Three transgenic lines were established. It was determined by Southern blot analyses that 5–6 copies of the human prototype c-Ha-*ras* genes were integrated into the genome of each transgenic mouse in a tandem array (data not shown). These transgenes in the rasH2, rasH7 and rasH8 lines were stably transmitted to the off-

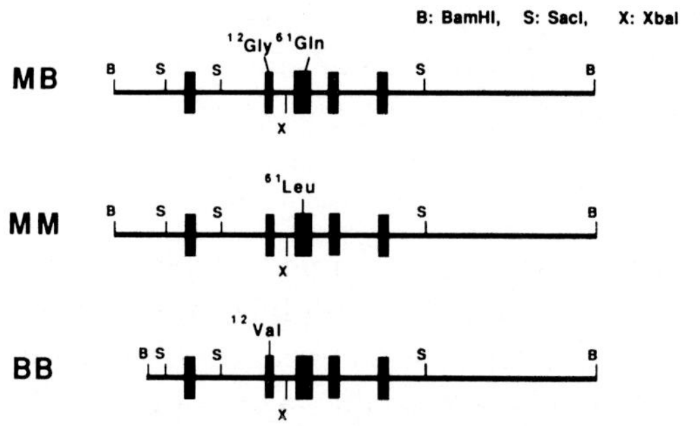

FIG. 1. Structure of the injected human c-Ha-*ras* gene. MB: human prototype c-Ha-*ras* gene which was constructed by ligating the normal part of the activated (BB and MM) genes.

TABLE 1. Natural Tumor Incidences in Transgenic *ras* Mice

Observation period	6 months	18 months
Number of Tg. mice	24	50
Tg. mice with tumors	0	24 (6)
Angiosarcomas	0	13
Lung adenocarcinomas	0	8
Harderian gland adenocarcinomas	0	4
Skin papillomas	0	3
Lymphomas	0	2

Number in parentheses is the number of mice that developed double tumors. Tg.: rasH2 transgenic mice.

spring in accordance with Mendel's law. Since the rasH2 line was the most extensively analyzed of these three lines, we report in this paper the experimental results of tumorigenesis using rasH2 mice. The other lines seemed to have almost the same characters as those of the rasH2 line.

High Tissue-specific Tumor Incidence in Transgenic Mice

The rasH2 founder mouse suddenly died of massive bleeding in the abdominal cavity four months after birth. It was diagnosed as an angiosarcoma of the spleen after being stained by the anti-factor VIII antibody. This tumor was transplantable into a nude mouse. Two of the 20 transgenic offspring developed angiosarcomas just like the founder mouse within five months and one developed a skin papilloma in three months. Because there seemed an extraordinarily high incidence of natural tumors in F1 mice within a very short period, we produced 74 transgenic progenies and separated them into two groups (Table 1). The first group showed neither tumors nor preneoplastic stages histologically when sacrificed at six months of age (Table 1). In the second group, 24 of 50 transgenic mice developed tumors within 18 months. Thirteen transgenic mice had angiosarcomas, especially of the spleen and the dermis. Eight had lung adenocarcinomas, three skin papillomas, four adenocarcinomas of the Harderian glands and two lymphomas. Six of 24 transgenic mice with tumors developed double tumors, each of which occurred independently (Table 1). None of the non-transgenic littermates analyzed so far have developed any tumors. In the rasH7 and rasH8 lines, angiosarcomas, lung adenocarcinomas, adenocarcinomas of the Harderian glands, skin papillomas and lymphomas were also observed. Since the tumors in these mice with human prototype c-Ha-*ras* genes seemed to develop tissue-specifically, we expected the tissue-specific or tumor-specific overexpression of the transgenes that induced the tumors. Therefore, we next investigated the expression pattern of the transgenes in several tissues.

Expression of the Transgenes

It was revealed by RNA blot analyses that the transgene mRNA was expressed at various levels both in tumor cells and in all normal tissues examined (Fig. 2). The RNA expression pattern of the transgenes was the same in transgenic mice with and without tumors. The RNA expression was highest in the brain and the

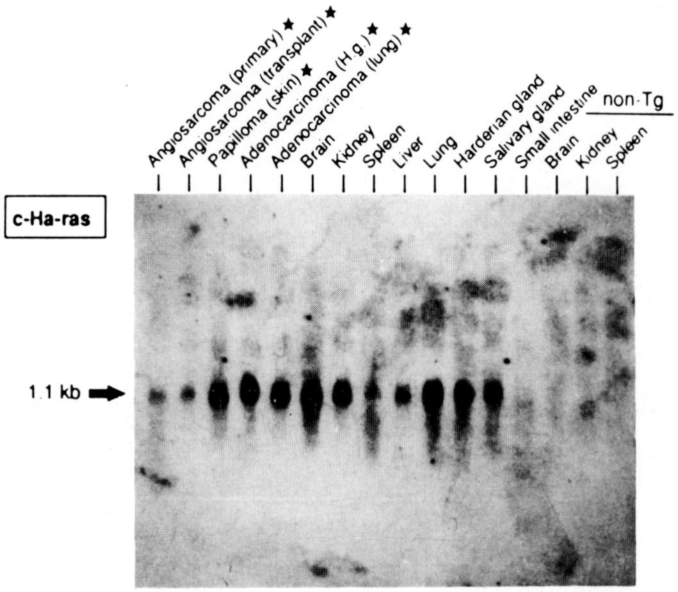

FIG. 2. RNA expression patterns from the transgenes in tumors and several normal tissues of rasH2 transgenic mice. Total RNAs were extracted from tumors and from normal tissues of affected transgenic mice. RNA blot analyses were performed as described in the text. These RNAs were probed with human c-Ha-*ras* cDNA.

kidney that never developed tumors. Therefore, it seems that the overexpression of the transgene was not the only reason for the tumorigenesis.

Somatic Point Mutational Activation of the Transgenes

A somatic mutation of the transgenes in these tumor cells was examined by polymerase chain reaction (PCR) followed by oligonucleotide hybridization (*15*). The DNA fragment of 63 bp including the 12th codon or that of 73 bp including the 61st codon of both human and murine c-Ha-*ras* genes was amplified in DNA samples. PCR products were analyzed by Southern blot hybridization using mutation-specific oligonucleotide probes. A spontaneous point mutation of the transgenes, at least one of the 5–6 copies, was detected only in the tumors and not at all in the normal tissue samples. In angiosarcomas, a somatic point mutation was detected at the 61st codon from CAG (Gln) to CTG (Leu), whereas in skin papillomas, the somatic mutation was detected at the 12th codon from GGC (Gly) to GTC (Val) (Fig. 3). The RNA expression of both the somatically mutated transgene(s) and the normal transgenes was also detected in tumors using cDNA synthesis followed by PCR and oligonucleotide hybridization. In the rasH2 line, somatic point mutation of the transgene in the spontaneous tumors was detected in all 16 angiosarcomas, two of eight lung adenocarcinomas and two of four Harderian gland adenocarcinomas at the 61st codon and two of four skin papillomas at the 12th codon, but was not detected in normal tissues at all (Table 2). Interestingly, the single point mutations detected in tumors other than skin papillomas were restricted to one specific site:

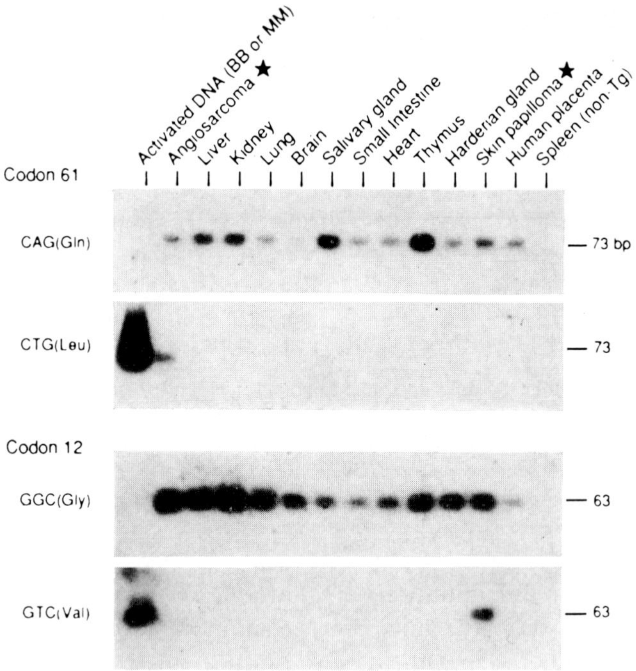

FIG. 3. Identification of somatic point mutation of the transgenes in tumors. A 63 bp DNA fragment was amplified with exon 1 amplimers, subjected to Southern blot analysis, and probed with oligonucleotides specific for mutations at the 12th codon. The activated transgenes were detected only in tumors and not at all in normal tissues.

TABLE 2. Somatic Point Mutations in Natural Tumors of rasH2 Transgenic Mice

Site of mutation	Number of mice	12th GGC→GTC	61st CAG→CTG
Angiosarcomas	13	0	13
Lung adenocarcinomas	8	0	2
Harderian gland adenocarcinomas	4	0	2
Skin papillomas	3	1	0
Lymphomas	2	0	0

Somatic mutations in the transgenes are detected at the 12th and 61st codons.

the 61st codon with transversion from CAG (Gln) to CTG (Leu) which has the highest transforming activity among the amino acids substituted by a single nucleotide change. However, in skin papillomas, point mutation was detected at the 12th codon with transversion from GGC (Gly) to GTC (Val). Almost the same results were obtained in the rasH7 and rasH8 lines. No somatic mutations of murine endogenous c-Ha-*ras* genes were detected in tumors at the 12th codon or 61st codon (data not shown).

Tumor Induction in Transgenic Mice by MNU or DMBA Administration

To examine whether these rasH2 transgenic mice were susceptible to chemical carcinogens, we chose two carcinogens, MNU and DMBA, since they have been

TABLE 3. Tumor Incidences in Transgenic rasH2 Mice by MNU

MNU dose (mg/kg)	Tg. or non-Tg.	Number of mice	Forestomach papillomas	Skin papillomas	Lymphomas
0	Tg.	11	0	0	0
	Non-Tg.	13	0	0	0
0.5	Tg.	19	1	0	0
	Non-Tg.	24	0	0	0
5.0	Tg.	19	2	0	0
	Non-Tg.	25	0	0	0
50	Tg.	56	56 (55)	9 (9)	4
	Non-Tg.	77	1	0	11

MNU was administered intraperitoneally only once to transgenic mice and their nontransgenic littermates. Twelve weeks after administration, systemic observation was performed in each mouse. Only papillomas and lymphomas were found. Number in parentheses is the number of tumors which had the point mutation at the 12th codon of the transgenes. All mutations were from GGC (Gly) to GAC (Asp). Tg.: Transgenic mice carrying human c-Ha-*ras* genes (rasH2 line).

known to induce specific point mutations on the c-Ha-*ras* genes. Firstly, the dose-response effects of MNU on these mice were examined. Mice were divided into four groups; 24, 43, 44, and 133 of them were given a single injection of 0, 0.5, 5 or 50 mg/kg of MNU intraperitoneally (i.p.) at 8 weeks of age, respectively. Twelve weeks after administration, all mice were sacrificed for systemic pathological observation.

Interestingly, forestomach papillomas developed in all transgenic mice when they received 50 mg/kg of MNU. Total tumor incidences and types observed are shown in Table 3. These results clearly indicated that the tumor incidence by MNU administration is dose dependent; when administered 50 mg/kg of MNU i.p., all 56 transgenic mice developed forestomach papillomas, whereas only one of 77 non-transgenic mice developed forestomach papillomas. These results demonstrate that the development of forestomach papillomas was due to the effects of both transgenes and MNU. Skin papillomas were developed in nine out of 56 mice and the incidence was clearly higher than the 0/77 in the controls ($p<0.0001$). No papillomas developed at all in nontransgenic littermates used as control.

Lymphomas were observed in four of 56 transgenic mice and 11 of 77 non-transgenic littermates. The difference of the incidcnces was not significant. Therefore, it was concluded that lymphomas were not due to the effects of the transgene.

An introduction of DMBA into rasH2 transgenic mice also induced tumors 8 weeks after i.p. injection at a rate of about 80%. These were squamous cell carcinomas of the forestomach, adenocarcinomas of the lung and angiosarcomas of the spleen.

Somatic Point Mutation of the Transgene in Tumors

To determine whether the transgene in the tumors became activated, we employed the PCR method followed by oligonucleotide hybridization (*15*). Fifty-six forestomach papillomas, 9 skin papillomas and 4 lymphomas that developed in rasH2 mice receiving 50 mg/kg of MNU were analyzed. The frequency and position of the mutation of the transgenes are shown in Table 3. All the forestomach papillomas except one, 9 of the 9 skin papillomas and one of the 4 lymphomas contained GC to AT transition at the 12th codon in the transgene, which had a point mutation from GGC (Gly) to GAC (Asp). We never detected the mutational activation by MNU at the 61st codon in the transgene that was detected in angiosarcomas occurring spontaneously in this rasH2 line. Mutations at the 12th and 61st codons in the murine c-Ha-*ras* gene have never been detected at all. One forestomach papilloma did not show any mutations at the 12th and 61st codons of the transgene and murine c-Ha-*ras* gene.

All DMBA-induced tumors had the point mutation at the 61st codon of the transgenes from CAG (Gln) to CTG (Leu).

As in the previous study (*13*), we demonstrated that the transgene mRNA and protein product (p21) were expressed in all tissues examined in rasH2 transgenic mice. All the tumors induced by MNU or DMBA, which had somatically mutated transgenes, expressed the mutationally activated transgenes.

ras Transgenic Mice as Models for Tissue-specific Tumorigenesis

Three transgenic mouse lines (rasH2, rasH7, and rasH8) were established with 5–6 copies of human prototype c-Ha-*ras* transgenes independently. In these lines, tumors developed spontaneously in about 50% of transgenic mice within 18 months, and only in restricted tissues (endothelium, squamous epithelium of the skin, bronchioloalveolar epithelium, epithelium of the Harderian gland, and lymphocytes). Moreover, in rasH2 transgenic mice, a single intraperitoneal injection of MNU (50 mg/kg) induced forestomach papillomas at a very high incidence (100%) within 12 weeks, and an i.p. injection of DMBA also induced squamous cell carcinomas of the forestomach, lung adenocarcinomas and spleen angiosarcomas at a rate of about 80%.

RNA blot analyses showed that the RNA expression pattern of the transgene during oncogenesis and among several tissues was similar to that of the endogenous murine c-Ha-*ras* gene (*16*). Thus, it was revealed that mRNAs of the transgenes were expressed in both tumors and normal tissues. Neoplastic cells have therefore never developed solely by the expression of the prototype human c-Ha-*ras* transgenes in combination with the murine endogenous c-Ha-*ras* gene in transgenic mice.

Next, the point mutational activation of the transgenes in the tumors was examined using PCR followed by oligonucleotide hybridization. Somatic point mutational activation at the 61st codon of the transgene was detected in angiosarcomas, lung adenocarcinomas and Harderian gland adenocarcinomas, but mutation at the 12th codon of the transgenes was detected in skin papillomas. Compared with spontaneous tumors, there are some differences in the nature of MNU- and DMBA-induced tumors. The first is the pattern of tissue-specificity of tumor development. MNU administration seemed to promote tumorigenesis in the forestomach epithelium and skin epidermis, and DMBA injection in the squamous cells of the forestomach, epithelial cells of the lung and the vascular endothelium of the spleen. It is therefore suggested that somatic mutational activation of the human c-Ha-*ras* genes might be a causative and tissue-specific tumorigenic event in transgenic mice.

These results raise some questions, however. Is the somatic point mutational activation of transgenes the only cause of the tumors which developed in these lines? It has been suggested that tumors might develop following multiple genetic events (*17*, *18*). However, from these results we could not rule out the possibility that the tumors which developed in these lines were caused by somatic mutational activation of the transgenes associated with other tumorigenic event(s). Furthermore, the frequent occurrence of double or triple tumors developed multiclonally suggest that a single somatic mutation of human prototype c-Ha-*ras* transgenes may have a marked effect on tissue-specific tumorigenesis. If multiple events are always necessary in tumorigenesis, other events should occur as frequently as the specific site point mutations. If they occur only rarely, it is not very likely that secondary events occur simultaneously during tumorigenesis together with somatic point mutational activation of the transgenes.

The reason mutational activation was found only in the transgene and not in the murine c-Ha-*ras* gene is not clear. One possibility is that the transgene is more labile spontaneously and susceptible to alkylation by MNU and DMBA or less efficiently repaired after alkylation than the murine c-Ha-*ras* gene. Another possibility is that tumors produced by the activated transgene grow more rapidly than those produced by activated murine c-Ha-*ras*.

Although the transgene was activated by MNU administration and expressed in various tissues, tumors developed in our system exclusively in the skin epidermis and forestomach epithelium, both of which consisted of keratinocytes. Furthermore, point mutation at codon 61 by DMBA induced only squamous cell carcinomas, lung adenocarcinomas and angiosarcomas of the spleen that were observed in spontaneous tumors having the point mutation at codon 61 of the transgenes. This suggested that all cell types are not equally susceptible to transformation by the activated transgene.

Our results offer good evidence that somatic point mutational activation of the human c-Ha-*ras* gene is an initiating event of tumorigenesis in transgenic mice. The very high incidence of tumorigenesis within a short latent period (8–12 weeks) in our system provides a good animal model for the study of chemical carcinogenesis and the function of the c-Ha-*ras* gene in tumorigenesis.

Acknowledgments

We thank Mrs. K. Katsuki, Miss A. Morita, Messrs K. Nakao, K. Kaseda and K. Nakamura for their excellent technical assistance and animal care in this work. The work was supported in part by a Grant-in-Aid for Cancer Research and a Grant-in-Aid for Scientific Research on Priority Areas (to M. Katsuki) from the Ministry of Education, Science and Culture, Japan and by a Grant-in-Aid (to M. Katsuki) from the Ministry of Health and Welfare for the Comprehensive 10 year Strategy for Cancer Control, Japan.

REFERENCES

1. Barbacid, M. *ras* Genes. Annu. Rev. Biochem., *56*: 779–827, 1987.
2. Bos, J. L. The *ras* gene family and human carcinogenesis. Mutat. Res., *195*: 255–271, 1988.
3. Guerrero, I. and Pellicer, A. Mutational activation of oncogenes in animal model systems of carcinogenesis. Mutat. Res., *185*: 293–308, 1987.

4. Balmain, A. and Brown, K. Oncogene activation in chemical carcinogenesis. Adv. Cancer Res., *51*: 147–182, 1988.
5. Sukumar, S. An experimental analysis of cancer: Role of *ras* oncogenes in multistep carcinogenesis. Cancer Cell, *2*: 199–204, 1990.
6. Zarbl, H., Sukumar, S., Arthur, A. V., Martin-Zanca, D., and Barbacid, M. Direct mutagenesis of Ha-*ras*-1 oncogenes by N-nitroso-N-methylurea during initiation of mammary carcinogenesis in rats. Nature, *315*: 382–385, 1985.
7. Eadie, J. S., Conrad, M., Toorchen, D., and Topal, M. D. Mechanism of mutagenesis by O^6-methylguanine. Nature, *308*: 201–203, 1984.
8. Quintanilla, M., Brown, K., Ramsden, M., and Balmain, A. Carcinogen-specific mutation and amplification of Ha-*ras* during mouse skin carcinogenesis. Nature, *322*: 78–80, 1986.
9. Hanahan, D. Dissecting multistep tumorigenesis in transgenic mice. Annu. Rev. Genet., *22*: 479–519, 1988.
10. Cory, S. and Adams, J. Transgenic mice and oncogenesis. Annu. Rev. Immunol., *6*: 25–48, 1988.
11. Quaife, C. J., Pinkert, C. A., Ornitz, D. M., Palmiter, R. D., and Brinster, R. L. Pancreatic neoplasia induced by *ras* expression in acinar cells of transgenic mice. Cell, *48*: 1023–1034, 1987.
12. Bailleul, B., Surani, M. A., White, S., Barton, S. C., Brown, K., Blessing, M., Jorcano, J., and Balmain, A. Skin hyperkeratosis and papilloma formation in transgenic mice expressing a *ras* oncogene from a suprabasal keratin promoter. Cell, *62*: 697–708, 1990.
13. Saitoh, A., Kimura, M., Takahashi, R., Yokoyama, M., Nomura, T., Izawa, M., Sekiya, T., Nishimura, S., and Katsuki, M. Most tumors in transgenic mice with human c-Ha-*ras* gene contained somatically activated transgenes. Oncogene, *5*: 1195–1200, 1990.
14. Sekiya, T., Prassolov, V. S., Fushimi, M., and Nishimura, S. Transforming activity of the c-Ha-*ras* oncogene having two point mutations in codons 12 and 61. Jpn. J. Cancer Res. (Gann), *76*: 851–855, 1985.
15. Verlaan-de Vries, M., Bogaard, M. E., van den Elst, H., van Boom, J. H., van der Eb, A. J., and Bos, J. L. A dot-blot screening procedure for mutated *ras* oncogenes using synthetic oligodeoxynucleotides. Gene, *50*: 313–320, 1986.
16. Katsuki, M., Kimura, M., Hata, J., Takahashi, R., Nozawa, S., Yokoyama, M., Izawa, M., Sekiya, T., Nishimura, S., and Nomura, T. Embryonal tumors from transgenic mouse zygotes carrying human activated c-Ha-*ras* genes. Mol. Biol. Med., *6*: 567–572, 1989.
17. Land, H., Parada, L. F., and Weinberg, R. A. Tumorigenic conversion of primary embryo fibroblasts requires at least two cooperating oncogenes. Nature, *304*: 596–602, 1983.
18. Brown, K., Buchmann, A., and Balmain, A. Carcinogen-induced mutations in the mouse c-Ha-*ras* gene provide evidence of multiple pathways for tumor progression. Proc. Natl. Acad. Sci. U.S.A., *87*: 538–542, 1990.

MULTISTAGE CARCINOGENESIS, C. C. HARRIS ET AL. (EDS.),
JAPAN SCI. SOC. PRESS, TOKYO/CRC PRESS, BOCA RATON, PP. 259–274, 1992

Transgenic Models of Human Cancer

Steven H. HINRICHS,[*1] Joseph D. FONTES,[*1] Nathan D. BILLS,[*1]
and Philip D. SCHNEIDER[*2]

Departments of Pathology and Microbiology, University of Nebraska Medical Center, Omaha, Nebraska 68198[*1]
and Department of Surgery, University of California, Davis, California 95616[*2], *U.S.A.*

Abstract: Transgenic animal technology has been useful for the direct demonstration of the tumorigenic potential of oncogenes *in vivo*. Over the past eight years a wide variety of oncogenes and proto-oncogenes from viral and cellular sources have been inserted into the germline of mice with subsequent development of neoplasia. Many of the published reports describe similarities between morphologic features of the transgenic mice tumors and those occurring naturally in humans. We discuss the morphologic features of selected transgenic models carrying viral genes and review their applicability to investigations directed toward understanding cancer in general and specifically gastric cancer, neurofibromatosis and leukemia. Examples of the impact of nutrition, interaction with growth factors and initiation with chemical carcinogens are presented. In one of the models functional similarities to the mechanism of oncogenesis in human T-cell leukemia virus type-1 (HTLV-1) lymphoma may exist with activation of cytokine production and subsequent autocrine stimulation. The transgenic model of proximal gastric cancer demonstrates features similar to those seen in carcinogen-induced neoplasia.

These studies underscore the vast potential of transgenic models for inquiry into the genetic and epigenetic basis of human carcinogenesis. However, many features of transgenic cancer models differ from cancer in humans and the specific criteria for judging the value of transgenic models remain unclarified. For example, although the tumors arising in the HTLV-1 Tax transgenic mice show numerous similarities to human neurofibromatosis including development of lesions of the iris, the similarities do not necessarily extend to the molecular involvement of neurofibromatosis-1 (NF-1), a gene with structural and functional homology to GTPase activating proteins. Transgenic experiments of the future will ask questions beyond whether a particular gene is capable of initiating the neoplastic process. The ability to construct systems *in vivo* with a defined starting point that facilitate further controlled manipulation of events resulting in cancer provide great opportunities to dissect the various molecular pathways involved in such a process. Therefore, gene knockout experiments and disruption of gene function will further enhance our ability to understand the multi-factorial process of tumor development.

Transgenic animals hold great promise as models for human cancer. However, numerous issues must first be addressed before the full applicability of these tumor models are realized. The purpose of this paper is to present observations and data associated with selected transgenic animal systems and discuss the relationship between molecular mechanism, pathogenesis, and morphology. The importance of each of these specific issues may differ depending upon the focus of the individual cancer researcher. For a transgenic model to be maximally useful it should mimic the molecular events known to occur in human neoplasia, demonstrate the identical morphological features of the developing tumor and respond to therapeutic interventions in the same manner as the human counterpart. These goals may eventually be achievable as more is discovered about the basic biology of cancer and we learn to modify transgene constructs to reflect this new knowledge. At present, it is possible to use the described transgenic systems to identify promising and meaningful avenues of new research into the biological phenomenon associated with the multi-stage progression of benign to malignant cells.

Transgenic mice are useful for the study of multi-stage carcinogenesis because they represent *in vivo* models where systems known to play a role in tumorigenesis remain intact and integrated (reviewed in *1*). The neurologic, immune, and endocrine system, vascular supply and normal cell to cell interactions are retained in a fully functional manner. In addition, the animals genetic background or susceptibility may be selected. Environmental conditions, including dietary manipulation, and the introduction of chemical carcinogens, can be studied upon the basic background of an activated onco-transgene. Further, the ability to perform a morphologic analysis is of particular value since the histologic appearance of the lesions as they develop may be used to guide the molecular biologist in identification of important molecular phenomenon associated with the transition to neoplasia. Morphologic study may identify important clues in identifying the cellular effect of the gene used in the transgene construct.

A limited number of studies to date have used transgenic animals to address questions beyond the determination of the oncogenic potential of a given gene. Transgenic animals provide an unique opportunity to dissect the changes in cellular physiology that follow the initial, defined genetic insult that the onco-transgene represents. Insight into the susceptibility of various cell types and tissues may be gained by studying the response of different tissue types to the presence of the introduced oncoprotein. A wide variety of projects in transgenic animals utilizing various approaches have been described and are summarized in Table 1.

TABLE 1. Selected Transgenic Experiments Investigating General Issues Regarding Oncogenesis and the Multi-stage Progression to Neoplasia

Mutations, spontaneous or induced	Disruption of int-1	ref. *2*
Over-expression/amplification of oncogene	c-myc expression	ref. *3*
Transcriptional changes	Zinc finger bmi-1	ref. *4*
Epigenetic phenomenon	Obligate wounding	ref. 5
Environmental factors	v-Ha-ras and carcinogen	ref. *6*
	Carcinogen and pim-1	ref. *7*
	Folate deficiency/tax	ref. *8*
Combination of events	Oncogene cooperation	ref. *9*

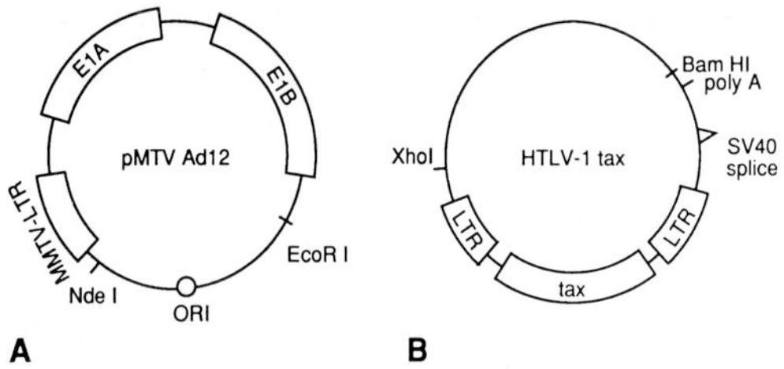

FIG. 1. Schematic representation of the transgenes expressing adenovirus early genes E1A, E1B, and HTLV-1 Tax.

Work begun originally in the laboratory of Dr. Gilbert Jay focused on the cellular effect of specific viral genes including the Tax gene from human T-cell leukemia virus type-1 (HTLV-1) and the early genes E1A, E1B from adenovirus type 12. The role of these genes in viral physiology has been studied extensively, and the ability of these genes to modify or disrupt cellular pathways *in vitro* leading to transformation was known. However, the specific cellular pathways through which these genes interact *in vivo* was unclear and they were therefore selected for use in transgenic mice (Fig. 1). The phenotypes that resulted in the transgenic mice were unexpected and have fostered many lines of interesting research. We have selected to present the findings from the HTLV-1 and adenovirus systems and discuss their clinical and basic mechanistic implications.

Contrasts between Mesenchymal and Epithelial Tumor Models

We are interested in the use of transgenic models to gather data regarding the overall mass of tissue involved in the proliferative phenomenon and determine the relative risk of malignant transformation for specific tissues. Certain anatomical sites such as transitions occurring at the squamous columnar junction or areas subject to trauma and tissue damage may be at higher risk for tumor development than other locations in the same organism.

Transgenic experiments may be able to directly demonstrate that unique mechanisms are involved in malignant transformation of tissues with different embryonic origins. The identification of such mechanisms may be useful in the correlation of histologic and biochemical properties with clinical determinations of whether a tumor is benign or malignant. In epithelial cancers, the criteria for malignancy are usually met by the demonstration of invasion of the adjacent connective tissue. However, for mesenchymal tumors the distinction is much more difficult because the adjacent stroma has morphologic similarities to the tumor.

The initial discovery of transforming genes made use of a relatively transformed mesenchymal cell line, NIH 3T3 cells. The now standard focus forming assay using these cells has led to the elucidation of many oncogenes, from both human tumor and viral sources. However, the potential for selecting oncogenes that are most active in transforming mesenchymal cells places a limitation on this assay. The same caveat applies to transgenic animal systems. The tumor types that arise may be the result of cellular susceptibility as well as oncogene activity. For example, mesenchymal tissues when mature retain their regenerative capability but are not generally constantly replicating as are epithelial surfaces. The repertoire of genes expressed in quiescent cells must be different from actively dividing cells. Beyond cell lineage issues, the role of normal physiologic pathways, which may promote tumor formation in the transgene expressing cells, must be carefully examined. The differences in the physiology of the cell lineages effected may have a role in the pattern of transgene expression. Several reports have documented the unexpected development of mesenchymal tumors in transgenic mice using viral genes typically associated in humans or other animals with epithelial lesions (*10*).

Much elegant work with epithelial tumors in transgenic mice has involved the mammary gland system (*3*). Transgenic mice expressing c-myc, c-ras, int-1, and int-2, as well as crosses of these animals, has provided a sound basis for the study of the pathways involved in mammary tumorigenesis (*11*). In most cases a clear progression of tumor development can be demonstrated. A demonstration of the correlation between genetic changes and morphologic progression to malignancy has been detailed in humans with familial polyposis (*12–14*). Characterizing analogous events in a transgenic mouse system would be of great value.

Background of the HTLV-1 Tax Transgenic System

HTLV-1 is considered to be the causative agent of adult T-cell leukemia (ATL) and is also associated with a chronic myelopathy known as tropical spastic paraparesis (TSP) in the Carribean as well as HTLV-1 associated myelopathy (HAM) in Japan (*15–17*). ATL typically develops after a long latency period and less than 1% of individuals with antibodies to HTLV-1 ever develop ATL (reviewed in *18*). The HTLV-1 genome codes for two proteins named Tax and Rex in addition to the structural genes. The transactivator protein, Tax (p40, pX) has been the focus of efforts to identify the oncogenic mechanism through which the virus works (*19*). *In vivo* experimental evidence showing how a single gene could potentially cause such disparate clinical symptoms was lacking prior to the derviation of transgenic mice expressing Tax.

Human neurofibromatosis (NF) is a condition consisting of a broad spectrum of disorders (20). NF is commonly a inherited but also has a high spontaneous mutation rate. The morphologic findings may include cafe au lait macules, neurofibromas, freckling, optic glioma, Lisch nodules and distinctive osseous lesions. There is an increased incidence of acute myelogenous leukemia (AML). Molecular genetic studies have implicated the involvement of NF-1, a gene with structural and functional homology to GTPase activating proteins (*21*).

Key Features of the HTLV-1 Tax Transgenic System

To determine the potential role of Tax in the development of HTLV-1 pathology a transgene was generated incorporating the coding sequence for Tax flanked by viral long terminal repeats (LTR's) on both the 5′ and 3′ ends (22). Through microinjection of pronuclear embryos several separate lines of transgenic animals were

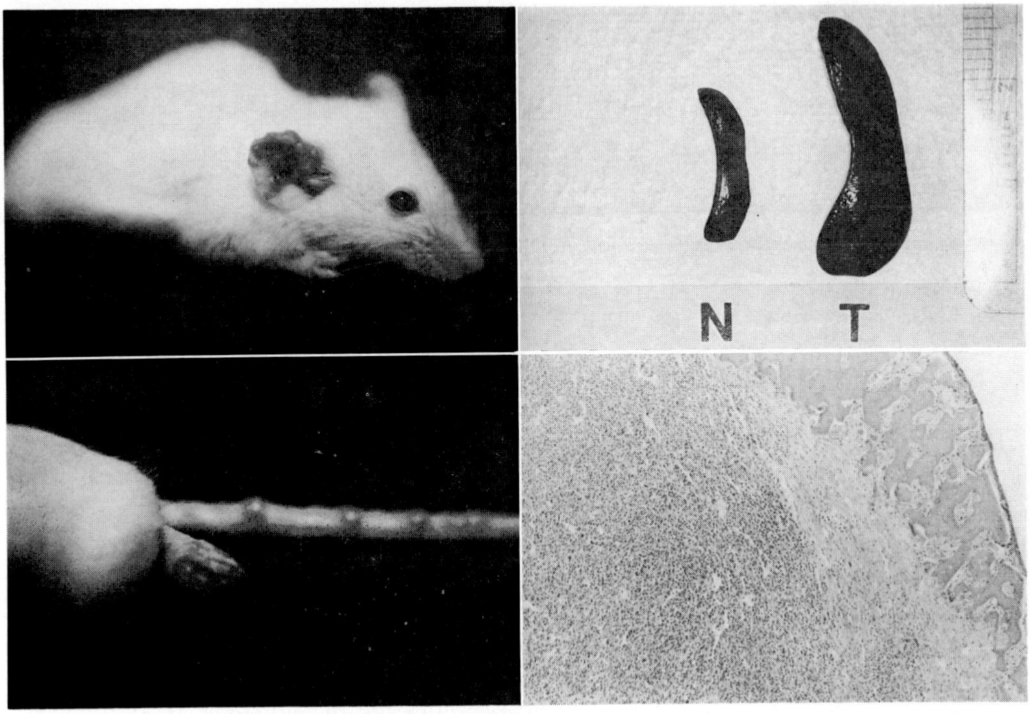

FIG. 2. Characteristic phenotype of HTLV-1 tax mice with multiple simultaneous nodules on ear, (upper left), hind foot, and tail (lower left). Bone lesions with expansion of the marrow and disruption of cortical bone (lower right). Spleen of transgenic Tax mouse (T) compared to non-transgenic control (N).

produced and two of these lines showing similar phenotypes have been studied continuously over the past 4 years. A second phenotype appearing in these animals (characterized by thymic expression of the tax gene and early death before reaching sexual maturity) has not been a subject of study in our laboratory. Issues which inpact on the significance of the system include: 1) in each of the two studied transgenic lines the site of integration of the transgene is unique as evidenced by different flanking sequences, 2) each of the transgenic lines incorporate approximately 20 to 50 copies of the transgene, 3) expression of the tax gene is detectable in mesenchymal tissues within the first four weeks of life, 4) there is a direct relationship between the levels of RNA and protein expression as demonstrated by Nerenberg *et al.*, 5) high levels of expression of Tax are present in muscle; however, no proliferative phenomenon results (*23*), and 6) no evidence of lymphoid expression or myeloid expression of the tax gene was found.

The characteristic feature in the HTLV-1 tax transgenic mice is the development of soft tissue tumors of peripheral neural sheath origin between 60 and 90 days of age (*24*). Of the over 200 mice studied from these lines, all mice with two notable exceptions have developed peripheral nerve sheaths tumors. The most frequent exception are those animals that develop intracranial tumors of the fifth cranial nerve ganglion and die before 60 days of age. In rare instances animals with intra-

TABLE 2. Theoretical Model of Steps Involved in Carcinogenesis in Transgenic Mice

Transgene expression
1 (cytokine, cAMP)
Tissue damage
2
Cell proliferation and angiogenesis
3
Benign neoplasia
4 (cytokines)
Malignant neoplasia

In the HTLV-1 Tax system, cytokines induced through expression of Tax may be markers of neoplastic progression.

cranial tumors will also develop peripheral nerve tumors. The second exception is two females that did not develop tumors until eight and nine months of age, respectively.

The tumors are typically peripheral and multifocal in distribution, affecting the forelimbs, ears, snout, and tail (Fig. 2). Forelimb tumors may appear in the metacarpal or tarsal areas as well as weight-bearing surfaces. Ear tumors first become apparent as hypervascular papules adjacent to an ear punch site. Frequently, tumor development in the tail is at the amputation site where tissue had been removed for genotype determination. A hypervascular patch also precedes the development of tumors on the tail and is typically present two weeks before the development of an obvious nodule. Studies by Green *et al.* have shown that approximately 70% of the tax mice develop adrenal tumors in addition to the peripheral soft tissue neoplasms (*25*). An additional characteristic feature develops in a third line of mice characterized by cellular proliferation in the iris and/or ciliary body. These are the characteristics that bear similarities to human neurofibromatosis which have been reviewed in *26*.

Evidence of the peripheral nerve sheath origin of the tumors has been obtained by electron micrograph studies of the lesions when becoming first apparent and measuring approximately 1 mm in size. The predominant cell type is the perineural fibroblast that in early lesions retains a discontinuous external laminae (*24*). Few or no differentiating features are seen in tumors that measure greater than 2 mm in size. Histologic and ultrastructural examination of the lesions in the adrenal medulla, cranial nerve ganglion and iris lesions show common features suggesting a similar origin from perineural fibroblast. Additional evidence for the origin of tumors in the tax transgenic mice coming from the peripheral nerves is the sequential sectioning of tumors and the deomonstration of continuity with major and minor nerve trunks.

One of the key advantages of a transgenic model of cancer is the reproducibility of the system in the generation of animals with a well defined onset and progression of neoplasia. A theoretical model can then be proposed in which specific stages are identified through which each tumor must pass in its progression from a benign to a malignant phenotype. We have attempted to identify such a model of multistage carcinogenesis for transgenic animal systems and will address this model in light of the observations from the HTLV-1 tax system and the MMTV E1A E1B system (Table 2).

Multi-stage Progression of Neoplasia

In the HTLV-1 transgenic system, Tax is expressed at an early age in mesenchymal tissues (*22*). Since non-transgenic control mice do not develop tumors, expression of tax is a key initial step in tumorigenesis and no evidence exists to suggest tax expression must first be induced. All peripheral nerve fibroblasts in a transgenic animal are potentially capable of expressing Tax at any one time, yet tumors develop in a relatively small percentage of these cells as evidenced by the development of fewer than ten neurofibromas in the typical transgenic mouse. Through immunohistochemical studies it has been shown that not all perineural fibroblasts in tumors or normal nerves express Tax simultaneously. Yet Tax expression persists in cell lines derived from the tumors and argues for Tax being essential for maintenance of the phenotype. We have shown that Tax transgene expression in tumor cells both *in vitro* and *in vivo* is inducible by 8-bromo-cAMP and isoproterenol, respectively. *In vitro*, this increase in tax expression is followed by the upregulation the c-fos and leukemia inhibitory factor (LIF) genes. These secondary responses follow the increase in Tax protein, and are not due to cAMP directly. We have therefore reconsidered the question of induction of the transgene and propose that neuroendrocrine stimulation *in vivo* may potentially trigger the initial proliferation of discreet populations of neurofibroblasts or raise the level of Tax above a threshold whereby other genes are activated. Other studies in transgenic animals have characterized expression of the transgene as an initiation step which requires subsequent promotion for the development of tumors (*6*).

In the Tax system a second phenomenon which appears to be required or enhances further development of tumors is tissue damage. We noted the presence of tumors at peripheral sites in the animals and considered several issues including temperature dependent pathways. However, the most convincing evidence for the requirement of tissue damage for progression of tumors in these animals is the identification and association of habits of specific animals with the development of tumors at specific sites. For example, the type of caging material and aggressiveness of the animal while feeding can determine whether tumors develop around the snout and male animals frequently develop tumors on the tail in cages where multiple aggressive males are maintained. In experiments where a single incision was made in the tail, no tumors were induced. This is consistent with a model where multiple and repetitive tissue damage is essential for tumorigenesis. However, it is not appropriate to consider trauma as the sole explanation. In keeping with the above mechanism of cAMP induction, gene expression may be enhanced by Tax in cells that are beginning to proliferate as a result of injury. This process has been described in transgenic studies conducted by others where investigator initiated tissue damage is a necessary step for tumor formation (*5*). This finding is significant in light of reports of humans with neurofibromatosis who developed tumors at the site of recent trauma (*20*). As a result of this observation anti-inflammatory agents are being examined as experimental therapeutics.

Focal hyperemia is also predictive of subsequent tumor development. In keeping with the overall concept of tissue damage and repair it is possible to predict the development of subsequent tumor when a hyperemic area is identified on the tail or ears. It is still undetermined in the LTR-tax mouse whether these erythremic foci represent simple inflammatory activity, with increased vascular perfusion, or whether angiogenesis is occurring prior to tumor development. Other studies in transgenics have clearly defined the importance of angiogenesis in the development of pancreatic tumors.

Two considerations led us to investigate the role that cytokine induction might play in the development of pathology in this transgenic mouse systems. The tax gene has been shown to transactivate several cellular genes that include hematopoietic growth factors (HGF) or growth factor receptors including interleukin-2 (IL-2), the IL-2 receptor and the granulocyte macrophage colony stimulating factor (GM-CSF) in human ATL (*27, 28*). A key morphologic feature of the transgenic animals is the early infiltration of tumors by granulocytes. This infiltration occurs even when the tumors are collections of eight to ten cells. It is also at this stage that the origin of the tumors from perineural fibroblast is best demonstrated. The molecular correlation of this histologic finding is the expression of GM-CSF in early transgenic animal tumors and in cell lines derived from these tumors (29). *In vivo*, GM-CSF has been shown to cause increases in macrophages, eosinophils, and at high enough concentration, megakaryocytes. It is remarkable, however, that in the absence of additional trauma the granulocytes show no evidence of degranulation and there is no ultra-structural evidence of necrosis or membrane destruction in the early tumors. Typically GM-CSF is thought to have a local effect; however it has been shown that other HGFs act systemically as well, in the maintenance of normal leukocyte populations (*30*). In the transgenic animals there is a roughly doubling in the size of the spleen with a clear-cut hyperplasia of the bone marrow, which may very well be due to tumor produced GM-CSF (Fig. 2). Maturation and release of these granulocytes from the marrow or spleen is not certain since in over 50% of cases only slightly elevated levels of circulating granulocytes are found. In other animals, the circulating granulocyte level is markedly elevated.

For cancer researchers the characterization of the tumors in the mice as benign or malignant is important. The morphologic and histologic similarity between the tumors developing in the transgenic mice and human neurofibromatosis is striking. Specific comparisons of the transgenic model with human neurofibromatosis have been made. For purposes of this discussion it is not easy to characterize the tumors as malignant from a histologic viewpoint. Although one criteria, that of increased mitotic figures can be used to categorize a tumor as malignant in some cases this results in the animal in only a rapidly enlarging tumor without impinging on any critical organs and causing early death. In other situations a small tumor arising in the fifth cranial nerve ganglion can result in significant morbidity and still be characterized as histologically benign. These same difficulties are encountered in humans with neurofibromatosis. In the transgenic system we have used chromosome analysis and tissue culture growth characteristics to characterize the malignant nature of the tumor cells. In addition, metastases of tumor cells has occurred to neck lymph nodes with the primary presumably being the large tumors along the snout and along facial cranial nerves. The large majority of tumors characterized as benign have a diploid chromosome content without gross abnormalities. Tumor cells collected from tumors approaching 1 cm in diameter grow well in tissue culture and can be established as long term cell lines. Chromosome analysis of these well established cells in culture show an aneuploid karyotype with chromosome counts in the hypotetraploid range. Several abnormal chromosomes derived from translocations are currently under study. Several other findings are found in animals with large tumors, the most consistent being bony lesions and in rare occasions bone tumors.

If an animal model were to mimic the phenomenon of disease found in HTLV-1 associated leukemia or lymphoma then the model should reasonably demonstrate how the gene could be present in an animal for a long period of time with only the infrequent development of a malignant phenotype. In humans infected with HTLV-1 less than 1% eventually develop leukemia or lymphoma. Presumably this conversion to a malignant phenotype in humans is through acquired mutations in a proliferating cell driven by the cytokine growth factor pathway involving IL-2 and IL-2 receptor. A similar phenomenon may occur in the transgenic animals as inferred from recent *in vitro* data. We have analyzed the supernatants of the tumor cell lines and found not only the abundant expression of GM-CSF but also M-CSF, IL-6, and LIF. Assigning a causative role in the development of the malignant phenotype to the expression of these various cytokines is speculative; however, at both steps one and four indirect data lend support to this hypothesis. Two of the three factors identified as being capable of transactivation *via* the Tax protein have also been shown to be produced in mouse and human fibroblasts in response to inflammatory mediators. These factors include IL-6, granulocyte macrophage colony stimulating factor and transforming growth factor beta. Our reason for implicating the additional factors colony stimulating factor (CSF-1) and LIF is their role in hematopoiesis and their effect upon osteoclasts and marrow stromal elements, respectively. Studies have shown that while these cytokines stimulate myeloid proliferation they also are involved in myeloid differentiation. In approximately two to three per cent of animals we have seen the development of lesions arising within the bone marrow characterized by a nodular elevation of the cortex and replacement of the bone marrow spicules by primitive mesenchymal cells admixed with large numbers of bone marrow progenitors. There is considerable bone remodeling and replacement by stromal cells, and only rarely do lesions develop meeting minimal criteria for neoplasia.

Proximal Gastric Cancer: Molecular and Clinical Issues

Gastric neoplasia presents many theoretical problems for the cancer biologist and has considerable importance as a human disease in general. The incidence of gastric cancer has been declining in the West since the 1950's with a similar decline noted in Japan in more recent years (*31–33*). The worldwide prevalence, however, still makes gastric cancer the most lethal visceral malignancy. Carcinomas of the esophagogastric junction in humans are becoming common gastric malignancies accounting for up to 40% of all gastric cancers. A report from the USA National Cancer Institute suggests that in the ten years prior to 1987, the incidence of proximal gastric cancer has become the most rapidly increasing cancer in the United States (*34*). In addition, because of the well recognized progression of benign changes associated with reflux esophagitis including metaplasia, columnar heterotopia, dysplasia and progression to malignancy, this entity constitutes a fascinating morphological and molecular problem (*35–37*).

The specific clinical as well as molecular questions may be related to phenomenon associated with the development and maintenance of epithelium at transitions from columnar to squamous epithelium. Similar questions may be raised about the biology of Human Papillomavirus associated carcinoma arising in the uterine cervix and Nasopharyngeal Carcinoma associated with Epstein Barr Virus arising in the nasopharynx.

In contrast to humans the transition from squamous to columnar epithelium does not occur at the esophogastric junction but rather in the mid portion of the stomach in mice. The squamous lined forestomach therefore exists as a reservoir and the cardiac glands found at the squamous columnar esophageal gastric junction in humans are found immediately distal to the squamous columnar junction in the mid-portion of the stomach in mice.

Key Features of the MMTV E1A, E1B System

Human adenoviruses can transform a variety of cell types through the effect of the early genes E1A and E1B (*38*). These genes cooperate to elevate levels of expression and subsequent transforming activity in order to accomplish a fully transformed phenotype. The adenovirus E1A and E1B genes were selected for use in the transgene construct under the regulation of the mouse mammary tumor virus (MMTV) long terminal repeat rather that the homologous promoter. This alternative promoter was required because introduction of adenovirus early genes under its own regulatory control would likely result in early developmental abnormalities leading to death *in utero*. The MMTV LTR appears to direct expression sometime after the early stages of embryogenesis and development (*39*). In addition, the MMTV LTR may be hormonally regulated. The adenovirus E1B gene has been shown to interact with the p53 gene which in many systems shows features consistent with an anti-oncogene (*40*). EiA interacts with cellular genes and also binds to the retinoblastoma gene product (*41*).

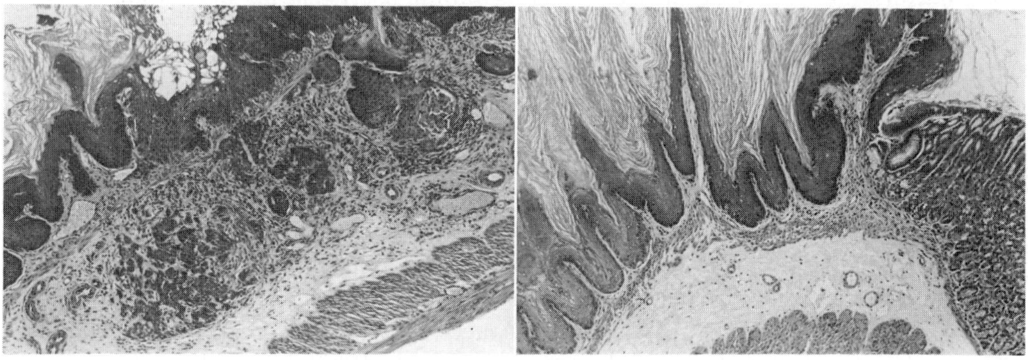

FIG. 3. Morphologic similarity between proximal gastric lesions in E1A, E1B transgenic mice and methylbenzyl nitrosamine. Hyperplastic changes occurring at the squamous side of the squamocolumnar junction (upper left). Invasive carcinoma arising at the squamocolumnar junction.

Of the 23 mice carrying the MMTV E1A, E1B transgene, 11 developed neoplastic proliferations in the gastric forestomach (*42*). Expression of the early genes was not detected in gastric epithelium in the transgenic animals before the development of carcinoma. Presumably those animals carrying the transgene that did not develop transformation did not undergo activation of the promoter. Therefore in contrast with the HTLV-1 system, activation of expression was a key step in development of the phenotype. None of the animals that developed tumor survivied to sexual maturity. The inability to derive a continuously breeding line of mice greatly limited the ability to study progressive events in these animals. However, sufficient numbers were available to identify several morphologic stages and recently a new model has become available which shows essentially identical features to those obtained in the transgenic system.

Morphologic features of the transgenic Ad 12 mice include papillary and multinodular appearance of the forestomach correlated histologically by an epithelial hyperplasia (Fig. 3). A second feature of the lesions was an expanded squamous submucosa with nests of atypical cells forming glandular structures. The origin of this glandular epithelium is unknown; however, it may be from submucosal glands. There was a clear progression from the hyperplastic and dysplastic overlying squamous epithelium to atypical and infiltrating squamous nests and gland forming tumors into the underlying submucosa and muscularis. Although the squamous component appeared histologically malignant only the glandular component of the tumors showed evidence of metastases to lymph nodes and lungs. Metastases is an infrequent observation in transgenic systems but is critical evidence for characterizing a tumor as malignant.

Studies of expression of the E1A and E1B genes by Northern blot showed expression of both genes in the stomach with tumor, metastatic tumors, and testes with low levels of expression in the brain. Although brain and testes showed no evidence of neoplasia it is important to note that all male mice were unable to transmit the transgene. Exceptions to this pattern of expression were seen in two animals of which one was capable of transmitting the transgene with subsequent development of tumors within the olfactory epithelium (*43*). A parallel experiment attempted to show whether or not the adenovirus genes when expressed separately in transgenic mice would be capable of causing transformation. When transgenic mice were derived expressing either but not both of the E1A and E1B genes, no tumors developed. Induction of E1B or E1A expression was accomplished by treatment with dexamethasone however no tumors were observed over a period of one year.

Since it has not been possible to derive a breeding colony of the MMTV Ad-12 mice, data relevant to the early issues involved in development of gastric neoplasia and morphologic appearance is minimal. The number of gene affected by or interacting with Ad-12 E1A does not appear to be as numerous as in the HTLV-1 Tax system however more may be found (*44*). It is known that Ad-12 E1A can down-regulate the expression of major histocompatibility complex (MHC) class I genes *in vitro* and the suppression of class I antigens may be important for the lack of recognition of Ad-12 transformed cells by the immune system. The levels of class I gene expression were therefore studied in the transgenic system using a probe which identified the class I K, D, and L genes mRNA. The stomach containing carcinoma showed a decrease of class I gene expression in comparison to a normal littermate when equal amounts of RNA were studied. Importantly, no differences in class I gene expression were noted between liver and testes in transgenic mice with or without tumors.

Tissue damage and angiogenesis have not been directly implicated in the role of tumor development in the Ad-12 transgenic system. However, the morphologic features encountered in progression from benign to malignant tumors has been more fruitful. Previous studies have been identified from the literature in which gastric tumors were generated in mice given the carcinogen methylbenzylnitrosamine (*45*). By adjusting the dosage and route of administration we have been able to confirm these findings with the development of forestomach adeno and squamous carcinomas. These carcinogen-induced tumors bear a striking a morphologic similarity to those seen in the transgenic Ad-12 mice although with a greater preponderance of squamous carcinoma. It has also been possible to study the morphologic appearance of early lesions which could not be done in large numbers in the transgenic system. In the carcinogen induced model there is florid squamous hyperplasia of the epithelium immediately adjacent to the squamous columnar junction and the appearance of dysplastic glands within the expanded submucosa are again found.

The normal physiologic proliferation associated with the continual cycling of gastric mucosae is a potential pathway for transgene perturbation leading to transformation analogous to the issues that may be important in the mammary system. This is in contrast to the mesenchymal neurofibromas of the LTR-Tax mouse, where a discreet, crisis-oriented physiologic pathway (inflammation and tissue repair) is a likely contributor to tumor development.

Conclusions

Our interest has focused not only on the initiating effects that lead to transgene expression but also on correlating the morphologic and molecular features associated with neoplasia. Molecular events at the squamous columnar junction is a topic of considerable interest and questions have been raised as to whether there is an anatomic basis for the increased risk for neoplasia. Studies in our laboratory and elsewhere have shown that there is a slight increase in the rate of mitotic division in the squamous epithelium immediately adjacent to the transition zone. This observation has relevance when considering the importance of the interaction of E1A with retinoblastoma gene product as well as p53 and the control of cell cycle. We have considered the concept that progression from benign to malignant neoplasia may occur through the acquisition of mutations by either of two mechanisms: 1) increasing the rate of mitoses in a system with a defined mutation rate, or 2) increasing the mutation rate per cell division (*46*). If the mutation rate per division is constant then increasing the number of divisions will increase the eventual mutation rate. Increasing the number of stem cells in division will also affect the mutation rate. If a transgene acts through the cell cycle by increasing the number of stem cells in division then a hyperplastic epithelium should precede the development of a fully malignant neoplasm. The morphologic observations in the transgenic Ad-12 system as well as in the carcinogen induced system are consistent with both mechanisms causing an increase in the number of proliferating cells. Some researchers have noted the mechanistic similarities between E1A and Tax (Chen, 1985 #50).

It is important then to ask how observations from the HTLV-1 Tax system impact on these concepts. Why can either the transgenes E1A, E1B or carcinogen act to rapidly convert normal epithelium to benign hyperplastic epithelium with a near 100% transformation to malignant epithelium whereas in the HTLV-1 Tax system prolonged driving of the myeloid monocytic series by numerous cytokines results only in a hyperplastic or pre-leukemic state. Similarly, the neurofibromas are most frequently benign with malignant features occurring only rarely. Our conclusion is that the risk for a mutation or event leading to a fully malignant phenotype is different for each of the tissues of the animal. In such a model, tissues that are quiescent rather than proliferative would be expected to have a different rate of transformation to a malignant phenotype.

A second issue is that transcriptional factors may work through different types of regulatory pathways that are tissue specific. One type of pathway may involve interaction with multiple regulatory proteins and necessarily results in the increased expression of several different genes that are cytokines or cytokine receptors. The transgenic HTLV-1 system may be such a model. Transcriptional factors that directly influence cell cycle regulation would be expected to result in a more rapid rate of transformation. The MMTV Ad-12 system may be such an example however much additional work is needed. Transgenic animals will be useful to explore these and many other issues relevant to the mutli-stage progression of carcinogenesis.

REFERENCES

1. Hanahan, D. Dissecting multistep tumorigenesis in transgenic mice. Annu. Rev. Genet., *22(479)*: 479–519, 1988.
2. Thomas, K. and Capecchi, M. Targeted disruption of the murine int-1 protooncogene resulting in severe abnormalities in midbrain and cerebellar development. Nature, *346*: 847–850, 1990.
3. Leder, A., Pattengale, P., Kuo, A., Stewart, T., and Leder, P. Consequences of widespread deregulation of the c-myc gene in transgenic mice: multiple neoplasms and normal development. Cell, *45*: 485–495, 1986.
4. Haupt, Y., Alexander, W., Barri, G., Klinken, S., and Adams, J. Novel zinc finger gene implicated as myc collaborator by retrovirally accelerated lymphomagenesis in Eu-myc transgenic mice. Cell, *65*: 753–763, 1991.
5. Schuh, A., Keating, S., Monteclaro, F., Vogt, P., and Breitman, M. Obligatory wounding requirement for tumorigenesis in v-jun transgenic mice. Nature, *346*: 756–759, 1990.
6. Leder, A., Kuo, A., Cardiff, R., Sinn, E., and Leder, P. v-Ha-ras transgene abrogates the initiation step in mouse skin tumorigenesis: Effects of phorbol esters and retinoic acid. Proc. Natl. Acad. Sci. U.S.A., *87*: 9178–9182, 1990.
7. Breuer, M., Slebos, R., Verbeek, S., Van Lohuzien, M., Wientjiens, E., and Berns, A. Very high frequency of lymphoma induction by a chemical carcinogen in pim-1 transgenic mice. Nature, *340*: 61–63, 1989.
8. Bills, N., Hinrichs, S., Morgan, R., and Clifford, A. Delayed tumor onset in transgenic mice fed a low folate diet. J. Natl. Cancer Inst., in press.

9. Alexander, W. S., Adams, J. M., and Cory, S. Oncogene cooperation in lymphocyte transformation: malignant conversion of E mu-myc transgenic pre-B cells *in vitro* is enhanced by v-H-ras or v-raf but not v-abl. Mol. Cell. Biol., *9(1)*: 67–73, 1989.
10. Lindgren, V., Sippola, T. M., Skowronski, J., Wetzel. E., Howley, P. M., and Hanahan, D. Specific chromosomal abnormalities characterize fibrosarcomas of bovine papillomavirus type 1 transgenic mice. Proc. Natl. Acad. Sci. U.S.A., *86(13)*: 5025–5029, 1989.
11. Sinn, E., Muller, W., Pattengale, P., Tepler, I., Wallace, R., and Leder, P. Coexpression of MMTV/v-Ha-ras and MMTV/c-myc genes in transgenic mice: synergistic action of oncogenes *in vivo*. Cell, *49(4)*: 465–475, 1987.
12. Nishisho, I., Nakamura, Y., Miyoshi, Y., Miki, Y., Ando, H., Horii, A., Koyama, K., Utsunomiya, J., Baba, S., Hedge, P., Markham, A., Krush, A., Petersen, M., Hamilton, M. S., Nilbert, M., Levy, D. B., Preisinger, A., Smith, K., Su, L., Kinzler, K., and Vogelstein, B. Mutations of chromosome 5q21 genes in FAP and colorectal cancer patients. Science, *253*: 665–669, 1991.
13. Vogelstein, B., Fearon, E. R., Kern, S. E., Hamilton, S. R., Preisinger, A. C., Nakamura, Y., and White, R. Allelotype of colorectal carcinomas. Science, *244(4901)*: 207–211, 1989.
14. Vogelstein, B., Fearon, E. R., Hamilton, S. R., Kern, S. E., Preisinger, A. C., Leppert, M., Nakamura, Y., White, R., Smits, A. M., and Bos, J. L. Genetic alterations during colorectal-tumor development. N. Engl. J. Med., *319(9)*: 525–532, 1988.
15. Hinuma, Y., Nagata, K., Hanaoka, M., Nakai, M., Matsumoto, T., Kinoshita, K., Shirakawa, S., and Miyoshi, I. Adult T-cell leukemia: antigen in an ATL cell line and detection of antibodies to the antigen in human sera. Proc. Natl. Acad. Sci. U.S.A., *78(6476)*: 6476–6480, 1981.
16. Gessain, A., Vernant, J. C., Maurs, L., Barin, F., Gout, O., Calendar, A., and de The, G. Antibodies to human T-lymphotropic virus type 1 in patients with tropical spastic paraparesis. Lancet, *ii*: 407–410, 1985.
17. Osame, M., Igata, A., Matsumoto, M., Izumo, S., Usuku, K., Rosales, R. L., and Tara, M. HTLV-1 associated myelopathy (HAM). Kansenshogaku Zasshi, 1988 (in Japanese).
18. Gallo, R. C. The first human retrovirus. Sci. Am., *256*: 88–98, 1987.
19. Ballad, D. W., Bohnlein, E., Lowenthal, J. W., Wano, Y., Franza, B. R., and Greene, W. C. HTLV-I tax induces cellular proteins that activate the kB element in the IL-2 receptor gene. Science, *241*: 1652–1655, 1988.
20. Riccardi, V. and Eichler, J. Neurofibromatosis: Phenotype, Natural History, and Pathogenesis, The Johns Hopkins University Press, Baltimore, 1986.
21. Xu, G., O'Connell, P., Viskochil, D., Cawthon, R., Robertson, M., Culver, M., Dunn, D., Stevens, J., Gesteland, R., White, R., and Weiss, R. The neurofibromatosis type 1 gene encodes a protein related to GAP. Cell, *62*: 599–608, 1990.
22. Nerenberg, M., Hinrichs, S., Reynolds, R., Khoury, G., and Jay, G. The tat gene of human T-lymphotropic virus type 1 induces mesenchymal tumors in transgenic mice. Science, *237*: 1324–1329, 1987.
23. Nerenberg, M. and Wiley, C. Degeneration of oxidative muscle fibers in HTLV-1 tax transgenic mice. Am. J. Pathol., *135*: 251–259, 1989.
24. Hinrichs, S. H., Nerenberg, M., Reynolds, R. K., Khoury, G., and Jay, G. A transgenic mouse model for human neurofibromatosis. Science, *237(4820)*: 1340–1343, 1987.
25. Green, J., Baird, A., Hinrichs, S., Klintworth, G., and Jay, G. Adrenal medullary tumors and iris proliferation in a transgenic mouse model of neurofibromatosis. Submitted.

26. Baird, A., Green, J., Jay, G., and Hinrichs, S. Neurofibromatosis: Key features of the transgenic mouse model. Comp. Pathol. Bull. AFIP, in press.
27. Cross, S. L., Feinberg, M. B., Wolf, J. B., Holbrook, N. J., Wong-Staal, F., and Leonard, W. J. Regulation of the human interleukin-2 receptor a chain promoter: activation of a non-functional promoter by the transactivator gene of HTLV-I. Cell, *49*: 466–469, 1987.
28. Chan, J. Y., Slamon, D. J., Nimer, S. D., Golde, D. W., and Gasson, J. C. Regulation of expression of human granulocyte/macrophage colony stimulating factor. Proc. Natl. Acad. Sci. U.S.A., *83*: 8669–8673, 1986.
29. Green, J., Begley, D., Wagner, T., and Jay, G. Trans-activation of granulocyte-macrophage colony-stimulating factor and the interleukin-2 receptor in transgenic mice carrying the human T-lymphotropic virus type 1 tax gene. Mol. Cell. Biol., *9*: 4731–4737, 1989.
30. Maekawa, T., Metcalf, D., and Gearing, D. Enhanced suppression of human myeloid leukemic cell lines by combinations of IL-6, LIF, GM-CSF and G-CSF. Int. J. Cancer, *45*: 353–358, 1990.
31. Meyers, W. C., Damiano, R. J., Rotolo, F. S., and Postlethwait, R. W. Adenocarcinoma of the stomach. Changing patterns over the last 4 decades. Ann. Surg., *205(1)*: 1–8, 1987.
32. Cady, B., Rossi, R. L., Silverman, M. L., Piccione, W., and Heck, T. A., Gastric adenocarcinoma. A disease in transition. Arch. Surg., *124(3)*: 303–308, 1989.
33. Kampschoer, G., Nakajima, T., and van de Velde, C. Changing patterns in gastric adenocarcinoma. Br. J. Surg., *76*: 914–916, 1989.
34. Blot, W., Kneller, R., and Fraumeni, J. Rising incidence of adenocarcinoma of the esophagous and gastric cardia. JAMA, *265*: 1287–1289, 1991.
35. Correa, P. Precursors of gastric and esophageal cancer. Cancer, *50*: 2554–2565, 1982.
36. Goyal, R. Columnar cell-lined (Barrett's) esophagus: a historical perspective. Barrett's Esophagus: Pathophysiology, Diagnosis, and Management. *In*; I. Spechler and R. Goyal (eds.), pp. 1–17, Elsevier, New York, Amsterdam, 1985.
37. Hameeteman, W., Tytgat, G., Houthoff, H., and van den Tweel, J. Barrett's esophagus: development of dysplasia and adenocarcinoma. Gastroenterology, *96*: 1249–1256, 1989.
38. Bernards, R., Houweling, A., Schrier, P., Bos, J., and Van der Eb, A. Characterization of cells transformed by Ad5/Ad12 hybrid early region 1 plasmids. Virology, *120*: 422–432, 1982.
39. Stewart, T., Hollingshead, P., and Pitts, S. Multiple regulatory domains in the mouse mammary tumor virus long terminal repeat revealed by analysis of fusion genes in transgenic mice. Mol. Cell. Biol., *8*: 473–479, 1988.
40. Sarnow, P., Ho, Y., Williams, J., and Levine, A. Adenovirus E1b-58kd tumor antigen and SV450 large tumor antigen are physically associated with the same 54 kd cellular protein in transformed cells. Cell, *28*: 387–394, 1982.
41. Whyte, P., Buchkovich, K., Horowitz, J., Friend, S., Raybuck, M., Weinberg, R., and Harlow, E. Association between an oncogene and an anti-oncogene: The adenovirus E1A proteins bind to the retinoblastoma gene product. Nature, *334*: 124–129, 1988.
42. Koike, K., Hinrichs, S. H., Isselbacher, K. J., and Jay, G. Transgenic mouse model for human gastric cancer. Proc. Natl. Acad. Sci. U.S.A., *86*: 5615–5619, 1989.
43. Koike, K., Jay, G., Hartley, J. W., Schrenzel, M. D., Higgins, R. J., and Hinrichs, S. H. Activation of retrovirus in transgenic mice: association with development of olfactory neuroblastoma. J. Virol., *64*: 3988–3991, 1990.

44. Webster, K. A., Muscat, G. E., and Kedes, L. Adenovirus E1A products suppress myogenic differentiation and inhibit transcription from muscle-specific promoters. Nature, *332(6164)*: 553–557, 1988.
45. Sander, J. and Schweinsberg, F. Tumorinduktion bei Mausen durch N-Methyl-nitrosamine in niedriger Dosierung (German). Z. Krebsforsch., *79*: 157–161, 1973.
46. Cohen, S. M. and Ellwein, L. B. Cell proliferation in carcinogenesis. Science, *249*: 1007–1011, 1990.

PROMOTION, PROGRESSION, INVASION, AND METASTASIS

MULTISTAGE CARCINOGENESIS‘ C. C. HARRIS ET AL. (EDS.),
JAPAN SCI. SOC. PRESS, TOKYO/CRC PRESS, BOCA RATON, PP. 227–283, 1992

The Roles of Specific Isoforms of Protein Kinase C in Growth Control and Human Colon Cancer

I. Bernard WEINSTEIN

Comprehensive Cancer Center, Institute of Cancer Research, and Department of Genetics and Development, Columbia University, New York, New York 10032, U.S.A.

Abstract: Protein kinase C (PKC) consists of a family of lipid-regulated enzymes which play a pivotal role in signal transduction. Studies with the cell line R6-PKC3, a derivative of R6 rat fibroblasts that overexpresses $PKC_{\beta 1}$, provide direct evidence that this isoform of PKC influences cell morphology, growth control, the production of an autocrine growth factor, and the action of an activated H-*ras* oncogene. Analysis of ^{32}P-labelled phosphoproteins indicates that R6-PKC cells display increased phosphorylation of a 80/87 kDa protein (designated MARCKS), and after treatment with TPA they display a dramatic prolongation in the phosphorylation and in the cytosolic accumulation of this protein. These alterations in MARCKS may be responsible, at least in part, for the altered growth properties of R6-PKC3 cells. We have also examined the expression of endogenous isoforms of PKC in R6 cells and oncogene-transformed derivatives. Normal R6 cells express four isoforms of PKC, cPKCα, nPKCε, nPKCδ, and nPKCζ; nPKCδ and nPKCε are the most abundant. nPKCε and nPKCδ have an unusual distribution since 60–80% is membrane-bound. In response to TPA, the cytosolic levels of all four PKC isozymes were recruited to the membrane fraction. Prolonged treatment of R6 cells with TPA caused total loss of cPKCα, nPKCδ, and nPKCζ but only a 60% reduction in nPKCε. Transformation of R6 cells by an activated c-H-*ras*, v-*src*, or v-*fos* oncogene caused a marked increase in expression, at both the mRNA and protein levels of cPKCα and nPKCδ, decreased expression of nPKCε, and no significant effect on nPKCζ. No major changes in the expression of these four PKC isoforms occurred in cells transformed by a v-*myc*, *neu* or v-*mos* oncogene. Nuclear run-on assays and studies using actinomycin D revealed that the increased expression of cPKCα in *ras*-transformed cells is due to increased transcription. Taken together these results indicate that the expression of PKC isoforms in rodent fibroblasts is more complex than previously thought, and suggest that each of these isoforms plays a distinct role in growth control and neoplastic transformation. In studies on colon carcinogenesis we have found that primary human colon tumors display decreased expression of specific isoforms of PKC and decreased cellular levels of diacylglycerol. Furthermore, overexpression of $PKC_{\beta 1}$ in HT29 colon cancer cells inhibits growth and tumorigenicity. Thus, specific isoforms of PKC can have reciprocal effects on growth in different cell systems. These findings are discussed within the context of multistage carcinogenesis as "progressive disorder in signal transduction."

Clinical, epidemiological and experimental evidence indicate that carcinogenesis is a multistage process. It is appropriate, therefore, that this symposium highlights recent advances in this important area of cancer research. In certain experimental systems three distinct stages can be identified, initiation, promotion and progression. There is evidence that on mouse skin both the initiation and progression stages involve mutagenic events, while tumor promotion appears to involve epigenetic alterations in gene expression that lead to the selective outgrowth of initiated cells (for review see refs. *1*, *2*). At the same time it should be emphasized that under conditions of repeated exposure to carcinogens, for example cigarette smoking or certain chronic dietary or occupational exposures, the carcinogenic process is more likely to be represent a continuum of repetitive mutagenic events and clonal outgrowths. Indeed, the genetic analysis of human colon cancer and certain other forms of cancer indicate that the multistage carcinogenic process is associated with the progressive acquisition of mutations, including activating mutations in oncogenes, inactivating mutations in putative suppressor genes, and other genetic changes (*2*, also see other papers in this volume). Thus, the evolution of a fully malignant tumor is a highly complex process that can involve multiple exogenous agents, multiple biochemical mechanisms and mutiple disturbances in cellular genes (*1*, *2*). Nevertheless, recent studies on the molecular mechanisms of action of chemical carcinogens and tumor promoters, coupled with developments in the fields of tumor virology, oncogenes, growth factors and receptors, provide a unitary concept for understanding the multistage carcinogenic process, a concept we have termed "a progressive disorder in signal transduction" (*3*, *4*). This paper describes recent studies from our laboratory on the enzyme protein kinase C (PKC) that illustrate this concept, and the relevance of PKC to human colon carcinogenesis.

A number of years ago our laboratory and others obtained evidence that the tumor promoter 12-O-tetradecanoyl-phorbol-13-acetate (TPA) is a potent modulator of growth, differentiation and gene expression, and that its earliest effects are exerted at the level of the plasma membrane (*1*, *2*). A major advance in our understanding of mechanisms of tumor promotion came when it was demonstrated that TPA directly activates PKC, a phospholipid-dependent serine/threonine protein kinase of central importance in signal transduction, and that PKC is also the major cellular receptor for TPA (*5*, *6*). Eight distinct subspecies of PKC, encoded by 7 distinct genes, have been identified, which are designated α, β_1, β_2, γ, δ, ε, ζ, and η (for review see *6*, *7*). The δ, ε, ζ, and η, isoforms constitute a distinct subfamily that lacks a putative Ca^{2+} binding domain present in the α, β, and γ isoforms.

Effects of Overexpression of PKC on Growth Control, Oncogene-induced Transformation and Gene Expression

To gain further insight into the role of PKC in signal transduction and multistage carcinogenesis, and to better define the biochemical properties and physiologic effects of a specific isoform of PKC, our strategy has been to construct a series of cell lines that constitutively overproduce high levels of the β_1 isoform of PKC. R6 rat embryo fibroblast cells transduced with a retrovirus vector pMV7-PKC$_{\beta 1}$ vector express a 20–50 fold greater PKC enzyme activity than control vector-infected cells.

Detailed studies on one of these overexpressors, R6-PKC3, indicated that it displays several disturbances in growth control (*8*). These findings, as well as results obtained with derivatives of both the murine fibroblast cell line C3H $10T^{1/2}$ (*9*) and rat liver epithelial cell lines (*10*), that also overexpress $PKC_{\beta1}$, provide direct evidence that this isoform of PKC can alter cell morphology, disturb growth control, and alter gene expression, particularly in the presence of TPA.

Although the R6-PKC3 cells are not fully transformed, they display a marked increase in susceptibility to transformation by an activated c-H-*ras* oncogene (*11*), thus providing genetic evidence for a cooperative interaction between PKC and a *ras* oncogene in the process of cell transformation. One can rationalize this interaction by the fact that *ras* transformed cells often display increased levels of diacylglycerol (DAG) (*11*). The increased levels of DAG would provide continuous activation of the high levels of $PKC_{\beta1}$ present in our overproducer cells. These findings provide a model in which multiple disturbances in a signal transduction pathway act together to enhance cell transformation.

More recently, we have developed derivatives of the R6 cell line that overexpress PKC_{α} at a level of PKC enzyme activity approximately equal to that of the R6-PKC3 cells that overexpress $PKC_{\beta1}$. Both types of overexpressor cells display an altered morphology. In contrast to the R6-PKC3 cells, however, the cells that overexpress PKC_{α} do not display an increased saturation density in monolayer culture, they fail to grow in agar and they are not tumorigenic in nude mice (*12* and unpublished studies). To our knowledge, these results provide the first definitive evidence that two different isoforms of PKC, in this comparison PKC_{α} and PKC_{β}, have different phenotypic effects even when expressed in the same cell type. We are currently carrying out a similar analysis with PKC_{ε}.

Expression of Multiple Isoforms of PKC in Normal and Oncogene-transformed R6 Cells

In recent studies we have examined the expression of endogenous isoforms of PKC in normal R6 cells and the effects of oncogene-induced transformation on the expression of these specific isoforms (*13, 14*). We have found that normal R6 cells express four isoforms of PKC, PKCα, PKCε, PKCδ, and PKCζ at both the mRNA and protein levels. To our surprise, PKCε and PKCδ are the most abundant when quantitated by Western immunoblot analysis. In agreement with these results both Ca^{2+}-dependent and Ca^{2+}-independent PKC activities are detected in extracts of these cells. Subcellular fractionation in the presence of EGTA revealed predominant localization of PKCα and PKCζ in the cytosol. Cell lysis in the presence of Ca^{2+} caused the redistribution of $>50\%$ of PKCα to the membrane fraction, whereas PKCζ remained in the cytosol. PKCε and PKCδ have an unusual distribution with 60–80% being in a Ca^{2+}-insensitive, membrane-bound form. In response to treatment of R6 cells with TPA, the cytosolic levels of all four PKC isozymes were recruited to the membrane fraction. Membrane-bound PKCδ also underwent a shift in molecular mass consistent with modification by phosphorylation. Prolonged treatment of R6 cells with TPA caused total loss of PKCα, PKCδ, and PKCζ but only a 60% reduction in PKCε.

We have found that transformation of R6 cells by an activated c-H-*ras*, v-*src*, or v-*fos* oncogene causes a marked increase in the expression of PKCα and PKCδ, decreased expression of PKCε and no significant alteration in the expression of PKCζ (*13, 14*). These changes occurred at both the mRNA and protein levels, but did not significantly affect the subcellular distribution of the particular isoform. No major changes in the expression level of any of the four PKC isoforms occurred in cells transformed by a v-*myc*, *neu*/v-*erb*B, or v-*mos* oncogene. Nuclear run-on assays and studies using actinomycin D revealed that the increased expression of PKCα in *ras*-transformed cells is the consequence of enhanced transcription of the PKCα gene.

Taken together, these results indicate that the expression of PKC isoforms in rodent fibroblasts is more complex than previously thought. The four individual isoforms of PKC that are co-expressed in R6 cells differ in their subcellular distribution, their responses to Ca^{2+} and TPA, and their expression following cell transformation by specific oncogenes. These findings suggest that each of these isoforms play distinct roles in growth control and neoplastic transformation. Our findings also raise the possibility that differential expression of specific isoforms of PKC may play an important role in the multistage carcinogenic process. It will be of interest, therefore, to determine whether human tumors display alterations in their profiles of PKC isoforms when compared to the normal tissues of origin.

Role of PKC in Colon Cancer

Despite the fact that colon cancer is the second most common cause of cancer deaths in the United States, the etiology of this disease is not known. Factors that have been implicated include a high fat and low fiber diet; mutagens (*i.e.*, fecapentaene) produced by the intestinal microflora; bile acids, which in experimental systems have a tumor promoting effect; and genetic predisposition (for review see *4, 15*). The following evidence indicates that the PKC signal transduction pathway plays a role in colon carcinogenesis: 1) the bile acid deoxycholic acid (DOC) stimulates PKC activity *in vitro* (*16*), and in intact cells it induces PKC translocation and the expression of PKC-responsive genes (*15*); 2) human colon tumors have decreased levels of PKC enzyme activity (*17, 18*), and decreased levels of PKC_β RNA (unpublished studies); and 3) human colon tumors display decreased intracellular levels of DAG, the normal physiologic activator of PKC (*19, 20*).

In view of the above findings, it was of interest to determine the effects of overexpression of PKC on the growth properties of colon carcinoma cells. The pMV7-$PKC_{\beta 1}$ vector was introduced into the human colon cancer cell line HT29 by using an amphotropic packaging system. This procedure yielded derivatives that display an 11–15 fold increase in PKC activity (*21*). These cells grow normally but, in contrast to control HT29 cells, when treated with TPA they display dramatic changes in morphology and their growth in both monolayer culture and in agar suspension is markedly inhibited. Also in contrast to the control cells, the HT29 cells that overproduce $PKC_{\beta 1}$ fail to differentiate when exposed to sodium butyrate. Of greatest interest is the fact that the cells that overproduce $PKC_{\beta 1}$ display a marked reduction in tumorigenicity in nude mice. Thus, in HT29 cells high expression of $PKC_{\beta 1}$ acts as a tumor suppressor.

It is curious that overexpression of $PKC_{\beta 1}$ in HT29 colon cancer cells produces effects on growth which are exactly the opposite of those produced by overexpression of $PKC_{\beta 1}$ in rodent fibroblast and rodent liver epithelial cells (see above). It is apparent, therefore, that the biologic effects of a specific isoform of PKC depend on the cell in which it is expressed. These findings are consistent with what we believe is emerging as a general theme, namely that the biologic effects of certain oncogenes, growth factors and various components of signal transduction pathways are highly context dependent (*3*, *4*). Our findings with PKC are also consistent with previous evidence indicating that TPA (which acts through PKC) can stimulate the differentiation and inhibit the growth of some cell types, whereas in other cell types it can inhibit differentiation and stimulate cell growth (*1*, *2*). The effects of PKC activation on cell growth may also depend on the stage of differentiation of colonic epithelial cells.

A Holistic View of Signal Transduction

Our studies on the overexpression of the β_1 isoform of PKC indicate that a single isoform of PKC can produce highly pleiotropic effects on cellular morphology, gene expression, growth control and suceptibility to malignant transformation by diverse types of oncogenes. Some of these effects depend upon the specific cell type in which this enzyme is expressed and the environment in which the cells are grown. Studies are in progress to determine whether overexpression of the other isoforms of PKC produce similar or different effects. It is difficult to rationalize the present findings in terms of simple linear pathways of signal transduction. Results obtained with various hormones, neurotransmitters, growth factors, receptors, ion channels, protein kinases, protein phosphatases, second messengers, and transcription factors lead to similar conclusions (*1–4*, *6*). It is apparent, therefore, that the signal transduction pathways of mammalian cells constitute a dynamic and highly interactive network, that includes considerable "cross-talk" and both positive and negative feedback circuitry. In a sense, all components of the system have the potential of influencing each other. Specific components of signal transduction pathways might be thought of as transistors whose biologic effects depends on the "wiring diagram" of the particular cell type in question.

The complexity in signal transduction probably explains why multiple types of exogenous agents, multiple steps, multiple mechanisms and multiple genes are involved in the carcinogenic process. This complexity also explains why the genotypes and phenotypes of tumors can be highly heterogeneous, even when they are induced by the same agent and in the same tissue. It is for these reasons that we have defined multistage carcinogenesis as a "progressive disorder in signal transduction" (*1*, *4*).

Acknowledgments

The author wishes to acknowledge the valuable contributions to this paper made by numerous colleagues who have worked in his laboratory, especially: Christoph M. Borner, Paul M. Choi, Sarah Nichols Guadagno, Jose Guillem, Sadayori Hoshina, Gerard H. Housey, Wendy Hsiao, Ling-Ling Hsieh, Mark D. Johnson, Paul Kirschmeier, Robert S. Krauss, Masami Moritomi, Kevin O'Driscoll, Kam-Meng Tchou-Wong, and Marius Ueffing. He also appreciates the technical support of Miriam F. Levy and the collaboration with Drs. P. LoGerfo, and K. Forde on colon cancer. Sheila M. Washington provided valuable assistance in preparing this manuscript. This research was supported by NCI Grant CA 02656 and awards from the Aaron Diamond Foundation and the Markey Charitable Trust (to I.B.W.). Sections of this paper are modified from previously published papers from this laboratory.

REFERENCES

1. Weinstein, I. B. Growth factors, oncogenes and multistage carcinogenesis. J. Cell Biochem., *33*: 213–224, 1987.
2. Weinstein, I. B. The origins of human cancer: molecular mechanisms of carcinogenesis and their implications for cancer prevention and treatment. Cancer Res., *48*: 4135–4143, 1988.
3. Weinstein, I. B. The role of protein kinase C in growth control and the concept of carcinogenesis as a progressive disorder in signal transduction. *In*; Y. Nishizuka (ed.), The Biology and Medicine of Signal Transduction, 307–316, Raven Press, New York, 1990.
4. Weinstein, I. B., Borner, C. M., Krauss, R. S., O'Driscoll, K., Choi, P. M., Morotomi, M., Hoshina, S., Hsieh, L.-L., Tchou-Wong, K.-M., Guadagno Nichols, S., Ueffing, M., and Guillem, J. G. Pleiotropic effects of protein kinase C and the concept of carcinogenesis as a progressive disorder in signal transduction. *In*; J. Brugge, T. Curran, E. Harlow, and F. McCormick (eds.), Origins of Human Cancer: A Comprehensive Review, pp. 113–124, Cold Spring Harbor Laboratory Press, Cold Spring Harbor, 1991.
5. Castagna, M., Takai, Y., Kaibuchi, K., Sano, K., Kikkawa, U., Nishizuka, Y. Direct activation of calcium-activated phospholipid-dependent protein kinase by tumor-promoting phorbol esters. J. Biol. Chem., *257*: 7847–7851, 1982.
6. Kikkawa, U., Kishimoto, A., and Nishizuka, Y. The protein kinase C family: heterogeneity and its implications. Annu. Rev. Biochem., *58*: 31–44, 1989.
7. Pears, C. J. and Parker, P. J. Domain interactions in protein kinase C. J. Cell Science, *100*: 683–686, 1991.
8. Housey, G. M., Johnson, M. D., Hsiao, W.-L. W., O'Brian, C. A., Murphy, J. P., and Kirschmeier, P. T. Overproduction of protein kinase C causes disordered growth control in rat fibroblasts. Cell, *52*: 343–354, 1988.
9. Krauss, R. S., Housey, G. M., Johnson, M. D., and Weinstein, I. B. Disturbances in growth control and gene expression in a C3H10T1/2 cell line that stably overproduces protein kinase C. Oncogene, *4*: 991–998, 1989.
10. Hsieh, L. L., Hoshina, S., and Weinstein, I. B. Phenotypic effects of overexpression of $PKC_{\beta 1}$ in rat liver epithelial cells. J. Cell. Biochem., *41*: 179–188, 1989.
11. Hsiao, W.-L. W., Housey, G. M., Johnson, M. D., and Weinstein, I. B. Cells that overproduce protein kinase C are hypersensitive to transformation by an activated H-*ras* oncogene. Mol. Cell. Biol., *9*: 2641–2647, 1989.
12. Borner, C. Filipuzzi, Weinstein, I. B., and Imber, R. Failure of wild-type of a mutant form or kinase C-α to transform fibroblasts. Nature, *353*: 78–80, 1991.
13. Borner, C., Nichols, S. F., Hsieh, L. L., Hsiao, W.-L. and Weinstein, I. B. Transformation by a ras oncogene causes increased expression of $PKC_{\alpha 1}$ and decreased expression of PKC_{ε}. Cell Growth Diff., *1*: 653–660, 1990.
14. Borner, C., Guadagno, S. N., Hsiao, W. W.-L., Fabbro, D., Barr, M., and Weinstein, I. B. Expression of four protein kinase C isoforms in rat fibroblasts. II. Differential alterations in *ras*-, *src*-, and *fos*-transformed cells. J. Biol. Chem., *267*: 12900–12910,

1992.

15. Guillem, J. G., Morotomi, M., Kahn, S., Johnson, M. D., Wei, J., and Weinstein, I. B. The Molecular Biology of Colorectal Cancer, Semin. Colon Rectal Surg., *2*: 58–63, 1991.
16. Fitzer, C. J., O'Brian, C. A., Guillem, J. G., and Weinstein, I. B. The regulation of protein kinase C by chenodeoxycholate, deoxycholate and several related bile acids. Carcinogenesis, *8*: 217–220, 1987.
17. Guillem, J. G., O'Brian, C. A., Fitzer, C. J., Forde, K. A., LoGerfo, P., Treat, M., and Weinstein, I. B. Altered levels of protein kinase C and Ca^{2+}-dependent protein kinases in human colon carcinomas. Cancer Res., *47*: 2036–2039, 1987.
18. Kopp, R., Noelke, B., Sauter, G., Schildberg, F. W., Paumgartner, G., and Pfeiffer, A. Altered protein kinase C activity in biopsies of human colon adenomas and carcinomas. Cancer Res., *51*: 205–210, 1991.
19. Phan, S.-C., Morotomi, M., Guillem, J. G., LoGerfo, P., and Weinstein, I. B. Decreased levels of 1,2-sn-diacylglycerol in human colon tumors. Cancer Res., *51*: 1571–1573, 1991.
20. Sauter, G., Nerlich, A., Spengler, U., Kopp, R., and Pfeiffer, A. Low diacylglycerol values in colonic adenomas and colorectal cancer. Gut, *31*: 1041–1045, 1990.
21. Choi, P., Tchou-Wong, Kam-Meng, and Weinstein, I. B. Overexpression of protein kinase C in HT29 colon cancer cells causes growth inhibition and tumor suppression. Mol. Cell. Biol., *10*: 4650–4657, 1990.

MULTISTAGE CARCINOGENESIS, C. C. HARRIS ET AL. (EDS.),
JAPAN SCI. SOC. PRESS, TOKYO/CRC PRESS, BOCA RATON, PP. 285–292, 1992

Mutations of the Adenomatous Polyposis Coli Gene in Familial Polyposis Coli Patients and Sporadic Colorectal Tumors

Yusuke NAKAMURA,*[1] Isamu NISHISHO,*[1] Kenneth W. KINZLER,*[2] Bert VOGELSTEIN,*[2] Yasuo MIYOSHI,*[1] Yoshio MIKI,*[1] Hiroshi ANDO,*[1] Akira HORII,*[1] and Hiroki NAGASE*[1]

Department of Biochemistry, Cancer Institute, Tokyo 170, Japan[1] and Oncology Center, The Johns Hopkins University School of Medicine, Baltimore, Maryland 21231, U.S.A.*[2]*

Abstract: We have isolated several genes in the chromosome 5q21 region tightly linked to hereditary familial polyposis coli (FAP) and Gardner's syndrome (GS). Two of these genes (MCC and APC) were found to be somatically altered by point mutation, deletion or insertion in tumors of sporadic colorectal cancer patients. One of them (adenomatous polyposis coli; APC) was also found to mutate in the germ-line of both APC and GS patients. The identification of these genes has significant implications for understanding the pathogenesis of colorectal neoplasia and for the diagnosis and counseling of individuals with inherited predispositions to colorectal cancer. Furthermore, in one colon carcinoma, we identified an interesting mechanism causing dysfunction of the APC gene. This gene was disrupted by a somatic insertion of a long interspersed repetitive element (LINE-1 sequence: L1) into the last exon. As an insertional sequence contains a 3′ portion of the L1 consensus sequence including the poly(A) tract and an 8 bp target-site duplication was observed, this insertion is suspected to be caused by a retrotranscriptional insertion of one of the L1 sequences. This is the first case of the disruption of a tumor suppressor gene by the insertion of a movable genetic element.

Two genetic disorders, familial polyposis coli (FAP) and Gardner's syndrome (GS), which predispose patients to the development of hundreds to thousands of adenomatous polyps in colon and rectum are important for identifying genes responsible for adenoma formation. As one or more of these adenomatous polyps progress to carcinoma if not surgically treated, they are also significant materials with which to study several genetic changes associated with colorectal tumorigenesis. FAP is the most common autosomal disease leading to cancer predisposition, affecting one in 0.01%–0.02% of the American and Japanese populations (*1*). GS is a related disorder in which multiple lipomas, fibromas, osteomas, and desmoid tumors develop as well as a large number of polyps of the colon and rectum. Patients with FAP and GS are also susceptible to the development of carcinomas of other organs, especially gastric cancers in Japanese patients (*1*). The gene(s) responsible for FAP and GS have been assigned to chromosome 5q21 by cytogenetics and linkage analysis (*2–5*). Although FAP and GS are relatively rare causes of colorectal cancer (*1*), the gene(s) responsible for them is considered to be important for tumor development in patients with non-inherited forms of colorectal cancer as this region was suggested as a commonly deleted region in sporadic colorectal carcinoma (*6, 7*). Moreover, as these losses of 5q21 alleles were observed in very small adenomas (*8*), this genetic alteration is considered an early event for tumorigenesis. Such losses are generally thought to indicate the presence of a tumor suppressor gene in the deleted region.

We used the "positional cloning" method to isolate this tumor suppressor gene on 5q21 and identified two genes which are mutated in germ-line DNA in FAP patients and tumor DNAs from sporadic colorectal cancer patients.

Isolation of the Adenomatous Polyposis Coli (APC) and Mutated in Colorectal Carcinoma (MCC) Genes

Our approach to identifying the gene(s) responsible for colorectal neoplasia was based on information from findings on the germ line DNAs of FAP and GS patients and the DNAs of sporadic colorectal carcinomas. In particular, we used DNA markers, which showed tight linkage to FAP and GS by linkage analysis, as anchor points for seeking genes expressed in normal colonic mucosa. By examining a large number of cosmid and yeast artificial chromosome (YAC) clones from the locus, five genes expressed in normal and neoplastic colon were isolated (*9*). Among these five genes, we focused on two of particular interest because of particular lines of evidence. First, Southern blots to examine genetic changes in tumor DNAs from patients with FAP and sporadic colorectal carcinomas with these two cDNAs as probes, detected somatic changes in two tumors of more than 200 tumors studied—a rearrangement/deletion whose centromeric end was located within the MCC gene (*10*) and a nearly 750 bp insertion in the coding region of the APC gene (*11*). Second, allelic deletions of chromosome 5q21 in sporadic colorectal tumors appeared to be centered in this region (*12, 13*). Based on such information, we attempted to examine alterations of the MCC or APC genes in patients with APC and GS, and in sporadic colorectal carcinomas. As the first step to facilitate the identification of such alterations, the intron/exon structure of the MCC and APC genes was determined. The coding region of MCC consisted of 17 exons and that of APC of 16 exons. These sequences were used to design primers for polymerase chain reaction (PCR) analysis and RNase protection assay of constitutional DNAs from APC and GS patients, and DNAs of sporadic colorectal carcinomas.

Somatic Mutations in the MCC Gene

First, we amplified exons of the MCC gene in 95 FAP patients and 50 colorectal cancers by PCR method (*14*). These DNAs were analyzed by a ribonuclease (RNase) protection assay (*10*) as shown in Fig. 1. The PCR products were denatured and then hybridized to *in vitro* transcribed RNA products, representing normal genomic sequences. The DNA-RNA hybrids were digested with RNase A, which can digest

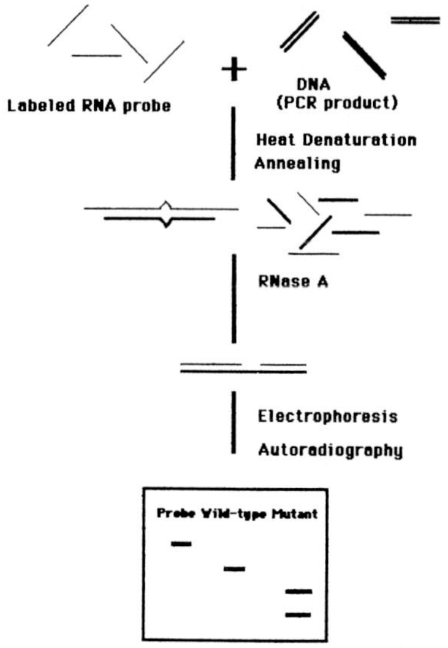

FIG. 1. Principle of RNase protection analysis.

TABLE 1. Somatic Mutations of the MCC Gene in Sporadic Colorectal Carcinomas

Tumor	Codon	Nucleotide change	Amino acid change
1	12	GAG/gtaaga—GAG/gtaaaa	Splice donor
2	145	ctcag/GGA—atcag/GGA	Splice acceptor
3	267	CGG—CTG	Arg—Leu
4	490	TCG—TTG	Ser—Leu
5	506	CGG—CAG	Arg—Gln
6	698	GCT—GTT	Ala—Val

RNA at base pair mismatches, and these products were visualized by autoradiography after gel electrophoresis. Both sense and antisense RNA products were made and RNase protection analysis done for the two strands of each exon because approximately 30–50% of all mismatches are detectable by this method (*15*). Although we found no change in FAP or GS patients, somatic mutations in sporadic colorectal carcinomas were detected (*10*). The PCR products revealing abnormal patterns were then subcloned and the DNA sequences determined. Table 1 presents the results of somatic mutations in the 50 sporadic colorectal tumors examined (*16*).

Germ Line Mutations in the APC Gene in APC and GS Patients

We next examined exons of the APC gene. By RNase protection assay, one variant (FAP21) was detected in exon 8 among 74 unrelated APC and GS patients as shown in Fig. 2. Cloning and subsequent DNA sequencing of the PCR product of the patient revealed a C to T transition in codon 414 that resulted in an amino acid change from arginine to cysteine (shown in Fig. 3A), which was suspected to be responsible for drastic dysfunction of the protein encoded by the APC gene. This was not observed in any of 200 DNA samples from patients without colon cancer.

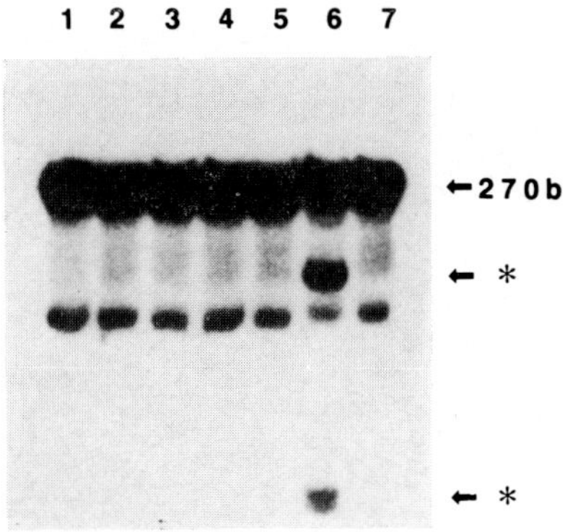

Fig. 2. PCR and RNase protection analysis of the APC gene in FAP patients.

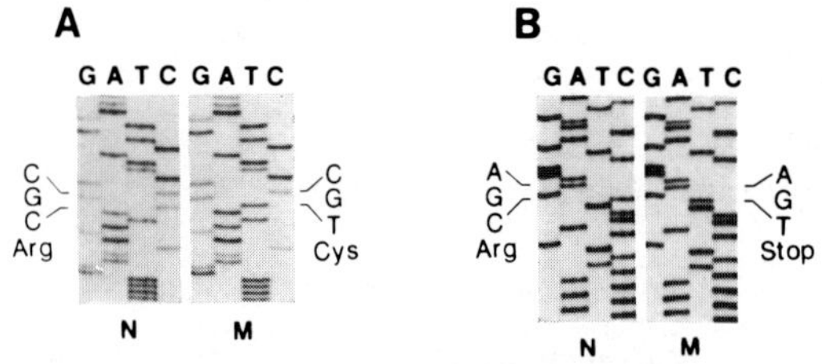

Fig. 3. Sequence analysis of variant PCR products from FAP patients. (A) A C (in normal allele, N) to T (in mutated allele, M) transition in APC codon 414 that resulted in a change from arginine to cysteine in patient P21. (B) A C to T transition in APC codon 302 that resulted in a change from arginine to a stop codon in patient P24.

TABLE 2. Germ Line Mutations of the APC Gene in FAP Patients

Patient	Codon	Nucleotide change	Amino acid change
P102	213	CGA—TGA	Arg—Stop
P93	280	TCA—TGA	Ser—Stop
P24	302	CGA—TGA	Arg—Stop
P34	302	CGA—TGA	Arg—Stop
P21	414	CGC—TGC	Arg—Cys
P60	713	TCA—TGA	Ser—Stop
P100	932	TCA—TAA	Ser—Stop

(*16* and author's unpublished data).

RNase protection analysis of exon 6 also revealed an identical variant pattern in two FAP patients (FAP24 and 34). Cloning and sequencing of these variants indicated that both had a C to T transition at codon 301 that resulted in a change from arginine (CGA) to stop codon (TGA) (Fig. 3B). This C to T transition generating early termination of the gene product has strongly suggested that mutation in the APC gene is the cause of FAP. Seven significant changes (6 terminations and one amino acid change) in the APC gene are summarized in Table 2 (*16* and author's unpublished data).

Somatic Mutations in the APC Gene in Sporadic Colorectal Carcinomas

Nearly 100 sporadic colorectal carcinomas were also examined. The abnormal patterns, which were not seen in DNA isolated from normal colonic mucosa from the same patient, were detected in two tumors (T27 and T135) by RNase protection assay. This indicates that the altered RNase protection patterns were the results of somatic mutations. DNA sequencing of T27 indicated a somatic mutation of CGA (arginine) to TGA (stop codon) at codon 331, resulting in early termination of the gene product. The result of DNA sequence in T135 revealed a GT to GC change at the splice donor site (Fig. 4). Moreover, this tumor showed loss of heterozygosity at one of the polymorphic marker loci (L5.71) of the MCC gene, which is less than 150 kb apart from the APC gene (*10*). This result indicated that the normal gene product encoded by APC was completely lost in tumor 135. Furthermore, one case of colon cancer (T34) also showed a 5 bp insertion (CAGCC) between codons 288 and 289, resulting in a stop at codon 291 due to frame shift. Somatic mutations in the APC gene so far identified are summarized in Table 3.

Somatic Insertion of the L1 Sequence into the APC Gene in a Colon Carcinoma

During an investigation of somatic mutations of the APC gene in 45 colorectal carcinomas, we found a 4.1 kb *Bgl*II fragment in addition to the 3.4 kb *Bgl*II normal size fragment in one colon cancer using the last exon of the APC gene as a probe (Fig. 5). An extra fragment was also detected by other restriction endonucleases including *Msp*I, *Hin*dIII, *Eco*RI and *Pst*I (data not shown). All extra bands were approximately 750 bp larger than normal fragments. On the basis of these data, it

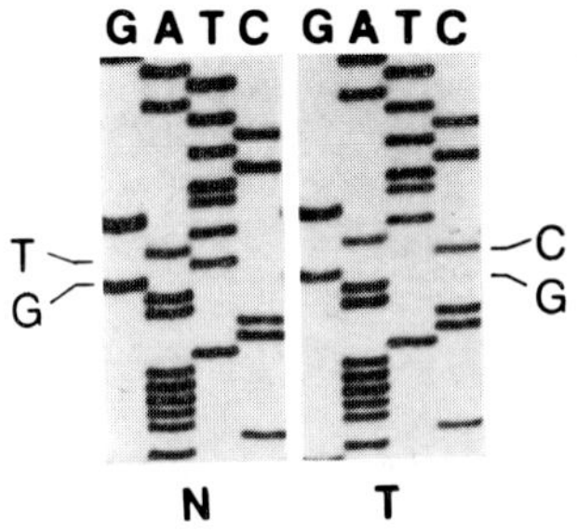

FIG. 4. Sequence analysis of sporadic colon cancer T135. (A) Sequence analysis of the T135 PCR product shows a T (in normal allele) to C (in mutated allele) transition in the splice donor site.

TABLE 3. Somatic Mutations of the APC Gene in Sporadic Colorectal Carcinomas

Tumor	Codon	Nucleotide change	Amino acid change
T34	289	CCAGT—CCCAGCCAGT	Insertion
T27	332	CGA—TGA	Arg—Stop
T135	438	CAA/gtaa—CAA/gcaa	Splice donor
T201	1338	CAG—TAG	Gln—Stop

Ref. *16*.

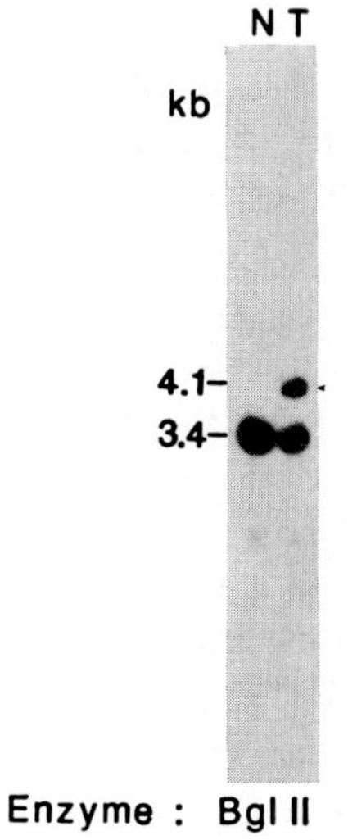

FIG. 5. Southern blot analysis of the APC gene from normal tissue (N) and colon cancer (T) of the same patient. The restriction endonuclease *Bgl*II was used for DNA digestion.

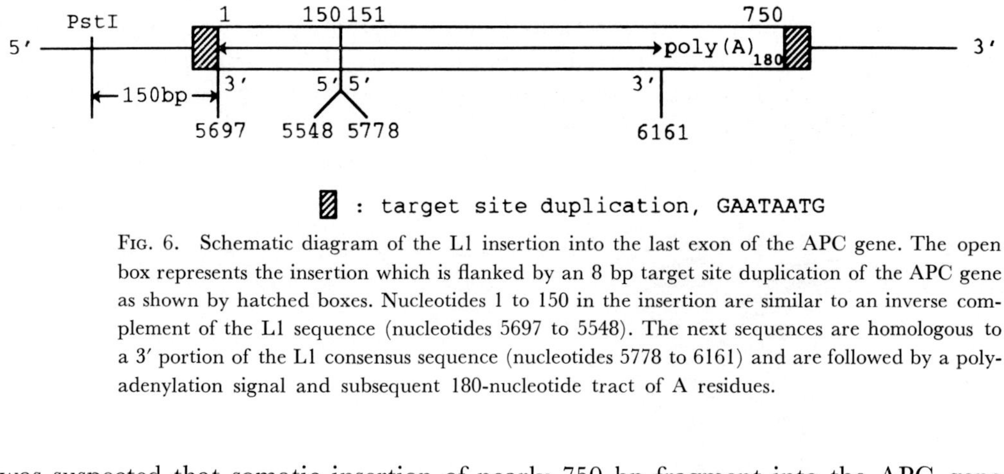

FIG. 6. Schematic diagram of the L1 insertion into the last exon of the APC gene. The open box represents the insertion which is flanked by an 8 bp target site duplication of the APC gene as shown by hatched boxes. Nucleotides 1 to 150 in the insertion are similar to an inverse complement of the L1 sequence (nucleotides 5697 to 5548). The next sequences are homologous to a 3′ portion of the L1 consensus sequence (nucleotides 5778 to 6161) and are followed by a polyadenylation signal and subsequent 180-nucleotide tract of A residues.

was suspected that somatic insertion of nearly 750 bp fragment into the APC gene occurred in this colon cancer. To characterize the insertional sequence, a 4.1 kb *Bgl*II fragment containing the insertion was subcloned from tumor DNA and sequenced (*11*). The insertional sequence consisted of two blocks which were highly homologous with the L1 consensus sequence (*17*). The first fifth of the insertional sequence was very similar to an inverse complement of the L1 consensus sequence (nucleotides 5697 to 5548). The next half was highly homologous to the 3′ portion of the L1 consensus sequence (nucleotides 5778 to 6161, L1 sequence), and was followed by a polyadenylation signal and 170 bp of poly(A) as shown in Fig. 6. The insertional event resulted in perfect duplication of at least 8 nucleotides of the target site in the APC gene without loss of APC sequences (*11*).

The results described above demonstrate that the APC gene was mutated in the germline of APC and GS patients as well as in some sporadic cancers. The prevalence of such mutations cannot yet be fully assessed, because only a portion of the gene product has been examined in detail. However, the finding of the several mutations detected here indicates a profound effect on the predicted gene product (creating stop codons by point mutation or frameshift, or destroying a donor site of the splicing junction), and strongly suggests that the APC gene is involved in the generation of FAP patients as well as sporadic colon cancers. A second gene, MCC, located close to the APC gene has so far been found to be mutated only in sporadic colorectal carcinomas.

Although the biological role of L1 elements is unclear, the mobility of some Ll elements in humans was also reported (*18*, *19*). *De novo* insertions of Ll sequences in the factor VIII gene resulted in hemophilia A (*18*), and an insertional mutation of the *myc* locus by a LINE-1 sequence was found in a human breast carcinoma (*19*). In the latter case, the effect of L1 insertion for tumorigenesis was unclear because the insertion was into the intron. In our case, however, insertion of the L1 element into the APC gene in a carcinoma clearly caused the disruption of the tumor suppressor gene; this is the first case showing that the L1 sequence plays a role in the somatic mutagenesis of a tumor suppressor gene.

The inserted L1 sequence presented here is homologous with the 3′ portion of the L1 consensus sequence including ORF-2, but it is unclear whether this element merely induces the somatic mutation of the APC gene resulting in loss of the tumor suppressor function, or functions positively in tumorigenesis as described for retroviruses or retrotransposons. In either case, these results demonstrated that certain L1 elements can act as mutagens disrupting a tumor suppressor gene as well as an oncogene at the somatic level, and are involved in tumor induction and/or progression by insertional mutagenesis.

Acknowledgments

This work was supported partly by a grant from the Ministry of Education, Science and Culture, Japan and grants from the Princess Takamatsu Research Foundation, the Clayton Fund, the McAshan Fund, the Damon Runyon-Walter Winchell Cancer Research Fund, and NIH.

REFERENCES

1. Utsunomiya, J. and Lynch, H. T. (eds.). Hereditary Colorectal Cancer, Springer-Verlag, Tokyo, 1990.
2. Herrera, L., Kakati, S., Gibas, L., Pietrzak, E., and Sandberg, A. Brief clinical report: Gardner syndrome in a man with an interstitial deletion of 5q. Am. J. Med. Genet., *25*: 473–476, 1986.
3. Bodmer, W., Bailey, C., Bodmer, J., Bussey, H., Ellis, A., Gorman, P., Lucibello, F., Murday, V., Rider, S., Scambler, P., Sheer, D., Solomon, E., and Spurr, N. Localization of the gene for familial adenomatous polyposis on chromosome 5. Nature, *328*: 614–616, 1987.
4. Nakamura, Y., Lathrop, M., Leppert, M., Dobbs, M., Wasmuth, J., Wolff, E., Carlson, M., Fujimoto, E., Krapcho, K., Sears, T., Woodward, S., Hughes, J., Burt, R., Gardner, E., Lalouel, J.M., and White, R. Localization of the genetic defect in familial adenomatous polyposis within a small region of chromosome 5. Am. J. Hum. Genet., *43*: 638–644, 1988.

5. Dunlop, M. G., Steel, C. M., Wyllie, A. H., Bird, C. C., and Evans, H. J. Linkage analysis in familial adenomatous polyposis: order of C11P11 (D5S71) and pi227 (D5S37) loci at the APC gene. Genomics, *5*: 350, 1989.
6. Solomon, E., Voss, R., Hall, V., Bodmer, W., Jass, J., Jeffreys, A., Lucibello, F., Patel, I., and Rider, S. Chromosome 5 allele loss in human colorectal carcinomas. Nature, *328*: 616–619, 1987.
7. Fearon, E. R. and Vogelstein, B. A genetic model for colorectal tumorigenesis. Cell, *61*: 759–767, 1990.
8. Vogelstein, B., Fearon, E. R., Hamilton, S. R., Kern, S. E., Preisinger, A. C., Leppert, M., Nakamura, Y., White, R., Smits, A. M. M., and Bos, J. L. Genetic alterations during colorectal-tumor development. N. Eng. J. Med., *319*: 525–532, 1988.
9. Kinzler, K. W., Nilbert, M. C., Su, L-K., Vogelstein, B., Bryan, T. M., Levy, D. B., Smith, K. J., Preisinger, A. C., Hedge, P., McKechnie, D., Finniear, R., Markham, A., Groffen, J., Boguski, M. S., Altschul, S. F., Horii, A., Ando, H., Miyoshi, Y., Miki, Y., Nishisho, I., Nakamura, Y. Identification of FAP locus genes from chromosome 5q21. Science, *253*: 661–665, 1991.
10. Kinzler, K. W., Nilbert, M. C., Vogelstein, B., Bryan, T. M., Levy, D. B., Smith, K. J., Preisinger, A. C., Hamilton, S. R., Hedge, P., Markham, A., Carlson, M., Joslyn, G., Groden, J., White, R., Miki, Y., Miyoshi, Y., Nishisho, I., and Nakamura, Y. Identification of a gene located at chromosome 5q21 that is mutated in colorectal cancers. Science, *251*: 1366–1370, 1991.
11. Miki, Y., Nishisho, I., Horii, A., Miyoshi, Y., Utsunomiya, J., Kinzler, K., Vogelstein, B., and Nakamura, Y. Disruption of the APC gene by retrotransposal insertion of L1 sequence in a colon cancer. Cancer Res., *82*: 1003–1007, 1991.
12. Ashton-Rickardt, P.G., Wyllie, A. H., Bird, C. C., Dunlop, M. G., Steel, C. M., Morris, R. G., Piris, J., Romanowski, P., Wood, R., White, R., and Nakamura, Y. MCC, a candidate familial polyposis gene in 5q21, shows frequent allele loss in colorectal and lung cancer. Oncogene, *6*: 1881–1886, 1991.
13. Miki, Y., Nishisho, I., Miyoshi, Y., Horii, A., Ando, H., Nakajima, T., Utsunomiya, J., and Nakamura, Y. Frequent loss of heterozygosity at the MCC locus on chromosome 5q21-22 in sporadic colorectal carcinomas. Jpn. J. Cancer Res., *82*: 1003–1007, 1991.
14. Baker, S. J., Preisinger, A. C., Jessup, J. M., Paraskeva, C., Markowitz, S., Willson, J. K. V., Hamilton, S., and Vogelstein, B. p53 gene mutations occur in combination with 17p allelic deletions as late events in colorectal tumorigenesis. Cancer Res., *50*: 7717–7722, 1990.
15. Myers, R. M. and Maniatis, T. Cold Spring Harbor Symp. Quant. Biol., *51*: 275, 1986.
16. Nishisho, I., Nakamura, Y., Miyoshi, Y., Miki, Y., Ando, H., Horii, A., Koyama, K., Utsunomiya, J., Baba, S., Hedge, P., Markham, A., Krush, A. J., Petersen, G., Hamilton, S. R., Nilbert, M. C., Levy, D. B., Bryan, T. M., Preisinger, A. C., Smith, K. J., Su, L-K., Kinzler, K. W., and Vogelstein, B. Mutations of chromosome 5q21 genes in FAP and colorectal cancer patients. Science, *253*: 665–669, 1991.
17. Fanning, T. G. and Singer, M. F. LINE-1: a mammalian transposable element. Biochim. Biophys. Acta, *910*: 203–212, 1987.
18. Kazazian, H. H. Jr., Wong, C., Youssoufian, H., Scott, A. F., Phillips, D. G., and Antonarakis, S. E. Hemophilia A resulting from *de novo* insertion of L1 sequences represents a novel mechanism for mutation in man. Nature, *332*: 164–166, 1988.
19. Morse, B., Rotherg, P. G., South, V. J., Spandorfer, J. M., and Astrin, S. M. Insertional mutagenesis of the *myc* locus by a LINE-1 sequence in a human breast carcinoma. Nature, *333*: 87–90, 1988.

MULTISTAGE CARCINOGENESIS, C. C. HARRIS ET AL. (EDS.),
JAPAN SCI. SOC. PRESS, TOKYO/CRC PRESS, BOCA RATON, PP. 293–305, 1992

Role of *src*-like Protooncogenes in Lymphocyte Proliferation

Tadashi YAMAMOTO,*[1] Yuji YAMANASHI,*[1] Masakazu TAKEUCHI,*[1]
Noemi FUSAKI,*[1] Fumiaki UCHIUMI,*[1] Takuya KATAGIRI,*[1]
Kentaro SEMBA,*[1] and Kumao TOYOSHIMA*[2]

The Institute of Medical Science, The University of Tokyo, Tokyo 108, Japan[1] and*
Research Institute for Microbial Diseases, Suita, Osaka 565, Japan[2]*

Abstract: Cross-linking of membrane-bound immunoglobulins, which are B cell antigen receptors, causes proliferation and differentiation of B cells or the inhibition of their growth. The receptor-mediated signalling involves tyrosine phosphorylation of cellular proteins. The Src-like protein-tyrosine kinase Lyn is expressed preferentially in B cells and is an intracytoplasmic constituent of the B cell antigen receptor complex. Cross-linking of membrane-bound immunoglobulin M with antibody induced rapid increases in the kinase activities of Lyn and Lyn-associated phosphatidylinositol-3 kinase. Cross-linking of B-cell antigen receptor also induced association of Lyn with an 85 kDa non-catalytic subunit of phosphatidylinositol-3 kinase. Thus, Lyn is functionally associated with membrane-bound immunoglobulin M, and seems to participate in B cell antigen receptor-mediated signalling. On the other hand, accumulating evidence shows that Fyn and Lck are involved in T-cell activation. Co-immunoprecipitation experiments showed that Fyn was physically associated with T cell antigen receptor-CD3 complex. Transient expression of actively mutated Fyn, having Phe-528 instead of Tyr-528, in Jurkat T cells stimulated the *fos* promoter and serum response element (SRE), suggesting that the Fyn kinase stimulates c-*fos* expression through SRE. An analogous set of experiments showed that introduction of the active Fyn alone had little effect on *IL-2* promoter. However, it could stimulate transcription from this promoter when transfected cells were stimulated by a combination of Concanavalin A (ConA) and 12-O-tetradecanoylphorbol-13-acetate (TPA). Under the same conditions, normal Lck and Lyn could not stimulate *IL-2* promoter.

Protein-tyrosine kinases are involved in signal transduction systems that control cell proliferation and differentiation (*1–4*). These kinases can be divided into receptor-type kinases and nonreceptor-type kinases (or Src-like kinases). The Src-like kinases are generally associated with the internal portion of the plasma membrane, and may act as signal transducers in association with surface receptors that lack an intracellular catalytic domain (*3, 4*). This concept was originally established by the observation that the Src-like kinase Lck is physically and functionally associated with T cell surface antigens CD4 and CD8, receptors for major histocompatibility complex molecules (*5–7*). Successively, associations of the lymphocyte antigen receptor with the Src-like kinases Lyn, Blk and Fyn, and of IL-2 receptor with Lck were also reported (*8–11*). However, the physiological substrates or targets of these Src-like kinases in receptor-mediated signalling have yet to be identified.

In recent studies on the targets of the tyrosine kinases, much information has been obtained about the platelet-derived growth factor receptor (PDGF-R). The binding of PDGF to PDGF-R (β-type) activates the receptor's kinase activity and induces its association with tyrosine-phosphorylated proteins such as phosphatidylinositol-3 kinase (PI-3 kinase), ras GTPase activating protein (GAP) and phospholipase C-γ (PLC-γ) upon the ligand-mediated signalling (*11*). PI-3 kinase is also associated with ligand-stimulated receptors for colony-stimulating factor 1 and insulin (*11–13*) and with an activated form of Src, $p60^{v\text{-}src}$ (*14*). These proteins, PI-3 kinase, GAP, and PLC-γ, are assumed to be involved in shifting cells from G_0 to G_1 (*15*) and therefore are likely to also be relevant to antigen-receptor mediated signalling that results in activation of resting lymphocytes in G_0 state and shifting them to enter into cell cycle. However, stimulation of lymphocytes induces tyrosine phosphorylation of at least 10 cellular proteins (*8*), suggesting the presence of more target proteins that are yet to be characterized. Some of them would open up a cascade specific to lymphocyte signalling. In addition, T cell activation is accompanied by transactivation of a number of cellular genes (*16*). Here, we show evidences that support a notion that Fyn and Lyn are directly involved in these processes.

Activation of Lyn on mIgM Cross-linking

WEHI-231 and Daudi cells are murine and human B-lymphoblastoid cells, respectively, and carry membrane-bound immunoglobulin M (mIgM) on their surface (*17–20*). Both lines behave as normal B cells in terms of initial biochemical events such as PI turnover, Ca^{2+} mobilization and tyrosine phosphorylation of proteins after mIgM cross-linking (*8, 17, 18, 21, 22*, and Fig. 3). The physical association of Lyn with mIgM (*8*) suggests that Lyn plays a role in mIgM-mediated signalling. This possibility was tested by incubating WEHI-231 cells with goat antibody to IgM (μ chain) for 1 min and measuring kinase activity of Lyn by immune-complex kinase assay using monoclonal antibody Lyn-8, which reacts with both murine and human Lyn. The cross-linking of mIgM resulted in about 2- to 3-fold increase in activity as measured by *in vitro* autophosphorylation (Fig. 1, A). The amount of Lyn protein immunoprecipitated with Lyn-8 did not increase during the incubation period (data not shown). Similar activation of the Lyn kinase was observed when splenic B cells of a BALB/c mouse were incubated with antibody to IgM (unpublished observation). Goat antibody to human IgG (γ chain) had no effect on the kinase activity of Lyn of WEHI-231 cells (Fig. 1, A). Curiously, however, the level of phosphorylation of enolase, which was added to the reaction mixture as an exogenous substrate, was not increased following antibody-mediated stimulation (unpublished observation). To test whether this discrepancy depended on the nature of the monoclonal antibody used, we examined the effect of mIgM cross-linking on Lyn kinase using the human B cell line Daudi and the monoclonal antibody Lyn-9, which is specific for human Lyn. One minute of mIgM cross-linking resulted in 4- to

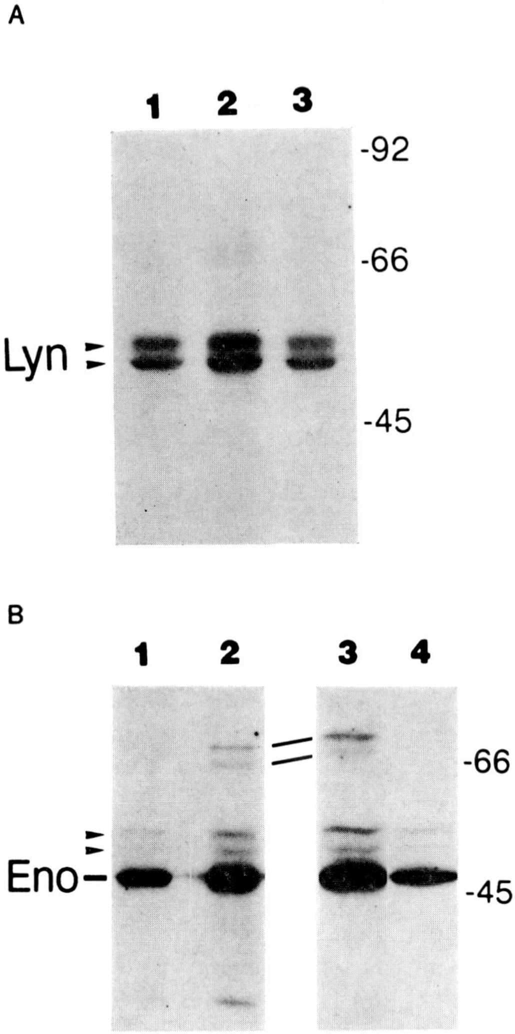

FIG. 1. Activation of Lyn kinase after mIgM cross-linking. (A) Murine WEHI-231 B cells (3×10^6) were incubated in the absence (lane 1) or presence of antibody to murine IgM (lane 2) or human IgG (lane 3) and lysed with TNE buffer. The lysates were subjected to immunoprecipitation with monoclonal antibody Lyn-8, which reacts with both human and murine Lyn, and immune-complex kinase assay without enolase was performed. (B) Human Daudi B cells (3×10^6) were incubated in the absence (lane 1) or presence of antibody to human IgM (lanes 2 and 3) or murine IgG (lane 4) and lysed with TNE buffer (1% (vol/vol) Nonidet P-40/50 mM Tris-HCl, pH 8.0/20 mM EDTA/0.2 mM sodium orthovanadate with aprotinin at 10 μg/ml. The lysates were subjected to immunoprecipitation with monoclonal antibody Lyn-9, which is specific to human Lyn, and immune-complex kinase assay with enolase. Positions of Lyn (arrowheads), enolase (Eno), and protein standard markers ($M_r\times10^{-3}$) are indicated.

5-fold increase of Lyn kinase activity, as measured by both *in vitro* autophosphorylation and phosphorylation of the exogenous substrate enolase (Fig. 1, B), with no change in the amount of Lyn (data not shown). Antibody to murine IgG (γ chain) had no effect on Lyn kinase activity (Fig. 1, B). Thus Lyn-8 seems to inhibit mIgM-mediated

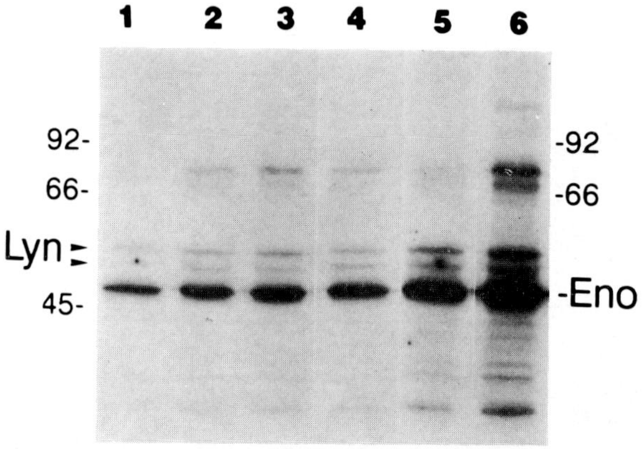

FIG. 2. Rapid activation of Lyn kinase by mIgM cross-linking. Daudi cells (3×10^6) were incubated with antibody to IgM for various times and then the kinase activity of Lyn was examined as described for Fig. 1B, Lane 1, untreated control; lane 2, 15-sec incubation; lane 3, 1-min incubation; lane 4, 5-min incubation; lanes 5 and 6, longer exposure of lanes 1 and 3, respectively. Positions of Lyn, enolase (Eno), and protein markers ($M_r \times 10^{-3}$) are indicated.

activation of Lyn kinase to phosphorylate enolase *in vitro* by some unknown mechanism. From the above findings, we conclude that the cross-linking of mIgM activates Lyn kinase.

In parallel with the mIgM-mediated activation of Lyn kinase, about 70 kDa phosphoproteins were detected after mIgM cross-linking of both WEHI-231 cells (Fig. 1, A, lane 2) and Daudi cells (Fig. 1, B, lanes 2 and 3, and Fig. 2). This suggests that the stimulation induces association of Lyn with these 70 kDa proteins in B cells. Since faint bands of about 70 and 75 kDa proteins were also detected before the treatment (Fig. 2, lane 5), very small amount of these molecules may be associated before the stimulation.

Tyrosine phosphorylation of cellular proteins reaches a peak within 2 to 15 min after cross-linking of the B cell antigen receptor (*8*, *21*, *22*). Moreover, the level of tyrosine phosphorylation of PLC-γ of Daudi cells is increased 2-fold within 90 sec and 4-fold (the peak activity) within 30 min after mIgM cross-linking (*18*). We analyzed the time course of the activation of Lyn kinase after mIgM cross-linking (Fig. 2). The *in vitro* kinase activity of Lyn was increased 2- to 3-fold within 15 sec, and 4- to 5-fold (the peak activity) within 1 min of the cross-linking. This rate of activation is rapid enough to explain up-regulation of cellular tyrosine phosphorylation, which suggests that Lyn transduces at least part of the mIgM-mediated signals to intracellular targets. Veillette *et al.* showed that only Lck co-immunoprecipitated with CD4 is activated after CD4 cross-linking, while non-CD4 associated Lck is not activated (*5*). We have previously shown that Lyn is co-immunoprecipitated with mIgM from 1% digitonin lysates of B cells (*8*). However, the level of Lyn co-immunoprecipitated with mIgM after mIgM cross-linking is very low, because mIgM changed rapidly (more than 90% within 1 min) to a digitonin-insoluble form after the stimulation (unpublished observation). Thus, it was difficult to evaluate the kinase activity of Lyn co-immunoprecipitated with mIgM after the cross-linking.

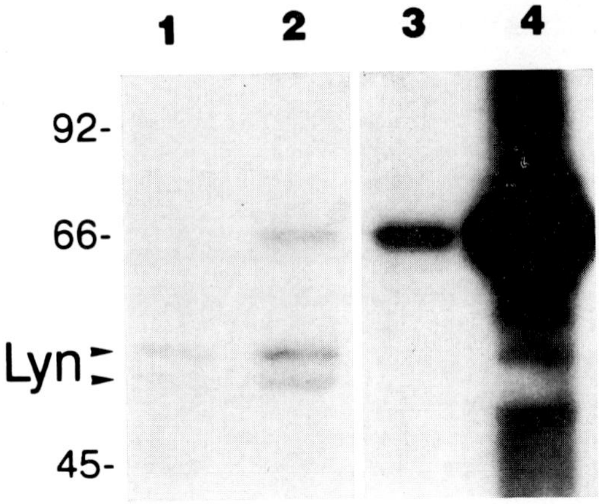

FIG. 3. Effect of mIgM cross-linking on tyrosine phosphorylation of Lyn and other proteins. WEHI-231 cells, 10^7 (lanes 1 and 2) or 5×10^6 (lanes 3 and 4), were incubated in the absence (lanes 1 and 3) or presence (lanes 2 and 4) of antibody to IgM and lysed with TNE buffer. The lysates were subjected to immunoprecipitation with Lyn-8 (lanes 1 and 2) or Py-20 anti-phosphotyrosine antibody (lanes 3 and 4) coupled covalently to protein A-Sepharose. The immunoprecipitates were washed five times with TNE buffer, and their phosphotyrosine-containing proteins were examined by immunoblotting.

Tyrosine Phosphorylation of Lyn and Its Associated Proteins

We then evaluated tyrosine phosphorylation of anti-Lyn immunoprecipitates before and 1 min after mIgM cross-linking. Western blotting of the immunoprecipitates from WEHI-231 cells with antibody to phosphotyrosine revealed 2- to 3-fold increase of tyrosine phosphorylation of Lyn upon mIgM cross-linking (Fig. 3). This is consistent with our previous data suggesting that the tyrosine phosphorylations of 53 kDa and 56 kDa protein are induced by mIgM cross-linking (*8*). Interestingly, 66 kDa (WEHI-231, Fig. 3) or 70 kDa (Daudi, data not shown) protein containing phosphotyrosine was found in Lyn-8 or Lyn-9 immunoprecipitates only after the cross-linking (Fig. 3). Either the 66 kDa or the 70 kDa protein co-migrated with a phosphotyrosine-containing protein that gave the most intense band in immunoprecipitates with PY-20, monoclonal antibody to phosphotyrosine, after mIgM cross-linking of each B cell (Fig. 3, lane 4). It must be noticed that a fraction of phosphotyrosine-containing proteins are immunoprecipitated with PY-20, because the phosphoproteins detected by immunoblotting are larger than those immunoprecipitated (*8*). In addition, 45 kDa, 73 kDa, 80 kDa, and 100 kDa phosphotyrosine-containing proteins were detected in Lyn-9 immunoprecipitates after mIgM cross-linking of Daudi cells, and bands co-migrating with these phosphoproteins were also detected in the PY-20 immunoprecipitate after cross-linking. A similar set of phosphoproteins (40 kDa, 45 kDa, 70 kDa, 75 kDa, 100 kDa, and 130 kDa) was found by *in vitro* phosphorylation of Lyn-9 immunoprecipitates from the lysates of antibody-treated Daudi cells (Fig. 1, B, and Fig. 2). 66 kDa and 70 kDa phosphoproteins were also found by *in vitro* phosphorylation of Lyn-8 immunoprecipitates from the lysates of antibody-treated WEHI-231 cells (Fig. 1, A). Thus, some signals of mIgM cross-linking may be transduced to these phosphoproteins *via* Lyn kinase.

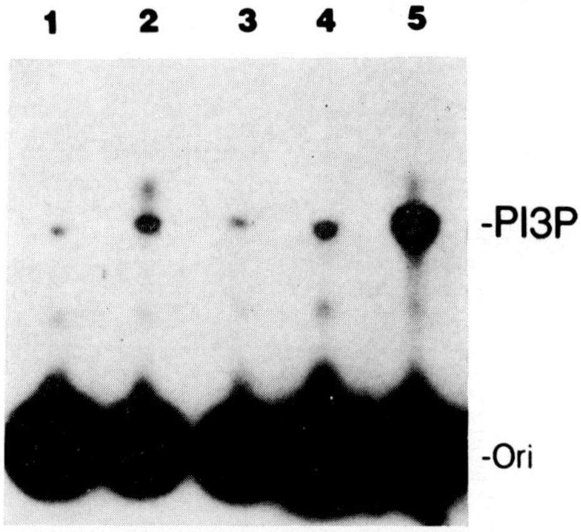

FIG. 4. Activation of Lyn-associated PI3-kinase by mIgM cross-linking. Daudi cells, 10^7 (lanes 1–3) or 5×10^6 (lanes 4 and 5), were incubated in the absence (lanes 1 and 4) or presence of antibody to IgM (lanes 2 and 5) or to murine IgG (lane 3) and lysed with TNE buffer. The lysates were subjected to immunoprecipitation with Lyn-9 (lanes 1–3) or PY-20 (lanes 4 and 5), and PI3-kinase in the immunoprecipitates was assayed.

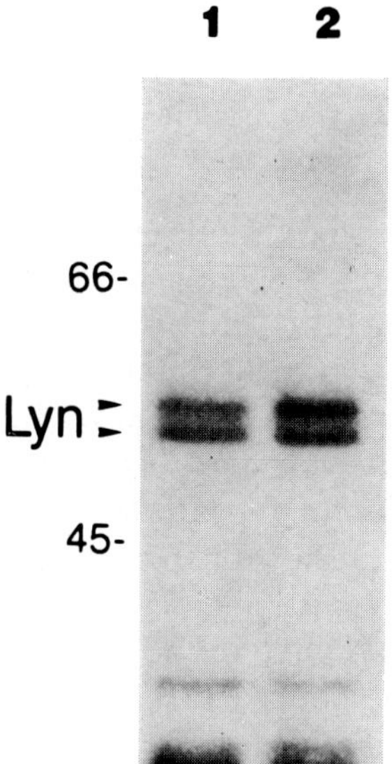

FIG. 5. Association of Lyn with mIgM and mIgD in splenic B cells. B cells (10^7) from BALB/c mice were lysed with lysis buffer and the lysates were subjected to coimmunoprecipitation with monoclonal antibody to IgM (lane 1) or to IgD (lane 2) and *in vitro* phosphorylation. The phosphoproteins were reimmunoprecipitated with rabbit antibody to Lyn.

Up-regulation of the Association of Lyn with PI3-Kinase

To test whether PI-3 kinase is one of the targets of Lyn kinase in mIgM-mediated signalling, we examined Lyn-associated PI-3 kinase activity before and 1 min after mIgM cross-linking of Daudi cells (Fig. 4). The PI-3 kinase activity in anti-Lyn immunoprecipitates was increased about 5-fold after mIgM cross-linking of Daudi cells (Fig. 4, lanes 1 and 2). However, stimulation of Daudi cells, which does not express mIgG, with antibody to murine IgG (γ chain) did not increase the Lyn-associated PI-3 kinase activity (Fig. 4, lane 3). PI-3 kinase apparently consists of an 85 kDa noncatalytic subunit (p85) and 110 kDa catalytic subunit (*23–26*). The p85 subunit could bind to several tyrosine kinases by interaction between the SH2 domain and phosphotyrosine-containing peptides (*11*, *27*, *28*). We examined the association of the p85 with Lyn using antibodies to human p85. The level of Lyn-associated p85 was increased 4- to 5-fold 1 min after mIgM cross-linking (data not shown). Since the increase in Lyn-associated PI-3 kinase activity was proportional to that of p85 associated with Lyn, it is unlikely that an individual PI-3 kinase associated with Lyn becomes activated upon mIgM cross-linking. Moreover, both the PI-3 kinase activity and the amount of the p85 in PY-20 immunoprecipitates increased 7- to 9-fold after mIgM cross-linking (Fig. 4, lanes 4 and 5), which suggests that a certain fraction of phosphotyrosine-containing PI-3 kinase is associated with Lyn. Thus, interaction of PI-3 kinase with active Lyn may cause tyrosine phosphorylation of p85, which in turn would induce their stable association, as in the case of association of $p60^{v\text{-}src}$ with PI-3 kinase (*27*).

All the above data support the notion that Lyn is an intracytoplasmic signal transducing molecule of B cell antigen receptor and that PI-3 kinase is important in the signalling. Therefore, we examined whether Lyn is also associated with mIgD, another major B cell antigen receptor. The results clearly showed that Lyn is a constituent of mIgD and mIgM complexes of murine splenic B cells (Fig. 5). Interestingly, the smallest of the three Lyn-associated 30–40 kDa phosphoproteins, which exist as disulfide linked dimers (*8*) of mIgM and mIgD complexes differ in molecular mass by 1kDa. This may reflect the difference between mIgM-α and mIgD-α (*29*, *30*). A recent study on the mIg-associated molecules revealed that mIgM/D-α and mIg-β were tyrosine phosphorylated rapidly (within 1 min) after mIgM/D cross-linking (*31*). The activated Lyn kinase may be responsible for this phosphorylation. Another line of study has suggested that CD45, membrane-bound tyrosine phosphatase, regulates mIgM-mediated signalling (*32*). It is important to examine possible functional or physical interactions between Lyn and CD45, G-proteins, GAP, PLC-γ or another regulators/substrates.

Possible Involvement of Fyn in T Cell Activation

T lymphocytes recognize antigens that are physically associated with self major histocompatibility complex (MHC) molecules on the surface of the antigen presenting cells. The antigen-MHC receptor on T cells (TCR) is a heterodimer of two covalently linked polypeptide chains designated α and β. The cell-surface expression and the function of $\alpha\beta$ heterodimer requires its association with the CD3 complex that consists of at least five distinct integral membrane proteins, γ, δ, ε, ζ, and η chains. The response of T cells to the antigen-major MHC complex consists of a series of cellular events collectively called T cell activation, which includes activation of protein-tyrosine kinase (*33*) and induction of a number of genes whose products are essential

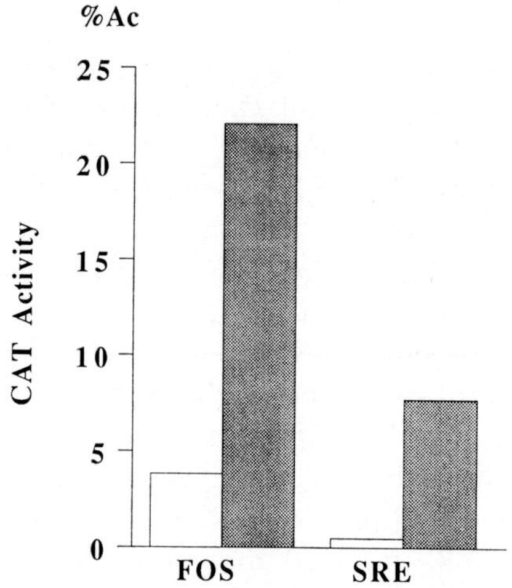

FIG. 6. Activation of c-*fos*CAT and SRECAT by cotransfection with active T-*fyn* cDNA to Jurkat cells. c-*fos*CAT or SRECAT plasmids were cotransfected with pβAM vector plasmid or pβT*fyn*F plasmid into Jurkat cells. Then, the CAT activity of the cell lysates was measured, the activity being shown as the percentage of conversion of chloramphenicol into acetylated form. Open and solid bars represent CAT activity with pβAM and pβT*fyn*F, respectively.

for the function of T cells. Among these the *fos* and *IL-2* genes are of particular interest because of their pivotal roles in regulation of T cell growth. We and others have previously shown that Fyn is associated with T-cell antigen receptor (*9* and our unpublished data). Then, we analyzed if Fyn is involved in T cell antigen receptor-mediated transactivation of the *fos* and *IL-2* genes.

Transactivation of the c-fos Promoter through SRE by Active T-Fyn Kinase

To examine the effect of the Fyn kinase on c-*fos* expression in T cells, we first cloned the cDNA of active T-*fyn* that encoded the thymus-type Fyn protein (*34*) with Phe-528 instead of Tyr-528 (T-fynF) into the expression plasmid (pβAM) containing chicken β-actin promoter. A reporter plasmid (c-*fos*CAT) containing the bacterial *CAT* gene for the chloramphenicol acetyl transferase downstream of the 445-bp 5′-flanking sequence of the c-*fos* gene (*35*) was used as a monitor for its transcriptional activity. These plasmids were cotransfected into Jurkat T cells. Jurkat cells were chosen because of the similarity to normal resting T-cells in their response to the TCR stimulation. As shown in Fig. 6, transfection of T-fynF enhanced the c-*fos* promoter activity by 5.5-fold as compared with that of the control plasmid.

Since the c-*fos* promoter contains SRE, TRE, and CRE, we examined which element was responsible for the T-fynF-mediated stimulation of the c-*fos* promoter. To this end, the T-fynF construct was transfected into Jurkat cells together with SRECAT, TRECAT, or CRECAT reporter plasmids. The result clearly showed that T-fynF greatly stimulated SRE while less stimulation of TRE and CRE was observed by the expression of T-fynF (Fig. 6, and data not shown). The degrees of stimulation of SRE, TRE, and CRE by T-fynF were about 18-, 4-, and 3-folds as compared with control experiments. These data showed that the c-*fos* promoter

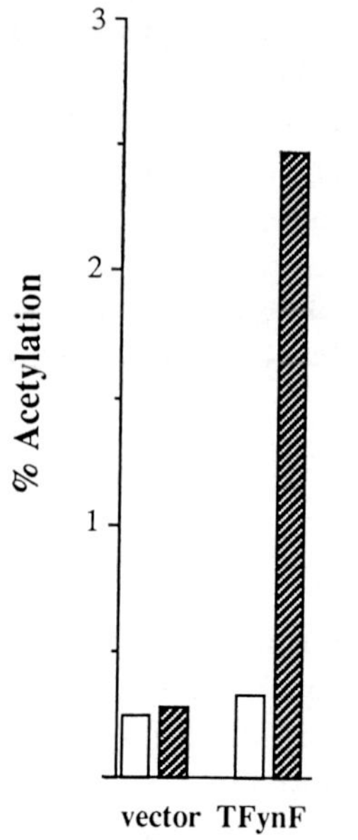

FIG. 7. Activation of *IL-2*CAT by active T-*fyn*. *IL-2*CAT was cotransfected with pME18S vector plasmid or pMT*fyn*F into Jurkat cells. TPA and ConA (striped bars) were added to the transfectants eight hours before the cell harvest. Then the CAT activity was measured.

was activated by T-fynF primarily through SRE.

Transactivation of IL-2 Promoter by Active T-Fyn

Within an hour of binding of the ligands to the TCR/CD3 complex, T cell begins transcribing the *IL-2* gene. In order to examine whether the Fyn kinase is involved in the TCR-mediated transactivation of the *IL-2* gene, a reporter plasmid (*IL-2* CAT) in which the promoter region of the *IL-2* gene was ligated upstream of the CAT gene was prepared. The promoter of the *IL-2* gene consists of a 584-bp 5′ flanking sequence and a 52-bp sequence from the first exon containing the initiator ATG of the *IL-2* gene (*36*). Expression of the CAT activity of this *IL-2*CAT has been shown to be specific to the activated T-cells and paralleled with expression of the endogenous *IL-2* gene (*36*). Cotransfection of T-fynF construct in which *fyn* cDNA coding for T-fynF was ligated under the chimeric promoter of SV40 and HTLV-1 promoters (SRα) into Jurkat cells showed only a slight activation of CAT activity of *IL-2*CAT as compared with that from cells cotransfected with the vector plasmid (Fig. 7). This result indicates that elevated tyrosine kinase activity alone is not sufficient for the induction of the *IL-2* gene.

Then, T cells cotransfected with *IL-2*CAT and the T-fynF construct were stimulated by 12-O-tetradecanoylphorbol-13-acetate (TPA) and/or mitogens such as Concanavalin (Con A) or phytohemaglutinin (PHA). In this system phorbol ester TPA provides a second signal that is required for TCR-mediated mitogenesis. The effect of the elevated kinase activity of T-fynF on *IL-2* promoter was remarkable when the transfectants were treated with a combination of TPA and ConA (Fig. 7). On the other hand, treatment of the transfectants with TPA alone or with ConA alone had little effect on the expression of the *IL*-2CAT (data not shown). Next, we cross-linked the CD3 molecule by anti-CD3ε antibodies on the surface of the Jurkat T cells that had been transfected with the *IL-2*CAT and T-fynF constructs. When TPA treatment was accompanied by the CD3 cross-linking, significant transactivation of the *IL-2* promoter was observed. Treatment with TPA and anti-CD3 without exogenous T-fynF had little effect (data not shown). These data showed that active Fyn kinase could transactivate the *IL-2* promoter in combination with extracellular mitogenic stimulants of the T cells.

Prospects

Recently, Burkhardt *et al.* reported that Blk and Fyn were activated after either mIgM or mIgD cross-linking by using rabbit polyclonal antibodies to these Src-like kinases (*11*). Thus, Lyn, Blk, and Fyn may share pathway(s) in B cell antigen receptor-mediated signalling, and comparison of their role(s) in the signalling should be made. They also reported that mIgM cross-linking did not result in reproducible changes in the activity of Lyn. The apparent discrepancy between this and our observations may reflect differences of antibodies and/or cells used in the experiments.

Our data also provide evidence that Fyn plays an important role in signalling upon stimulation of T cells. First, elevated kinase activity of Fyn stimulated the c-*fos* promoter most likely through SRE. Second, transactivation of *IL-2* promoter was augmented in T cells with higher activity of Fyn kinase when the cells received mitogenic stimulation that mimicked TCR-mediated activation. This suggests a critical importance of Fyn in transducing membrane signals into more distal cellular events. This is consistent with the observation that overexpression of Fyn in thymocytes of transgenic mice results in an augmented TCR response (*37*).

There are several binding sites for transcription factors in the upstream region of the *IL-2* gene (*36*). Among these the putative NF-κB binding site and NF-AT1 site are candidates for Fyn-responsive sequence, because our preliminary study showed that Fyn kinase could stimulate the promoter activity in the long terminal repeat (LTR) of human immuno-deficiency virus (HIV) type I that contains NF-κB and NF-AT1 sites (*38*, and references therein).

The CD3 ζ chain has been implicated in T-cell signalling via TCR. We have evidence that Fyn interacts with the CD3 ζ chain (unpublished data). This interaction would be a prerequisite for tyrosine phosphorylation of ζ by the Fyn kinase. The ζ chain thus phosphorylated might, in turn, recruit SH2-containing signalling molecules such as PLC-γ, GAP, and PI3-kinase as insulin receptor-associated p185, which becomes tyrosine phosphorylated by the insulin receptor upon insulin stimulation, interacts with PI3-kinase (*39*). Recently a molecule termed Zap was shown to interact with the ζ chain (*40*). This interaction might be important to specify T-cell specific response to antigenic activation. In this context it would be important to examine whether Zap can be a target of Fyn kinase, although data in ref. *40* do not support this particular condition. It is also necessary to identify a target protein of Lyn and/or Blk in B lymphocytes which would specify B cell response to antigenic activation.

REFERENCES

1. Hunter, T. and Cooper, J. A. Protein-tyrosine kinases. Annu. Rev. Biochem., *54*: 897–930, 1985.
2. Ullrich, A. and Schlessinger, J. Signal transduction by receptor with tyrosine kinase activity. Cell, *61*: 203–212, 1990.
3. Cooper, J. A. The *src* family of protein-tyrosine kinases. *In*; B. E. Kemp and P. F. Alewood (eds.), Peptides and Protein Phosphorylation, pp. 85–113, CRC Press, Boca Raton, Florida, 1990.
4. Semba, K. and Toyoshima, K. Structure and function of *src* family kinases. *In*; K. Sikora and D. Carney (eds.), Genes and Cancer, pp. 73–83, John Wiley & Sons, Chichester, 1990.
5. Veillette, A., Bookman, M. A., Horak, E. M., Samelson, L. E., and Bolen, J. B. Signal transduction through the CD4 receptor involves the activation of the internal membrane tyrosine-protein kinase $p56^{lck}$. Nature, *338*: 257–259, 1989.
6. Barber, E. K., Dasgupta, J. D., Schlossman, S. F., Trevillyan, J. M., and Rudd, C. E. The CD4 and CD8 antigens are coupled to a protein-tyrosine kinase ($p56^{lck}$) that phosphorylates the CD3 complex. Proc. Natl. Acad. Sci. U.S.A., *86*: 3277–3281, 1989.
7. Abraham, N., Miceli, M. C., Parnes, J. R., and Veillette, A. Enhancement of T-cell responsiveness by the lymphocyte-specific tyrosine protein kinase $p56^{lck}$. Nature, *350*: 62–66, 1991.
8. Yamanashi, Y., Kakiuchi, T., Mizuguchi, J., Yamamoto, T., and Toyoshima, K. Association of B cell antigen receptor and protein-tyrosine kinase $p56^{lyn}$. Science, *251*: 192–194, 1991.
9. Samelson, L. E., Phillips, A. F., Luong, E. T., and Klausner, R. D. Association of the fyn protein-tyrosine kinase with T-cell antigen receptor. Proc. Natl. Acad. Sci. U.S.A., *87*: 4358–4362, 1990.
10. Hatakeyama, M., Kono, T., Kobayashi, N., Kawahara, A., Levin, S. D., Perlmutter, R. M. and Taniguchi, T. Interaction of the IL-2 receptor with the *src*-family kinase $p56^{lck}$: Identification of novel intermolecular association. Science, *252*: 1523–1528, 1991.
11. Burkhardt, A. L., Brunswick, M., Bolen, J. B., and Mond, J. J. Anti-immunoglobulin stimulation of B lymphocytes activates *src*-related protein-tyrosine kinases. Proc. Natl. Acad. Sci. U.S.A., *88*: 7410–7414, 1991.
12. Varticovski, L., Druker, D., Morrison, D., Cantley, L., and Roberts, T. The colony stimulating factor-1 receptor associates with and activates phosphatidylinositol-3 kinase. Nature, *342*: 699–702, 1989.
13. Ruderman, N. B., Kapreller, R., White, M. F., and Cantley, L. C. Activation of phosphatidylinositol 3-kinase by insulin. Proc. Natl. Acad. Sci. U.S.A., *87*: 1411–1415, 1990.
14. Fukui, Y., Kornbluth, S., Jong, S.-M., Wang, L.-H., and Hanafusa, H. Phosphatidylinositol kinase type I activity associates with various oncogene products. Oncogene Res., *4*: 283–292, 1989.
15. Cantley, L. C., Auger, K. R., Carpenter, C., Duckworth, B., Graziani, A., Kapeller, R., and Soltoff, S. Oncogenes and signal transduction. Cell, *64*: 281–302, 1991.
16. Crabtree, G. R. Contingent genetic regulatory events in T lymphocyte activation. Science, *243*: 355–361, 1989.
17. Ales-Martinez, J. E., Cuende, E., Martinez, A. C., Parkhouse, R. M. E., Pezzi, L., and Scott, D. W. Signalling in B cells. Immunol. Today, *12*: 201–205, 1991.

18. Carter, R. H., Park, D. J., Rhee, S. G., and Fearon, D. T. Tyrosine phosphorylation of phospholipase C induced by membrane immunoglobulin in B lymphocytes. Proc. Natl. Acad. Sci. U.S.A., *88*: 2745–2749, 1991.
19. Adams, V. E., Lieberman, R., Sandlund, J., Kiwanuka, J., Novikovs, L., Kirsch, I., Hollis, G., and Magrath, I. T. Antiimmunoglobulin inhibition of Burkitt's lymphoma cell proliferation and concurrent reduction of c-*myc* and μ heavy chain gene expression. Cancer Res., *49*: 3235–3241, 1989.
20. Reth, M., Hombach, J., Wienands, J., Campbell, K. S., Chien, N., Justement, L. B., and Cambies, J. C. The B-cell antigen receptor complex. Immunol. Today, *12*: 196–201, 1991.
21. Campbell, M.-A. and Sefton, B. M. Protein-tyrosine phosphorylation is induced in murine B lymphocytes in response to stimulation with anti-immunoglobulin. EMBO. J., *9*: 2125–2131, 1990.
22. Gold, M. R., Law, D. A., and DeFranco, A. L. Stimulation of protein-tyrosine phosphorylation by the B lymphocyte antigen receptor. Nature, *345*: 810–813, 1990.
23. Skolnik, E. Y., Margolis, B., Mohammadi, M., Lowenstein, E., Fischer, R., Drepps, A., Ullrich, A., and Schlessinger, J. Cloning of PI3 kinase-associated p85 utilizing a novel method for expression/cloning of target proteins for receptor tyrosine kinases. Cell, *65*: 83–90, 1991.
24. Shibasaki, F., Homma, Y., and Takenawa, T. Two types of phosphatidylinositol kinase from bovine thymus: monomer and heterodimer forms. J. Biol. Chem., *266*: 8108–8114, 1991.
25. Escobedo, J. A., Navankasattusasa, S., Kavanaugh, W. M., Milfay, D., Fried, V. A., and Williams, T. cDNA cloning of a novel 85 kd protein that has SH2 domain and regulates binding of PI3-kinase to the PDGF β-receptor. Cell, *65*: 75–82, 1991.
26. Otsu, M., Hiles, I., Gout, I., Fry, M. J., Ruiz-Larrea, F., Panayotou, G., Thompson, A., Dhand, R., Hsuan, J., Totty, N., Smith, A. D., Morgan, S. J., Courtneidge, S. A., Parker, P. J., and Waterfield, M. D. Characterization of two 85 kd proteins that associate with receptor tyrosine kinases, middle-T/pp60$^{c\text{-}src}$ complexes, and PI3-kinase. Cell, *65*: 91–104, 1991.
27. Fukui, Y. and Hanafusa, H. Phosphatidylinositol kinase activity associates with viral p60^{src} protein. Mol. Cell. Biol., *11*: 1972–1979, 1991.
28. Matsuda, M., Mayer, B. J., Fukui, Y., and Hanafusa, H. Binding of transforming protein p47$^{gag\text{-}crk}$ to a broad range of phosphotyrosine-containing proteins. Science, *248*: 1537–1539, 1990.
29. Campbell, K. S. and Cambier, J. C. B lymphocyte antigen receptors (mIg) are non-covalently associated with a disulfide linked, inducibly phosphorylated glycoprotein complex. EMBO, J., *9*: 441–448, 1990.
30. Campbell, K. S., Hager, J. H., Friedrich, R. J., and Cambier, J. C. IgM antigen receptor complex contains phosphoprotein products of B29 and *mb-1* genes. Proc. Natl. Acad. Sci. U.S.A., *88*: 3982–3986, 1991.
31. Gold, M. R., Matsuuchi, L., Kelly, R. B., and DeFranco, A. L. Tyrosine phosphorylation of components of the B-cell antigen receptors following receptor crosslinking. Proc. Natl. Acad. Sci. U.S.A., *88*: 3436–3440, 1991.
32. Justement, L. B., Campbell, K. S., Chien, N. C., and Cambier, J. C. Regulation of B cell antigen receptor signal transduction and phosphorylation by CD45. Science, *252*: 1839–1842, 1991.
33. June, C. H., Fletcher, M. C., Ledbetter, J. A., and Samelson, L. E. Increase in the tyrosine phosphorylation are detectable before phospholipase C activation after T cell receptor activation. J. Immunol., *144*: 1591–1599, 1990.

34. Cooke, M. P. and Perlmutter, R. M. Expression of a novel form of the *fyn* proto-oncogene in hematopoietic cells. New Biologist, *1*: 66–74, 1989.
35. Deschamps, J., Meijlink, F., and Verma I. M. Identification of a transcriptional enhancer element upstream from the proto-oncogene *fos*. Science, *230*: 1174–1177, 1985.
36. Fujita, T., Shibuya, H., Ohashi, T., Yamanishi, K., and Taniguchi, T. Regulation of human interleukin-2 gene: Functional DNA sequences in the 5′ flanking region for the gene expression in activated T lymphocytes. Cell, *46*: 401–407, 1986.
37. Cooke, M. P., Abraham, K. M., Forbush, K. A., and Purlmutter, R. M. Regulation of T-cell receptor signaling by a *src* family protein-tyrosine kinase. Cell, *65*: 281–291, 1991.
38. Ching, L., Lai, C., Sigman, D. S., and Gaynor, R. B. Cloning of a cellular factor, interleukin binding factor, that binds to NFAT-like motifs in the human immunodeficiency virus long terminal repeat. Proc. Natl. Acad. Sci. U.S.A., *88*: 7739–7743, 1991.
39. Sun, X. J., Rothenberg, P., Kahn, C. R., Backer, J. M., Araki, E., Wilden, P. A., Cahill, D. A., Goldstein, B. J., and White, M. F. Structure of the insulin receptor substrate IRS-1 defines a unique signal transduction protein. Nature, *352*: 73–77, 1991.
40. Chan, A. C., Irving, B. A., Fraser, J. D., Weiss, A. The ζ chain is associated with a tyrosine kinase and upon T-cell antigen receptor stimulation associates with ZAP-70, a 70-kDa tyrosine phosphoprotein. Proc. Natl. Acad. Sci. U.S.A., *88*: 9166–9170, 1991.

MULTISTAGE CARCINOGENESIS, C. C. HARRIS ET AL. (EDS.),
JAPAN SCI. SOC. PRESS, TOKYO/CRC PRESS, BOCA RATON, PP. 307–318, 1992

myc, *max*, and a Novel *rlf*-L-*myc* Fusion Protein in Small-cell Lung Cancer

Imre Västrik, Tomi P. Mäkelä, Päivi J. Koskinen, Kalle Saksela, and Kari Alitalo

Laboratory of Cancer Biology, Departments of Virology and Pathology, University of Helsinki, Haartmaninkatu 3, 00290 Helsinki, Finland

Abstract: The functional properties of Myc proteins are likely to be modulated by interactions with other nuclear proteins. One such protein called Max has already been characterized (*1*). Through their homologous helix-loop-helix and leucine zipper structures, Myc and Max proteins form heterodimers that bind to specific DNA sequences more efficiently than Myc or Max alone. We have recently identified ΔMax, a naturally occurring truncated version of Max, which is also able to dimerize with Myc in the nucleus, but is cytoplasmic in the absence of Myc. These two forms of Max can act either as enhancers or suppressors of co-transformation by c-*myc* and *ras*.

Oncogenic activation of *myc* genes in human cancer involves deregulated *myc* expression. Oncogenes of the *myc* family are activated in several types of human tumors as a result of gene amplification or chromosomal translocation. We have recently characterized a gene fusion and a chimeric protein product formed by L-*myc* and part of a novel gene called *rlf* in small-cell lung cancer (SCLC) cell lines. Although the chimeric mRNAs were shown to be identical, they result from distinct DNA rearrangements. We have also established a physical linkage between normal *rlf* and L-*myc* using pulsed field gel electrophoresis. Thus, the *rlf*-L-*myc* gene fusions are due to similar but not identical intrachromosomal rearrangements at 1p32. Similar *in vivo* rearrangements involving *rlf* and L-*myc* have been found in at least one primary SCLC tumor. The presence of independent genetic lesions that cause the formation of identical chimeric *rlf*-L-*myc* proteins suggests a role for the fusion protein in the development of these SCLC tumors.

Members of the *myc* gene family (c-*myc*, N-*myc*, and L-*myc*) have been implicated in neoplasia and in the control of normal cell proliferation (reviewed in *2–4*). In addition to sporadic activations in various tumors, the *myc* genes are commonly activated in Burkitt's lymphomas, neuroblastomas, and small-cell lung cancer (reviewed in *5–7*). Moreover, at least in the case of neuroblastoma, amplification of the N-*myc* gene correlates with treatment failure (*8*, *9*), and therefore provides an important diagnostic tool in this disease.

A more direct oncogenic role for Myc proteins has been demonstrated by their ability to transform primary rat embryo fibroblasts in association with a c-Ha-*ras* oncogene (*10–13*). All Myc proteins can also cause lymphoid malignancies in transgenic mice when expressed under the control of an immunoglobulin enhancer (*14–17*). Differentiation of several cell types is associated with downregulation of *myc* gene expression (*18*), and differentiation can be induced (*19*) or inhibited (*20*) by transfection of antisense or sense constructs of the *myc* genes, respectively.

Although the normal functions of the Myc proteins remain to be solved, several recent clues suggest that these proteins, like so many other nuclear oncoproteins, will turn out to be transcription factors. Especially the identification of Max and ΔMax, the proteins that form sequence-specific DNA-binding complexes with Myc should prove useful in studies on Myc function.

Characteristics of Myc Proteins

Sequence comparison of Myc proteins reveals several conserved domains, which might be expected to be indispensable for *myc* activity (reviewed in *2, 3, 7, 21, 22*). Figure 1 depicts the c-Myc protein with these conserved domains shown as white areas. Mutational studies of the c-*myc* gene have defined large regions of the c-Myc protein that are completely or partly dispensable for transformation (*23*), and for the negative autoregulation of c-*myc* (*24*). Even some of the very conserved regions were dispensable in both assays (*e.g.*, domains IV and V in Fig. 1), suggesting that the Myc proteins perform several distinct functions. In these studies, a large part in the N-terminal region (in addition to domain VI) was critical for transformation (Fig. 1). Interestingly, chimeric constructs containing similar domains from c-Myc (Fig. 1; *25*) or corresponding regions from L-Myc (K. Saksela, unpublished experiments) activate transcription in heterologous systems. It is also worth noting that domains II-III appear to be responsible for the interactions with the protein product of the retinoblastoma (RB) tumor suppressor gene, suggesting that Myc and Rb can function cooperatively in controlling cell proliferation (Fig. 1; *26*).

Other characterized functional regions in the Myc proteins include the nuclear localization signal of c-Myc (*27*), which is fairly well conserved in N-Myc but not in L-Myc, two casein kinase II (CK-II) phosphorylation sites (*28*), and a Mitogen activated protein kinase-2 (MAP-2)-related kinase/glycogen synthase kinase-3 site

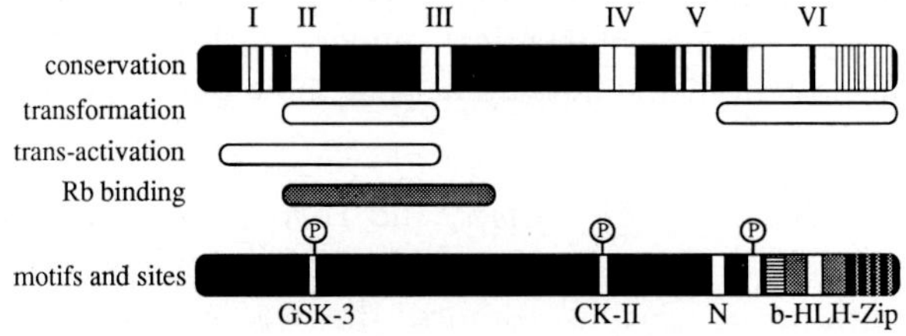

FIG. 1. Structural characteristics of the c-Myc protein. Conserved domains (deduced from an alignment of 20 Myc protein sequences) are shown in white on the top (I–VI). Deletions deleterious for rat embryo fibroblast (REF) transformation or retinoblastoma protein binding, and the region sufficient for transactivation in a heterologous system are indicated as white bars in the middle. Characterized phosphorylation sites (the more C-terminal CK-II site is only marked with the P), the nuclear localization signal (N), and the DNA-binding and oligomerization motif (bHLH/Zip) are shown on the bottom. See text for references.

v-Myc	MC-29 retrovirus	Pan-Myc box-P-M-P-P-L-S-P-S-R
c-Myc	Xenopus 1	Pan-Myc box-P-T-P-P-L-S-P-S-R
	Xenopus 2	-"-
	Rainbow trout	-"-
	Chick	-"-
	Cat	-"-
	Human	-"-
	Mouse	-"-
	Woodchuck	-"-
	Rat	-"-
Rat B-Myc		-P-T-P-R-P-S-P-G-H
N-Myc	Canary	Pan-myc box-P-T-P-P-L-S-P-S-R
	Chick	-"-
	Human	-"-
	Mouse	-"-
	Woodchuck-1	-"-
	Woodchuck-2	Pan-myc box-P-T-P-P-L-S-P-S-C
Rat s-Myc		Pan-myc box-P-T-P-R-L-S-P-G-R
L-Myc	Mouse	Pan-myc box-P-S-P-P-T-S-P-P-W
	Human	-"-
	Human-2	Pan-myc box-P-..................P-P-W

FIG. 2. Amino acid sequence of the MAP2-related kinase/GSK-3 phosphorylation sites in Myc proteins. Shown are the homologous sequences deduced from sequenced c-*myc*, N-*myc*, and L-*myc* genes. Note that L-Myc does not have the P-L-S/T-P sequence suggested as the consensus for the MAP2-related kinase target sequence, but instead a P-S-P-P-T-S-P sequence, which fits with the consensus of the GSK-3 kinase (*29, 30*).

(GSK3; Fig. 2; refs. *29, 30*). The role of these phosphorylations in Myc functions is not clear; comparison of the transforming efficiencies of CKII phosphorylation-negative mutants with wild-type Myc did not indicate differences (*31*). Interestingly, however, phosphorylation of the MAP-2-related kinase/GSK-3 kinase site is stimulated by serum and protein kinase C-activating phorbol esters (*29, 30*).

The C-terminal domain VI of the Myc proteins share several structural domains with transcriptional regulators (reviewed in *3, 21*). These include the basic-helix-loop-helix (*32*) and leucine zipper (*33*) DNA binding and dimerization motifs, which have been identified from various activators. Besides all three Myc proteins, adjacent helix-loop-helix and leucine repeat domains preceded by a basic motif (bHLH/Zip) have been identified from TFE-3 (*34*), USF (*35*), and AP-4 (*36*) transcription factors.

The structural homology of c-Myc with USF and TFE-3, which both bind an immunoglobulin enhancer core consensus sequence CANNTG (E-box; *32, 37*), led to the prediction that the basic domain of c-Myc would also recognize an E-box elements. This was found to be true for both bacterially produced c-Myc (*38, 39*) and a chimera containing the c-Myc basic domain linked to a E12/E47 dimerization interface (*40*). Utilizing a polymerase chain reaction (PCR)-based selection technique (*38*), Blackwell and coworkers identified the optimal c-Myc binding oligonucleotide to contain the CACGTG core. In addition to the core consensus sequence, a preferable flanking sequence has been identified as GAC-CACGTG-GTC, although there were no absolute requirements in the flanks (*41*).

High concentrations of bacterially produced c-Myc proteins (*42*) and viral v-Myc proteins (*43*) have been shown to form homo-oligomers. However, the high number of charged residues at the coiled-coiled interface of the c-Myc leucine zipper suggested heterodimer formation by c-Myc (*44*).

Functional Partners of Myc: Max and ΔMax

Screening of a bacterial expression library with a glutathione S-transferase-Myc hybrid has led to the identification of a protein called Max (*1*), which forms a stable hetero-dimer with c-Myc. Structural analysis of Max and its murine homologue (Myn; 45) revealed yet another bHLH/Zip protein closely related to the C-terminal part of c-Myc. In addition to the bHLH/Zip region (which in Max is at the N-terminal end), Max contains a C-terminal domain suggested to have a regulatory role (*1*). Although Max forms complexes with all three Myc proteins and with itself, if does not associate with several other bHLH/Zip proteins (*1*).

Polymerase chain reaction cloning has revealed an additional longer form of *max* cDNA containing a 101 bp extra exon in the middle of the long open reading frame. Due to a translation termination in the insert, this cDNA was predicted to result in the formation of a truncated Max protein called ΔMax. ΔMax contains an almost intact bHLH/Zip domain, but lacks the carboxy terminus (Fig. 3). ΔMax protein can still form sequence-specific DNA-binding complexes with c-Myc. Experiments with the C-terminal part of c-Myc show that Myc/Max and Myc/ΔMax hetero-dimeric complexes bind DNA with greater affinity than any of the components alone. Interestingly, immunofluorescence studies showed that a ΔMax protein is almost exclusively cytoplasmic in COS cells. However, when coexpressed with c-Myc, ΔMax shifts to the nucleus, suggesting an efficient *in vivo* association of the two proteins.

Coexpression of ΔMax in c-*myc*/*ras* transfected rat embryo fibroblasts enhanced transformation 2–5 fold, whereas coexpression of Max in the same assay had an opposite, suppressing effect on transformation. We have proposed the following hypothesis to explain these observations:

The Max protein is capable of forming homo-dimeric complexes which bind DNA (*1*, *45*). High level expression of Max is therefore likely to lead to the formation of Max homo-dimers, which may be responsible for the observed suppression of transformation. In contrast to the nuclear Max homo-dimers, the ΔMax homo-dimers are cytoplasmic, and thus cannot bind DNA. In this model ΔMax could augment transformation by Myc by forming functional hetero-dimeric c-Myc/ΔMax complexes which go into the nucleus, whereas the ΔMax homo-dimers would be retained in the cytoplasm. Probably the c-Myc/Max hetero-dimer functions in a similar manner, but can possibly be negatively regulated by *e.g.* phosphorylation/dephosphorylation events in the regulatory domain lacking from ΔMax. Thus ΔMax would represent a constitutively active form of Max. On the other hand,

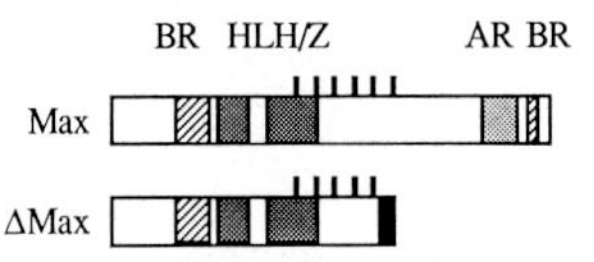

FIG. 3. Schematic comparison of the Max and ΔMax proteins. The five amino acid sequence GESES encoded by the internal exon specific to ΔMax is shown in black. Positions of amino acids contributing to the leucine zipper are denoted by spikes. BR, basic region; HLH/Z, helix-loop-helix-leucine zipper domain; AR acidic region.

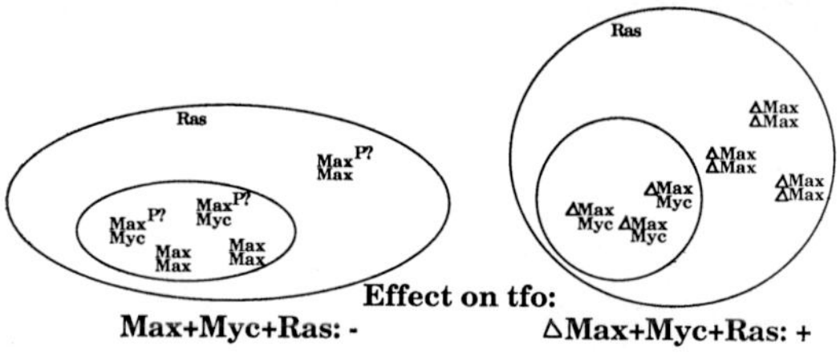

FIG. 4. A model for the effects of Max and ΔMax proteins in Myc+Ras cotransformation assay. See the text for details.

the Max/Max homo-dimer has a negative effect in the cotransformation assay, which could be due to competition for the same *in vivo* binding sites. Figure 4 illustrates essential features of this model.

Function of Myc

Although structural characteristics strongly suggest that Myc functions as a transcriptional regulator, at least one critical link is still missing, namely characterization of direct *in vivo* targets of Myc. Several studies are presently under way to investigate whether one of the genes known to be regulated by Myc would be such a target. Genes suggested to be either positively or negatively regulated by *myc* genes include the c-*myc* itself (*24, 46*), the α-prothymosin gene (*47*), the HSP70 gene (*48*), the plasminogen activator inhibitor 1 (PAI-1; *49*), the LFA-1 adhesion receptor (*50*), and the major histocompatibility complex (MHC) class I molecule (*51–53*). Another candidate for a direct Myc target is the p53 gene; the promoter region of p53 has an E-box binding site (CACGTG), which is essential for high expression of p53 (*54*). In a meeting report this site was claimed to mediate trans-activation of p53 by direct binding of the c-Myc protein (*55*).

A Fusion Protein Formed by L-myc and a Novel Gene in SCLC

Small-cell lung cancer cell lines with amplified *myc* genes provide a useful system to analyze the *myc* proteins (reviewed in *56*), and may also prove fruitful in *in vivo* studies of *myc* binding proteins, such as the recently identified Max protein (*1*). During analysis of such cell lines (*57, 58*), an abnormally large L-*myc* protein was observed in the GLC28 SCLC cell line. Comparison of this protein with a previously identified abnormal L-*myc* protein identified from the CORL47 SCLC cell line (*59*) revealed these proteins to be virtually identical (*60*). Characterization of L-*myc* cDNA clones from the GLC28 cell line indicated that the abnormal protein resulted from a gene fusion between L-*myc* and a previously uncharacterized gene, which has been termed *rlf* (for rearranged L-*myc* fusion; *60*). As shown schematically in Fig. 5, the *rlf*-L-*myc* fusion gene directs the synthesis of a fusion mRNA with the first exon of *rlf* spliced either to the second (3.7 kb mRNA) or to the third exon of L-*myc* (3.2 kb mRNA). The first exon of L-*myc* is not included in either mRNA, because it does not contain a splice acceptor. The 3.7 kb mRNA produces the observed N-terminally extended L-*myc* protein of 446 aa instead of the normal L-*myc* protein of 364 aa.

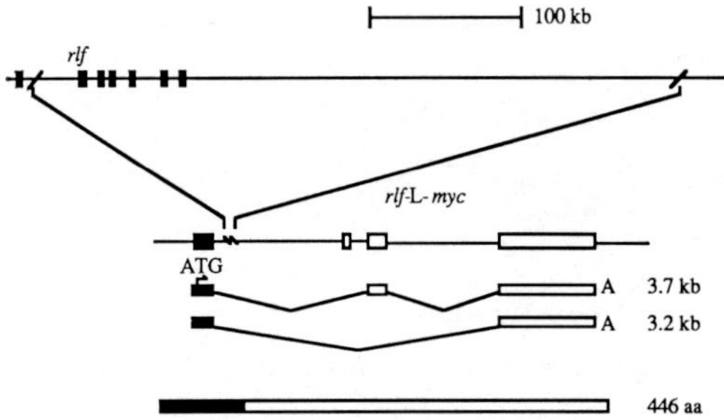

FIG. 5. *rlf* and L-*myc* genes are located within 500 kb of each other on chromosome 1 at 1p32. The *rlf*-L-*myc* rearrangements characterized in several cases of small-cell lung cancer are due to intrachromosomal rearrangements joining (at least) exon I of *rlf* upstream of L-*myc*. This results in the production of two alternatively spliced *rlf*-L-*myc* fusion transcripts and a 446 amino acid protein with 79 N-terminal amino acids from *rlf*. The exact number and size of *rlf* exons is not known.

TABLE 1. Different Types of DNA Rearrangements Involving *rlf* and L-*myc* Genes in SCLC

Class	T/C	Tumor/cell line	Rearrangement		Amplification
			rlf	L-*myc*	
I	C	CORL47	+	+	+
	C	GLC28	+	+	+
	T	LuC194	+	+	+
	C	ACC-LC-49[a)]	+	+	+
	C	ACC-LC-48	+	+	+
	C	SK-LC-17	+	+	+
II	C	CORL88	—	—	+
	T	RO	—	—	+
	T	AS	—	—	+
	T	PA	—	—	+
	C	ACC-LC-177	—	—	+
	C	ACC-LC-178	—	—	+
	C	ACC-LC-52	—	—	+
III	C	U1690	—	+	+
	C	ACC-LC-49[a)]	—	+	+
IV	T	LuC49	+	—	—
	T	LuC26	—	+	—

T: primary tumor. C: tumor cell line. [a)] The ACC-LC-49 line has other rearrangements involving L-*myc* besides the *rlf*-L-*myc* rearrangement as described in (*65*).

In all cases identified to date the *rlf*-L-*myc* rearrangement has been associated with gene amplification. The breakpoints differ considerably on both the L-*myc* and *rlf* sides (*61, 62*). However, in all cases the rearrangements occur upstream of the L-*myc* gene, and in the first intron of the *rlf* gene, and they would thus be expected to encode similar fusion proteins.

The rlf-myc Fusions Are Caused by Intrachromosomal Rearrangements

A previous cytogenetic study indicated that one of the cell lines (CORL47) did not contain abnormalities of chromosome 1 (*63*). Because L-*myc* is located at 1p32 (*64*), this suggested that at least in this case the rearrangement is not due to a chromosomal translocation. Accordingly, *rlf* locus maps to chomosome 1 and PFGE analysis shows that the *rlf* and L-*myc* genes are both present in a 780 kb MluI DNA fragment (*61*). A refined long-range restriction map surrounding these two loci shows that the first exon of *rlf* is approximately 480 kb upstream of L-*myc* (Fig. 5). This physical linkage has since been confirmed by the finding of coamplification of unrearranged *rlf* and L-*myc* in several SCLCs (*62, 65*; Table 1).

Relationship of Rearrangement and Gene Amplification

All intrachromosomal rearrangements leading to the *rlf*-L-*myc* fusions have also been involved in DNA amplification. However, in all cases the rearrangement has occurred before DNA amplification. In addition to the *rlf*-L-*myc* rearrangements, the L-*myc* gene has been found involved in two other amplification-associated rearrangements (cell lines ACC-LC-49 and U1690; see Table 1). Both of these cell lines produce apparently normal L-*myc* mRNAs (*60, 65*).

Homogenous rearranged amplified DNA has been described for the N-*myc* gene in a primary neuroblastoma (*66*), and for the c-*myc* gene in the COLO320 DM cell line (the *pvt-myc* fusion; *67*), although in both cases amplified copies of the unrearranged gene can also be found (*66, 68, 69*). In all *rlf*-L-*myc* rearrangements, in the *pvt-myc* rearrangement, and in several neuroblastomas with amplifications and rearrangements (*70*) the rearranged DNA has been located in the vicinity of the corresponding *myc* gene in the normal genomic configuration, suggesting that specific local rearrangements occur as initial amplification steps. Such a concept is inherent in the currently held models for gene amplification (*71–73*).

A Recombinogenic DNA Region Upstream of L-myc

Because the breakpoints in the different *rlf*-L-*myc* fusions differ considerably on both the *rlf* and the L-*myc* side, the rearrangement mechanism probably is not sequence-specific. Sequence analysis of the region surrounding the L-*myc* breakpoint in the GLC28 cell line indicated that it contains an Alu repeat sequence. Further mapping and sequencing of the L-*myc* upstream region has revealed a large DNA region clustered with repeated sequences (*74*). The characterized breakpoint in the ACC-LC-49 cell line does not involve *rlf*, but another novel locus (EX) instead (*65*). However, the ACC-LC-49 cell line also contains a less well characterized *rlf*-L-*myc* rearrangement. The U1690 breakpoint also involves a new locus and not *rlf* (see above). All three mapped breakpoint regions are located in the cluster of repeats which thus represents a recombinatorial hotspot of repetitive sequences (*62*), and the rearrangements may have occurred as homologous recombinations as described previously (*75*). Interestingly, a recombinogenic A+T-rich region containing Alu-repeats is frequently involved in early amplification-associated rearrangements of the Chinese hamster adenylate deaminase gene (*76*).

Table 1 contains a summary of the different configurations of the L-*myc* and/or *rlf* genes in SCLC cell lines and tumors. Several classes can be distinguished according to the amplification and rearrangement status of L-*myc* and *rlf*. Class I SCLCs contain a *rlf*-L-*myc* rearrangement associated with DNA amplification. All analyzed cases (excluding the LuC194 tumor, from which material was not available) have also been found to produce the chimeric *rlf*-L-*myc* mRNAs. Class II contains SCLCs with coamplification of *rlf* and L-*myc* with no rearrangements detected in conventional Southern analysis. They also appear to produce normal L-*myc* transcripts. Class III represents cases where the L-*myc* gene is rearranged with another locus. The ACC-LC-49 cell line appears to have two distinct rearrangements, and therefore is included in both Class I and Class III. Class IV SCLCs contain rearrangements of either *rlf* or L-*myc* without DNA amplification. According to the material analyzed (14 cases) it would appear that the *rlf* gene is commonly involved in coamplification with L-*myc*. This might be expected due to the short distance between the two genes. Interestingly, rearrangements fusing intron I of *rlf* to the upstream region of L-*myc* and leading to the production of chimeric *rlf*-L-*myc* mRNAs are found in six out of fourteen analyzed cases.

The finding of *rlf*-L-*myc* rearrangements in five SCLC cell lines and importantly also in a primary SCLC tumor (*62*) suggests the presence of a selective pressure for this rearrangement during tumor growth. This could be attributed either to the switch from the L-*myc* transcriptional control elements to those of *rlf*, resulting in deregulation of the normally strictly controlled expression of L-*myc*. Deregulation by a similar promoter switch has been suggested to be the activating mechanism of c-*myc* in a woodchuck liver tumor, where the *hcr* locus fuses upstream of c-*myc* (*77*).

Alternatively, the alteration of the amino terminus of L-*myc* could affect the activity or substrate specificity of the L-*myc* protein. Concerning this, it is interesting to note that the N-terminal region of the c-*myc* (*25*) and L-*myc* (K. Saksela, unpublished results) proteins are involved in transcription activation in a heterologous system. In addition, N-terminal domains of both *c-myc* and N-*myc* have recently been shown to associate with the retinoblastoma protein (see above; *26*). Therefore, it will be interesting to explore the possibility that the abnormal N-terminal sequences in the *rlf*-L-*myc* fusion protein interfere with this association.

REFERENCES

1. Blackwood, E. M. and Eisenman, R. N. Max: a helix-loop-helix zipper protein that forms a sequence-specific DNA-binding complex with Myc. Science, *251*: 1211–1217, 1991.
2. Penn, L. J. Z., Laufer, E. M., and Land, H. C-MYC: evidence for multiple regulatory functions. Semin. Cancer Biol., *1*: 69–80, 1990.
3. Lüscher, B. and Eisenman, R. N. New light on Myc and Myb. Part I. Myc. Genes Dev., *4*: 2025–2035, 1990.
4. Alitalo, K. and Schwab, M. Oncogene amplification in tumor cells. Adv. Cancer Res., *47*: 235–281, 1986.
5. Cory, S. Activation of cellular oncogenes in hemopoietic cells by chromosome translocation. Adv. Cancer Res., *47*: 189–234, 1986.
6. Schwab, M. Amplification of N-*myc* in human neuroblastomas. Trends Genet., *1*: 271–275, 1985.
7. Saksela, K. *myc* genes and their deregulation in lung cancer. J. Cell. Biochem., *42*: 153–

180, 1990.
8. Brodeur, G. M., Seeger, R. C., Schwab, M., Varmus, H. E., and Bishop, J. M. Amplification of N-*myc* in untreated human neuroblastomas correlates with advanced disease stage. Science, *224*: 1121–1124, 1984.
9. Seeger, R. C., Brodeur, G. M., Sather, H., Dalton, A., Siegel, S. E., Wong, K. Y., and Hammond, D. Association of multiple copies of the N-*myc* oncogene with rapid progression of neuroblastomas. N. Engl. J. Med., *313*: 1111–1118, 1985.
10. Land, H., Parada, L. F., and Weinberg, R. A. Tumorigenic conversion of primary embryo fibroblasts requires at least two cooperating oncogenes. Nature, *304*: 596–602, 1983.
11. Schwab, M., Varmus, H. E., and Bishop, J. M. Human N-*myc* gene contributes to neoplastic transformation of mammalian cells in culture. Nature, *316*: 160–162, 1985.
12. Yancopoulos, G. D., Nisen, P. D., Tesfaye, A., Kohl, N. E., Goldfarb, M. P., and Alt, F. W. N-*myc* can cooperate with *ras* to transform normal cells in culture. Proc. Natl. Acad. Sci. U.S.A., *82*: 5455–5459, 1985.
13. Birrer, M. J., Segal, S., DeGreve, J. S., Kaye, F., Sausville, E. A., and Minna, J. D. L-*myc* cooperates with *ras* to transform primary rat embryo fibroblasts. Mol. Cell. Biol., *8*: 2668–2673, 1988.
14. Adams, J. M., Harris, A. W., Pinkert, C. A., Corcoran, L. M., Alexander, W. S., Cory, S., Palmiter, R. D., and Brinster, R. L. The c-*myc* oncogene driven by immunoglobulin enhancers induces lymphoid malignancy in transgenic mice. Nature, *318*: 533–538, 1985.
15. Rosenbaum, H., Webb, E., Adams, J. M., Cory, S., and Harris, A. W. N-*myc* transgene promotes B lymphoid proliferation, elicits lymphomas and reveals cross-regulation with c-*myc*. EMBO J., *8*: 749–755, 1989.
16. Dildrop, R., Ma, A., Zimmerman, K., Hsu, E., Tesfaye, A., DePinho, R., and Alt, F. W. IgH enhancer-mediated deregulation of N-*myc* gene expression in transgenic mice: generation of lymphoid neoplasias that lack c-*myc* expression. EMBO J., *8*: 133–136, 1989.
17. Möröy, T., Fisher, P., Guidos, C., Ma, A., Zimmerman, K., Tesfaye, A., DePinho, R., Weissman, I., and Alt, F. W. IgH enhancer regulated expression of L-*myc*: abnormal T lymphocyte development and T cell lymphomagenesis. EMBO J., *9*: 3659–3666, 1990.
18. Thiele, C. J., Reynolds, C. P., and Israel, M. Decreased expression of N-*myc* precedes retinoic acid induced morphological differentiation of human neuroblastoma. Nature, *313*: 404–406, 1985.
19. Griep, A. E. and Westphal, H. Antisense Myc sequences induce differentiation of F9 cells. Proc. Natl. Acad. Sci. U.S.A., *85*: 6806–6810, 1988.
20. Larsson, L. G., Ivhed, I., Gidlund, M., Pettersson, U., Vennström, B., and Nilsson, K. Phorbol ester-induced terminal differentiation is inhibited in human U-937 monoblastic cells expressing a v-*myc* oncogene. Proc. Natl. Acad. Sci. U.S.A., *85*: 2638–2642, 1988.
21. Collum, R. G. and Alt, F. W. Are *myc* proteins transcription factors? Cancer Cells, *2*: 69–75, 1990.
22. DePinho, R. A., Hatton, K. S., Morgenbesser, S. D., and Torres, R. The *myc* family of nuclear oncoproteins: structure, biochemistry and activities. *In*; W. R. Paukovits (ed.), Growth Regulation and Carcinogenesis, Vol. 1, pp. 195–206, CRC Press, Boca Raton, Florida, 1991.
23. Stone, J., de Lauge, T., Ramsay, G., Jakobovits, E., Bishop, J. M., Varmus, H., and Lee, W. Definition of regions in human c-*myc* that are involved in transformation and

nuclear localization. Mol. Cell. Biol., *7*: 1973–1977, 1987.
24. Penn, L. J., Brooks, M. W., Laufer, E. M., and Land, H. Negative autoregulation of c-*myc* transcription. EMBO J., *9*: 1113–1121, 1990.
25. Kato, G. J., Barrett, J., Villa-Garcia, M., and Dang, C. V. An amino-terminal c-*myc* domain required for neoplastic transformation activates transcription. Mol. Cell. Biol., *10*: 5914–5920, 1990.
26. Rustgi, A. K., Dyson, N., and Bernards, R. Amino-terminal domains of c-*myc* and N-*myc* proteins mediate binding to the retinoblastoma gene product. Nature, *352*: 541–544, 1991.
27. Dang, C. V. and Lee, W. M. Identification of the human c-*myc* protein nuclear translocation signal. Mol. Cell. Biol., *8*: 4048–4054, 1988.
28. Lüscher, B., Kuenzel, E. A., Krebs, E. G., and Eisenman, R. N. Myc oncoproteins are phosphorylated by casein kinase II. EMBO J., *8*: 1111–1119, 1989.
29. Saksela, K., Mäkelä, T. P., Hughes, K., Woodgett, J. R., and Alitalo, K. Activation of PKC increases phosphorylation of the L-*myc* trans-activator domain at a GSK-3 target site. Oncogene, *7*: 347–353, 1992.
30. Alvarez, E., Northwood, I. C., Gonzalez, F. A., Latour, D. A., Seth, A., Abate, C., Curran, T., and Davis, R. J. Pro-Leu-Ser/Thr-Pro is a consensus primary sequence for substrate protein phosphorylation. J. Cell. Biochem., *266*: 15277–15285, 1991.
31. Street, A. J., Blackwood, E., Lüscher, B., and Eisenman, R. N. Mutational analysis of the carboxy-terminal casein kinase II phosphorylation site in human c-*myc*. Curr. Top. Microbiol. Immunol., *166*: 251–258, 1990.
32. Murre, C., McCaw, P. S., and Baltimore, D. A new DNA binding and dimerization motif in immunoglobulin enhancer binding, daughterless MyoD, and *myc* proteins. Cell, *56*: 777–783, 1989.
33. Landschulz, W. H., Johnson, P. F., and McKnight, S. L. The leucine zipper: a hypothetical structure common to a new class of DNA binding proteins. Science, *240*: 1759–1764, 1988.
34. Beckmann, H., Su, L. K., and Kadesch, T. TFE3: a helix-loop-helix protein that activates transcription through the immunoglobulin enhancer μE3 motif. Genes Dev., *4*: 167–179, 1990.
35. Gregor, P. D., Sawadogo, M., and Roeder, R. G. The adenovirus major late transcription factor USF is a member of the helix-loop-helix group of regulatory proteins and binds to DNA as a dimer. Genes Dev., *4*: 1730–1740, 1990.
36. Hu, Y.-F., Lüscher, B., Admon, A., Mermod, N., and Tjian, R. Transcription factor AP-4 contains multiple dimerization domains that regulate dimer specificity. Genes Dev., *4*: 1741–1752, 1990.
37. Sen, R. and Baltimore, D. Multiple factors interact with the immunoglobulin enhancer sequences. Cell, *46*: 705–716, 1986.
38. Blackwell, T. K., Kretzner, L., Blackwood, E. M., Eisenman, R. N., and Weintraub, H. Sequence-specific DNA binding by the c-*myc* protein. Science, *250*: 1149–1151, 1990.
39. Kerkhoff, E., Bister, K., and Klempnauer, K. H. Sequence-specific DNA binding by Myc proteins. Proc. Natl. Acad. Sci. U.S.A., *88*: 4323–4327, 1991.
40. Prendergast, G. C. and Ziff, E. Methylation-sensitive sequence-specific DNA binding by the c-*myc* basic region. Science, *251*: 186–189, 1991.
41. Halazonetis, T. D. and Kandil, A. N. Determination of the c-MYC DNA-binding site. Proc. Natl. Acad. Sci. U.S.A., *88*: 6162–6166, 1991.
42. Dang, C. V., McGuire, M., Buckmire, M., and Lee, W. M. Involvement of the 'leucine zipper' region in the oligomerization and transforming activity of human c-*myc* protein.

Nature, *337*: 664–666, 1989.

43. Bader, J. P. and Ray, D. A. MC29 virus-coded protein occurs as monomers and dimers in transformed cells. J. Virol., *53*: 509–514, 1985.
44. O'Shea, E. K., Rutkowski, R., Stafford, W. III, and Kim, P. S. Preferential heterodimer formation by isolated leucine zippers from Fos and Jun. Science, *245*: 646–647, 1989.
45. Prendergast, G. C., Lawe, D., and Ziff, E. B. Association of Myn, the murine homolog of Max, with c-Myc stimulates methylation-sensitive DNA binding and Ras cotransformation. Cell, *65*: 395–407, 1991.
46. Grignani, F., Lombardi, L., Inghirami, G., Sternas, L., Cechova, K., and Dalla-Favera, R. Negative autoregulation of c-*myc* gene expression is inactivated in transformed cells. EMBO J., *9*: 3913–3922, 1990.
47. Eilers, M., Schirm, S., and Bishop, J. M. The MYC protein activates transcription of the alpha-prothymosin gene. EMBO J., *10*: 133–141, 1991.
48. Kaddurah-Daouk, R., Greene, J. M., Baldwin A. S. Jr., and Kingston, R. E. Activation and repression of mammalian gene expression by the c-*myc* protein. Genes Dev., *1*: 347–357, 1987.
49. Prendergast, G. C., Diamond, L. E., Dahl, D., and Cole, M. D. The c-*myc*-regulated gene mrl encodes plasminogen activator inhibitor 1. Mol. Cell. Biol., *10*: 1265–1269, 1990.
50. Inghirami, G., Grignani, F., Sternas, L., Lombardi, L., Knowles, D. M., and Dalla-Favera. R. Down-regulation of LFA-1 adhesion receptors by C-*myc* oncogene in human B lymphoblastoid cells. Science, *250*: 682–686, 1990.
51. Versteeg, R., Noordermeer, I. A., Krüse-Wolters, M., Ruiter, D. J., and Schrier, P. I. *c-myc* down-regulates class I HLA expression in human melanomas. EMBO J., *7*: 1023–1029, 1988.
52. Lenardo, M., Rustgi, A. K., Schievella, A. R., and Bernards, R. Suppression of MHC class I gene expression by N-*myc* through enhancer inactivation. EMBO J., *8*: 3351–3355, 1989.
53. Bernards, R., Dessain, S. K., and Weinberg, R. A. N-*myc* amplification causes down-modulation of MHC class I antigen expression in neuroblastoma. Cell, *47*: 667–674, 1986.
54. Ronen, D., Rotter, V., and Reisman, D. Expression from the murine p53 promoter is mediated by factor binding to a downstream helix-loop-helix recognition motif. Proc. Natl. Acad. Sci. U.S.A., *88*: 4128–4132, 1991.
55. Reisman, D., Ronen, D., and Rotter, V. Site specific binding by c-Myc to the p53 promoter: a target for trans-activation by c-Myc. Report at the Seventh Annual Oncogene Meeting, Frederick, Maryland, 1991.
56. Alitalo, K., Mäkelä, T. P., Saksela, K., Hirvonen, H., and Koskinen, P. Oncogene amplification: analysis of *myc* oncoproteins. *In*; R. Kellems (ed.), Gene Amplification in Mammalian Cells: Techniques and Applications, Marcel Dekker, Inc., New York, in press.
57. Mäkelä, T. P., Saksela, K., and Alitalo, K. Two N-*myc* polypeptides with distinct amino termini encoded by the second and third exons of the gene. Mol. Cell. Biol., *9*: 1545–1552, 1989.
58. Saksela, K., Mäkelä, T. P., Evan, G., and Alitalo, K. Rapid phosphorylation of the L-*myc* protein induced by phorbol ester tumor promoters and serum. EMBO J., *8*: 149–157, 1989.
59. Evan, G. Unpublished results.
60. Mäkelä, T. P., Saksela, K., Evan, G., and Alitalo, K. A fusion protein formed by L-*myc* and a novel gene in SCLC. EMBO J., *10*: 1331–1335, 1991.

61. Mäkelä, T. P., Kere, J., Winqvist, R., and Alitalo, K. Intrachromosomal rearrangements fusing rlf and L-*myc* in SCLC. Mol. Cell. Biol., *11*: 4015–4021, 1991.
62. Mäkelä, T. P., Shiraishi, M., Borrello, M. G., Sekiya, T., and Alitalo, K. Rearrangement and coamplification of L-*myc* and rlf in primary lung cancer. Oncogene, *7*: 151–157, 1992.
63. Waters, J. J., Ibson, J. M., Twentyman, P. R., Bleehen, N. M., and Rabbitts, P. H. Cytogenetic abnormalities in human small cell lung carcinoma: cell lines characterized for *myc* gene amplification. Cancer Genet. Cytogen., *30*: 213–223, 1988.
64. Nau, M. M., Brooks, B. J., Battey, J., Sausville, E., Gazdar, A. F., Kirsch, I. R., McBride, O. W., Bertness, V., Hollis, G. F., and Minna, J. D. L-*myc*, a new *myc*-related gene amplified and expressed in human small cell lung cancer. Nature, *318*: 69–73, 1985.
65. Sekido, Y., Takahashi, T., Mäkelä, T. P., Obata, Y., Ueda, R., Hida, T., Kenja, H., Shimokata, K., Alitalo, K., and Takahashi, T. Complex intrachromosomal rearrangement in the process of amplification of the L-*myc* gene in small cell lung cancer. Mol. Cell. Biol., *12*: 1747–1754, 1992.
66. Hiyama, E., Hiyama, K., and Yokoyama, T. Neuroblastoma with DNA amplification and rearrangement in the N-*myc* gene region. Cancer Res., *51*: 1946–1951, 1991.
67. Shtivelman, E. and Bishop, J. M. The PVT gene frequently amplifies with MYC in tumor cells. Mol. Cell. Biol., *9*: 1148–1154, 1989.
68. Alitalo, K., Schwab, M., Lin, C. C., Varmus, H. E., and Bishop, J. M. Homogeneously staining chromosomal regions contain amplified copies of an abundantly expressed cellular oncogene (c-*myc*) in malignant neuroendocrine cells from a human colon carcinoma. Proc. Natl. Acad. Sci. U.S.A., *80*: 1707–1711, 1983.
69. Schwab, M., Klempnauer, K. H., Alitalo, K., Varmus, H., and Bishop, M. Rearrangement at the 5′ end of amplified c-*myc* in human COLO 320 cells is associated with abnormal transcription. Mol. Cell. Biol., *6*: 2800–2806, 1986.
70. Shiloh, Y., Shipley, J., Brodeur, G. M., Bruns, G., Korf, B., Donlon, T., Schreck, R. R., Seeger, R., Sakai, K., and Latt, S. A. Differential amplification, assembly, and relocation of multiple DNA sequences in human neuroblastomas and neuroblastoma cell lines. Proc. Natl. Acad. Sci. U.S.A., *82*: 3761–3765, 1985.
71. Kinzler, K. W., Zehnbauer, B. A., Brodeur, G. M., Seeger, R. C., Trent, J. M., Meltzer, P. S., and Vogelstein, B. Amplification units containing human N-*myc* and c-*myc* genes. Proc. Natl. Acad. Sci. U.S.A., *83*: 1031–1035, 1986.
72. Trask, B. J. and Hamlin, J. L. Early dihydrofolate reductase gene amplification events in CHO cells usually occur on the same chromosome arm as the original locus. Genes Dev., *3*: 1913–1925, 1989.
73. Stark, G. R., Debatisse, M., Giulotto, E., and Wahl, G. M. Recent progress in understanding mechanisms of mammalian DNA amplification. Cell, *57*: 901–908, 1989.
74. Mäkelä, T. P., Saksela, K., and Alitalo, K. Amplification and rearrangement of L-*myc* in small cell lung cancer. Mutat. Res., *276*: 307–315, 1992.
75. Lehrman, M. A., Goldstein, J. L., Russell, D. W., and Brown, M. S. Duplication of seven exons in LDL receptor gene caused by Alu-Alu recombination in a subject with familial hypercholesterolemia. Cell, *48*: 827–835, 1987.
76. Hyrien, O., Debatisse, M., Buttin, G., and de Saint Vincent, B. R. A hotspot for novel amplification joints in a mosaic of Alu-like repeats and palindromic A+T-rich DNA. EMBO J., *6*: 2401–2408, 1987.
77. Etiemble, J., Möröy, T., Jacquemin, E., Tiollais, P., and Buendia, M.-A. Fused transcripts of c-*myc* and a new cellular locus, hcr in a primary liver tumor. Oncogene, *4*: 51–57, 1989.

MULTISTAGE CARCINOGENESIS, C. C. HARRIS ET AL. (EDS.),
JAPAN SCI. SOC· PRESS, TOKYO/CRC PRESS, BOCA RATON, PP. 319–337, 1992

Molecular Inhibition of Cancer Cell Invasion and Metastasis

Vincent CASTRONOVO, William G. STETLER-STEVENSON, Mark E. SOBEL, and Lance A. LIOTTA

Laboratory of Pathology, National Cancer Institute, National Institutes of Health, Bethesda, Maryland 20892, U.S.A.

Abstract: A group of coordinated cellular processes, not just one gene product, is responsible for invasion and metastasis, the most life-threatening aspect of cancer. It is now recognized that negative factors may be just as important as positive elements. Genetic changes causing an imbalance of growth regulation lead to uncontrolled proliferation necessary for both primary tumor and metastasis expansion. However, unrestrained growth does not, by itself, cause invasion and metastasis. This phenotype may require additional genetic changes. Thus, tumorigenicity and metastatic potential have both overlapping and separate features. Invasion and metastasis can be facilitated by proteins which stimulate tumor cell attachment to host cellular or extracellular matrix determinants, tumor cell proteolysis of host barriers, such as the basement membrane, tumor cell locomotion, and tumor cell colony formation in the target organ for metastasis. Facilitory proteins may act at many levels both intracellularly and extracellularly, but are counterbalanced by factors which can block their production, regulation or action. A common theme has emerged: in addition to loss of growth control, an imbalanced regulation of adhesion, proteolysis, and motility appears to be required for invasion and metastasis. Re-equilibrating the expression of the genes involved in these tumor invasion related events could potentially constitute the basis for new anti-cancer therapeutic strategies.

Metastatic Cells Can Dominate the Primary Tumor Population

Metastasis is a cascade of linked sequential steps involving multiple host-tumor interactions (*1–3*). To successfully create a metastatic colony, a cell or group of tumor cells must be able to leave the primary tumor, invade the local host tissue, enter the circulation, arrest at the distant vascular bed, extravasate into the target organ interstitium and parenchyma, and proliferate as a secondary colony. Angiogenesis is required for the expansion of the primary tumor mass, and new blood vessels penetrating the tumor are frequent sites for tumor cell entry into the circulation (*4, 5*). Angiogenesis is also required for expansion of the metastatic colony. At any stage, tumor cells must overcome host immune cell killing (*2*). A very small percentage ($<0.01\%$) of circulating tumor cells ultimately initiate successful metastatic colonies. Consequently, metastasis has been viewed originally by Fidler and Hart (*1*) as a highly selective competition favoring the survival of a subpopulation of metastatic tumor cells that pre-exist within the heterogeneous primary tumor.

Fidler's metastatic subpopulation concept is well accepted, but the relative size of this subpopulation in the primary tumor may vary with time and among tumors. Estimating the size of the metastatic subpopulation is of clinical significance since a prognostic assay based on a sample of the primary tumor would be highly inaccurate if the aggressive subpopulation was only a very small proportion of the total number of tumor cells being sampled. Recently, Kerbel (*6*) has addressed the subpopulation question experimentally using genetic markers. He determined that the metastatic subpopulation dominates the primary tumor mass early in its growth. The dominance may be due to selective growth of the metastatic subpopulation in response to local cytokines. Thus, measurement of the average level of a molecular marker in a primary tumor sample is likely to reflect the general metastatic propensity of the entire tumor. Indeed, this has been borne out by a number of clinical studies indicating that the average level of specific protein markers or amplified oncogenes measured in the primary tumor can be correlated with clinical aggressiveness parameters of metastasis and recurrence (*7–10*).

Tumor Cell Interaction with the Extracellular Matrix

During the development of invasive tumors, tumor cells disobey the social order of organ boundaries and cross into tissues where they don't belong. The mammalian organism is divided into a series of tissue compartments separated by extracellular matrix units consisting of the basement membrane and its underlying interstitial stroma (*3, 11*). The basal cells of the epithelium or organ parenchymal side of this unit are attached to the basement membrane. On the opposite side, the interstitial stroma contains stromal cells, fibroblasts, and myofibroblasts. The nervous system, muscle cells, and blood vessels are also surrounded by a continuous basement membrane. During all types of benign tissue remodeling, proliferative disorders, and carcinoma *in situ*, the cell populations on either side of this connective tissue unit do not intermix. Only during the transition from *in situ* to invasive carcinoma, do tumor cells penetrate the epithelial basement membrane and enter the underlying interstitial stroma to interact with the stromal cells. Thus, a definition of the behavior of the metastatic tumor cell is the tendency to cross tissue compartment boundaries and intermix with opposite cell types (*1, 12*).

The continuous basement membrane is a dense meshwork of collagen, glycoproteins, and proteoglycans which normally does not contain any pores large enough for passive tumor cell traversal. Consequently, invasion of the basement membrane must be an active process. Once the tumor cells enter the stroma, they gain access to lymphatics and blood vessels for further dissemination. Tumor cells must cross basement membranes to invade nerves and muscle. During intravasation or extravasation, the tumor cells of any histologic origin must penetrate the subendothelial basement membrane. As a general feature of all types of carcinomas (12), defects in the basement membrane are associated with invasion. In contrast, benign proliferative disorders are all characterized by a continuous basement membrane separating the epithelium from the stroma. The general observation of defective basement membranes associated with cancer invasion and progression indicates that aggressive tumor cells may interact with basement membranes in a manner fundamentally different from normal cells. This general feature of malignant tumors provides the foundation for investigation of molecular mechanisms.

Interactions of the tumor cell with the basement membrane can be separated into three steps: attachment, matrix dissolution, and migration. The first step is binding of the tumor cell to the basement membrane mediated by cell surface receptors of the integrin (*13, 14*) and non-integrin (*15, 16*) variety. Matrix receptors recognize glycoproteins such as laminin, type IV collagen, and fibronectin in the basement membrane. Two to eight hours after attachment, a localized zone of lysis is produced in the basement membrane at the point of tumor cell contact. Tumor cells directly secrete degradative enzymes (*17*) or induce the host to elaborate proteinases to degrade the matrix and its component adhesion molecules. Matrix lysis takes place in a highly localized region close to the tumor cell surface (*18*), where the amount of active enzyme outbalances the natural proteinase inhibitors that are present in the serum and/or the matrix, or that are secreted by normal cells in the vicinity. Locomotion is the third step of invasion which propels the tumor cell across the basement membrane and stroma through the zone of matrix proteolysis. An early step in locomotion is pseudopodial protrusion at the leading edge of the migrating cell (*19, 20*). The induction of pseudopodia is directional, is regulated by cell surface ligand binding, and involves a coordinated mobilization of cytoskeletal elements which interact with the inner membrane surface. The cellular machinery of tumor cell locomotion is a fertile topic for future study, and will undoubtedly benefit from insights learned from studies of immune cells (*2*) and non-mammalian organisms (*20*). It is now recognized that random tumor cell motility can be regulated by tumor cell cytokines ("autocrine motility factors" and "scatter factors") (*19, 21, 22*). Autocrine motility factors act through a receptor activated G protein susceptible to inhibition by pertussis toxin. Augmented random motility by tumor cells causes dispersion at the primary site. In addition, the direction and site of the tumor cell locomotion may be influenced by host organ-derived chemoattractants. Such chemoattracts could play a role in the organ selective homing of metastasis. This could complement other mechanisms of organ homing which include preferential adhesion to organ specific endothelium and preferential growth in selected organs due to local growth factors (*23*).

Interactions of Cancer Cells with Laminin: a Critical Step of the Metastatic Cascade

Laminin, a major component of basement membranes, is a large glycoprotein composed of many distinct domains which exhibit a variety of biological properties including attachment, spreading, migration, proliferation, and differentiation of normal and neoplastic cells (*24, 25*). Laminin is the first extracellular matrix protein synthesized in early development and can be detected at the two-cell stage in the mouse embryo (*24*). Laminin was first purified and characterized from a mouse fibrosarcoma, the Engelbreth-Holm-Swarm (EHS) tumor (*26*). Rotary shadowing replicas of laminin molecules appear under the electron microscope as a cross-structure with three short arms and a long arm (*24, 25*). It is composed of three polypeptides designated as chain A, chain B1 and chain B2 which are linked together by disulfide bonds (*24, 25*). Most of the structural and biochemical studies have been performed using EHS laminin, considered as the prototype molecule. However, recent studies have identified various isoforms of laminin with distinct polypeptides chains, chain composition and structure (*24*). The specific functions of these different isoforms of laminin have not been completely elucidated. These variants of laminin are considered, along with the well known EHS laminin, as members of a large family of extracellular matrix molecules, the laminins.

There is a growing body of evidence indicating that interactions between cancer cells and laminin play a key role at several steps of the metastatic cascade. Tumor cells exposed to laminin produce ten times more experimental metastases than control cells (*27*). Highly malignant cell lines express laminin or laminin-like moieties on their surface (*28*). Preincubation of murine melanoma cells with laminin dramatically enhanced experimental metastasis (*29*). Highly metastatic fibrosarcoma cells expressed much more laminin on their cell surface than tumor cells with low metastatic potential (*30*). A short amino acid sequence from the B1 chain of laminin was reported to inhibit experimental metastasis (*31*). Furthermore, incubation of metastatic tumor cells with anti-laminin antibodies inhibited their further attachment to perfused umbilical endothelium (*32*) in an *ex vivo* assay and reduced experimental metastasis in mice *in vivo* (*33*). Incubation of cancer cells with laminin enhances their secretion of type IV collagenase, a proteolytic enzyme that digests the backbone molecules of basement membrane: type IV collagen.

Interactions between laminin and malignant cells are mediated through a variety of cell surface proteins including a 67 kDa laminin receptor (*34–36*), several members of the integrin family (*37*), galactosyltransferase (*38*), members of the β-galactoside binding lectin family (*39, 40*) and several other molecules not yet fully characterized (*41*). The specific physiological roles of each of these laminin-binding proteins as well as the domains of laminin with which they interact represent a complex puzzle, the pieces of which are slowly falling into place.

The 67 kDa Laminin Receptor, Basis for Potential New Diagnostic and Prognostic Markers and for New Anti-cancer Therapeutic Strategies

Among the several laminin-binding proteins identified, our laboratory has been studying a 67 kD laminin receptor (67 LR) purified from several cell lines as well as from normal and neoplastic tissues (*34–36*). The 67 LR appears to be responsible for the strong affinity of cells for laminin ($K_d = 10^{-9}$) since antibodies raised against the 67 kD laminin receptor specifically inhibit high affinity binding of laminin to cells in binding assays (*42*). The 67 LR is present at the surface of normal and cancer cells and appears to mediate strong attachment and motility response of cells to laminin (*43, 44*). The expression of the 67 LR was shown, in several *in vitro* and *in vivo* systems, to be dramatically increased in highly metastatic cells (*44–48*). This has been shown both at the protein level and at the mRNA level. To better understand the molecular mechanisms that regulate the expression of the 67 LR, cDNA clones of the receptor were obtained by screening a human endothelial cell lambda gt11

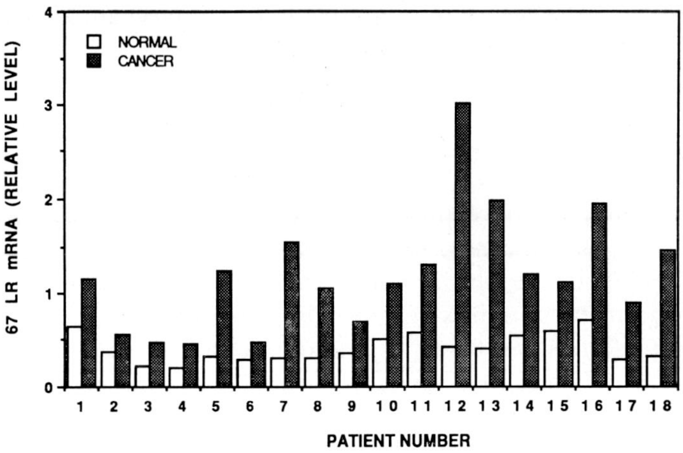

FIG. 1. Increased laminin receptor mRNA levels in human colon cancers. Relative laminin receptor mRNA level in matched colon cancer/normal mucosa samples analyzed by Northern blot hybridization. Each column represents laminin receptor mRNA level in cancer tissue and normal adjacent colon mucosa quantified by densitometry and expressed as a ratio of laminin receptor mRNA/actin mRNA. Numbers correspond to specific patients.

cDNA library with a monoclonal antibody raised against purified 67 LR (*42*). The anti-67 LR antibody recognized the 67 LR on immunoblots and specifically inhibited the binding of laminin to cell membranes (*42*). Full length human and mouse cDNA clones have been obtained (*15, 49*). Verification of the clones included homology between the cDNA deduced amino acid sequence of the laminin receptor and amino acid sequences obtained from purified human placental 67 LR (*42*). Unexpectedly, the full length clones were found to encode a 295 amino acid polypeptide with a calculated molecular mass of 32 kDa. The nascent polypeptide obtained by *in vitro* translation of mRNA purified by select-hybridization using the 67 LR cDNA exhibited an apparent molecular mass of 37 kDa on SDS-PAGE (*15*). This 37 kDa polypeptide (37 LRP) was shown by pulse chase experiments to be the precursor of the mature 67 LR (*50*).

Scatchard analysis of laminin binding studies, immunocytochemical localization of the 67 LR using monoclonal and polyclonal antibodies to the 67 LR and immunoblot experiments have demonstrated that the expression of the 67 LR is increased in human carcinomas (*27*). Studies on human breast carcinoma-derived cell lines indicated that the increased expression of the 67 LR is due to an increased steady state level of laminin receptor mRNA (*42*). These data suggested that assessing the 67 LR mRNA level of human carcinoma cells may be of diagnostic and prognostic value. This possibility was strengthened by the work of Yow *et al.* (*49*), who isolated a 67 LR cDNA clone by screening colon carcinoma cDNAs on the basis of increased expression of specific genes. We have also shown that estradiol and progestins, two steroid hormones known to modulate the progression of human breast cancers, increase the expression of the 67 LR in steroid receptor positive breast cancer cells up to the level observed in the more clinically aggressive receptor negative breast cancer cells (*51*). A stimulation of the expression of the 67 LR was also observed when human breast cancer cells or melanoma cells were in contact with laminin or fibronectin, suggesting the existence of a positive feedback mechanism that provides the cells with a continuous supply of 67 LR (*52*). These data suggested that the 67 LR is differentially regulated in metastatic cells. We examined the expression of the 67 LR both at the protein level (using immunoperoxidase and immunoblot techniques) and at the mRNA level (using Northern and *in situ* hybridization techniques), in a variety of human cancers including breast, colon, and gastric carcinoma. In colon cancer, we found that the expression of the 67 LR was dramatically increased in the cancer tissue in comparison to the adjacent normal colonic mucosa (Fig. 1). The expression of 67 LR, both at the protein and mRNA level, was higher in primary colon carcinoma with metastases than in those with local invasion (*47*, *48*). Immunoperoxidase studies performed on breast aspiration biopsies showed that the 67 LR was detected in cells obtained from breast cancer and not in cells obtained from benign lesions including fibroadenoma, cyst and fibrocystic disease (*46*). In gastric cancer, the expression of the 67 LR was found to increase as the stage of the disease progresses (*48*). These data strongly suggest that the 67 LR is a gene product which plays a critical role in the constitution of the invasive and metastatic phenotype. Detection of the 67 LR in human carcinoma could therefore be a valuable adjunct in the diagnostic and prognostic evaluation of malignancies.

The increased expression of 67 LR in cancer cells, particularly in breast carcinoma, led us to investigate the possibility that antibody directed against this receptor could specifically target cancer cells. To test this possibility, an IgM monoclonal antibody was generated to a synthetic peptide from the cDNA-predicted ligand binding domain of the 67 LR (*53*). The disulfide bond of the IgM molecules was employed to couple the antibodies to the surface of liposomes that contained encapsulated adriamycin. The anti-67 LR liposomes bound to the surface of human breast carcinoma cells which contained high numbers of 67 LR, and exhibited a low degree of binding to human breast epithelial cells which expressed a low number of 67 LR. The anti-67 LR liposomes also competed for the binding of free laminin to the tumor cell surface, and excess laminin competed for the binding of the anti-67 LR liposomes. Adriamycin-encapsulated liposomes coupled to anti-67 LR monoclonal antibodies were more efficient in the inhibition of colony formation by human breast carcinoma cells compared to free adriamycin or to liposomes which were coupled to control antibodies (*53*). Thus, anti-67 LR liposomes may represent a new strategy for selective targeting of chemotherapeutic agents to carcinoma cells with exposed laminin receptors.

The original 37 LRP cDNA clones were isolated using a monoclonal antibody raised against purified 67 LR that specifically inhibited laminin binding to cell membranes and amnion (*42*). Therefore, we investigated the possibility that the 37 LRP contains within its sequence a domain that binds to laminin. To evaluate this hypothesis, a series of synthetic peptides (Table 1) were produced and tested in a variety of laminin binding assays. Among the peptides tested, peptide G was considered to be a potential candidate for a laminin binding domain because: (a) computer analysis predicted that the sequence of amino acids constituting peptide G had a high probability for reverse turn configuration (*15*), (b) the sequence of peptide G was contained within the common domain of six cDNA clones identified by an anti-67 LR monoclonal antibody that inhibited cell binding to laminin (*42*);

TABLE 1. Laminin Receptor Synthetic Peptides Derived from the cDNA Sequence and Their Corresponding Antibodies

Peptide	Sequence	Position[a)]	pI[b)]	HP[c)]
E	TPGTFTNQIQAAFREPRLLV	104–123	10.1	0.02
F	ALCNTDSPLRYVDIAIPCNN	146–164	3.9	0.06
G	IPCNNKGAHSVGLMWWMLAR	161–180	11.1	0.19
H	AAAEKAVTKEEFQGEWTAPA	216–234	4.3	0.02
GX	PMLRWGCHIAMVNKLSWGNA		11.0	0.19

[a)] The numbers indicate the position of the first and the last amino acid of the designated peptide, numbered from the amino terminus of the laminin receptor sequence; peptide GX contains a scrambled sequence of peptide G. [b)] pI was calculated by the IBI Pustell Analysis Software using the Henderson-Hasselbach equation. [c)] HP: hydrophobicity. Average hydrophobicity was calculated by the Helwheel Program of PC/gene.

(c) a peptide containing this sequence inhibited haptotaxis of cancer cells toward laminin (*44*); (d) a monoclonal antibody directed against a peptide overlapping the sequence of peptide G competed with laminin for binding to metastatic human breast cancer cells (*53*). We demonstrated that peptide G contains a high affinity binding domain (K_d=51.8 nM) for laminin (*54*). The observation that peptide G is able to elute the 67 LR from a laminin affinity column indicates that the binding domain contained within peptide G is utilized, at least in part, in the binding of the 67 LR to laminin. Peptide G therefore may be a potential inhibitor of the interactions between laminin and the 67 LR and could be very useful in determining the specific role played by this receptor in a variety of biological events in which cell-laminin interactions are involved.

Stable attachment of tumor cells to the endothelium, the first step of extravasation, is particularly critical for the success of hematogenous metastasis (*1*, *55*, *56*). The identification of the specific mechanism(s) leading to the anchorage of metastatic cancer cells to the vasculature offers the potential for selectively interfering with the metastatic cascade. Previous reports have implicated the basement membrane component laminin in blood-borne metastasis formation (*28–30*, *33*). The specific interactive pathway by which laminin participates in the formation of blood borne metastases is not clear. Some studies indicate that it is laminin present on the surface of malignant cells that plays a significant role in their interactions with the endothelium (*28*, *30*) while other reports suggest that it is the increase of unoccupied laminin receptors on the cancer cell surface, and not the increase of cell surface laminin, that correlates with metastatic potential (*43*). This latter assertion supposes that the initial contact of circulating cancer cells with the vasculature is with exposed subendothelial matrix and not with the endothelial cell surface itself. The exact pathway(s) relevant *in vivo* to the genesis of blood-borne metastasis has(have) not been established. Several scenarios, which are not mutually exclusive, could take place, including: (a) interaction between laminin present on the cancer cell surface and accessible to type IV collagen in exposed areas of the subendothelial matrix area (Fig. 2A); (b) interaction between unoccupied cancer cell laminin receptors and laminin that is accessible in exposed areas of the subendothelial matrix (Fig. 2B); (c) interaction between laminin present on the surface of cancer cells and unoccupied laminin receptors on the endothelial cell surface (Fig. 2C). Although previous studies

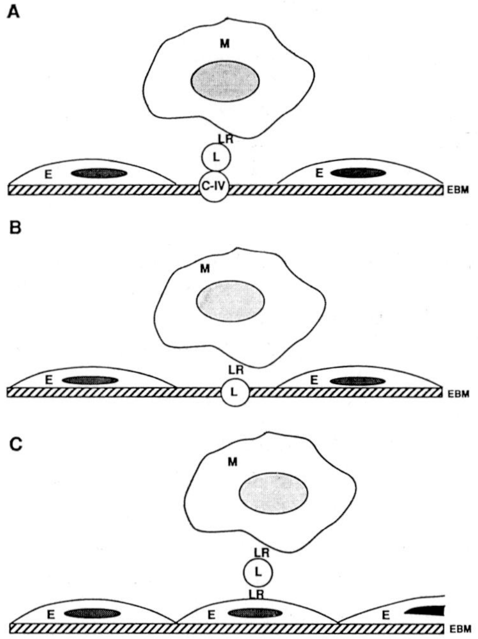

FIG. 2. Schematic representation of possible laminin interactive pathways that melanoma cells may use to attach to the vascular wall. (A) Melanoma cells (M) use the laminin (L) that is bound to their cell surface LR to interact with the type IV collagen (C-IV) that is accessible in exposed areas of the endothelial basement membrane (EBM); (B) melanoma cells use their unoccupied cell surface laminin receptors to interact with the laminin accessible in exposed areas of the endothelial basement membrane; (C) melanoma cells use the laminin that is bound to their cell surface laminin receptor(s) to interact with unoccupied laminin receptor(s) present on the surface of endothelial cells (E).

have provided evidence for the first two pathways, the relevance of the third pathway has not been examined until now.

We proposed the hypothesis that the 67 LR that are present on the surface of endothelial cells could play a critical role in the stable anchorage of cancer cells to the endothelium, using the bovine aortic endothelial cell (BAEC) monolayer model. The BAEC monolayer is a very useful *in vitro* model to study interactions between malignant cells and vascular endothelial cells (*56*, *57*). We demonstrated that BAEC exhibit 11,000 67 LR per cell (*52*) and that the strong attachment of melanoma cells to the endothelium is mediated, at least in part, by laminin present on the surface of the malignant cells (*52*). We tested the hypothesis that peptide G, a synthetic peptide that contains a high affinity laminin binding site for laminin, could inhibit melanoma cell attachment to BAEC monolayers. As expected, peptide G specifically interfered with the attachment of A2058 cells to the endothelial cells in a dose dependent manner (*58*). Neither peptide GX, containing a scrambled sequence of peptide G, nor other peptides containing sequences adjacent to peptide G on the 67 LR, had modulatory activity. These experiments specifically implicate the 67 LR as playing a crucial role in the attachment of cancer cells to the endothelium. To our knowledge, this is the first demonstration that a synthetic extracellular matrix receptor peptide containing the ligand binding site can interface with ligand-receptor interactions. Peptide G also specifically and significantly inhibited the attachment of human melanoma cells to human umbilical vein endothelium, indicating that the 67 LR mediates, at least in part, the attachment of human cancer cells to human endothelium. These data represent the first demonstration of the involvement of a specific laminin receptor in a crucial step of the metastatic cascade and identify a potential mechanism for the attachment of cancer cells to endothelial cells. The relevance of this pathway in blood-borne metastasis will be established by testing the effect of peptide G of the metastatic potential of melanoma cells. Such experiments should reveal whether peptide G, as a potential inhibitor of this process, could be used as an anti-metastatic agent to inhibit cancer cell arrest in the vasculature, preventing extravasation and the subsequent formation of metastatic foci.

Proteinases: From Correlation to Causality

A general aspect of malignant neoplasms may be an imbalance of proteolysis which favors invasion. However, proteolysis of tissue barriers is not a property unique to tumor cells. It is utilized for example during trophoblast implantation, embryo morphogenesis, tissue remodeling, parasitic and bacterial invasion, and angiogenesis. Furthermore, the defect in the tumor cell can not be simply unbridled production of degradative enzymes. This is because cell migration during invasion requires attachment and deattachment of the cell as it moves forward. Lysis of all matrix components around the tumor cell would simply remove the substratum necessary for proper cell traction. Thus, it is probable that the invading tumor cell uses proteolysis in a highly organized manner both spatially and temporally which does not differ functionally from the operating mode of normal cells which migrate through tissue barriers. The difference is that tumor cells couple proteolysis with motility to achieve invasion at times and places which would be inappropriate for normal cells.

The metastasis field has progressed from establishing a correlation between proteolysis and malignant progression to the finding that the actual blockade of certain proteinases will prevent invasion and metastasis. A positive association with tumor aggressiveness has been noted for a variety of classes of degradative enzymes including heparanases (*59*), serine (*60*), thiol (*61, 62*), and metal dependent (*63–65*) enzymes. Indeed, a cascade including all these enzymes is probably involved in the invasive process, and more than one enzyme is necessary but not sufficient. This conclusion is justified by the finding in multiple labs that inhibitors for metalloproteinases *or* inhibitors of serine proteinases can each block tumor cell invasion of native or reconstituted connective tissue barriers *in vitro* (*66–69*). Thus, the enzymes involved in tumor invasion and metastasis may well resemble the proteolytic cascades involved in blood coagulation.

Plasminogen activator, specifically urokinase type plasminogen activator (uPA), has been closely linked to the metastatic phenotype (*70, 71*). Anti-uPA antibodies block human HEP-3 cell invasion in the chick chorioallantoic membrane assay and murine B16F10 melanoma cell metastasis following tail vein injection (*72, 73*). Over expression of uPA in Ha-ras transformed 3T3 cells enhanced lung invasion

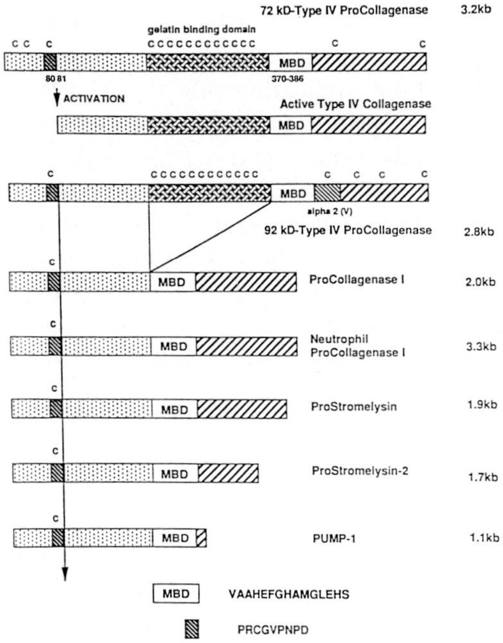

FIG. 3. Matrix metalloproteinase family. Type IV procollagenase (72 kDa and 92 kDa forms), interstitial procollagenase, neutrophil procollagenase, prostromelysin, prostromelysin-2, and PUMP-1 are represented diagrammatically and aligned to show regions of protein sequence homology. MBD: active site metal ion binding domain. Type IV procollagenases contain a cysteine rich, substrate binding domain which shows homology to fibronectin, but is absent from the other matrix metalloproteinase enzymes. Upon treatment with organomercurial compounds *in vitro*, all seven enzymes are activated with the concomitant removal of an amino terminal segment of the latent enzyme. The removed segment contains an unpaired cysteine residue within the conserved amino acid sequence PRCGVPDV located immediately adjacent to the proenzyme cleavage site. Site directed mutagenesis studies have shown that alterations in this sequence result in spontaneous activation of transin, the rat homologue of stromelysin. In the latent proenzyme, this sequence interacts with the metal ion through the unpaired cysteinyl residue to block activity. Pertubation of this interaction affects activation.

and experimental metastasis formation (*74*, *75*). Serine proteinase inhibitors also block tumor cell invasion through human amniotic membranes (*68*).

Among the list of enzymes involved in cancer, a large body of information has been accumulated concerning the matrix metalloproteinase gene family (Fig. 3). These enzymes have been subgrouped into three broad categories based on substrate preference: interstitial collagenases, type IV collagenases (gelatinases) and stromelysins (*75*). The interstitial collagenase is the best characterized and specifically degrades type I collagen (*65*). Neutrophil collagenase, which has recently been cloned appears very similar in substrate specificity (*76*). The stromelysins are three related gene products, stromelysin, stromelysin-2 and PUMP-1 which degrade a variety of matrix components including proteoglycans and non-collagenous glycoproteins such as laminin and fibronectin, as well as the non-collagenous domains of type IV collagen. The role of stromelysin in squamous carcinoma progression has recently been recognized (*77*). The type IV collagenases are named for their selective ability to cleave type IV collagen in a pepsin resistant triple-helical domain thus generating characteristic 1/4 amino terminal and 3/4 carboxyl terminal fragments (*78*). Both a 72 kD and 92 kD type IV collagenase exist and cDNA cloning has demonstrated that each is a unique gene product (*79, 80*).

All classes of matrix metalloproteinases are secreted as inactive zymogens and enzyme activation is an important control step in prteolysis. A new model for matrix metalloproteinase proenzyme activation has been proposed (*81–83*). The essential feature of this model is that all the latent forms of the matrix metalloproteinase enzymes have a metal atom-sulfhydryl side chain interaction that results in a catalytically inert active center. The sulfhydryl group in this interaction is donated by the CYS-73 residue which is contained in a highly conserved peptide present in all known members of this metalloproteinase family. The metal atom is presumably the zinc atom of the active site. Disruption of this interaction results in conformational rearrangement and rapid attainment of protease activity. The implication of this model is that mutations in the CYS-73 residue would result in intrinsic enzyme activation and thus could play a role in tumor progression. The *in vivo* mechanism of normal metalloproteinase activation is unknown but may involve the action of other proteinases either in solution or via a cell surface dependent mechanism (*18, 84, 85*). The latter would allow for precise cellular control at the point of matrix interaction.

Among the matrix metalloproteinase family members, an accumulating body of evidence supports a positive correlation between type IV collagenase activity and tumor cell invasion (*59, 86, 87*). Augmented type IV collagenase activity is associated with the genetic induction of a metastatic phenotype (*88–91*). Furthermore, use of agents which specifically inhibit type IV collagenase activity or block collagenase secretion prevent tumor cell invasion *in vitro* (*60, 92*). Immunohistochemical studies using affinity purified anti-72 kDa type IV collagenase antibodies (*81*) demonstrate that low levels of this enzyme are produced by normal, non-tumorigenic, non-metastatic cells such as the myoepithelial cells of the human breast (*93*). Benign proliferative lesions of the breast, benign polyps of the colon, normal colorectal and gastric mucosa all show negligible immunoreactivity for 72 kDa type IV collagenase. In contrast, almost all invasive colonic and gastric adenocarcinomas are positive for this antigen (*48, 94*). Down regulation of type IV collagenolytic activity by retinoic acid treatment of human melanoma cells has been correlated with a loss of the invasive phenotype (*59*). Studies of the mechanism of this effect reveal that retinoic acid treatment of these human melanoma cells results in a reduction of the steady state level of the 72 kDa type IV collagenase mRNA and loss of the invasive capacity (*65*). These results suggest that the 72 kDa type IV collagenase enzyme is a normal cell component that is dramatical y over-expressed in many invasive and metastatic human cancers.

Natural Proteinase Inhibitors Suppress Invasion

The secretion and activation of metalloproteinases is not enough to insure that they will degrade the target matrix substrate (*17*). This is because natural inhibitor proteins, produced either by the host, or by the tumor cell itself, can block the latent or the active metalloproteinases (*17*). Natural proteinase inhibitor proteins, such as tissue inhibitor of metalloproteinases (TIMPs) (*96*) or plasminogen activator inhibitors (PAIs) may therefore function as metastasis suppressor proteins which act to inhibit tumor cell invasion of the extracellular matrix. TIMP-1, the original member of the TIMP family (*97*), is a glycoprotein with an apparent molecular size of 28.5 kDa which forms a complex of 1: 1 stoichiometry with activated interstitial collagenase, activated stromelysin, or the 92 kDa type IV collagenase. It has been reported that transfection of antisense RNA which blocks TIMP-1 expression enhances the malignant phenotype (*98*). One explanation for this result is that the antisense RNA blocked the production of TIMP-1 which normally prevented the malignant phenotype. In animal models, administration of recombinant TIMP-1 blocks metastasis (*99, 100*).

Recently, Stetler-Stevenson *et al.* (*101, 102*) have isolated, purified, determined the complete primary structure, and cloned the first new member of the TIMP family, TIMP-2. An identical inhibitor was isolated from endothelial cells by DeClerk (*103, 104*). TIMP-1 and TIMP-2 are regulated independently and oppositely by 12-O-tetradecanoylphorbol-13-acetate (TPA), transforming growth factor β (TGF-beta), and other cytokines. TIMP-2 is a 21 kDa protein which selectively forms a complex with the latent proenzyme form of the 72 kDa type IV collagenase. The secreted protein has 194 amino acid residues and is not glycosylated. TIMP-2 shows 37% identity and overall 65.6% homology to TIMP-1 at the deduced amino sequence level. The position of the twelve cystein residues in TIMP-2 are conserved with respect to those present in TIMP-1, as are three of the four tryptophan residues; yet the two proteins are immunologically distinct. TIMP-2 inhibits at a 1: 1 ratio the type IV collagenolytic activity and the gelatinolytic activity associated with the 72 kDa enzyme. Unlike TIMP-1, TIMP-2 is capable of binding to both the latent and activated forms of the 72 kDa type IV collagenase and will abolish the hydrolytic activity of all members of the metalloproteinase family (*101, 105*). The 92 kDa type IV procollagenase can be found as a complex with TIMP-1 (79). Activation of either the latent 72 kDa or 92 kDa type IV collagenase-TIMP complex can be reversed by binding of a second role of TIMP-1 or TIMP-2. This suggests that on these enzymes there are two separate TIMP binding sites, and that binding of TIMP-1 or TIMP-2 to the latent proenzymes serves a different function than the inactivation that occurs following binding to the active species. The areas of the two proteins which differ in homology may contain the regions responsible for the functional differences (*101*). The net 72 kDa type IV collagenase activity consequently depends upon the balance between the levels of activated enzyme and TIMP-2. TIMP-2 is a potent inhibitor of cancer cell invasion through reconstituted extracellular matrix (*106*). TIMP-2 produced by the same tumor cells which make collagenase, therefore, exists as a natural suppressor of invasion.

REFERENCES

1. Fidler, I. J. and Hart, I. R. Biologic diversity in metastatic neoplasms—origins and implications. Science, *217*: 998–1001, 1982.
2. Schirrmacher, V. Experimental approaches, theoretical concepts, and impacts for

treatment strategies. Adv. Cancer Res., *43*: 1–32, 1985.

3. Liotta, L. A., Rao, C. N., and Barsky, S. H. Tumor invasion and the extracellular matrix. Lab. Invest., *49*: 636–642, 1983.
4. Folkman, J. and Klagsbrun, M. Angiogenic factors. Science, *235*: 442–447, 1987.
5. Folkman, J. Endothelial cells and angiogenic growth factors in cancer growth and metastasis. Cancer Metast. Rev., *9*: 171–174, 1990.
6. Kerbel, R. S. Growth dominance of the metastatic cancer cell: cellular and molecular aspects. Adv. Cancer Res., *55*: 87–131, 1990.
7. McGuire, W. L., Tandon, A. K., Allred, D. C., Chamness, G. C., and Clark, G. M. How to use prognostic factors in axillary node-negative breast cancer patients. J. Natl. Cancer Inst., *82*: 1006–1015, 1990.
8. Slamon, D. J., Godolphin, W., Jones, L. A., Holt, J. A., Wong, S. G., Keith, D. E., Levin, W. E., Stuart, S. G., Udove, J., Ullrich, A., and Press, M. F. Studies of the HER-2/*neu* proto-oncogene in human breast and ovarian cancer. Science, *244*: 707–713, 1989.
9. Lidereau, R., Callahan, R., Dickson, C., Peters, G., Escot, C., and Ali, I. U. Amplification of the *int-2* gene in primary human breast tumors. Oncogene Res., *2*: 285–291, 1988.
10. Tandon, A. K., Clark, G. M., Chamness, G. C., Chirgwin, J., and McGuire, W. L. Cathepsin D and prognosis in breast cancer. N. Engl. J. Med., *322*: 297–302, 1990.
11. Yurchenco, P. D. and Schittny, J. C. Molecular architecture of basement membranes. FASEB J. *4*: 1577–1590, 1990.
12. Barsky, S. H., Siegal, G. P., Jannotta, F., and Liotta, L. A. Loss of basement membrane components by invasive tumors but not by their benign counterparts. Lab. Invest., *49*: 140–146, 1983.
13. Hynes, R. O. Integrins: a family of cell surface receptors. Cell, *48*: 549–554, 1987.
14. Humphries, M. J., Olden, K., and Yamada, K. M. A synthetic peptide from fibronectin inhibits experimental metastasis of murine melanoma cells. Science, *233*: 467–469, 1986.
15. Rao, C., Castronovo, V., Schmitt, M. C., Wewer, U., Claysmith, A., Liotta, L. A., and Sobel, M. E. Evidence for a precursor of the high-affinity metastasis associated murine laminin receptor. Biochemistry, *28*: 7476–7486, 1989.
16. Aznavoorian, S., Stracke, M. L., Krutztch, H., Schiffman, E., and Liotta, L. A. Signal transduction for chemotaxis and haptotaxis by matrix molecules in tumor cells. J. Cell Biol., *110*: 1427–1438, 1990.
17. Gottesman, M. The role of proteases in cancer. Sem. Cancer Biol., *1*: 97–160, 1990.
18. Brown, P. D., Levy, A. T., Margulies, I., Liotta, L., and Stetler-Stevenson, W. G. Independent expression and cellular processing of the 72-kDa type IV collagenase and interstitial collagenase in human tumorigenic cell lines. Cancer Res., *50*: 6184–6191, 1990.
19. Guirguis, R., Margulies, I. M. K., Taraboletti, G., Schiffman, E., and Liotta, L. A. Cytokine-induced pseudopodial protrusion is coupled to tumor cell migration. Nature, *329*: 261–263, 1987.
20. Luna, E. J., Wuestehube, L. J., Ingalls, H. M., and Chia, C. P. The *Dictyostelium discoideum* plasma membrane: A model system for the study of actin-membrane interactions. Adv. Cell Biol., *3*: 1–33, 1989.
21. Liotta, L. A., Mandler, R., Murano, G., Katz, D. A., Gordon, R. K., Chiang, P. K., and Schiffmann, E. Tumor cell autocrine motility factor. Proc. Natl. Acad. Sci. U.S.A., *83*: 3302–3306, 1986.
22. Gherardi, E., Gray, J., Stoker, M., Perryman, M., and Furlong, R. Purification of

scatter factor, a fibroblast derived basic protein that modulates epithelial interactions and movement. Proc. Natl. Acad. Sci. U.S.A., *86*: 5844–5848, 1989.
23. Nicolson, G. L. Organ specificity of tumor metastasis: role of preferential adhesion, invasion, and growth of malignant cells at specific secondary sites. Cancer Metast. Rev., *7*: 143–188, 1988.
24. Beck, K., Hunter, I., and Engel, J. Structure and function of laminin: anatomy of a multidomain glycoprotein. FASEB J., *4*: 148–160, 1990.
25. Kleinman, H. K., Cannon, F. B., Laurie, G. W., Hassell, J. R., Aumailley, M., Terranova, V. P., and Martin, G. R. Biological activities of laminin. J. Cell Biochem., *27*: 317–325, 1982.
26. Timpl, R., Rhode, H., Gehron-Robey, S., Rennard, J., Foidart, M., and Martin, G. R. Laminin, a glycoprotein from basement membranes. J. Biol. Chem., *254*: 9933–9937, 1979.
27. Terranova, V. P., Rao, C. N., Kabelic, T., Margulies, I. M. K., and Liotta, L. A. Laminin receptor on human breast carcinoma cells. Proc. Natl. Acad. Sci. U.S.A., *80*: 444–448, 1983.
28. Varani, J., Lovett, E. J., McCoy, J. P., Shibata, S., Maddox, D. E., Goldstein, I. J., and Wicha, M. Differential expression of a laminin-like substance by high and low metastatic cells. Am. J. Pathol., *111*: 27–34, 1983.
29. Barsky, S. H., Rao, C. N., Williams, J. E., and Liotta, L. A. Laminin molecular domains which alter metastasis in a murine model. J. Clin. Invest., *74*: 843–848, 1984.
30. Malinoff, H. L., McCoy, J. P., Jr., Varani, J., and Wicha, M. S. Metastatic potential of murine fibrosarcoma cells is influenced by cell surface laminin. Int. J. Cancer, *33*: 651–655, 1984.
31. Iwamoto, Y., Robey, F. A., Graf, J., Sasaki, M., Kleinman, H. K., Yamada, Y., and Martin, G. R. YIGSR, a synthetic laminin pentapeptide, inhibits experimental metastasis formation. Science, *238*: 1132–1134, 1987.
32. Castronovo, V., Parent, B., Foidart, J. M., Heynen, E., Goffinet, G., Lambotte, R., and Mahieu, P. Perfusion of human umbilical veins. A new approach to study the interactions of circulating malignant cells with vascular wall and their modulation. Invasion Metast., *8*: 332–350, 1988.
33. Vollmers, H. P., Imhof, B. A., Braun, S., Waller, C. A., Schirrmacher, V., and Birchmeier, W. Monoclonal antibodies which prevent experimental lung metastases. Interference with adhesion of tumor cells to laminin. FEBS Lett., *172*: 17–20, 1984.
34. Lesot, H., Kuhl, U., and von der Mark, K. Isolation of a laminin-binding protein from muscle cell membranes. EMBO J., *2*: 861–865, 1983.
35. Malinoff, H. and Wicha, M. S. Isolation of a cell surface protein for laminin from murine fibrosarcoma cells. J. Cell Biol., *96*: 1475–1480, 1983.
36. Rao, C. N., Barsky, S. H., Terranova, V. P., and Liotta, L. A. Isolation of a tumor laminin receptor. Biochem. Biophys. Res. Commun., *111*: 804–808, 1983.
37. Albelda, S. M. and Buck, C. A. Integrins and other cell adhesion molecules. FASEB J., *4*: 2868–2880, 1990.
38. Ruynan, R. B., Versalovic, J., and Shur, B. D. Functionally distinct laminin receptors mediate cell adhesion and spreading: the requirement for surface galactosyl-transferase in cell spreading. J. Cell Biol., *107*: 1863–1871, 1988.
39. Woo, H. J., Shaw, L. A., Messier, J. M., and Mercurio, A. M. The major non-integrin laminin binding protein of macrophages is identical to carbohydrate binding protein 35 (Mac-2). J. Biol. Chem., *265*: 7097–7099, 1990.
40. Zhou, Q. and Cummings, R. D. The S-type lectin from heart tissue binds selectively

to the carbohydrate chains of laminin. Arch. Biochem. Biophys., *281*: 27–35, 1990.
41. Kleinman, H. K., Ogle, R. C., Cannon, F. B., Little, C. D., Sweeney, T. M., and Luckenbill-Edds, L. Laminin receptors for neurite formation. Proc. Natl. Acad. Sci. U.S.A., *83*: 8182–8186, 1988.
42. Wewer, U. M., Liotta, L. A., Jaye, M., Ricca, G. A., Drohan, W. N., Claysmith, A. P., Rao, C. N., Wirth, P., Coligan, J. E., Albrechtsen, R., Mudryj, M., and Sobel, M. E. Altered levels of laminin receptor mRNA in various human carcinoma cells have different abilities to bind laminin. Proc. Natl. Acad. Sci. U.S.A., *83*: 7137–7141, 1986.
43. Terranova, V. P., Rao, C. N., Kabelic, T., and Liotta, L. A. Laminin receptor on human breast cancer cells. Proc. Natl. Acad. Sci. U.S.A., *80*: 444–448, 1983.
44. Horan Hand, P., Thor, A., Schlom, J., Rao, C. N., and Liotta, L. A. Expression of laminin receptor in normal and carcinomatous tissues as defined by a monoclonal antibody, Cancer Res., *45*: 2713–2719, 1985.
45. Mafune, K., Ravikumar, T. S., Wong, J. M., Yow, H., Chen, L. B., and Steele, G. D. Expression of a Mr 32,000 laminin-binding protein messenger RNA in human colon carcinoma correlates with disease progression. Cancer Res., *50*: 3888–3891, 1990.
46. Castronovo, V., Colin, C., Claysmith, A. P., Chen, P. H. S., Lifrange, E., Lambotte, R., Krutzsch, H., Liotta, L. A., and Sobel, M. E. Immunodetection of the metastasis-associated laminin receptor in human breast cancer cells obtained by fine needle aspiration biospy. Am. J. Pathol., *137*: 1373–1381, 1990.
47. Cioce, V., Castronovo, V., Shmookler, M. B., Garbisa, S., Grigione, W. F., Liotta, L. A., and Sobel, M. E. Increased expression of the laminin receptor in human colon cancer. J. Natl. Cancer Inst., *83*: 29–36, 1991.
48. D'Errico, A., Garbisa, S., Liotta, L. A., Castronovo, V., Stetler-Stevenson, W. G., and Grigioni, W. F. Augmentation of type IV collagenase, laminin receptor and Ki67 proliferation antigen associated with human, gastric and breast carcinoma progression. Modern Pathol., *4*: 239–246, 1991.
49. Yow, H., Wong, J. M., Chen, H. S., Lee, C., Steele, G. D., Jr., and Chen, L. B. Increased mRNA expression of a laminin-binding protein in human colon carcinoma: complete sequence of a full-length cDNA encoding the protein. Proc. Natl. Acad. Sci. U.S.A., *85*: 6394–6398, 1988.
50. Castronovo, V., Claysmith, A. P., Barker, K. T., Cioce, V., Krutzsch, H., and Sobel, M. E. Biosynthesis of the 67 kDa laminin receptor. Biochem. Biophys. Res. Commun., *177*: 177–183, 1991.
51. Castronovo, V., Taraboletti, G., Liotta, L., and Sobel, M. Estrogen and progestins modulate laminin receptor expression in human breast cancer cell lines. J. Natl. Cancer Inst., *81*: 781–786, 1989.
52. Castronovo, V. and Sobel, M. E. Laminin and fibronectin increase the steady state levels of the 67 kD high affinity metastasis-associated laminin receptor mRNA in human cancer cells. Biochem. Biophys. Res. Commun., *168*: 1110–1117, 1990.
53. Rahman, A., Pannerselvam, M., Guirguis, R., Dodanna, P., Castronovo, V., Sobel, M., and Liotta, L. A. Anti-laminin receptor antibody targeting of liposomes with encapsulated doxorubicin to human breast cancer cells *in vitro*. J. Natl. Cancer Inst., *81*: 1794–1800, 1989.
54. Castronovo, V., Taraboletti, G., and Sobel, M. E. Functional domains of the 67 kDa laminin receptor precursor. J. Biol. Chem., *266*: 20440–20446, 1991.
55. Poste, G. and Fidler, I. J. The pathogenesis of cancer metastasis. Nature, *283*: 139–146, 1980.
56. Nicolson, G. L. Metastatic tumor cell attachment and invasion assay utilizing vascular

endothelial cell monolayers. J. Histochem. Cytochem., *3*: 214–220, 1982.
57. Kramer, R. H. and Nicolson, G. L. Interactions of tumor cells with vascular endothelial cell monolayers. A model for metastatic invasion. Proc. Natl. Acad. Sci. U.S.A., *76*: 5404–5408, 1979.
58. Castronovo, V., Taraboletti, G., and Sobel, M. E. Laminin receptor cDNA deduced synthetic peptide inhibits cancer cell attachment to endothelium. Cancer Res., *51*: 5672–5678, 1991.
59. Nakajima, M., Welch, D., Belloni, P. N., and Nicolson, G. L. Degradation of basement membrane type IV collagen and lung subendothelial matrix by rat mammary adenocarcinoma cell clones of differing metastatic potentials. Cancer Res., *47*: 4869–4876, 1987.
60. Reich, R., Thompson, E., Iwamoto, Y., Martin, G. R., Deason, J. R., Fuller, G. C., and Miskin, R. Effects of inhibitors of plasminogen activator, serine proteinases, and collagenase IV on the invasion of basement membranes by metastatic cells. Cancer Res., *48*: 3307–3312, 1988.
61. Recklies, A. D., Poole, A. R., and Mort, J. S. A cysteine proteinase secreted from human breast tumours is immunologically related to cathepsin B. Biochem. J., *207*: 633–636, 1982.
62. Sloane, B. R. and Honn, K. V. Cysteine proteinases and metastasis. Cancer Metast. Rev., *3*: 249–263, 1984.
63. Ostrowski, L. E., Rinch, J., Kreig, P., and Matrisian, L. Expression pattern of a gene for a secreted metalloproteinase during late stages of tumor progression. Mol. Carcinogen., *1*: 13–19, 1988.
64. Liotta, L. A., Abe, S., Robey, P., and Martin, G. Preferential digestion of basement membrane collagen by an enzyme derived from a metastatic murine tumor. Proc. Natl. Acad. Sci. U.S.A., *76*: 2268–2272, 1979.
65. Templeton, N. S., Brown, P. D., Levy, A. T., Margulies, I. M. K., Liotta, L. A., and Stetler-Stevenson, W. G.: Cloning and characterization of human tumor cell interstitial collagenase. Cancer Res., *50*: 5431–5437, 1990.
66. Thorgeirsson, U. P., Turpeenniemi-Hujanen, T., Neckers, L. M., Johnson, P. W., and Liotta, L. A. Protein synthesis but not DNA synthesis is required for tumor cell invasion *in vitro*. Invasion Metast., *4*: 73, 1984.
67. Wang, M. and Stearns, M. E. Blocking of collagenase secretion by estamustine during *in vitro* tumor cell invasion. Cancer Res., *48*: 6262–6271, 1988.
68. Mignatti, P., Robbins, E., and Rifkin, D. Tumor invasion through the human amniotic membrane: requirement for a proteinase cascade. Cell, *47*: 487–498, 1986.
69. Liotta, L. A. and Stetler-Stevenson, W. G. Metalloproteinases and cancer invasion. Semin. Cancer Biol., *1*: 99–106, 1990.
70. Dano, K., Andreasen, P. A., Grondahl-Hansen, J., Kristensen, P., Nielsen, L. S., and Skriver, L. Plasminogen activators, tissue degradation and cancer. Adv. Cancer Res., *44*: 139–266, 1985.
71. Sappino, A.-P., Busso, N., Belin, D., and Vassali, J.-D. Increase of urokinase type plasminogen activator gene expression in human lung and breast carcinomas. Cancer Res., *47*: 4043–4046, 1987.
72. Ossowski, L. and Reich, E. Antibodies to plasminogen activator inhibit human tumor metastasis. Cell, *35*: 611–619, 1983.
73. Esheicher, A., Wohlwend, A., Belin, D., and Vassalli, J. D. Characterization of the cellular binding site for the urokinase type plasminogen activator. J. Biol. Chem., *264*: 1180–1189, 1989.
74. Axelrod, J. H., Reich, R., and Mishkin, R. Expression of human recombinant plas-

minogen activators enhance invasion and experimental metastasis of Ha-ras transformed NIH 3T3 cells. Mol. Cell. Biol., *9*: 2133–2141, 1989.

75. Wilhelm, S., Collier, I., Kronberg, A., Eisen, A., Marmer, B., Grant, G., Bauer, E., and Liotta, L. A. Human skin fibroblast stromelysin: structure, glycosylation, substrate specificity, and differential expression in normal and tumorigenic cells. Proc. Natl. Acad. Sci. U.S.A., *84*: 6725–6729, 1987.
76. Hasty, K. A., Pourmotabbed, T. F., Goldberg, G. I., Thompson, J. P., Spinella, D. G., Stevens, R. M., and Mainardi, C. M.: Human neutrophil collagenase. J. Biol, Chem., *265*: 11421–11424, 1990.
77. Matrisian, L. and Bowden, T. Stromelysin/transin and tumor progression. Sem. Cancer Biol., *1*: 107–115, 1990.
78. Fessler, L., Duncan, K., and Tryggvason, K. Identification of the procollagen IV cleavage products produced by a specific tumor collagenase. J. Biol. Chem., *259*: 9783–9789, 1984.
79. Collier, I. E., Wilhelm, S. M., Eisen, A. Z., Marner, B. L., Grant, G. A., Seltzer, J. L., Kronberger, A., He, C., Bauer, E. A., and Goldberg, G. I. H-ras oncogene transformed human bronchial epithelial cells (TBE-1) secrete a single metalloproteinase capable of degrading basement membrane collagen. J. Biol. Chem., *263*: 6579–6587, 1989.
80. Wilhelm, S. M., Collier, I. E., Marmer, B. L., Eisen, A. Z., Grant, G. A., and Goldberg, G. I. SV40-transformed human lung fibroblasts secrete a 92-kDa type-IV collagenase which is identical to that secreted by normal human macrophages. J. Biol. Chem., *264*: 17213–17221, 1989.
81. Stetler-Stevenson, W. G., Krutzsch, H., Wacher, M. P., and Liotta, L. A. The activation of human type IV collagenase proenzyme. J. Biol. Chem., *264*: 1353–1356, 1989.
82. Vallee, B. L. and Auld, D. S. Zinc coordination, function and structure of zinc enzymes and other proteins. Biochemistry, *29*: 5647–5659, 1990,
83. Van Wart, H. E. and Birkedal-Hansen, H. The cysteine switch: A principle of regulation of metalloproteinase activity with potential applicability to the entire matrix metalloproteinase gene family. Proc. Natl. Acad. Sci. U.S.A., *87*: 5578–5582, 1990.
84. Herron, G. S., Banda, M. J., Clark, E. J., Gavrilovic, J., and Werb, Z. Secretion of metalloproteinases by stimulated capillary endothelial cells. II. Expression of collagenase and stromelysin activities is regulated by endogenous inhibitors. J. Biol. Chem., *261*: 2814–2818, 1986.
85. He, C., Wilhelm, S. M., Pentland, A. P., Marmer, B. L., Grant, G. A., Eisen, A. Z., and Goldberg, G. I. Tissue cooperation in a proteolytic cascade activating human interstitial collagenase. Proc. Natl. Acad. Sci. U.S.A., *86*: 2632–2636, 1989.
86. Liotta, L. A., Tryggvason, K., Garbisa, S., Hart, I., Foltz, C. M., and Shafie, S. Metastatic potential correlates with enzymatic degradation of basement membrane collagen. Nature, *284*: 67–68, 1980.
87. Turpeenniemi-Hujanen, T., Thorgeirsson, U. P., Hart, I. R., Grant, S., and Liotta, L. A. Expression of collagenase IV (basement membrane collagenase) activity in murine tumor cell hybrids that differ in metastatic potential. J. Natl. Cancer Inst., *75*: 99–108, 1985,
88. Muschel, R. J., Williams, J. E., Lowy, D. R., and Liotta, L. A. Harvey ras induction of metastatic potential depends upon oncogene activation and the type of recipient cell. Am. J. Pathol., *121*: 1–8, 1985.
89. Garbisa, S., Pozzatti, R., Muschel, R., Saffioti, V., Ballin, M., Goldfarb, R., Khoury, G., and Liotta, L. Secretion of type IV collagenolytic protease and metastatic pheno-

type: Induction by transfection with c-Ha-ras but not C-Ha-ras plus Ad2-Ela. Cancer Res., *47*: 1523–1528, 1987.

90. Bonfil, D. R., Reddel, R. R., Ura, H., Reich, R., Fridman, R., Harris, C. C., and Kleinszanto, A. J. P. Invasive and metastatic potential of a v-Ha-ras-transformed human bronchial epithelial cell line. J. Natl. Cancer Inst., *81*: 587–594, 1989.
91. Ura, H., Bonfil, R. D., Reich, R., Reddel, R., Pfeifer, A., Harris, C. C., and Klein, A. J. P. Expression of type IV collagenase and procollagen genes and its correlation with the tumorigenic, invasive, and metastatic abilities of oncogene-transformed human bronchial epithelial cells. Cancer Res., *49*: 4615–4621, 1989.
92. Wang, B. S., McLouglin, G. A., Richie, J. P., and Mannick, J. A. Correlation of the production of plasminogen activator with tumor metastasis in B16 mouse melanoma cell lines. Cancer Res., *40*: 288–292, 1980.
93. Monteagudo, C., Merino, M., San-Juan, J., Liotta, L., and Stetler-Stevenson, W. Immunohistologic distribution of type IV collagenase in normal, benign and malignant breast tissue. Am. J. Pathol., *136*: 585–592, 1990.
94. Levy, A., Cioce, V., Sobel, M. E., Garbisa, S., Griogioni, W. F., Liotta, L. A., and Stetler-Stevenson, W. G. Increased expression of the 72 kDa type IV collagenase in human colonic adenocarcinoma. Cancer Res., *51*: 439–444, 1991.
95. Hendrix, M., Wood, R., Seftor, E., Lotan, D., Nakajima, M., Misiorowski, R., Seftor, R. E. B., Stetler-Stevenson, W. G., Bevacqua, S. J., Liotta, L. A., Sobel, M. E., Raz, A., and Lotan, R. Retinoic acid inhibition of human melanoma cell invasion through a reconstituted basement membrane and its relation to decreases in the expression of proteolytic enzymes and motility factor receptor. Cancer Res., *50*: 4121–4130, 1990.
96. Carmichael, D. F., Sommer, A., Thomson, R., Anderson, D. C., Smith, C. G., Welgus, H. G., and Stricklin, G. P. Primary structure and cDNA cloning of human fibroblast collagenase inhibitor. Proc. Natl. Acad. Sci. U.S.A., *83*: 2407–2411, 1986.
97. Murphy, G., Cawston, T., and Reynolds, J. An inhibitor of collagenase from human amniotic fluid. Purification, characterization and action on metalloproteinases, Biochem. J., *195*: 167–170, 1981.
98. Khokha, R., Waterhouse, P., Yagel, S., Lala, P. K., Overall, C. M., Norton, G., and Denhardt, D. T. Antisense RNA-induced reduction in metalloproteinase inhibitor causes mouse 3T3 cells to become tumorigenic. Science, *243*: 947–950, 1989.
99. Schultz, R. M., Silberman, S., Persky, B., Bajkowski, A. S., and Carmichael, D. F. Inhibition by recombinant tissue inhibitor of metalloproteinases of human aminion invasion and lung colonization by murine B16-F10 melanoma cells. Cancer Res., *48*: 5539–5545, 1988.
100. Alvarez, O. A., Carmichael, D. F., and DeClerck, Y. A. Inhibition of collagenolytic activity and metastasis of tumor cells by a recombinant human tissue inhibitor of metalloproteinases. J. Natl. Cancer Inst., *82*: 589–595, 1990.
101. Stetler-Stevenson, W. G., Krutzsch, H. C., and Liotta, L. A. TIMP-2, a new member of the metalloproteinase inhibitor family. J. Biol. Chem., *264*: 17374–17378, 1989.
102. Stetler-Stevenson, W., Brown, P., Onisto, M., Levy, A., and Liotta, L. Tissue inhibitor of metalloproteinases-2 (TIMP-2) mRNA expression in tumor cell lines and human tumor tissues. J. Biol. Chem., *265*: 13933–13938, 1990.
103. DeClerck, Y., Yean, T., Ratzkin, B., Lu, H., and Langley, K. Purification and characterization of two related but distinct metalloproteinase inhibitors secreted by bovine aortic endothelial cells. J. Biol. Chem., *264*: 17445–17453, 1989.
104. Boone, T., Johnson, M., DeClerck, Y., and Langley, K. cDNA cloning and expression of a metalloproteinase inhibitor related to tissue inhibitor of metalloproteinases.

Proc. Natl. Acad. Sci. U.S.A., *87*: 2800–2804, 1990.

105. Goldberg, G. I., Marmer, B. L., Grant, G. A., Eisen, A. Z., Wilhelm, S., and He, C. Human 72-kDa type IV collagenase forms a complex with a tissue inhibitor of metalloproteinase inhibitor. Proc. Natl. Acad. Sci. U.S.A., *86*: 8207–8211, 1989.

106. Albini, A., Melchiori, A., Santi, L., Liotta, L. A., Brown, P. D., and Stetler-Stevenson, W. G. Tumor cell invasion inhibited by TIMP-2 J. Natl. Canc. Inst., *83*: 775–779, 1991.

MULTISTAGE CARCINOGENESIS, C. C. HARRIS ET AL. (EDS.),
APAN SCI. SOC. PRESS, TOKYO/CRC PRESS, BOCA RATON, PP. 339–347, 1992

Switch to the Angiogenic Phenotype during Tumorigenesis

Judah FOLKMAN*[1] and Douglas HANAHAN*[2]

The Department of Surgery, Children's Hospital of the Departments of Surgery and Anatomy and Cellular Biology, Harvard Medical School, Boston, Massachusetts 02115,[1] and The Department of Biochemistry, University of California, San Francisco, California 94143–0534,*[2] U.S.A.*

Abstract: Tumor growth and metastasis are angiogenesis-dependent. Virtually all solid tumors are neovascularized by the time they are detected. However, there is a *pre*vascular phase during early tumor development where few or no tumor cells are angiogenic and expansion of the tumor is restricted to a few mm^3. When enough tumor cells become angiogenic, the tumor can expand progressively and shed metastatic cells. This angiogenic switch has recently been quantitated for human breast cancer, as well as for prostate cancer. We have studied the problem of how tumors switch to the angiogenic phenotype by using transgenic mice in which tumors develop at a predictable time and in discrete *pre*vascular and vascular stages. When the transgene is the bovine papilloma virus (BPV) genome, angiogenic fibrosarcomas develop from non-angiogenic precursors called fibromatoses. The fibrosarcomas secrete growth factors for capillary endothelial cells. In contrast, the fibromatoses do not secrete endothelial cell growth factors. When the transgene consists of the large "T" antigen of SV40 under the control of the rat insulin promoter, 70% of pancreatic islets become hyperplastic and 4–10% of these become angiogenic at 6–7 weeks. Tumors arise from these neovascularized hyperplastic islets and reach $>1000\times$ the volume of the pre-angiogenic islets. The onset of angiogenic activity coincides with the secretion of acidic fibroblast growth factor (aFGF) and other growth factors not fully identified at this writing. These studies help to explain the switch to the angiogenic phenotype during tumorigenesis and provide models to discover antiangiogenic therapies directed at the *source* of angiogenic activity. Such therapy, when developed, may be co-administered with currently available angiogenesis inhibitors which are directed at the *target* of angiogenic activity, vascular endothelial cells.

Considerable evidence now exists in support of the hypothesis that tumor growth and metastasis are angiogenesis-dependent (*1*). In its simplest terms, this hypothesis states that the induction of new capillary blood vessels by a solid tumor is necessary for expansion of a tumor mass beyond a small volume of a few cubic millimeters (Fig. 1). New vessels carry nutrients and metabolites to and from tumors. Vascular endothelial cells within the new capillaries also contribute growth factors to the tumor. In the *absence* of angiogenesis, tumor growth is severely restricted. It is virtually

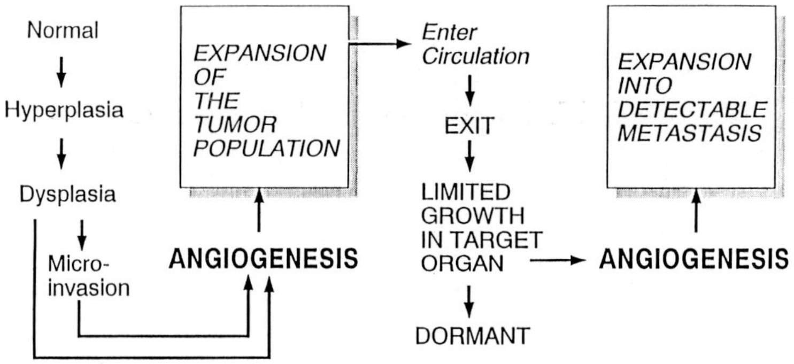

FIG. 1. Role of angiogenesis in tumor growth and metastasis. From ref. *40* with permission of the publisher.

impossible for most human or animal solid tumors to grow to a volume of 0.5 to 1 centimeter (*3*) without becoming vascularized. It must be kept in mind however that angiogenesis, while necessary for tumor growth is not sufficient. Certain tumors such as adrenal adenomas are highly angiogenic but the adenoma cells lack the proliferative potential to take advantage of this angiogenic activity. Also, some *in situ* carcinomas (especially breast) become angiogenic before they have acquired proliferative and invasive properties.

Recent evidence also suggests that angiogenesis is necessary but not sufficient for metastasis. The onset of angiogenesis is one of the earliest events of the metastatic cascade. Before a primary tumor has become vascularized, tumor cells rarely enter the circulation (*2*). After neovascularization has occurred, tumor cells are frequently shed into the circulation and in large numbers. A few tumor cells capable of surviving the circulation, arrest in a capillary vessel of a target organ, invade through the wall of the microvessel and form a microcolony of tumor within the extravascular space of the target organ. Such a micrometastasis is still not clinically detectable nor symptomatic unless it has the capacity to induce neovascularization. Lack of angiogenic activity by a micrometastasis may be one mechanism of tumor "dormancy". Thus, angiogenesis plays a critical role at the beginning and at the end of the metastatic cascade (*3*). We emphasize that while suppression of angiogenesis or its absence may severely restrict or prevent metastasis, the presence of angiogenesis in a tumor does not guarantee metastasis.

The Angiogenic Phenotype

It is now recognized that the development of a tumor from a normal cell is a multi-step process. The gradual de-regulation of cellular controls can be observed at the morphologic level (*4*). Thus, the events which often follow hyperplasia include dysplasia, invasiveness, angiogenesis and metastasis (Fig. 1). This multi-step progression during tumorigenesis can also be documented at the cellular level, *e.g.*, continuous growth *in vitro* (immortalization); at the chromosomal level, *e.g.*, aneuploidy; and at the genetic level *e.g.*, increased expression of oncogenes and/or sequential loss of tumor suppressor genes (*5*).

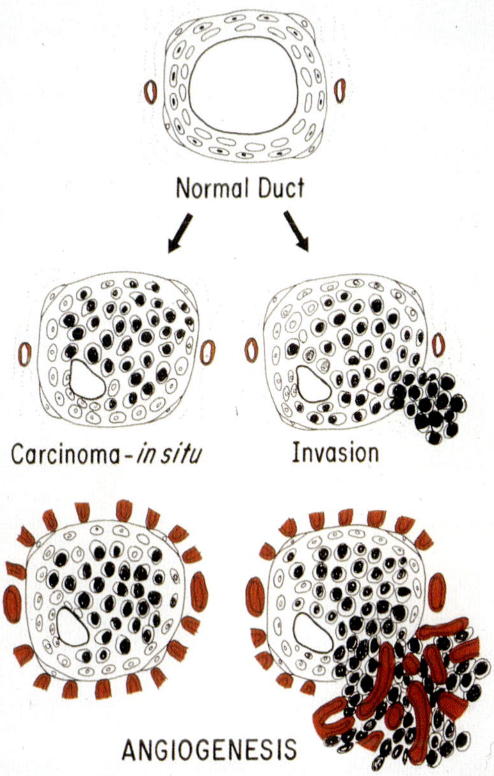

FIG. 2. Diagram of ducts in breast cancer after staining with antibody to factor VIII-related antigen, to show carcinoma *in situ* with and without angiogenesis. From ref. *40* with permission of the publisher.

The acquisition of angiogenic activity can now be recognized as a distinct step in the multi-step progression to neoplasia. Separable *pre*-vascular and vascular phases have been observed in human melanoma (*6*), carcinoma of the cervix (*7*), and in pharyngeal cancers. Recently, these two phases have been documented quantitatively in human breast cancer (*8*) and also in prostate cancer by staining histological sections with antibody to Factor VIII-related antigen, a marker unique to vascular endothelium. The prevascular and vascular phases can be clearly seen even in the same histological section of a breast cancer because of its multi-focal origin. The human breast contains between 6,000 and 10,000 ducts (*9*). A breast with a vascularized invasive tumor may harbor multiple carcinomas *in situ* that have not induced neovascularization and these may reside near other *in situ* carcinomas which are engulfed in intense neovascularization. One can also see ducts with microinvasive carcinoma before or after the onset of neovascularization. When microinvasion is accompanied by neovascularization, the tumor mass is usually found to be quite large (Fig. 2), suggesting that the induction of neovascularization has contributed to rapid expansion of the tumor population.

Factors That Mediate Angiogenesis

At least 7 polypeptides are now known to be angiogenic factors (*10, 11*). These include: the fibroblast growth factors (aFGF and bFGF); angiogenin; transforming growth factor-alpha (TGF-alpha); transforming growth factor-beta (TGF-beta); tumor necrosis factor-alpha (TNF-alpha); platelet-derived endothelial cell growth factor (PD-ECGF); and vascular endothelial cell growth factor (VEGF), also known as vasoproliferative factor (VPF). Basic fibroblast growth factor (bFGF), was the first angiogenic protein to be completely purified and it is the most potent of the known angiogenic polypeptides. It is also found in a wide variety of normal tissues and in many tumors.

Mechanisms of Switching to the Angiogenic Phenotype

While it can be demonstrated in human tumors that there is a switch to the angiogenic phenotype, and angiogenic factors which mediate this switch have been identified, very little is known about how the switch takes place. A major roadblock in studying its mechanism is the relative inaccessibility of the pre-angiogenic state in experimental animals. By the time a tumor can be detected after transplantation of tumor cells into a mouse, it is already highly vascularized. If the tumor cannot be detected this is often ascribed to "failure to take'. However, one of the causes of "no take" is failure of neovascularization.

Transgenic mouse models of multi-step tumorigenesis (*12, 13*) afford access to the developing tumor *prior* to the onset of neovascularization. In these mice, tumors arise at predictable times, and develop through a discrete *pre*-vascular and vascular stage.

In one system, the transgene is the bovine papilloma virus (BPV) genome (*14*). Highly angiogenic fibrosarcomas develop from non-angiogenic precursors called mild fibromatoses (*15*). The mild fibromatoses are thin, non-vascularized proliferations of fibroblasts in the dermis. They appear at approximately 6–8 months of age. They cannot be transplanted but, grow slowly *in vitro*. They are followed within a few months by aggressive fibromatosis characterized by greater cell density, increased numbers of mitoses and a thickened dermal layer of skin. These lesions are slightly angiogenic and induce the ingrowth of a few new capillaries. Fibrosarcomas usually arise out of the aggressive fibromatoses, beginning at about 12 months of age. The fibrosarcomas are highly angiogenic and grow into large masses which protrude from the skin and eventually kill the animals. Both aggressive fibromatoses and fibrosarcomas are transplantable.

When these three cell types were cultured *in vitro* and compared to normal skin fibroblasts from the same transgenic mice, all cells were found to express mRNA for bFGF and to synthesize this protein (*15*). No other proteins of the FGF family were expressed or synthesized by these cells. bFGF was found to be totally cell-associated in the normal cells and in the mild fibromatoses. No bFGF (or endothelial mitogenic activity) was found in their conditioned medium. In contrast, fibrosarcoma cells exported bFGF into the conditioned medium and it was biologically active (*i.e.*, it induced proliferation of capillary endothelial cells). Aggressive fibromatoses displayed an intermediate pattern, in which less bFGF activity was detected in the conditioned medium. All endothelial mitogenic activity was eliminated by neutralizing antibodies for bFGF (but not for aFGF), or by passing the medium over a heparin-affinity chromatographic column.

Thus, bFGF was a major mediator of endothelial mitogenic activity (and angiogenic activity) from these cells. Since the publication of this paper (*15*) we have found that the conditioned media of all four stages of this tumor also contain vascular endothelial cell growth factor (VEGF). The onset of angiogenic activity *in vivo* was highly correlated with the switch to export of bFGF from its cell-associated state. The export of bFGF was not due to cell lysis, nor to a general leakiness, because other cell associated proteins, such as lactate dehydrogenase did not increase in the conditioned medium. Of interest, is that exported bFGF had a molecular weight similar to the cell-associated bFGF (18,500). bFGF lacks a signal peptide. Thus, the molecular mechanism of the switch from cell-associated to exported bFGF is unknown. Nevertheless, the switch to exported bFGF in aggressive fibromatosis and fibrosarcoma correlates not only with histological neovascularization, but with the tumorigenicity of the cells themselves.

In another transgenic mouse system, the transgene consists of the large "T" antigen of SV40 sarcoma virus controlled by the rat insulin promoter (*16–18*). In these mice, approximately 70% of the pancreatic islets become hyperplastic and 4–10% of the hyperplastic islets become angiogenic at a predictable time (6–7 weeks). Tumors arise from these neovascularized hyperplastic islets and reach $>1{,}000\times$ the volume of the pre-angiogenic islets. The onset of angiogenic activity coincides with the export of aFGF accompanied by other growth factors not completely identified at this writing. The tumor cells also secrete VEGF.

In both models of switching to the angiogenic phenotype more than one angiogenic polypeptide may be involved (*18*). Certain human tumors such as melanoma have been reported to release more than one angiogenic factor (*19*).

Down-regulation of an Angiogenesis Suppressor Gene

The switch to the angiogenic phenotype cannot be simply explained by the export of one or more angiogenic factors out of tumor cells. Other components of the switch appear to be operating concomitantly. For example, in a hamster fibroblast cell line, a fragment of thrombospondin is normally secreted constitutively (*20*, *21*). Thrombospondin is an inhibitor of endothelial proliferation and of angiogenesis. However, during carcinogenesis of the fibroblasts, there is a 10-fold decrease in the secretion of thrombospondin, associated with inactivation of a suppressor gene which normally codes for this protein. An increase in angiogenic activity coincides with the decrease in secretion of the angiogenesis inhibitor. It is not known whether these tumor cells also release a separate angiogenic stimulator. Nevertheless, this model system may be a paradigm for other tumors where loss of negative regulators of angiogenesis is associated with increased angiogenicity and increased tumorigenicity.

Amplification of Angiogenic Activity

If the switch to the angiogenic phenotype depends upon export (or increased secretion) of an angiogenic polypeptide coupled with decreased secretion of an angiogenesis inhibitor, the resultant angiogenic activity may also be amplified or potentiated by other mechanisms. For example: (i) Certain tumors attract macrophages and activate them to secrete angiogenic factors (*22*). (ii) Other tumors release heparanases or collagenases which can mobilize bFGF from its storage sites in extracellular matrix (*23*, *39*). (iii) Some tumor cells are chemotactic to mast cells (*24*) which may release heparin. Heparin can mobilize FGF (*25*), protect FGF from degradation (*26*, *27*), increase endothelial cell motility and proliferation (*28*, *29*), and facilitate binding of FGF to its receptor on endothelial cells (*30*). (iv) The vascular endothelial cells of certain human tumors, such as colon carcinoma and neuroblastoma, contain an overabundance of bFGF compared to the endothelial cells in other tumors (*31*). This finding suggests that these tumors release some unknown mediator which stimulates excessive production of bFGF by local endothelial cells.

Inhibition of the Angiogenic Phenotype

Once the mechanisms for switching to the angiogenic phenotype are more completely understood, it may be possible to therapeutically interfere with this switch. Currently available angiogenesis inhibitors (*39*) are directed mainly at inhibition of endothelial proliferation or migration, *i.e.*, the principal target cell of angiogenic activity. There is as yet no known method to turn off the source of angiogenic activity. It may be fruitful, however, to review the possible points of attack for angiogenesis inhibitors in antiangiogenic therapy of cancer, in order to develop

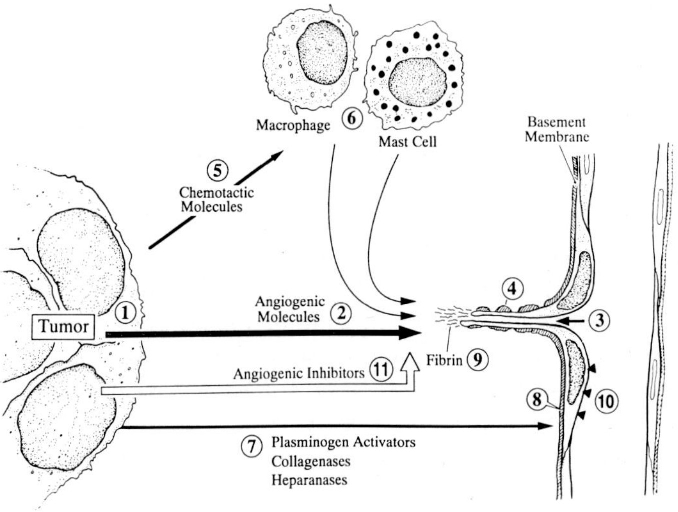

FIG. 3. Diagram of mechanisms likely to be involved in tumor angiogenesis and which may be targets for antiangiogenic therapy. See text for description. (From ref. *41* with permission of the publisher.)

drugs which operate at these points. Thus, an angiogenesis inhibitor could be directed against any of the following components of the angiogenic process (Fig. 3):

1. Pathways for export of angiogenic molecules from tumor cells.
2. Angiogenic molecules in transit.
3. Endothelial cell migration and/or proliferation.
4. Basement membrane production and degradation by endothelial cells of newly formed capillaries.
5. Tumor-derived factors that are chemotactic for macrophages or mast cells.
6. Angiogenic factors or angiogenic amplifiers secreted by macrophages and/or mast cells.
7. Tumor-derived (or endothelial-derived) plasminogen activators, collagenases, and heparanases (*32–35*).
8. bFGF stored in basement membrane (*36*).
9. Hypermeability of the neovascular bed (which leads to leakage of fibrin products into the extravascular space, among other effects) (*37*).
10. Endothelial markers by which to target tumor vasculature (*38*).
11. Endogenous inhibitors of endothelial cell growth secreted by the tumor (*20, 21*), or normally present in the circulation, or in adjacent tissues. (Augmentation of such endogenous inhibitors would be the antiangiogenic approach here).

To develop antiangiogenic therapy for clinical trial, it is useful to categorize these components under two central mechanisms of tumor angiogenesis: I) Switch to the angiogenic phenotype during tumorigenesis (*1, 2, 5–8, 11*) and II) Vascular endothelial cell response to stimulation by angiogenic factors (*3, 4, 9, 10*).

It is also apparent that pathological angiogenesis in non-neoplastic diseases such as psoriasis, ocular neovascularizations, hemangiomas, and arthritis may be treatable by the same angiogenesis inhibitors used for anti-cancer therapy. Therefore, the information gained from studying the switch to the angiogenic phenotype in neoplasia (*40*) may eventually help us to understand how angiogenesis is activated in angiogenic diseases, and how it may be controlled.

REFERENCES

1. Folkman, J. What is the evidence that tumors are angiogenesis dependent? J. Natl. Cancer Inst., *82(1)*: 4–6, 1990.
2. Liotta, L., Kleinerman, J., and Saidel, G. Quantitative relationships of intravascular tumor cells, tumor vessels, and pulmonary metastases following tumor implantation. Cancer Res., *34*: 997–1004, 1974.
3. Folkman, J. Tumor angiogenesis. *In*; Cancer Medicine, J. F., Holland, E. Frei, R. C. Bast, D. W. Kufe, D. L. Morton, and R. R. Weichselbaum, (eds.), Lea & Febiger, Melbourne, Pennsylvania, in press.
4. Studzinskie, G. P., Moore, D. C., and Carter, D. L. Suppressor genes: Restraint of growth or of tumor progression? Lab. Invest., *63(3)*: 279–282, 1990.
5. Vogelstein, B., Fearon, E. R., Kern, S. E., Hamilton, S. R., Preisinger, A. C., Nakamura, Y., and White, R. Allelotype of colorectal carcinomas. Science, *244(4901)*: 207–211, 1989.
6. Srivastava, A., Laidler, P., Hughes, L. E., Woodcock, J., and Shedden, E. J. Neovascularization in human cutaneous melanoma: a quantitative morphological and

Doppler ultrasound study. Eur. J. Cancer Clin. Oncol., *22(10)*: 1205–1209, 1986.

7. Sillman, F., Boyce, J., and Fruchter, R. The significance of atypical vessels and neovascularization in cervical neoplasia. Am. J. Obstet. Gynecol., *139*: 154–159, 1981.
8. Weidner, N., Semple, J. P., Welch, W. R., and Folkman, J. Tumor angiogenesis correlates with metastasis in invasive breast carcinoma. N. Engl. J. Med., *324*: 1–8, 1991.
9. Jensen, H. M. Angiogenesis induced by normal human breast tissue. *In*; Angiogenesis —Mechanisms and Pathobiology. Current Communications in Molecular Biology, D. B. Rifkin and M. Klagsbrun (eds.), pp. 155–157, Cold Spring Harbor Laboratory, New York, 1987.
10. Folkman, J. and Klagsbrun, M. Angiogenic factors. Science, *235*: 442–447, 1987.
11. Folkman, J. and Shing, Y. Angiogenesis. J. Biol. Chem., *267*: 10931–10934, 1992.
12. Hanahan, D. Dissecting multistep tumorigenesis in transgenic mice. Annu. Rev. Genet., *22*: 479–519, 1988.
13. Hanahan, D. Transgenic mice as probes into complex systems. Science, *246*: 1265–1275, 1989.
14. Lacey, M., Albert, S., and Hanahan, D. The bovine papilloma virus genome elicits skin tumours in transgenic mice. Nature, *322*: 609–612, 1986.
15. Kandel, J., Bossy-Wetzel, E., Radvanyi, F., Klagsbrun, M., Folkman, J., and Hanahan, D. Neovascularization is associated with a switch to the export of bFGF in the multistep development of fibrosarcoma. Cell, *65*: 1095–1104, 1991.
16. Hanahan, D. Heritable formation of pancreatic beta-cell tumors in transgenic mice expressing recombinant insulin/simian virus 40 oncogenes. Nature, *315(6015)*: 115–122, 1985.
17. Teitelman, G., Alpert, S., and Hanahan, D. Proliferation, senescence and neoplastic progression of β-cells in hyperplastic pancreatic islets. Cell, *52(1)*: 97–105, 1988.
18. Folkman, J., Watson, K., Ingber, D., and Hanahan, D. Induction of angiogenesis during the transition from hyperplasia to neoplasia. Nature, *339*: 58–61, 1989.
19. Herlyn, M., Clark, W. H., Rodeck, U., Mancianti, M. L., Jambrosic, J., and Koprowski, H. Biology of tumor progression in human melanocytes. Lab. Invest., *56(5)*: 461–474, 1987.
20. Rastinejad, F., Polverini, P. F., and Bouck, N. P. Regulation of the activity of a new inhibitor of angiogenesis by a cancer suppressor gene. Cell, *56*: 345–355, 1989.
21. Bouck, N. Tumor angiogenesis: the role of oncogenes and tumor suppressor genes. Cancer Cells, *2 (6)*: 179–185, 1990.
22. Polverini, P. J. and Leibovich, S. J. Induction of neovascularization *in vivo* and endothelial proliferation *in vitro* by tumor-associated macrophages. Lab. Invest., *51(6)*: 635–642, 1984.
23. Vlodavsky, I., Korner, G., Ishai-Michaeli, R., Bashkin, P., Bar-Shavit, R., and Fuks, Z. Extracellular matrix-resident growth factors and enzymes: possible involvement in tumor metastasis and angiogenesis. Cancer Metast. Rev., *9(3)*: 203–226, 1990.
24. Dethlefsen, S. M., Matsuura, N., and Zetter, B. R. Tumor growth and angiogenesis in wild type and mast cell deficient mice. FASEB J., *4(3)*: A263 (Abst. #2070), 1990.
25. Folkman, J., Klagsbrun, M., Sasse, J., Wadzinski, M., Ingber, D. E., and Vlodavsky, I. A heparin-binding angiogenic protein—basic fibroblast growth factor—is stored within basement membrane. Am. J. Pathol., *130*: 393–400, 1988.
26. Gospodarowicz, D. and Cheng, J. Heparin protects basic and acidic FGF from inactivation. J. Cell. Physiol., *128*: 474–484, 1986.
27. Rosengart, T. K., Johnson, W. V., Friesel, R., Clark, R., and Maciag, T. Heparin protects heparin-binding growth factor-I from proteolytic inactivation *in vitro*. Biochem.

Biophys. Res. Commun., *152(1)*: 432–440, 1988.
28. Azizkhan, R., Azizkhan, J., Zetter, B. R., and Folkman, J. Mast cell heparin stimulates migration of capillary endothelial cells *in vitro*. J. Exp. Med., *152*: 931–944, 1980.
29. Thornton, S. C., Mgeller, S. N., and Levine, E. M. Human endothelial cells: use of heparin in cloning and long-term serial cultivation. Science, *222 (4624)*: 623–625, 1983.
30. Yayon, A., Klagsbrun, M., Esko, J. D., Leder, P., and Ornitz, D. M. Cell surface, heparin-like molecules are required for binding of basic fibroblast growth factor to its high affinity receptor. Cell, *64*: 841–848, 1991.
31. Schulze-Osthoff, K., Risau, W., Vollmer, E., and Sorg, C. *In situ* detection of basic fibroblast growth factor by highly specific antibodies. Am. J. Pathol., *137(1)*: 85–92, 1990.
32. Herron, G. S., Banda, M. J., Clark, E. J., Gavrilovic, J., and Werb, Z. Secretion of metalloproteinases by stimulated capillary endothelial cells. J. Biol. Chem., *261*: 2814–2818, 1986.
33. Liotta, L., Steeg, P. S., and Stetlers, W. G. Cancer metastasis and angiogenesis—an imbalance of positive and negative regulation. Review. Cell, *64(2)*: 327–336, 1991.
34. Nakajima, M., Welch, D., Belloni, P. N., and Nicolson, G. L. Degradation of basement membrane type IV collagen and lung subendothelial matrix by rat mammary adenocarcinoma cell clones of differing metastatic potentials. Cancer Res., *47*: 4869–4876, 1987.
35. Pepper, M. S., Bellin, D., Montesano, R., Orci, L., and Vassalli, J. D. Transforming growth factor-beta 1 modulates basic fibroblast growth factor-induced proteolytic and angiogenic properties of endothelial cells *in vitro*. J. Cell Biol., *111(2)*: 743–755, 1990.
36. Vlodavsky, I., Folkman, J., Sullivan, R., Fridman, R., Ishai-Michaeli, R., Sasse, J., and Klagsbrun, M. Endothelial cell-derived basic fibroblast growth factor: synthesis and deposition into subendothelial matrix. Proc. Natl. Acad. Sci. U.S.A., *84*: 2292–2296, 1987.
37. Dvorak, H. F., Nagy, J. A., and Dvorak, A. M. Structure of solid tumors and their vasculature—implications for therapy with monoclonal antibodies (review). Cancer Cells, *3(3)*: 77–85, 1991.
38. Denekamp, J. and Hill, S. Angiogenic attack as a therapeutic strategy for cancer. Radiother. Oncol., *20* (Suppl.): 102–112, 1991.
39. Ingber, D., Fujita, T., Kishimoto, S., Sudo, K., Kanamaru, T., Brem, H., and Folkman, J. Synthetic analogues of fumagillin that inhibit angiogenesis and suppress tumour growth. Nature, *348(6301)*: 555–557, 1990.
40. Folkman, J. and Hanahan, D. Expression of the angiogenic phenotype during development of murine and human cancer. *In*; J. Brugge, T. Curran, E. Harrow, and F. McCormick (eds.), Origins of Human Cancer: A Comprehensive Review, pp. 803–814, Cold Spring Harbor Laboratory Press, New York, 1991.
41. Folkman, J. Angiogenesis—retrospect and outlook. *In*; R. Steiner, P. B. Weisz, and R. Langer (eds.), Angiogenesis. Key principles-Science-Technology-Medicine, pp. 4–13, Birkhauser-Verlag, Basel, Boston, 1992.

MULTISTAGE CARCINOGENESIS, C. C. HARRIS ET AL. (EDS.),
JAPAN SCI. SOC. PRESS, TOKYO/CRC PRESS, BOCA RATON, PP. 349–360, 1992

Multistep Hepatocarcinogenesis in Transgenic Mice Harboring SV40 T-Antigen Gene

Tomoyuki KITAGAWA,*1 Okio HINO,*2 Gang-Hong LEE,*1 Hong LI,*1 Jia LIU,*1 Kimie NOMURA,*1 Keiko OHTAKE,*1 Yasuhide FURUTA,*3 and Shinichi AIZAWA*3

*Department of Pathology,*1 Department of Experimental Pathology,*2 Cancer Institute, Tokyo 170, Japan and Laboratory of Molecular Oncology, Tsukuba Life Science Center, Institute of Physical and Chemical Research (Riken), Tsukuba, Ibaraki, 305, Japan*3*

Abstract: We have developed transgenic mice that inherit albumin promoter-regulated simian virus 40 (SV40) large T-antigen gene, expressed specifically in hepatocytes. These mice all develop multifocal hepatocellular carcinomas (HCCs) at around 5 months and die of liver insufficiency by 7 months in remarkable synchrony. The liver tissue appears normal in the initial 3 weeks, and thereafter rapid cytomegalic degeneration of original hepatocytes, proliferation of quasi-regenerative hepatocytes, neoplastic cell foci, nodules and finally HCCs develop in sequence. Considerable variation existed both in morphological and enzymatic features and in T-antigen expression among neoplastic lesions, including carcinomas. Oligonucleotide hybridization studies revealed activating point mutations of the c-H-*ras* oncogene in 40% (10/25) of tumors obtained at around 6 months. The positive signals were, however, considerably weaker in half of them suggesting that such tumors comprised cells both with and without *ras* mutation. Sequential observation of culture cell lines established from tumors also revealed the appearance of activated c-H-*ras* with time, which was associated with biological progression. Thus, in this model system, *ras* activation may be an event occurring in a relatively late phase of carcinogenesis associated with progression of tumors. Karyotype analysis of cell lines revealed remarkable chromosomal instability. In studies of sister chromatid exchange in hepatocytes, twice as frequent occurrence was demonstrated in transgenic mice as in their counterpart hepatocytes. Thus T-antigen may be contributing as a mutagen to the hepatocarcinogenesis, in addition to its cytotoxic and growth modifying activities.

Simian virus 40 (SV40) T-antigen is well known to be a very potent viral transforming protein which immortalizes and transforms cells in culture (*1–3*) and causes malignant tumors in transgenic mice (*4–7*). T-antigen alone, however, appears insufficient for causing true malignant change, because in culture a long period time is required for the immortalized cells to acquire true malignant potential and in transgenic mice there is a multistep carcinogenesis.

We also produced a transgenic mouse line carrying an albumin promoter-regulated SV40 T-antigen gene expressed specifically in hepatocytes. As described previously (*8*, *9*) this transgenic mouse (T-mouse) revealed a distinct multistep progression of hepatocarcinogenesis, resulting in mutiple hepatocellular carcinomas at around 6 months with amazing synchrony. Since no exogenous carcinogen is given in drastic fashion as seen in the "initiation" procedure in chemical carcinogenesis, this mouse provides a useful system for anlyzing the underlying mechanisms of multistep carcinogenesis.

Generation of Transgenic Mouse

A transgene of the structure illustrated in Fig. 1 was microinjected into male pronuclei of F2 zygote between B6 and SJL mice. The generated T-mouse has a single integration site of the transgene which specifically expressed in hepatocytes. Descendants of the T-mouse have been produced by crossing with normal B6 or C3H female.

Sequential Morphological and Biochemical Observation of Hepatocarcinogenesis

Up to the end of the 2nd week of age, no recognizable histological change was observed in the T-mouse liver in comparison with the normal counterpart (non-transgenic littermate), although T-antigen was clearly expressed in all of the hepatocyte nuclei (Fig. 2). Mitotic indices of T-mouse and normal mouse hepatocytes at the end of the 2nd week were about the same, 0.330+0.063 and 0.395+0.087%, respectively.

During the 3rd week, hepatocytes with enlarged nuclei began to appear randomly in the lobules, and this cytomegalic change became prominent in most hepatocytes in subsequent weeks (Fig. 3). Many abnormal mitoses and necrotic single cells were scattered, reflected in the high serum transaminase level (700–800 IU of GOT and GPT). Nuclei of the cytomegalic cells were huge and often bizarre in shape with coarse granular heterochromatin and multiple small nucleoli. Although the atypia of these cells was striking, they did not behave as malignant cells, and the normal architecture of the liver tissue was maintained. T-antigen was demonstrated weakly in the nuclei.

From 7 weeks onwards, foci of quasi-regenerative hepatocytes appeared ran-

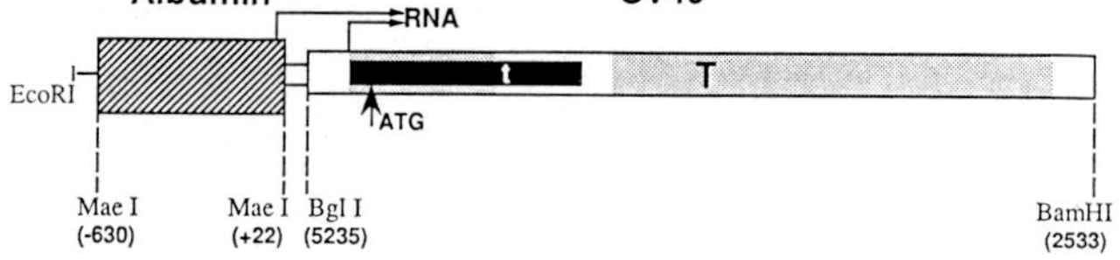

FIG. 1. Structure of the hybrid albumin-SV40 T-antigen gene. The hatched box denotes mouse albumin promoter gene and the open box SV40 early gene, in which the coding sequences of large T- and small t-antigen genes are indicated by the striped and the filled boxes, respectively. The restriction sites are given as the sites in the original DNA clones for each unit with base numbers in parenthesis. Transcription and translation start sites are also indicated.

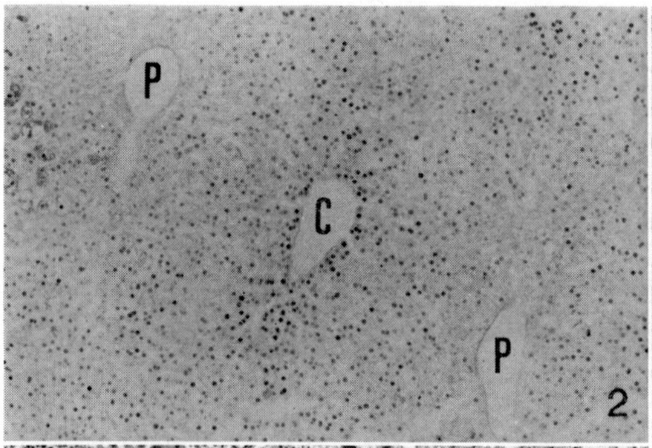

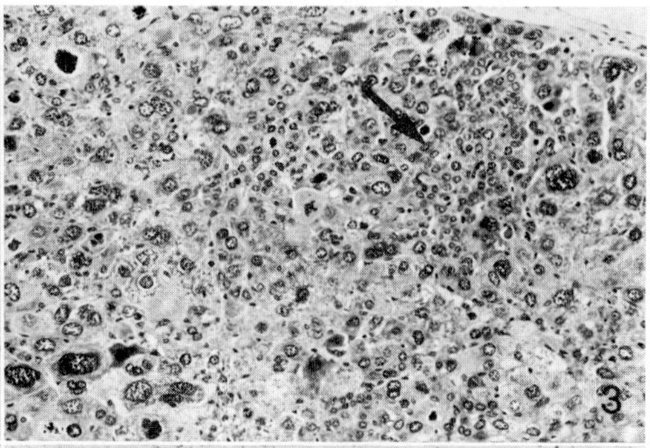

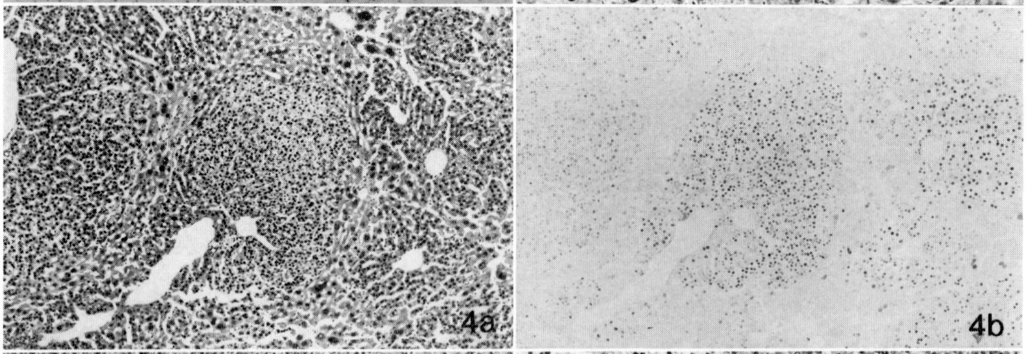

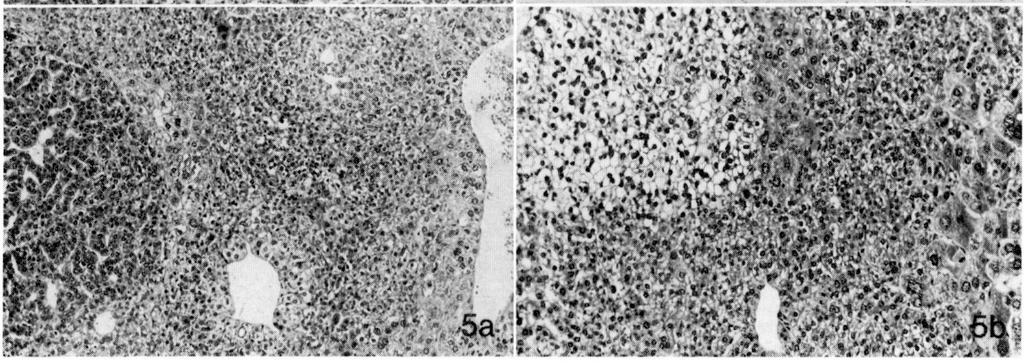

FIG. 2. Immunohistochemical demonstration of SV40 T-antigen in the liver of T-mouse at 3 weeks of age. Nuclei of all the hepatocytes are stained positive. Note the normality of the liver tissue with uniform size of hepatocyte nuclei. The nuclei located around the central vein (C) show stronger reaction. P indicates the portal vein. ×120.

FIG. 3. Liver of T-mouse at 7 weeks of age showing striking cytomegalic change of hepatocytes. Note scattered atypical mitotic figures and a tiny focus of quasi-regenerative hepatocytes with small nuclei (arrowhead). HE, ×150.

FIG. 4. (a) Liver of T-mouse at 12 weeks of age. Foci of quasi-regenerative hepatocytes are replacing the cytomegalic hepatocytes. HE, ×50. (b) A serial section showing distinct expression of T-antigen in quasi-regenerative hepatocytes and very weak reaction in cytomegalic original cells.

FIG. 5. Liver of T-mouse at 12 weeks of age showing foci comprised of basophilic cells (a) or clear cells (b), with background of regenerative and cytomegalic hepatocytes. HE, ×100 and ×150, respectively.

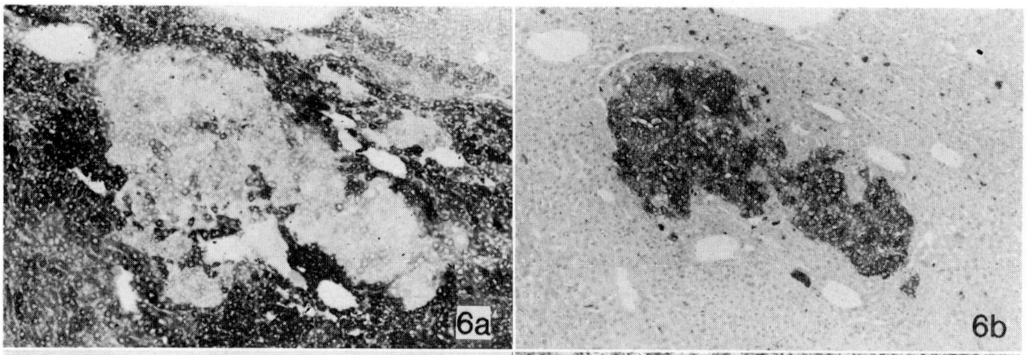

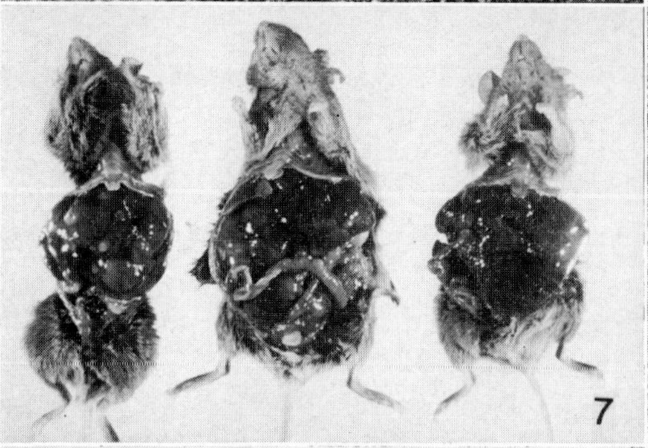

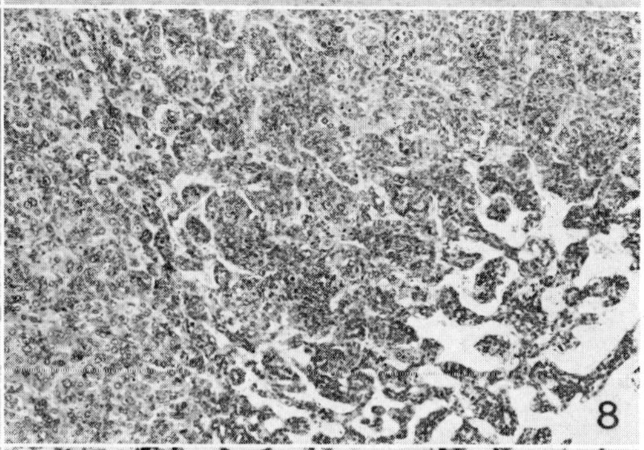

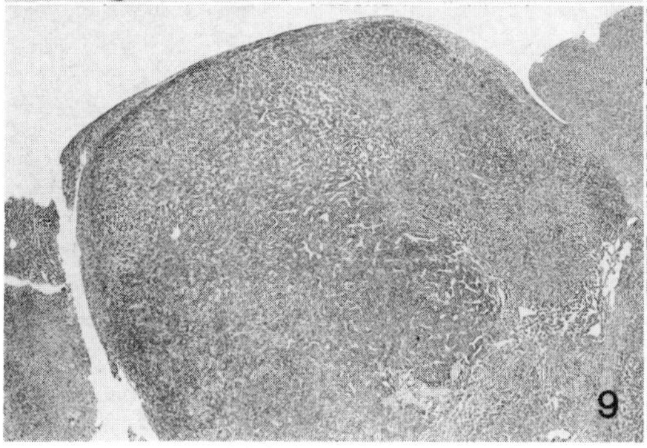

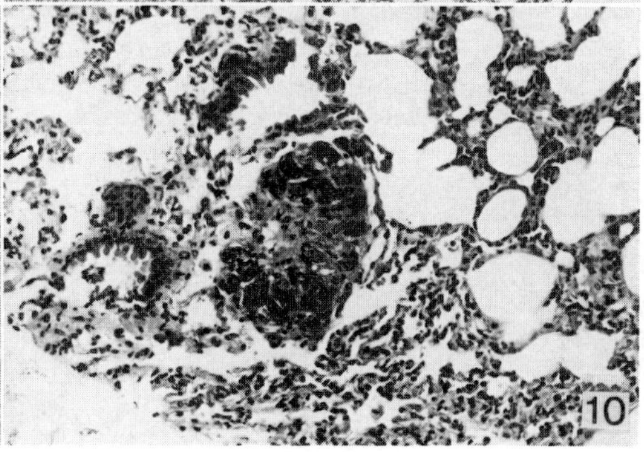

FIG. 6. Pictures showing a G-6-P-deficient (a) and GGT-positive focus (b) developed by 12 weeks of age. Serial section. HE, ×75.

FIG. 7. Macroscopical liver tumors developed in T-mice by 24 weeks of age.

FIG. 8. Histology of a hepatocellular carcinoma. HE, ×150.

FIG. 9. Hepatocellular carcinoma developing in a nodular lesion less malignant in histological appearance. HE, ×15.

FIG. 10. Microscopic foci of pulmonary metastasis seen in a mouse at 24 weeks of age. HE, ×200.

domly in the hepatic lobules (Fig. 3, arrowhead), rapidly replacing the cytomegalic hepatocytes so that most of the liver tissue was replaced by the new cells by 12 weeks (Fig. 4a). T-antigen was expressed in these cells to the same degree as seen in the original hepatocytes in the initial weeks, whereas it was very weak or not demonstrated in the original hepatocyte-derived cytomegalic cells at this phase (Fig. 4b). Neither ductal nor periportal "oval cell" proliferation was observed.

From 11 weeks of age, foci showing a distinctly nodular growth pattern appeared.

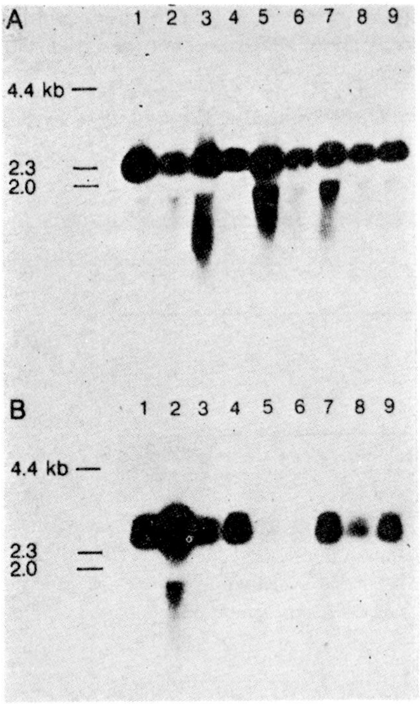

FIG. 11. Northern blot study on expression of albumin (A) and T-antigen (B) in HCCs. 1. Non-tumorous liver of a 24-week old transgenic mouse. 2–9. HCCs.

They were comprised of eosinophilic, basophilic, or clear cells with some structural atypia (Fig. 5a and 5b). While regenerative hepatocytes showed normal levels of glucose-6-phosphatase (G-6-P) activity, the cells of foci were characterized by reduced levels of this enzyme (Fig. 6a), or occasionally by the appearance of γ-glutamyltranspeptidase (GGT) activity (Fig. 6b), reminiscent of altered cell foci seen in rodent chemical carcinogenesis (*10*). In these foci, T-antigen was expressed generally at a moderate level but occasionally at higher or reduced levels. The lesions consisting of hepatocytes with eosinophilic hepatocytes tended to show reduced levels, or absence, of T-antigen expression.

From around 20 weeks of age, gross hepatic tumors developed and the animals died by 7 months with bulky liver, more than 10 times normal size, filled with numerous tumors measuring up to 30 mm in diameter (Fig. 7). Many of the tumors were composed of cells similar to those of foci, but there were also overt hepatocellular carcinomas (HCCs) showing distinct cellular and structural atypia (Fig. 8). Occasionally nodule-in-nodule and/or cancer-in-nodule patterns were observed (Fig. 9). Microscopic pulmonary metastases were detected, though infrequently (Fig. 10).

A tendency toward cytomegalic change was also seen in some of the quasi-regenerative and neoplastic cells, but it was generally much less conspicuous than that seen in the original hepatocytes. T-antigen measured by mRNA level was variable among gross nodules and HCCs (Fig. 11).

These sequential observations were consistent in subsequent generations and were not influenced by the sex of the host. Non-transgenic littermates did not show

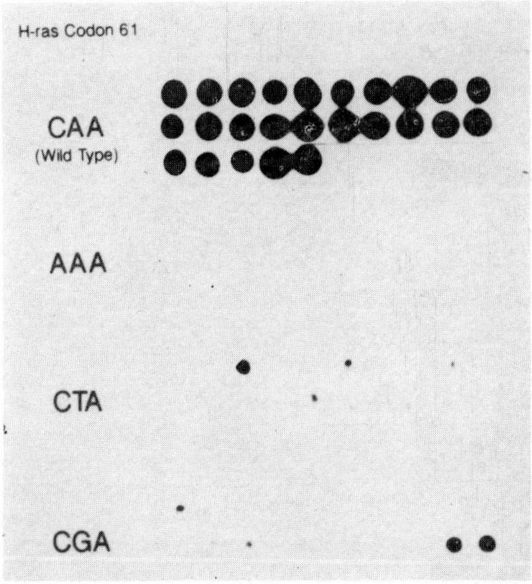

FIG. 12. Oligonucleotide hybridization analysis of c-H-*ras* codon 61. While all 25 HCC samples reacted strongly to wild type probe (CAA), 4 and 6 of them, respectively, gave positive signals when hybridized with probes having CTA or CGA type mutations.

any significant histological abnormalities up to at least one year of age.

The above observations are in good concert with others describing hepatocarcinogenesis in SV40 T- antigen-harboring mice (*4–7*), although the time span for development of tumors varied and in our system the initial "hyperplasia" described by others was not impressive.

H-ras Gene Activation during Carcinogenesis

Since activating point mutations of c-H-*ras* at codon 61 are very commonly seen in both spontaneous (*11*) and chemically induced (*12, 13*) mouse HCCs, we studied the *ras* gene mutation in HCCs developing in the T-mouse at around 24 weeks (*14*).

DNA fragments around codon 61 of mouse c-H-*ras* were amplified from 10 μ sections of formalin-fixed and paraffin-embedded HCC specimen by polymerase chain reaction (PCR) utilizing primers described by Buchmann *et al.* (*15*). Oligonucleotide hybridization was performed using synthetic 19 mer antisense single-stranded DNA probes according to the method described by Verlaan-de Vries *et al.* (*16*).

The results of the study are shown in Fig. 12. In total, 25 HCCs were analyzed. Strong signals were observed for the wild-type CAA probe for all samples. Activated forms of c-H-*ras* were detected in 10 HCCs. Four out of these 10 cases contained an A-to-T conversion at the second position of the codon 61, an A-to-G conversion at the same position being observed in the other six HCCs.

A noteworthy finding was that individual intensities of the mutated allele signals were significantly different among the positive samples even on one filter. To exclude the possibility that these differences were caused by amplification of one of the c-H-*ras* alleles, high molecular weight DNAs extracted from mutation-positive tumors

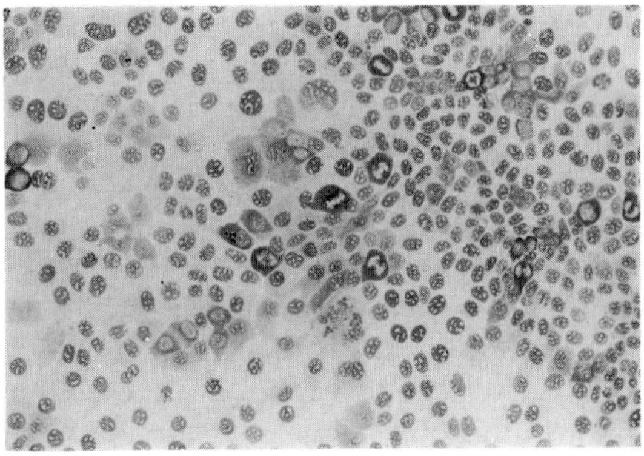

FIG. 13. T-antigen expression in a cell line derived from a HCC (TH-1). T-antigen is commonly localized in hepatocyte nuclei but at mitosis it shifts to cytoplasm. Immunohistochemistry utilizing monoclonal antibody against T-antigen (gift of Dr. N. Yamaguchi) and an ABC kit. ×30.

TABLE 1. Biological and Molecular Properties of SV40-T-mouse Liver Cell Lines in Early and Late Passages

Origin	No. of lines	Early passages				Late passages[a]			
		Soft agar	Nude	Tf.A[b]	*ras*	Soft agar	Nude	Tf.A	*ras*
HCC (24 weeks)	9: 4	+	+	+	+	+	+	+	+
	2	+	+	−	−	+	+	+	−
	3	−	−	−	−	+	+	+	+
Hepatocyte (3–12 weeks)	10: 9	−	−	−	−	−	−	−	−
	1	−	−	−	−	−	−	−	+[c]

[a] Over 20 passages (6 months). [b] Tf.A: transforming activity in SHOK transfection assay. [c] Very weak.

were digested with the restriction enzyme *Bam*HI and analyzed by Southern blotting using a v-H-*ras* probe. Neither amplification nor loss of c-H-*ras* was detectable in any of the samples (data not shown).

To confirm further the specificity and presence of the point mutations, oligonucleotide hybridization was performed for PCR products after digestion with the restriction enzymes *Xba*I or *Taq*I. An A-to-T or A-to-G conversion at the second position of c-H-*ras* codon 61 creates *Xba*I or *Taq*I sites, respectively (*13*), and the positive signals in each case disappeared after digestion with the appropriate enzyme (data not shown).

The study thus demonstrated that mutational activation of c-H-*ras* at codon 61 is also frequent in HCCs developed in T-mouse, the type of point mutation being not specifically different from those seen in spontaneous or chemically-induced mouse HCCs (*21, 22*). Since no amplification or loss of c-H-*ras* sequence was observed in the mutation positive tumors, the weak signal may imply that such tumors comprised cells both with and without *ras* mutation, in other words a mixed population of tumor cells at stages before and after "progression". We have previously shown that activated ras was not necessary for immortalization of mouse liver epithelial cells derived from "normal" C3H mouse but that it was able to convert the immortal cells into HCCs by transfection (*17, 18*).

In an attempt to confirm the ras activation-associated progression in HCCs, we made many hepatocytic cell lines derived from HCCs and liver of young animals (3–12 weeks) and carried out sequential observations over 20 passages (6 months) *in vitro* (*15*, *19*). A representative cell line derived from a HCC (TH-1), immunohistochemically stained for T-antigen, is shown in Fig. 13.

The results are summarized in Table 1. Among 9 cell lines established from HCCs, 4 showed growth capabilities in both soft agar and in nude mice from the beginning, as well as H-*ras* activation and transforming activity in the SHOK cell transfection assay (*20*). A further 2 HCC lines were positive in the two biological tests and also in transforming activity from the first, but remained negative for H-*ras* activation all along. In the case of the remaining 3 HCC cell lines which had been negative for all four features at early stages of culture, progression was evident in association with the appearance of ras point mutation in the later passages. Increment of the growth rate was seen not only in terms of passages but also in a shortening of the latent period required for tumor growth after transplantation. Progression was also evidenced by morphological changes. In contrast to the findings with the HCC cell lines, the 10 cell lines orignating from livers of young animals showed no growth capabilities in soft agar or nude mice throughout the experimental period. Only one of them revealed a weakly positive signal for H-*ras* point mutation at the 38th generation when the probe for CTA-type mutation was used.

The data from this study thus demonstrated the simultaneous occurrence of *ras* activation and appearance of transforming activity in HCC cell lines. Thus H-*ras* activation may be an event occurring in the late stage of hepatocarcinogenesis in the T-mouse.

Chromosomal Instability in T-mouse Hepatocytes

Karyotype analysis was carried out concerning 3 cell lines established from HCCs and 2 lines derived from young animal liver (*21*). Part of the results together with biological features of cell lines are shown in Table 2. About 10 metaphases were karyotyped from each cell line, in which modal chromosome numbers varied from one cell line to another with aneuploidies from pseudotriploid to pseudohexaploid. No cell demonstrated a normal chromosome pattern. Karyotype variation including a multitude of gains and losses of different chromosomes was remarkable not only between cell lines but also among cells from one and the same line. Among 60 karyotyped cells from the five cell lines, no two cells with exactly the same karyotype could be found. All of this indicated that genetic abnormalities occur very frequently in T-mouse hepatocytes.

It has been suggested that T-antigen may exert mutagenic effects, in addition to its cytotoxic and growth stimulating activities, which could contribute to the chromosomal instability and, further, to the multistep progression of carcinogenesis (*22*, *23*). In an attempt to assess the mutagenicity of T-antigen, we studied the rates of sister chromatic exchange (SCE) and gross chromosomal aberration in T-mouse hepatocytes at 16–18 days of age when no nuclear atypia are visible morphologically. Hepatocytes were obtained through collagenase perfusion from T-mouse and nontransgenic littermates and cultured in the presence of bromodeoxyuridine. A representative picture of SCEs seen in a tetraploid metaphase cell is shown in

TABLE 2. General Features of the Established SV40-T-mouse Liver Cell Lines

Cell line	Age of animals (weeks)[a]	Passage checked	Growth in nude mice	Growth in soft agar	H-*ras* activation	Karyotype	Translocation		Deletion	
							Type	Frequency	Incidence/cell	Frequency
T101	3	6	—	—	—	Pseudotriploid	t (15, 1)	6/9	1	8/9
T48-1	7	14	—	—	—	Pseudotriploid	—	—	—	—
TH22-1a	24	38	+	+	A^{182}-T	Pseudotetraploid	t (15, ?)	10/11	1	10/11
TH23-2a	24	30	+	+	A^{182}-T	Pseudotriploid	t (?, X)	3/14	1 or 2	10/14
TH-1	22	42	+	+	A^{182}-T	Pseudohexaploid	t (5, ?)	3/16	2–4	14/16

[a] The time at which the hepatocytes were obtained for culture.

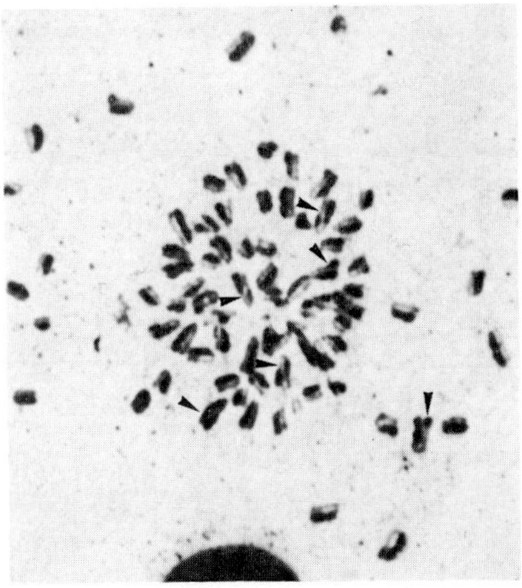

FIG. 14. Representative picture showing many SCEs, part of them pointed out by arrows, seen in tetraploid hepatocytes incubated with BrdU during the initial 24 hr in culture and maintained without BrdU for another 24 hr. ×180.

TABLE 3. Frequency of SCE and Karyotype Abnormality

Animal	SV40-T	Diploid cells		Tetraploid cells	
		SCE/cell	KA[a]	SCE/cell	KA[a]
1	+	12.6±4.2 (20)[b]	0	20.0±5.4 (12)[b]	0
2	+	13.3±6.8 (21)	0	23.0±6.3 (12)	0
3	+	12.3±3.6 (27)	0	21.3±3.6 (12)	0
4	+	13.4±3.7 (29)	0	20.3±4.5 (12)	0
Average[c]		13.0±4.6 (97)	0	21.2±4.9 (48)	0
1	—	7.9±3.0 (20)	0	10.8±2.0 (12)	0
2	—	7.4±2.9 (24)	0	12.0±1.5 (11)	0
3	—	7.1±3.0 (22)	0	10.1±3.3 (8)	0
4	—	7.1±4.2 (15)	0	11.1±3.7 (14)	0
Average[c]		7.4±3.3 (81)	0	11.0±2.6 (45)	0

[a] No. of cells with karyotype abnormality.
[b] Total metaphases analyzed.
[c] $p<0.01$.

Fig. 14 and the results of investigations are summarized in Table 3. SCE was seen in T-mouse hepatocytes twice as frequently as in the normal counterpart. No karyotype abnormalities in terms of numerical change or gross aberration were detected at this phase. The results thus indicated mutagenic properties of T-antigen.

Acknowledgments

This work was supported in part by Grants-in-Aid for Cancer Research from the Ministry of Education, Science and Culture and the Ministry of Health and Welfare of Japan, and Research Grants from the Princess Takamatsu Cancer Research Fund and the Vehicle Racing Commemorative Foundation.

REFERENCES

1. Woodworth, D. D., Kreider, J. W., Mengel, L., Miller, T., Meng, Y., and Isom, H. C. Tumorigenicity of simian virus 40-hepatocyte cell lines: effect of *in vitro* and *in vivo* passage on expression of liver-specific genes and oncogenes. Mol. Cell Biol., *8*: 4492–4501, 1988.
2. Rhim, J. S., Jay, G., Arnstein, P., Price, F. M., Sanford, K. K., and Aaronson, S. A. Neoplastic transformation of human epidermal keratinocytes by AD12-SV40 and Kirsten sarcoma viruses. Science, *227*: 1250–1252, 1985.
3. Lanford, R. E., Wong, C., and Butel, J. S. Differential ability of a T-antigen transport-defective mutant of simian virus 40 to transform primary and established rodent cells. Mol. Cell Biol., *5*: 1043–1050, 1985.
4. Dyer, K. R. and Messing, A. Metal-inducible pathology in the liver, pancreas, and kidney of transgenic mice expressing SV40 early region genes. Am. J. Pathol., *135*: 401–410, 1989.
5. Held, W. A., Mullins, J. J., Kuhn, N. J., Gallagher, J. F., Gu, D. G., and Gross, K. W. T antigen expression and tumorigenesis in transgenic mice containing a mouse major urinary protein/SV40 T antigen hybrid gene. EMBO J., *8*: 183–191, 1989.
6. Sepulveda, A. R., Finegold, M. J., Smith, B., Slagle, B. L., Demayo, J. L., Shen, R. F., Woo, S. L., and Butel, J. S. Development of a transgenic mouse system for the analysis of stages in liver carcinogenesis using tissue-specific expression of SV40 large T-antigen controlled by regulatory elements of the human α-1-antitrypsin gene. Cancer Res., *49*: 6108–6117, 1989.
7. Sandgren, E. P., Quaife, C. J., Pinkert, C. A., Palmiter, R. D., and Brinster, R. L. Oncogene-induced liver neoplasia in transgenic mice. Oncogene, *4*: 715–724, 1989.
8. Hino, O., Kitagawa, T., Nomura, K., Ohtake, K., Furuta, Y., and Aizawa, S. Sequential morphological observation of hepatocarcinogenesis in transgenic mice of albumin promoter-SV40 large T antigen gene. Proc. Jpn. Cancer Assoc., 48th Annu. Meet., 49, 1989.
9. Hino, O., Kitagawa, T., Nomura, K., Ohtake, K., Cui, L., Furuta, Y., and Aizawa, S. Hepatocarcinogenesis in transgenic mice carrying albumin-promoted SV40 T antigen gene. Jpn. J. Cancer Res., *82*: 1226–1233, 1991.
10. Moore, M.A. and Kitagawa, T. Hepatocarcinogenesis in the rat: the effect of promoters and carcinogens *in vivo* and *in vitro*. Int. Rev. Cytol., *101*: 125–173, 1986.
11. Reynolds, S. H., Stowers, S. J., Maronpot, R. R., Anderson, M. W., and Aaronson, S. A. Detection and identification of activated oncogenes in spontaneously occurring benign and malignant hepatocellular tumors of B6C3F1 mouse. Proc. Natl. Acad. Sci. U.S.A., *83*: 33–37, 1986.
12. Balmain, A. and Brown, K. Oncogene activation in chemical carcinogenesis. Adv. Cancer Res., *51*: 147–182, 1988.
13. Wiseman, R. W., Stewart, B. C., Grenier, D., Miller, E. C., and Miller, J. A. Characterization of c-H-*ras* proto-oncogene mutations in chemically induced hepatomas of the B6C3F1 mouse. Proc. Am. Assoc. Cancer Res., *28*: 147, 1987.
14. Lee, G-H., Li, H., Ohtake, K., Nomura, K., Hino, O., Furuta, Y., Aizawa, S., and Kitagawa, T. Detection of activated c-H-*ras* oncogene in hepatocellular carcinomas developed in transgenic mice harboring albumin promoter-regulated simian virus 40 gene. Carcinogenesis, *11*: 1145–1148, 1990.
15. Buchmann, A., Mahr, J., Bauer-Hofmann, R., and Schwarz, M. Mutations at codon 61 of the Ha-*ras* proto-oncogene in precancerous liver lesions of the B6C3F1 mouse. Mol. Carcinogen., *2*: 121–125, 1989.

16. Verlaan-de Vries, M., Bogaard, M. E., van den Elst, H., van Boom, J. H., van der Eb, A. J., and Bos, J. L. A dot-blot screening procedure for mutated ras oncogenes using synthetic oligodeoxynucleotides. Gene, *50*: 313–320, 1986.
17. Lee, G-H., Sawada, N., Mochizuki, Y., Nomura, K., and Kitagawa, T. Immortal epithelial cells of normal C3H mouse liver in culture: possible precursor populations for spontaneous hepatocellular carcinoma. Cancer Res., *49*: 403–409, 1989.
18. Lee, G-H., Sakai, R., Nagao, M., and Kitagawa, T. Role of activated c-H-ras oncogene in the induction and progression of immortal liver epithelium cell lines derived from normal C3H mice. Int. J. Cancer, *47*: 60–65, 1991.
19. Li, H., Liu, J., Nomura, K., Lee, G-H., Hino, O., Ohtake, K., Aizawa, S., and Kitagawa, T. *In vitro* progression-associated c-H-*ras* activation in neoplastic hepatocyte lines established from SV40-T antigen gene-harboring transgenic mice. Jpn. J. Cancer Res., *82*: 4–7, 1991.
20. Higashi, T., Sasai, H., Suzuki, F., Miyoshi, T., Ohuchi, T., Takai, A-I., Mori, T., and Kakunaga, T. Hamster cell line suitable for transfection assay of transforming genes. Proc. Natl. Acad. Sci. U.S.A., *87*: 2409–2413, 1990.
21. Liu, J., Li, H., Nomura, K., Dofuku, R., and Kitagawa, T. Cytogenetic analysis of hepatic cell lines derived from SV40-T antigen gene-harboring transgenic mice. Cancer Genet. Cytogenet., *55*: 207–216, 1991.
22. Ray, F. A., Peabody, D. S., Cooper, J. L., Cram, L. S., and Kraemer, P. M. SV40 T antigen alone drives karyotype instability that precedes neoplastic transformation of human diploid fibroblasts. J. Cell Biochem., *42*: 13–31, 1990.
23. Stewart, N. and Bacchetti, S. Expression of SV40 large T antigen, but not small t antigen, is required for the induction of chromosomal aberrations in transformed human cells. Virology, *180*: 49–57, 1991.

MULTISTAGE CARCINOGENESIS, C. C. HARRIS ET AL. (EDS.),
JAPAN SCI. SOC. PRESS, TOKYO/CRC PRESS, BOCA RATON, PP. 361–370, 1992

Hepatocarcinogenesis in the LEC Rat with Hereditary Hepatitis

Noritoshi TAKEICHI

Laboratory of Pathology, Cancer Institute, Hokkaido University School of Medicine, Sapporo 060, Japan

Abstract: A new mutant developing spontaneous hepatitis and hepatocellular carcinoma has been discovered among Long Evans rats. Hepatitis appears suddenly in the mutant, Long Evans Cinnamon (LEC) rats, three to four months after birth. Characteristic clinical signs of the hepatitis are jaundice, bilirubinuria, subcutaneous bleeding and loss of body weight. The affected rats showed a high mortality and histological changes with focal necrosis of hepatocytes and infiltration of a few inflammatory cells. Genetic studies indicate that a single autosomal recessive gene is responsible for the hepatitis. Long-surviving rats show chronic hepatitis, and subsequently develop hepatocellular carcinoma at one and a half years of age. We recently found an abnormal copper accumulation in the liver of LEC rats prior to development of the hepatitis. Copper concentration in the liver is over 40 times more than that of normal Long Evans Agouti (LEA) rats, whereas the serum ceruloplasmin and copper levels are lower. An excess of toxic-form copper, free copper, will cause DNA damage in the presence of free radicals and oxygen radicals. Such DNA damage by the radicals is considered to be responsible for hepatic necrosis and hepatocellular carcinoma in LEC rats.

The Long Evans Cinnamon (LEC) rat has drawn much attention as an experimental animal model for the study of human liver diseases since it was established at Hokkaido University in 1981. LEC rats offer a clinical course closely resembling that of human hepatic diseases from hepatitis, cirrhosis to fatal liver cancer (*1–3*).

It has been possible to induce hepatitis or liver cancer in the laboratory, which, however, has not enabled us to examine hepatic diseases as incidences in linear sequence. Since LEC rats follow a sequential course from acute hepatitis to chronic hepatitis, cholangiofibrosis (cirrhosis) and eventually to liver cancer, this clinical course gives us an opportunity to examine the liver diseases as they progress.

In this review, I describe the establishment of the LEC rat, its clinical and pathological features of acute hepatitis, chronic hepatitis and liver cancer, and also deal with our most recent finding of abnormal copper accumulation in the liver of the animal and its possible correlation with hepatocarcinogenesis.

TABLE 1. Incidence of Spontaneous Hepatitis between Two Substrains of Long Evans Rats, LEC and LEA Rats

Strain	Sex	No. of diseased rats / No. of rats examined[a] (%)	No. of rats dying / No. of diseased rats (%)	No. of rats / With remission (%)
LEC	F	75/83 (90)	41/75 (55) (128±38)[b]	35/75 (45)
	M	59/67 (88)	32/59 (48) (151±45)[b]	35/67 (52)
LEA	F	0/38	—	—
	M	0/36	—	—

[a] All rats showed jaundice and bilirubinuria. [b] Mean survival days±S.D.

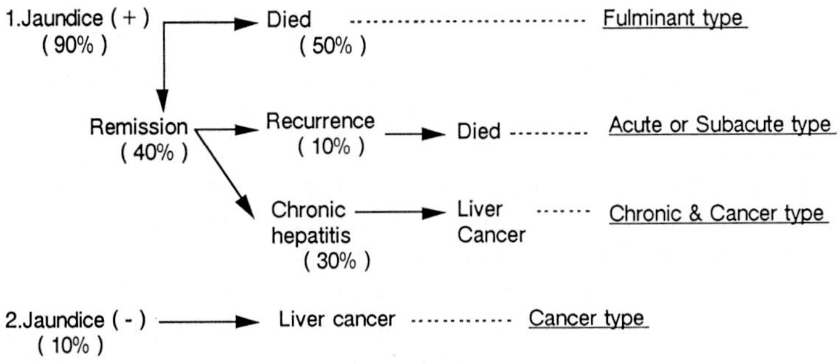

FIG. 1. Clinical course of hepatitis in LEC rats.

Establishment of LEC Rats

From a closed colony of Long Evans (LE) rats, two inbred strains, Long Evans Cinnamon (LEC) and Long Evans Agouti (LEA) rats were isolated according to coat color (*1*). We observed spontaneous development of acute hepatitis only in the LEC rats from the 24th generation onward. As shown in Table 1, between the 24th and 31st generation of brother-sister matings of LEC and LEA rats, 134 (90%) of 150 (male, 67; female, 83) LEC rats born from 26 pregnant mothers spontaneously developed acute hepatitis with predominant jaundice; the remaining 10% also showed subclinical signs of hepatitis.

Clinical Observations

The first conspicuous sign of hepatic disorder in LEC rats is severe jaundice which suddenly appears at the age of 4 months, particularly in the ear and the extremities, followed by body weight loss, anemia, hematurea, oliguria and subcutaneous bleeding. Fifty percent of the rats developing acute hepatitis suffer from complications of kidney failure and die within 2 weeks after hepatitis onset. The death rate is 70% for female and 40% for male. Autopsy reveals bilirubin sedimentation under the peritoneum, intestinal bleeding, atrophied reddish-brown liver, enlarged spleen, and yellowish kidneys. These clinical and pathological findings closely resemble those of human fulminant hepatitis. Forty percent of the LEC rats experience a recession of the disease, but 10% of those surviving die of a recurrence. Forty percent of all LEC rats survive longer than 1 year, and nearly all of the survivors develop hepatocellular carcinoma (Fig. 1).

Laboratory Data

LEC rat hepatitis can be diagnosed by urinary bilirubin test prior to onset of the disease. Chronological changes of urinary bilirubin closely correlate with clinical symptoms. Moreover, the decreased numbers of red blood cells, hemoglobin and platelets are most striking in fulminant cases. Blood coagulation is delayed due to the marked decrease of prothrombin activity in these fulminant cases. Although serum glutamic oxaloacetic transaminase (GOT) and glutamic pyruvic transaminase (GPT) levels remain within their normal ranges until the age of 3 months, they then suddenly rise: GOT level reaches over 2,000 units in all LEC rats with jaundice, and GPT levels also rise. Serum bilirubin levels rise at the onset of jaundice in most cases, some reaching over 60 mg/dl.

Histopathological Findings

Macroscopic and microscopic examinations before the age of 3 months reveal no evidence of either liver atrophy or necrosis of hepatocytes in the liver of LEC rats. Hepatitis-afflicted rats older than 4 months show atrophied livers, enlarged spleens and yellowish kidneys. Hemorrhages are frequently observed in organs, particularly in the gut and the lung. Histological features are: numerous necroses scattered throughout the liver, but only slight inflammatory reactions (Fig. 2); enlarged nuclei and cytoplasm of hepatocytes, some of which have Councilman bodies in the sinusoid area. Many Kupffer cells with phagocytized bile and red blood cells are seen in the sinusoid, whereas a small number of inflammatory cells infiltrate

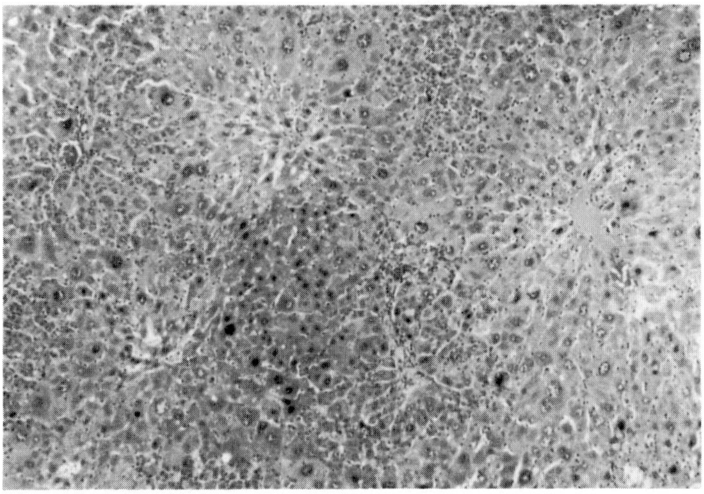

FIG. 2. Section of the liver of a 4-month-old LEC rat with severe jaundice. Focal hepatocyte necrosis with a few inflammatory reactions is seen. Hematoxylin and eosin stain (H&E), ×100

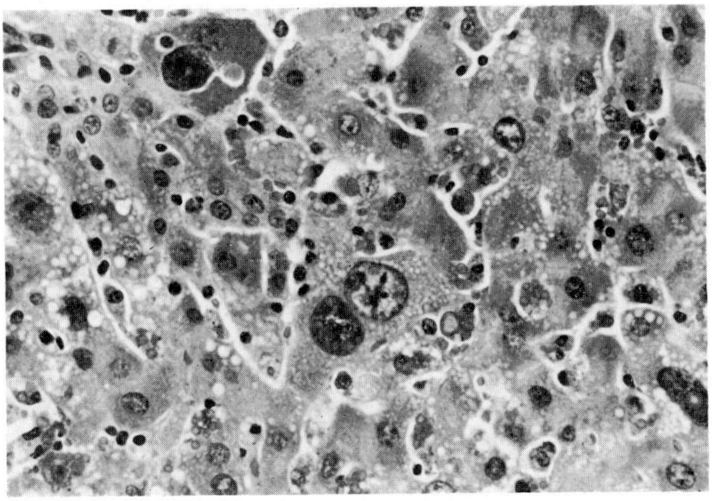

FIG. 3. High power magnification of Fig. 2. The nuclei of hepatocytes are extremely large. Some contain pseudo-inclusion bodies with Councilman bodies; activated Kupffer cells are also visible. H&E, ×200

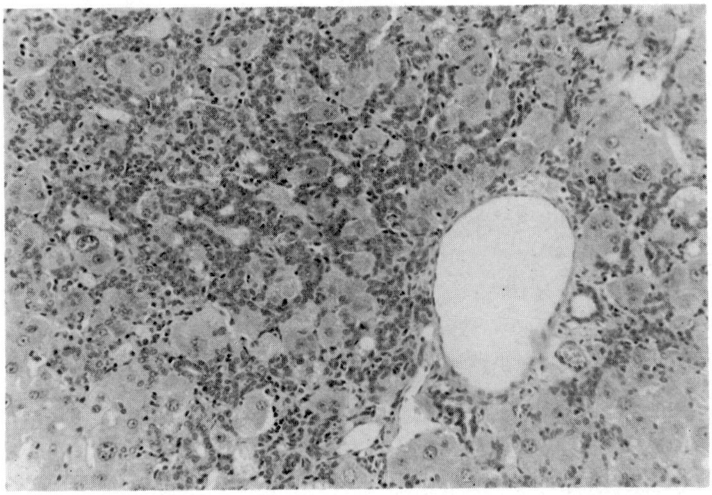

FIG. 4. Section of the liver of a 6-month-old LEC rat with chronic hepatitis. In the periportal areas are small hepatocytes and cholangio-epithelial cells with oval nuclei (oval cells). H&E, ×100

the Glisson's capsule or the sinusoid (Fig. 3). In LEC rats with jaundice in remission and which have survived over 6 months there are degenerative and regenerative changes: a number of inflammatory cells penetrate the Glisson's capsule, and beside the enlarged hepatocytes with huge nuclei, cholangioepithelial-like cells, small oval cells and pseudo-bile ducts proliferate in the periportal areas (Fig. 4). The regenerative changes become predominant throughout the liver after 8 months of age. Fibrous changes slowly extend to the surrounding liver tissues, and frequently occupy almost the entire surface of the liver by the age of 10 months. Histologically, these resemble

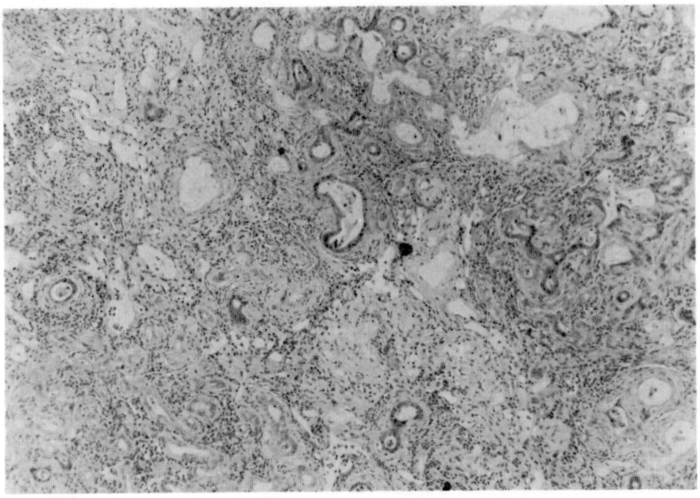

FIG. 5. Section of cholangiofibrosis in the liver of a 10-month-old LEC rat, showing various glandular structures surrounded by connective tissues. H&E, ×100

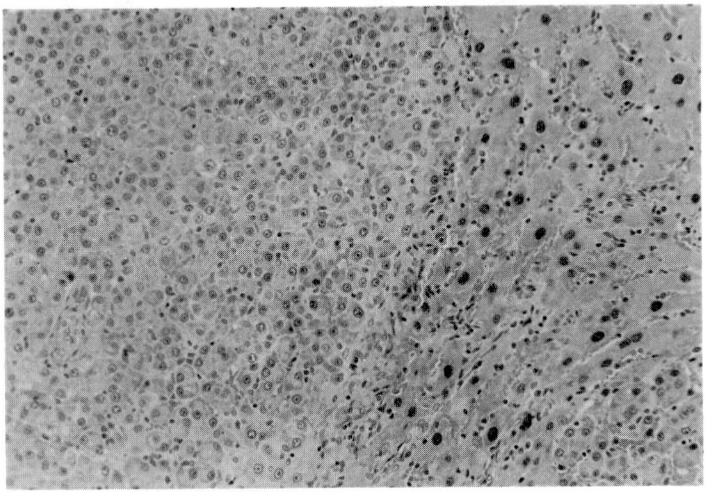

FIG. 6. Section of hyperplastic nodules in the liver of a 12-month-old LEC rat, showing well-developed adenoma (left) and degenerative hepatocytes (right). H&E, ×100

cholangiofibrotic tissues, consisting of columnar or cuboidal epithelial cells forming glandular structures with fibrous stroma (Fig. 5). In rats surviving longer than 1 year, soft, reddish tumors as well as hard whitish nodules develop. The nodules consist of well-developed and differentiated cells closely resembling the surrounding liver cells with trabecular structures. The tumors are hyperplastic nodules or benign adenomas (Fig. 6).

Those LEC rats that have either recovered from hepatitis or never shown any clinical sign of hepatitis are able to survive for long periods; however, around the age of one and a half year, they present palpable liver enlargement. The liver tumors observed at this stage are of roughly two types, hepatocellular carcinoma (HCC)

TABLE 2. Genetic Control of Development of Spontaneous Hepatitis[a] in LEC, LEA, F_1, F_2, and Backcross Rats

Generation	No. of rats examined (♀ : ♂)		% of hepatitis	χ^2	p[b]
	Jaundice (+)	Jaundice (−)			
LEC	50 (26: 24)	7 (3: 4)	88		
LEA	0	34 (18: 16)	0	0	NS
(LEC×LEA) F_1	0	38 (21: 17)	0	0	NS
(LEA×LEC) F_1	0	13 (6: 7)	0	0	NS
(LEC×LEA)×(LEC×LEA) F_2	14 (5: 9)	31 (15: 16)	31	0.89	NS
(LEA×LEC)×(LEA×LEC) F_2	13 (6: 7)	25 (11: 14)	34	1.72	NS
(LEC×LEA)×LEC	12 (6: 6)	18 (7: 11)	40	1.20	NS
(LEA×LEC)×LEC	17 (9: 8)	23 (10: 13)	43	0.90	NS

[a] Hepatitis was diagnosed by histological examination. [b] NS, not significant.

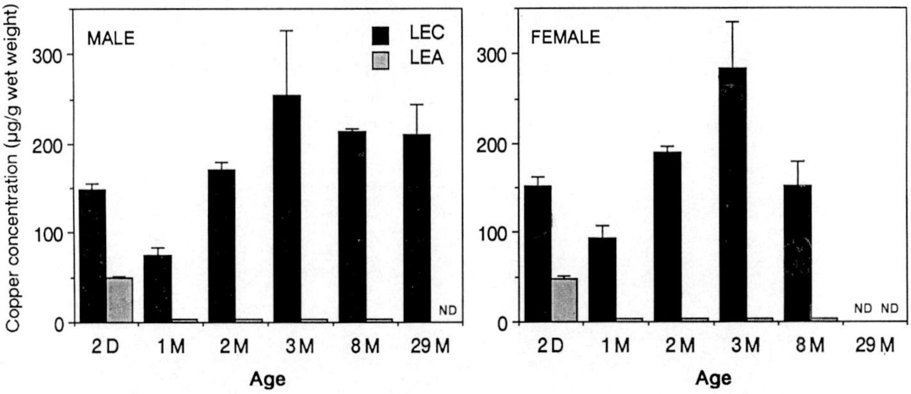

FIG. 7. Copper concentration in the liver of LEC and LEA rats aged 2 days (D) and 1, 2, 3, 8, and 29 months (M). ND, not done.

and/or cholangiofibrosis. Most of the HCCs are a well-differentiated type with a trabecular structure, according to Edmondson's classification, Types I & II (Fig. 9).

Pathogenesis of Hepatitis and Hepatocellular Carcinoma

1. Genetical study

A mutant developing jaundice was reported among laboratory rats and mice (*4, 5*). We first suspected that genetic factor(s) might be related to the occurrence of hepatitis. Therefore, to study the genetic background of hepatitis in LEC rats, LEC and LEA rats were crossbred, F_1, F_2, and backcross rats were produced, and the frequency of hepatitis was examined. None of the F_1 rats developed the condition, whereas 30% of F_2 and 40% of the backcrosses did (Table 2). The results prove that the hepatitis in LEC rats is inherited by a single autosomal recessive gene (designated *hts*) (*3, 6*). Although linkage of this gene with the development of hepatitis and HCC in LEC rats has not yet been determined, it has been shown that the gene is not linked with the coat color or sterility of the rats.

2. Discovery of abnormal copper accumulation

We recently found that copper is abnormally accumulated in the liver of LEC

TABLE 3. Spontaneous Hepatomas and Cholangiofibrosis in Long-surviving LEC Rats

Generation	Sex	No. with enlarged liver / No. surviving[a)] (%)	Incidence of (%) Hepatoma	Cholangiofibrosis
F26–	♀	48/52 (92) (521±91)[b)]	28/48 (58)	48/48 (100)
F32	♂	63/67 (94) (476±75)[b)]	57/63 (90)	63/63 (100)

a) All rats survived more than one year and were killed when they showed palpable enlargement of the liver.
b) Mean latent days±S.D.

rats, and that ceruloplasmin and copper in the serum levels are low (*7, 8*). The copper begins to accumulate at the age of 2 days, and reaches the hepatocytotoxic level at the age of 3 months, just before the onset of hepatitis (Fig. 7). These findings indicate that LEC rats congenitally have an abnormal copper metabolism, which consequently disturbs liver function and causes hepatitis.

The copper level in the brain of 8-month-old LEC rats is higher than that in LEA rats, which we suspect has a certain connection with spasms observed in the LEC rats between 6 and 12 months of age, though such cases are very rare.

The ceruloplasmin and the copper levels in the serum are both markedly low between 6 and 8 months. These features of LEC rats, hereditary mode by an autosomal recessive gene, acute hepatitis, copper accumulation in the liver before hapatitis onset and low ceruloplasmin and copper in the serum closely resemble the clinico-pathological features of Wilson's disease (*9–11*).

3. Abnormal copper metabolism in relation with liver cancer

Nearly 100% of the long-surviving LEC rats develop hepatocellular carcinoma after having suffered from chronic hepatitis and cholangiofibrosis (Table 3). This finding suggests that the abnormal copper metabolism is involved in the development of the HCC. Copper, as well as zinc, is an essential element in numerous metallo-enzymes, and is vital to a variety of biological and biochemical functions, including mitochondrial energy generation, scavenging oxygen radicals. The copper exists in protein-bound form, particularly binding to metallothionein. We suspect that non-protein-bound copper (free copper) causes damage to hepatocytes, whereas the metallothionein-bound copper is not cytotoxic.

We know that LEC rats have abnormalities in drug metabolism at the liver (*12*). It has also been observed that LEC rats have 10 times higher susceptibility to a small amount of chemical carcinogenic agents than LEA rats (*13*). These findings may be closely associated with the presence of a toxic form of copper in the LEC rats soon after birth.

4. Oxygen radicals and DNA damage

In 1983 Kasai and Nishimura (*14*) discovered the formation of an oxidative DNA-damaging product, 8-hydroxyguanine, during their study of DNA modification which they induced by heating carbohydrates. Various oxygen radical-forming agents such as radiation, cigarette smoking, metal compounds, *etc.* have been found to be effective in the formation of 8-hydroxydeoxyguanosine (8-OH-dG)

TABLE 4. Expression and Mutation of Oncogenes in Hepatocarcinogenesis of LEC Rats

1. Increased	
	c-*jun*, c-*myc*,[a] (c-*fos*)
2. Unchanged	
	c-*raf*, H-*ras*, N-*ras*, p53
3. Not detected	
	N-*myc*, *hst*
4. No mutation of *ras* genes[a]	
	H-*ras*, K-*ras*, N-*ras*

[a] Fujimoto *et al.*, 1991.

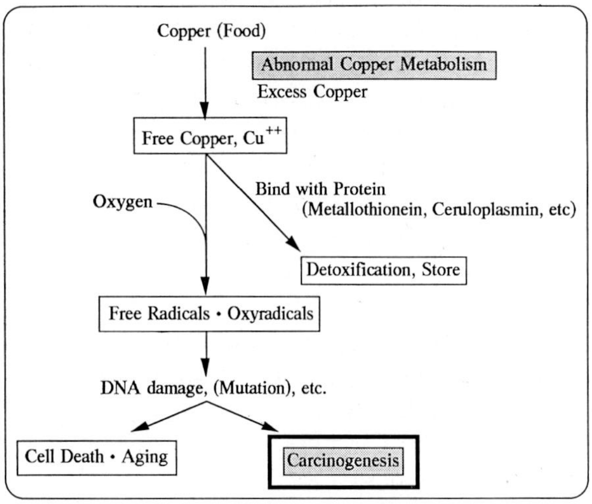

FIG. 8. Mechanisms of copper induced hepatic injury and hepatocarcinogenesis.

in DNA *in vitro*. Therefore, 8-OH-dG is a particularly useful marker for monitoring oxidative DNA damage in carcinogenesis studies of various oxygen radical-forming agents. Yamamoto *et al.* studied chronological changes of 8-OH-dG levels in DNA in the tissues of liver, kidney and brain of LEC and LEA rats (*15*). The levels in the DNA of LEC rat liver and kidney are higher than those of LEA rats at the age of 4 months when most LEC rats show clinical symptoms of acute hepatitis, and the higher levels are still maintained at the age of 8 months. These studies suggest that copper can induce DNA damage in the presence of hydrogen peroxide and reducing agents.

5. Expression of proto-oncogenes during hepatocarcinogenesis

Various proto-oncogenes have been found to play an essential role in the neoplastic process, including hepatocarcinogenesis. Fujimoto *et al.* (*16*) reported that 3 of 4 HCC had c-*myc* expression levels approximately 30-fold higher than that in LEA rats, whereas in the hyperplastic nodules and the non-tumorous portions of livers, c-*myc* expression was not elevated. We have also studied several proto-oncogenes during hepatocarcinogenesis in LEC rats (*17*). Expression of c-*jun* was significantly elevated in the liver tissues of LEC rats 8 months old, and decreased with the develop-

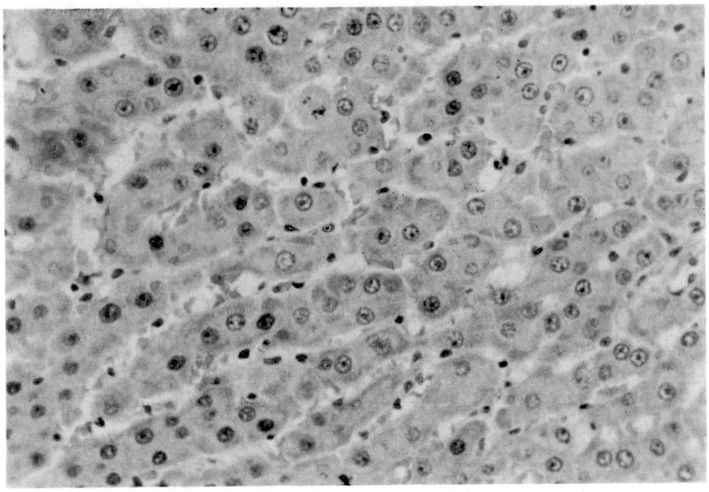

FIG. 9. Section of a well-differentiated hepatocellular carcinoma from an 18-month-old LEC rat, exhibiting the trabecular structure of tumorous hepatocytes. H&E, ×200

ment of HCC. Although the Ha-*ras* mutation has been found at high frequency in chemically induced and spontaneous liver tumors in mice, no *ras* (Ha-*ras*, Ki-*ras*, and N-*ras*) gene mutation has been observed in the HCC derived from LEC rats (Table 4). Based on these findings, we speculate that the highly expressed c-*myc* and c-*jun* might be involved in the hepatocarcinogenesis of LEC rats.

We therefore consider that in LEC rats the abnormal copper accumulation begins to disturb drug metabolism in the liver soon after birth, and that with the development of chronic hepatitis, necrosis and regeneration of hepatocytes are continuously repeated. During this process carcinogenic agents both environmental (food and water) and intrinsic factors may act as an initiator, and/while various growth factors may act as a promoter of cancer (Fig. 8).

Acknowledgments

The study was supported in part by Grants-in-Aid from the Princess Takamatsu Cancer Research Fund and the Ministry of Education, Science and Culture, Japan.

REFERENCES

1. Sasaki, M., Yoshida, M. C., Kagami, K. *et al.* Spontaneous hepatitis in an inbred strain of Long Evans rats. Rat News Lett., *14*: 4–6, 1985.
2. Yoshida, M. C., Masuda, R., Sasaki, M. *et al.* New mutation causing hereditary hepatitis in the laboratory rat. J. Hered., *78*: 361–365, 1987.
3. Takeichi, N., Kobayashi, H., Yoshida, M. C., Sasaki, M., Dempo, K., and Mori, M. Spontaneous hepatitis in Long-Evans Rats: A potential animal model for fulminant hepatitis in man. Acta. Pathol. Jpn., *38(11)*: 1369–1375, 1988.
4. Gunn, C. H. Hereditary acholuric jaundice in new mutant strain of rats. J. Hered., *29*: 137–139, 1939.
5. Saxton, A. M., Eisen, E. J., Johnson, B. H., and Burkhart, J. G. New mutation causing jaundice in mice. J. Hered., *76*: 441–446, 1985.

6. Masuda, R., Yoshida, M. C., Sasaki, M., Dempo, K., and Mori, M. Hereditary hepatitis in the LEC rat strain controlled by a single autosomal recessive gene. Lab. Anim., *22*: 166–169, 1988.
7. Li, Y., Togashi, Y., Sato, S., Emoto, T., Kang, J., Takeichi, N., Kobayashi, H., Kojima, Y., Une, Y., and Uchino, J. Spontaneous accumulation of copper in the liver of LEC rats with hereditary hepatitis: a model of Wilson's disease. J. Clin. Invest., *87*: 1858–1861, 1991.
8. Li, Y., Togashi, Y., Emoto, T., Kang, J., Takeichi, N., Kobayashi, H., Kojima, Y., Une, Y., and Uchino, J. Abnormal copper accumulation in non-cancerous and cancerous liver tissues of LEC rats developing hereditary hepatitis and spontaneous hepatoma. Jpn. J. Cancer Res., *82*: 490–492, 1991.
9. Wilson, S. A. K. Progressive lenticular degeneration of a familiar nervous disease associated with cirrhosis of the liver. Brain, *34*: 295–309, 1912.
10. Walshe, J. M. *In*; L. Shiff and E. R. Shiff (eds.), The liver in Wilson's disease (hepatolenticular degeneration). Disease of the Liver. pp. 1037–1050, Lippincott Co., Philadelphia, 1987.
11. Polio, J., Enrique, R. E., Chow, A., Wood, W. M., and Atterbury, C. E. Hepatocellular carcinoma in Wilson's disease. J. Clin. Gastroenterol., *11*: 220–224, 1989.
12. Sugiyama, T., Takeichi, N., Kobayashi, H. *et al.* Metabolic predisposition of a novel mutant (LEC rats) to hereditary hepatitis and hepatoma: alteration of the drug metabolizing enzymes. Carcinogenesis, *9*: 1569–1572, 1988.
13. Takahashi, H., Enomoto, K., Nakajima, Y., and Mori, M. High sensitivity of the LEC rat liver to the carcinogenic effect of diethyl-nitrosoamine. Cancer Lett., *51*: 247–250, 1990.
14. Kasai, H. and Nishimura, S. Hydroxylation of the C-8 position of deoxyguanosine by reducing agents in the presence of oxygen. Nucl. Acids Symp., *12*: 165–167, 1983.
15. Yamamoto, F., Kasai, H., Togashi, Y., Takeichi, N., Hori, T., and Nishimura, S. Analysis of 8-hydroxydeoxyguanosine (8-OH-dG) in LEC rats. Proc. Jpn. Cancer Res. Assoc. (Tokyo), 1991.
16. Fujimoto, Y., Ishizaka, Y., Tahira, T , Sone, H., Takahashi, H., Enomoto, K., Mori, M., Sugiyama, T., and Nagao, M. Possible involvement of c-*myc* but not *ras* genes in hepatocellular carcinomas developing after spontaneous hepatitis in LEC rats. Mol. Carcinogen., *4*: 269–274, 1991.
17. Suzuki, H., Fujita, H., Mullauer, L., Kuzumaki, N., Konaka, S., Togashi, Y., Takeichi, N., Kawamukai, Y., and Uchino, J. Increased expression of c-*jun* and glutathione S-transferase P genes during spontaneous hepatocarcinogenesis in LEC rats. Cancer Lett., *53*: 205–211, 1990.

MULTISTAGE CARCINOGENESIS, C C. HARRIS ET AL. (EDS.),
JAPAN SCI. SOC. PRESS, TOKYO/CRC PRESS, BOCA RATON, PP. 371–380, 1992

Biological Significance of Gene Amplification in Carcinogenesis

Masaaki TERADA, Hiromi SAKAMOTO, Yoshihisa OHMURA, Hiroyuki TSURUTA, Nobu AKIYAMA, Hiroki SASAKI, Masaru KATOH, Yutaka HATTORI, and Teruhiko YOSHIDA

National Cancer Center Research Institute, Tokyo 104, Japan

Abstract: K-*SAM* gene was originally isolated as an amplified gene in a stomach cancer cell line by in-gel DNA renaturation method. K-*SAM* encodes a membrane receptor with tyrosine kinase and is often amplified in poorly differentiated type of stomach cancer, while c-*ERBB-2* is often amplified in well differentiated type of stomach cancer. There are several forms of K-*SAM* mRNAs which are generated by alternative splicing, and two types of K-*SAM* protein without transmembrane region. The ligand of K-*SAM* is considered to be growth factor(s) belonging to fibroblast growth factor (FGF) or heparin binding growth factor (HBGF) family. We have also frequently found amplification of *HST-1* or *HSTF1* gene in esophageal cancer. *HST-1* gene, originally found as a transforming gene, is located on human chromosome 11q13, and it locates 35 kbp apart from its related gene, *INT-2*. Neither of the genes was expressed even in cancer cells with the co-amplification. By cosmid walking, we have identified at least two genes, designated tentatively as *EXP1* and *EXP2*, on the same amplicon as *HST-1* and *INT-2*, and the mRNAs for *EXP1* and *EXP2* genes were increased in amounts proportional to the degree of amplification.

One of the characteristics of cancer cells is chromosomal instability and fragility, including the presence of double minute chromosomes and homogeneous staining regions. Histochemical techniques have shown that the DNA content per cell is often increased in malignant cells, and that the increase in DNA content per cell is associated with more malignant cancers. However, amplification of only a limited number of oncogenes has been found in human cancers, and the incidence is relatively quite low. Amplification of genes other than known oncogenes, which give growth advantage, is expected to occur in cancers. We have, in fact, isolated an amplified gene, designated as K-*SAM* from a KATO III cells (*1*), a stomach cancer cell line derived from a schirrhous cancer. Nucleotide sequence analysis of K-*SAM* cDNA revealed that the K-*SAM* encodes a member receptor with ligand that belongs to fibroblast growth factor (FGF) or heparin binding growth factor (HBGF) family (*2*). We have also frequently found amplification of *HST-1* or *HSTF1* gene in esophageal cancer (*3, 4*), which was originally identified and characterized as a transforming gene (*5*). The *HST-1* gene, however, was not expressed even in the cells with its amplification. By cosmid walking, we have identified two genes on the same amplification unit as *HST-1*, and these two genes were expressed in amounts proportional to the degree of amplification. These results of our studies on amplified genes in cancer will be described and the biological significance of the gene amplification will be discussed.

General Method to Identify Gene Amplification

We intended to analyze for the presence of gene amplification in human cancer. However, most approaches to gene amplification so far have depended on Southern blot analysis using a known gene as a probe, especially oncogenes. Because a number of genes other than oncogenes are expected to be amplified in cancers, this candidate gene approach has its own limitation. A general strategy to identify amplified sequences had to be set up for cancer cells.

To identify gene amplification in cells, we employed the in-gel DNA denaturation-renaturation method, which was first developed by Dr. I. B. Roninson (*6*).

Amplified Sequences in Human Gastric Cancers

As expected, the in-gel DNA renaturation method visualized a normal common repetitive sequence, as shown by an arrow in Fig. 1. In contrast to the normal repetitive sequence, some fragments were found to be cancer-specific amplified sequences. KATO III and MKN7 cells showed an abundance of such amplified fragments (*7*). MKN7 cells are the cells from which c-*ERBB-2* was originally isolated and identified. KATO III is a cell line derived from a gastric signet-ring cell carcinoma and we determined to isolate an amplified gene from KATO III cells. The gel was excised, DNA was eluted, and a portion of the amplified sequences was cloned from the KATO III DNA (*1*).

Because the original DNA fragment did not contain an exon, a normal placental genomic library was screened to clone a neighboring fragment which hybridizes mRNA of KATO III. cDNA was cloned from the cDNA library prepared from mRNAs of KATO III cells. The corresponding gene was named K-*SAM*, which stands for KATO III stomach cells amplified gene (*2*).

KATO III cells are characterized by a large HSR (homogeneously staining region) on chromosome 11. K-*SAM* was mapped to the HSR by chromosomal *in situ* hybridization on KATO III cells, whereas the normal position of K-*SAM* was found to be on the long arm of chromosome 10 (unpublished data). Recently, a fragment on the KATO III HSR was cloned by phenol-enhanced reassociation technique. This fragment was derived from band q26 of chromosome 10 (*8*). It remains to be shown if this 10q26 fragment is in the same amplification unit as K-*SAM*.

K-SAM Amplification Is Not Restricted to a Cell Line

Southern blot analysis showed that the amplification of K-*SAM* was observed not only in KATO III, but also in other stomach cancer cells, including some clinical specimens of human stomach cancer. At least two patients with gastric cancer had

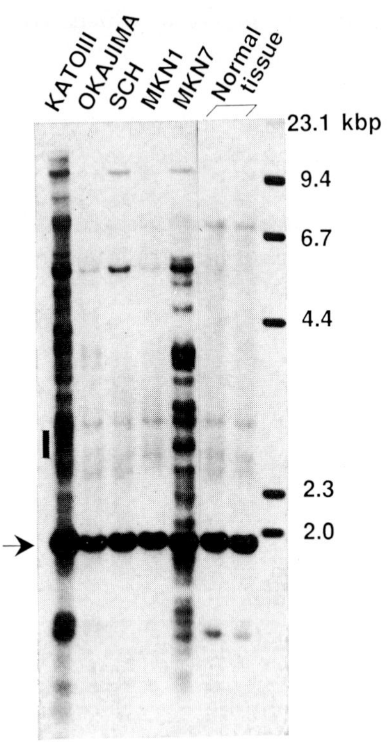

FIG. 1. Amplified sequences in gastric cancer cell lines detected by the in-gel DNA denaturation method (6). From left to right lanes: KATO III, a signet-ring cell carcinoma; OKAJIMA, a poorly-differentiated carcinoma; SCH, choriocarcinoma of the stomach; MKN1, an adenosquamous carcinoma; MKN7, a well-differentiated carcinoma; Normal tissue, normal spleen. An arrow points to one of the normal repetitive fragments. The original genomic fragment of K-*SAM* was isolated from the portion of the gel marked with a line. *Hin*dIII was used to restrict the DNAs.

TABLE 1. Amplification of K-*SAM* and c-*ERBB-2* in Gastric Cancers

	Poorly-differentiated type		Well-differentiated type	
	K-*SAM*	c-*ERBB-2*	K-*SAM*	c-*ERBB-2*
Fresh tumors	3/19	0/24	0/7	4/10
Xenografts	2/6	—	0/7	—
Cell lines	1/4	0/3	0/3	1/3
Total	6/29	0/27	0/17	5/13

There is in sharp contrast between K-*SAM* and c-*ERBB-2* amplification in two major categories of stomach cancers. The amplification of K-*SAM* has a strong tendency to occur in poorly-differentiated types, despite c-*ERBB-2* amplification occurring in well-differentiated types of stomach cancer.

amplified K-*SAM* genes in metastatic lesions, but not in primary tumors, suggesting a possible involvement of K-*SAM* amplification in the later stages of tumor progression.

K-*SAM* gene was overexpressed in these stomach cancer cells with K-*SAM* amplification. In contrast to stomach cancers, K-*SAM* amplification was rarely found in nongastric cancers. On the other hand, not all stomach cancer cells showed K-*SAM* amplification and overexpression. Consequently, we looked at which type of stomach cancer has K-*SAM* activation.

Table 1 summarizes our analysis of two major categories of stomach cancers: poorly-differentiated or diffuse types and well-differentiated or intestinal types. There is a strong tendency for K-*SAM* amplification to occur in poorly-differentiated types.

As described previously, this is in sharp contrast to c-*ERBB-2*, which is known to amplify preferentially in well-differentiated types of human stomach cancer (*9*).

K-SAM Is a Member of FGF Receptor Family

Figure 2 is a schematic presentation of the deduced K-*SAM* product. Like c-*ERBB-2*, K-*SAM* codes for a receptor type tyrosine kinase. The sequence analysis showed that K-*SAM* belongs to a family of FGF receptors or HBGF receptors. At least

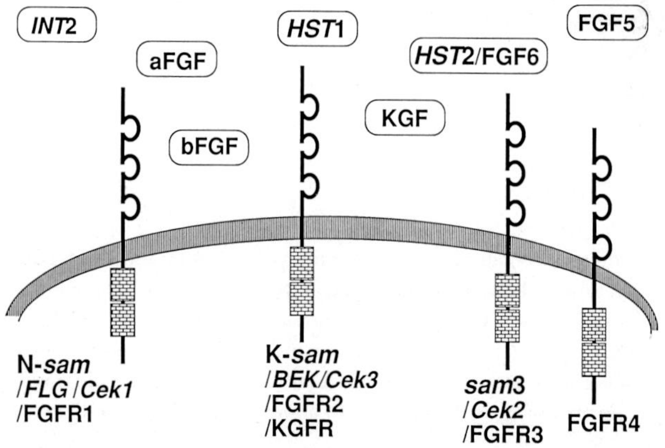

FIG. 2. Schematic illustration of FGF family of growth factor and FGF receptor family. Seven members of the FGF family, bFGF, aFGF, *INT-2*, *HST-1*, *FGF-5*, *HST-2*/FGF6, and KGF are presented together with 4 FGF-receptor family, including N-*SAM*, K-*SAM*, *SAM3*, and FGFR4. Ω, immunoglobulin like domain; ▒, membrane; ▦, tyrosine kinase domain.

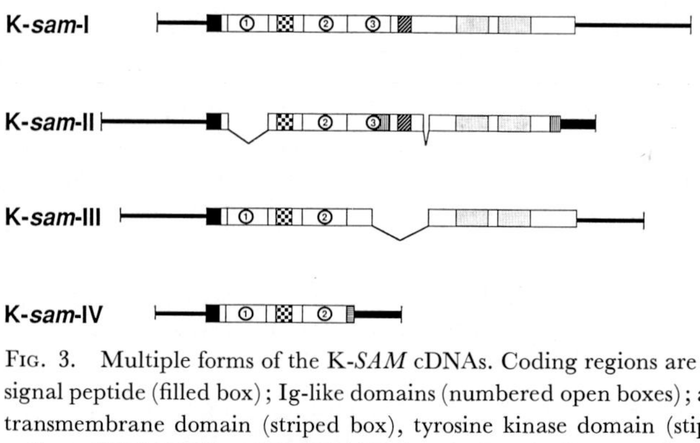

FIG. 3. Multiple forms of the K-*SAM* cDNAs. Coding regions are shown as boxes: hydrophobic signal peptide (filled box); Ig-like domains (numbered open boxes); acidic region (checkered box); transmembrane domain (striped box), tyrosine kinase domain (stippled box); divergent coding region of K-*SAM*-II and K-*SAM*-IV (hatched box). 3′ noncoding regions unique to K-*SAM*-II and K-*SAM*-IV are indicated by thick bars.

four distinct FGF receptor genes are known (Fig. 3) (*10–13*), and at least two of these four genes can give rise to multiple forms of the receptor by alternative splicing, especially at the extracellular domains of the receptors (*14, 15*).

Four different versions of K-*SAM* cDNAs were cloned from various sources as shown in Fig. 3. K-*SAM*-I was cloned from a normal brain cDNA library and represents a full-length transcript. K-*SAM*-I is identical with the human *bek*/FGFR2 product (*11*). K-*SAM*-II, which was cloned from a KATO III cell line, lacks the first immunoglobulin (Ig)-like domain of K-*SAM*-I, and its third Ig-like domain is modified. The carboxy terminus is also different from K-*SAM*-I. K-*SAM*-III and K-*SAM*-IV products do not have a transmembrane domain, suggesting that they are secreted. K-*SAM*-IV was also cloned from KATO III cells (*16*).

Functional significance of these variations remains to be elucidated. Receptors with different extracellular domains may show different affinity for ligands, as exemplified by *bek*/K-*SAM*-I (*11*) and the KGF receptor, which has a K-*SAM*-II-type extracellular domain (*17*). A secreted form of receptor tyrosine kinase lacking transmembrane intracellular domains has been identified for EGF (*18*) and basic FGF (*19*) receptors. They may act as a carrier or reservoir of ligands, or as a competitive inhibitor to the ligand-receptor interaction. In any case, the secreted form may be useful for development of a means of noninvasive diagnosis for gastric cancer.

Ligands for the FGF receptors also constitute a family of at least seven related heparin-binding growth factors (*20*). The combination of each FGF ligand and receptor is not a simple one-to-one, adding another level of complexity to the system. The diversity of these ligand-receptor families poses a number of exciting questions in biology. In the study of cancer, we have noticed that the amplification of the K-*SAM* gene is apparently specific to poorly-differentiated human stomach cancers. This specificity may argue the biological significance of the K-*SAM* product in the development of a subset of human stomach cancer.

Identification of HST-1 Gene

Along with the in-gel renaturation method, we have also tried a functional assay to identify cancer genes, an NIH3T3 focus formation assay to detect transforming genes.

Briefly, DNAs were isolated from human stomach cancer tissues, transfected to normal fibroblast cell line NIH3T3, and a gene which morphologically transforms NIH3T3 was cloned. One of the transforming genes we obtained from human stomach cancer was *HST-1*, which stands for human stomach (*5*). Surprisingly, the *HST-1* product was found to belong to an FGF or a HBGF family, the ligand family for the FGF receptors (*21*). We mapped *HST-1* to human chromosome 11 at band q13.3 (*22*). This region contains another member of the FGF family, the *INT-2* gene. The distance between *HST-1* and *INT-2* was determined to be less than 35 kb (*23*).

HST-1 and INT-2 Are Amplified but Not Expressed in Esophageal Cancers

We screened other types of human cancers by Southern blot analysis to look for the possible involvement of *HST-1*. We found that both *HST-1* and *INT-2* were

TABLE 2. Amplification of *HST-1* and *INT-2* Genes in Various Human Cancers

Esophageal cancers		
Fresh tumors	23/41	54%
Cell lines	5/13	38%
Breast cancers	21/176	12%
Gastric cancers	1/32	
Lung cancers	1/53	
Bladder cancers	1/18	
Renal cancers	0/13	

Coamplification of *HST-1* and *INT-2* was observed in almost half of the esophageal cancers.

amplified in almost half of the human esophageal cancer cases as summarized in Table 2. A subset of head and neck squamous cell carcinomas and breast cancers also showed amplification (*24–29*). The degree of amplification was usually two to ten fold.

Among 13 esophageal cancer cell lines established in Japan, five lines showed *HST-1* and *INT-2* coamplification. However, neither *HST-1* nor *INT-2* was expressed in these cell lines. This finding seems to be in contrast to breast cancers with *INT-2* amplification, where expression of *INT-2* has been reported (*29, 30*).

One of the explanations for the amplification without overexpression is the involvement of another cryptic cancer gene in this 11q13.3 amplification unit in the esophageal, but not breast, carcinogenesis. Therefore, we have started a chromosomal walking on this region.

Genomic Walking to Identify Amplified and Transcribed Sequences

By walking over 150 kb from *HST-1* to centromere, we have identified two genes which are coamplified together with *HST-1* and *INT-2* in the esophageal cancer cell lines. These new genes were designated *EXP1* and *EXP2*. Unlike *HST-1* and *INT-2*, *EXP1*, and *EXP2* were overexpressed in the cell lines with 11q13.3 amplification. Thus, these genes are strong candidates for the elusive genes wanted in human esophageal carcinogenesis.

Recently, another locus on 11q13, *BCL-1*, has been claimed to correspond to cyclin D (*31*), also referred to as *PRAD1* (*32*). The *BCL-1* locus is frequently coamplified with *HST-1*/*INT-2* (*33, 34*), and cyclin D/*PRAD1* was found to be overexpressed in esophageal cancers and head and neck carcinomas (*35, 36*). Thus, cyclin D is another strong candidate for the 11q13 esophageal cancer gene. Its relationship to *EXP1* and *EXP2* is under investigation.

Biological Significance

Multiple steps of initiation, promotion and progression are required for conversion of a normal cell to a fully malignant cell with metastatic and invasive capacity. During the course of the multi-step carcinogenesis, a number of genetic alterations occur involving oncogenes and tumor suppressor genes. There has been accumulating evidence that the scenario of multiple genetic alteration is specific to each type of cancer. Gene amplification probably occurs in the latest stage of the carcinogenic process, representing the results of genomic instability. The cells with amplified genes are considered to be selected out in the late stage of carcinogenesis, and the gene on the amplicon probably represents the one which provides the cells with growth advantage. Accordingly, cancer cells with amplified oncogenes are the ones in the latest stage of carcinogenesis and the ones with the most malignant phenotype: Presence of N-*MYC* amplification in neuroblastoma or that of c-*ERBB-2* amplification in breast carcinoma is a good marker for poor prognosis.

There are, however, only a limited number of oncogenes which have been reported to be amplified in cancer. Those include *MYC* oncogene family, *RAS* oncogene family, c-*ERBB-1*, c-*ERBB-2*, and *GLI*. It is likely that there are yet-to-be discovered oncogenes or genes providing cancer cells with growth advantage *in vivo*. As described in this paper, we have found many amplified DNA fragments in cancer cells by in-gel DNA renaturation method, and one of the genes on the amplicons was K-*SAM*. Judging from the results of analysis of cancer DNAs by the in-gel renaturation method, it was very likely that there are many different amplification units in a cancer cell. The presence of many different amplification units in a cancer cell was recently confirmed by analysis of amplified DNA fragments obtained by a genomic subtraction method (unpublished data). Isolation and characterization of frequently amplified genes in cancer will provide us with probes important for judging the prognosis of a patient with cancer. It also will lead to better understanding of the biology of cancer cells in the late stage of carcinogenesis.

Analysis of an amplification unit on 11q13 containing *HST-1* revealed that an amplification unit was at least 150 kbp in length, and contained several genes, some of which were not transcribed even in the cells with the amplification. There were also a few genes on the amplicon which express in amounts proportional to the degree of amplification of the gene, and the gene responsible for the progression of cancer should be determined by understanding of the biological function of the gene. Structural analysis on the amplification unit will also reveal the mechanisms involved in gene amplification in cancer and might lead to an understanding of the mechanisms involved in genomic instability in cancer.

Aknowledgments

This work was supported in part by a Grant-in-Aid for the Comprehensive 10-Year Strategy for Cancer Control from the Ministry of Health and Welfare and by Grants-in-Aid for Cancer Research from the Ministry of Health and Welfare, the Ministry of Education, Science and Culture, the Princess Takamatsu Cancer Research Fund and the Bristol-Myers Squibb Foundation.

REFERENCES

1. Nakatani, H., Sakamoto, H., Yoshida, T., Yokota, J., Tahara, E., Sugimura, T., and Terada, M. Isolation of an amplified DNA sequence in stomach cancer. Jpn. J. Cancer Res., *81*: 707–710, 1990.
2. Hattori, Y., Odagiri, H., Nakatani, H., Miyagawa, K., Naito, K., Sakamoto, H., Katoh, O., Yoshida, T., Sugimura, T., and Terada, M. K-sam, an amplified gene in stomach cancer, is a member of the heparin-binding growth factor receptor genes.

Proc. Natl. Acad. Sci. U.S.A., *87*: 5983–5987, 1990.

3. Tsuda, T., Nakatani, H., Matsumura, T., Yoshida, K., Tahara, E., Nishihira, T., Sakamoto, H., Yoshida, T., Terada, M., and Sugimura, T. Amplification of the hst-1 gene in human esophageal carcinomas. Jpn. J. Cancer Res., *79*: 584–588, 1988.
4. Tsuda, T., Tahara, E., Kajiyama, G., Sakamoto, H., Terada, M., and Sugimura, T. High incidence of coamplification of hst-1 and int-2 genes in human esophageal carcinomas. Cancer Res., *49*: 5505–5508, 1989.
5. Sakamoto, H., Mori, M., Taira, M., Yoshida, T., Matsukawa, S., Shimizu, K., Sekiguchi, M., Terada, M., and Sugimura, T. Transforming gene from human stomach cancers and a noncancerous portion of stomach mucosa. Proc. Natl. Acad. Sci. U.S.A., *83*: 3997–4001, 1986.
6. Roninson, I.B. Use of in-gel DNA renaturation for detection and cloning of amplified genes. Methods Enzymol., *151*: 332–371, 1987.
7. Nakatani, H., Tahara, E., Yoshida, T., Sakamoto, H., Suzuki, T., Watanabe, H., Sekiguchi, M., Kaneko, Y., Sakurai, M., Terada, M., and Sugimura, T. Detection of amplified DNA sequences in gastric cancers by a DNA renaturation method in gel. Jpn. J. Cancer Res., *77*: 849–853, 1986.
8. Mor, O., Messinger, Y., Rotman, G., Bar-Am, I., Ravia, Y., Eddy, R. L., Shows, T. B., Park, J. G., Gazdar, A. F., and Shiloh, Y. Novel DNA sequences at chromosome 10q26 are amplified in human gastric carcinoma cell lines: molecular cloning by competitive DNA reassociation. Nucl. Acids Res., *19*: 117–123, 1991.
9. Yokota, J., Yamamoto, T., Miyajima, N., Toyoshima, K., Nomura, N., Sakamoto, H., Yoshida, T., Terada, M., and Sugimura, T. Genetic alterations of the c-*erb*B-2 oncogene occur frequently in tubular adenocarcinoma of the stomach and are often accompanied by amplification of the v-*erb*A homologue. Oncogene, *2*: 283–287, 1988.
10. Lee, P. L., Johnson, D. E., Cousens, L. S., Fried, V. A., and Williams, L. T. Purification and complementary DNA cloning of a receptor for basic fibroblast growth factor. Science, *245*: 57–60, 1989.
11. Dionne, C.A., Crumley, G., Bellot, F., Kaplow, J. M., Searfoss, G., Ruta, M., Burgess, W. H., Jaye, M., and Schlessinger, J. Cloning and expression of two distinct high-affinity receptors cross-reacting with acidic and basic fibroblast growth factors. EMBO J., *9*: 2685–2692, 1990.
12. Keegan, K., Johnson, D. E., Williams, L. T., and Hayman, M. J. Isolation of an additional member of the fibroblast growth factor receptor family, FGFR-3. Proc. Natl. Acad. Sci. U.S.A., *88*: 1095–1099, 1991.
13. Partanen, J., Makela, T. P., Eerola, E., Korhonen, J., Hirvonen, H., Claesson-Welsh, L., and Alitalo, K. FGFR-4, a novel acidic fibroblast growth factor receptor with a distinct expression pattern. EMBO J., *10*: 1347–1354, 1991.
14. Johnson, D. E., Lu, J., Chen, H., Werner, S., and Williams, L. T. The human fibroblast growth factor receptor genes: a common structural arrangement underlies the mechanisms for generating receptor forms that differ in their third immunoglobulin domain. Mol. Cell Biol., *11*: 4627–4634, 1991.
15. Champion, A. P., Ronsin, C., Gilbert, E., Gesnel, M. C., Houssaint, E., and Breathnach, R. Multiple mRNAs code for proteins related to the BEK fibroblast growth factor receptor. Oncogene, *6*: 979–987, 1991.
16. Katoh, M., Hattori, Y., Sasaki, H., Tanaka, M., Sugano, K., Yazaki, Y., Sugimura, T., and Terada, M. K-*sam* gene encodes secreted as well as transmembrane receptor tyrosine kinase. Proc. Natl. Acad. Sci. U.S.A., *89*: 2960–2964, 1992.
17. Miki, T., Fleming, T. P., Bottaro, D. P., Rubin, J. S., Ron, D., and Aaronson, S. A. Expression cDNA cloning of the KGF receptor by creation of a transforming autocrine

loop. Science, *251*: 72–75, 1991.
18. Petch, L. A., Harris, J., Raymond, V. W., Blasband, A., Lee, D. C., and Earp, H. S. A truncated, secreted form of the epidermal growth factor receptor is encoded by an alternatively spliced transcript in normal rat tissue. Mol. Cell Biol., *10*: 2973–2982, 1990.
19. Johnson, D. E., Lee, P. L., Lu, J., and Williams, L. T. Diverse forms of a receptor for acidic and basic fibroblast growth factors. Mol. Cell Biol., *10*: 4728–4736, 1990.
20. Yoshida, T., Miyagawa, K., Sakamoto, H., Sugimura, T., and Terada, M. Identification and characterization of fibroblast growth factor-related transforming gene hst-1. Methods Enzymol., *198*: 124–138, 1991.
21. Yoshida, T., Miyagawa, K., Odagiri, H., Sakamoto, H., Little, P. F., Terada, M., and Sugimura, T. Genomic sequence of hst, a transforming gene encoding a protein homologous to fibroblast growth factors and the int-2-encoded protein (published erratum appears in Proc. Natl. Acad. Sci. U.S.A., *85* (6): 1967, 1988). Proc. Natl. Acad. Sci. U.S.A., *84*: 7305–7309, 1987.
22. Yoshida, M. C., Wada, M., Satoh, H., Yoshida, T., Sakamoto, H., Miyagawa, K., Yokota, J., Koda, T., Kakinuma, M., Sugimura, T., and Terada, M. Human HST1 (HSTF1) gene maps to chromosome band 11q13 and coamplifies with the INT2 gene in human cancer. Proc. Natl. Acad. Sci. U.S.A., *85*: 4861–4864, 1988.
23. Wada, A., Sakamoto, H., Katoh, O., Yoshida, T., Yokota, J., Little, P. F., Sugimura, T., and Terada, M. Two homologous oncogenes, HST1 and INT2, are closely located in human genome. Biochem. Biophys. Res. Commun., *157*: 828–835, 1988.
24. Zhou, D. J., Casey, G., and Cline, M. J. Amplification of human int-2 in breast cancers and squamous carcinomas. Oncogene, *2*: 279–282, 1988.
25. Merritt, W. D., Weissler, M. C., Turk, B. F., and Gilmer, T. M. Oncogene amplification in squamous cell carcinoma of the head and neck. Arch. Otolaryngol. Head Neck Surg., *116*: 1394–1398, 1990.
26. Somers, K. D., Cartwright, S. L., and Schechter, G. L. Amplification of the int-2 gene in human head and neck squamous cell carcinomas. Oncogene, *5*: 915–920, 1990.
27. Tsuda, H., Hirohashi, S., Shimosato, Y., Hirota, T., Tsugane, S., Yamamoto, H., Miyajima, N., Toyoshima, K., Yamamoto, T., Yokota, J., Terada, M., and Sugimura, T. Correlation between long-term survival in breast cancer patients and amplification of two putative oncogene-coamplification units: hst-1/int-2 and c-erbB-2/ear-1. Cancer Res., *49*: 3104–3108, 1989.
28. Adnane, J., Gaudray, P., Simon, M. P., Simony, L. J., Jeanteur, P., and Theillet, C. Proto-oncogene amplification and human breast tumor phenotype. Oncogene, *4*: 1389–1395, 1989.
29. Theillet, C., Le Roy, X., De Lapeyriere, O., Grosgeorges, J., Adnane, J., Raynaud, S. D., Simony-Lafontaine, J., Goldfarb, M., Escot, C., and Birnbaum, D. Amplification of FGF-related genes in human tumors: possible involvement of HST in breast carcinomas (published erratum appears in Oncogene, *4* (12): 1537, 1989). Oncogene, *4*: 915–922, 1989.
30. Liscia, D. S., Merlo, G. R., Garrett, C., French, D., Mariani, C. R., and Callahan, R. Expression of int-2 mRNA in human tumors amplified at the int-2 locus. Oncogene, *4*: 1219–1224, 1989.
31. Withers, D. A., Harvey, R. C., Faust, J. B., Melnyk, O., Carey, K., and Meeker, T. C. Characterization of a candidate bcl-1 gene. Mol. Cell Biol., *11*: 4846–4853, 1991.
32. Motokura, T., Bloom, T., Kim, H. G., Juppner, H., Ruderman, J. V., Kronenberg, H. M., and Arnold, A. A novel cyclin encoded by a bcll-linked candidate oncogene. Nature, *350*: 512–515, 1991.

33. Lammie, G. A., Fantl, V., Smith, R., Schuuring, E., Bookes, S., Michalides, R., Dickson, C., Arnold, A., and Peters, G. D11S287, a putative oncogene on chromosome 11q13, is amplified and expressed in squamous cell and mammary carcinomas and linked to BCL-1. Oncogene, *6*: 439–444, 1991.
34. Leonard, J. H., Kearsley, J. H., Chenevix, T. G., and Hayward, N. K. Analysis of gene amplification in head-and-neck squamous-cell carcinoma. Int. J. Cancer, *48*: 511–515, 1991.
35. Jiang, W., Kahn, S. M., Tomita, N., Zhang, Y. J., Lu, S. H., and Weinstein, I. B. Amplification and expression of the human cyclin D gene in esophageal cancer. Cancer Res., *52*: 2980–2983, 1992.
36. Schuuring, E., Verhoeven, E., Mooi, W. J., and Michalides, R. J. Identification and cloning of two overexpressed genes, U21B31/PRAD1 and EMS1, within the amplified chromosome 11q13 region in human carcinomas. Oncogene, *7*: 355–361, 1992.

MULTISTAGE CARCINOGENESIS, C. C. HARRIS ET AL. (EDS.),
JAPAN SCI. SOC. PRESS, TOKYO/CRC PRESS, BOCA RATON, PP. 381–391, 1992

A Population Perspective on Multistage Carcinogenesis

Suresh H. Moolgavkar

Fred Hutchinson Cancer Research Center, Seattle, Washington 98104, U.S.A.

Abstract: The concept of multistage carcinogenesis is one of the central dogmas of cancer research today. Recent laboratory work suggests that many specific genetic changes are associated with carcinogenesis. At the same time, there is increasing evidence that cell proliferation kinetics are important in carcinogenesis. In 1971, Knudson proposed his now celebrated two-mutation model for embryonal tumors. In fact, a two-mutation model that explicitly considers cell kinetics is the most parsimonious model consistent with the incidence of both childhood and adult cancer in human populations. This model has been known to be consistent, as well, with other epidemiologic and experimental data. But can such a model be reconciled with the laboratory evidence suggesting that many genetic alterations are required for malignant transformation?

In this paper, I examine multistage carcinogenesis from the population perspective. Can cancer incidence data in populations provide some insight into the number and nature of stages involved in malignant transformation? I focus attention on carcinoma of the colon because of the considerable amount of information that is now available on the genetics of these tumors. Also, as is the case with retinoblastoma, colon cancer occurs in sporadic and dominantly inherited forms. A comparison of the incidence of these two forms of colon cancer suggests that mutation at the familial adenomatous polyposis (FAP) locus is not necessary for colon cancer, and that inheritance of the gene for FAP is not equivalent to inheriting one of the essential steps on the pathway to colon cancer. Thus, colon cancer does not follow the retinoblastoma paradigm. The incidence of colon cancer in the general population and among polyposis subjects is consistent with two or three mutations on the pathway to malignancy. A three-mutation model is more consistent with the genetic alterations observed in colon carcinogenesis. I present and discuss a working model for colon cancer.

Recent laboratory data on the genetic alterations associated with malignant transformation appear to provide solid evidence in support of the concept of multistage carcinogenesis (*1*, *2*) first proposed in the 1950's. Yet important questions remain. Which of the many genetic alterations observed to be associated with carcinogenesis are actually required for malignant transformation? What is the mode of action of genes that confer a dominantly inherited predisposition to certain cancers? Can the number of mutations observed during malignant transformation be reconciled with the incidence rates of cancer in human populations in view of the available information on mutation rates?

For one particular tumor, retinoblastoma, the answers to these questions are known. Retinoblastoma is a rare tumor of the retina in children and occurs in both sporadic and dominantly inherited forms. It is now known that retinoblastoma is due to homozygous inactivation of a gene at the retinoblastoma locus on chromosome 13. This implies that two mutations (for homzoygous inactivation of the gene) are required for retinoblastoma, as first postulated by Knudson (*3–5*). In the dominantly inherited form of the disease, one inactivation event (*i.e.*, one of the two mutations) is inherited, so that every retinoblast carries an inactivated gene at the retinoblastoma locus on one of the two chromosomes 13. Thus, inheriting a predisposition to retinoblastoma is equivalent to inheriting the first step on the pathway to malignant transformation. Finally, by analyzing the incidence of retinoblastoma within the framework of a two-mutation model, Knudson and colleagues showed that the estimated mutation rates, approximately 10^{-7} per cell generation, were in good agreement with laboratory measurements of mutation rates.

Although retinoblastoma is a rare tumor in human populations, and therefore of little public health significance, its study provided some invaluable lessons. In particular, the central role of tumor suppressor genes in human carcinogenesis was underscored by the study of retinoblastoma. Further, as mentioned above, retinoblastoma provided a paradigm for one particular mode of inheritance of cancer susceptibility, *viz.*, inheritance of the first step in multistage carcinogenesis. In contrast to retinoblastoma, carcinoma of the colon is one of the commonest neoplasms of man, but it shares some parallels with retinoblastoma. Like retinoblastoma, it occurs both in sporadic and dominantly inherited forms, and, like retinoblastoma, the genetic alterations associated with malignant transformation have been extensively studied. To what extent can the lessons learnt from retinoblastoma be applied to colon cancer? In this paper I shall try to address that question from the population perspective. Can the study of the incidence of colon cancer in the general population and among polyposis cases give us some clues to the answer?

Multistage Carcinogenesis

The first formal multistage model of carcinogenesis was proposed by Armitage and Doll (*2*). They noted that the age-specific incidence rates of many human carcinomas increase roughly with a power of age, and showed that a multistage model predicted this behavior of the age-specific incidence curve. Explicitly, Armitage and Doll assumed that malignant tumors are clonal, arising from a single malignant cell that has arisen from a normal susceptible cell (presumably a stem cell) after a sequence of irreversible steps. Pictorially, the model may be represented as follows:

$$E_0 \xrightarrow{\lambda_0} E_1 \xrightarrow{\lambda_1} E_2 \xrightarrow{\lambda_2} \cdots \xrightarrow{\lambda_{n-1}} E_n.$$

Here, E_0 is a normal cell, E_n is a malignant cell, and each λ_j represents the rate at which a cell moves from one stage to the next. If the number of stem cells in the tissue of interest is N, then Armitage and Doll showed that the age-specific incidence rates per 100,000 individuals in the population are approximately given by the expression

$$I(t) = N\lambda_0\lambda_1 \cdots \lambda_n\, t^{n-1}/(n-1)!$$

where t represents age. Thus, the Armitage-Doll model predicts that incidence rates increase roughly with a power of age *i.e.*, $I(t)=ct^k$, where k, the exponent of age, is one less than the number of stages required for malignant transformation.

The importance of cell kinetics in carcinogenesis is now well appreciated, and a serious deficiency of the Armitage-Doll model is that it does not explicitly consider the kinetics of cell division and death. In contrast, Knudson's two-mutation model for embryonal cancers took explicit account of cellular kinetics. Indeed, it turns out that, when cell division and death are explicitly considered, a model postulating two mutations on the pathway to malignancy is consistent with the age-specific incidence curves of both childhood and adult tumors (*6*). Thus, the age-specific incidence curves of the adult tumors do not provide strong evidence in support of the notion that many steps are involved in the carcinogenic process. In fact, a two-

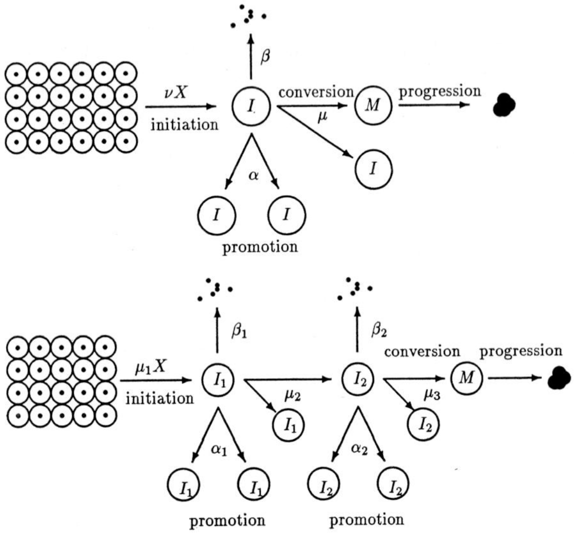

FIG. 1. Upper panel: two-mutation model for carcinogenesis. Rate of initiation depends upon the number of normal susceptible cells X and upon mutation rate v. Promotion results in clonal expansion of initiated cells with division rate α (per cell per year) and cell death (or differentiation) rate β (per cell per year). During cell division of initiated cells, one of the daughters may sustain the second mutation (with rate μ per cell per year) and become malignant. Subsequent changes are rapid and lead to tumor progression and metastasis. Lower panel: three-mutation model for carcinogenesis. Note that, in this model, promotion results in clonal expansion of cells in both intermediate compartments. Rate of initiation depends upon X and the first mutation rate μ_1. Rates of cell division in the two intermediate compartments I_1 and I_2 are denoted by α_1 and α_2. The rates of cell death or differentiation are β_1 and β_2. An I_1 cell may divide into one I_1 and one I_2 cell (*i.e.*, sustain the second mutation) with rate μ_2. Similarly, an I_2 cell may sustain the third mutation during cell division with rate μ_3, leading to a malignant daugher. Subsequent changes are rapid leading to tumor progression and metastasis. All rates are per cell per year as in the two-mutation model.

mutation model that explicitly incorporates cell kinetics is the most parsimonious model consistent with the incidence of cancer in human populations. This model has been shown to be consistent, as well, with other epidemiologic and experimental data (*7*). But can such a model be reconciled with the laboratory evidence suggesting that many genetic alterations are required for malignant transformation?

A two-mutation model for cancer, a generalization of Knudson's model for embryonal tumors, is shown in Fig. 1. This model incorporates two features: 1) transition of target stem cells into malignant cells *via* an intermediate stage in two rate-limiting, heritable and irreversible steps; 2) explicit consideration of cell division and cell death (or differentiation). In the parlance of chemical carcinogenesis, the first step may be identified with initiation, clonal expansion of initiated cells may be identified with promotion, and the second step may be identified with malignant conversion. A three-mutation model, an obvious extension of the two-mutation model, is also shown in Fig. 1.

The models in Fig. 1 take explicit account of cell division in the intermediate compartments, where the effect of perturbation of division kinetics is likely to be most important. Distinction probably should be made between two kinds of cell division. In the first kind of division, believed to be common in renewal tissue, division of stem cells is asymmetric, with one daughter cell remaining a stem cell and the other daughter being committed to differentiation. An increase in the rate of this type of division (type 1 division) will manifest itself as an increase in the mutation rate per unit of time. The second type of cell division is symmetric, with a stem cell dividing into two stem cells. An increase in this type of cell division results, not only in an increase in the mutation rate per unit of time, but also in an increase in the population of target stem cells if the increase in division rates is not compensated for by an increase in death rates. In Fig. 1, if $\alpha-\beta$ is greater than zero, then there is a net increase in the population of intermediate cells, and this, in turn, increases the probability of one of the cells becoming malignant. Thus, promotion, which increases $\alpha-\beta$, is particularly important in carcinogenesis.

Carcinoma of the Colon

This is one of the commonest neoplasms in Western populations. Recent laboratory work has shown that many specific genetic alterations are associated with colon cancer (*8*). It is not known which, or how many, of these genetic alterations are necessary for colon carcinogenesis. Like retinoblastoma, colon cancer occurs in sporadic and dominantly inherited forms (*9, 10*). I will show that a careful analysis of the incidence of these two types of colon cancer can shed some light on the number of rate-limiting events in colon cancer. Further, a comparison of colon cancer in the general population with that among polyposis subjects suggests that a mutation at the Familial Adenomatous Polyposis (FAP) locus is not one of the rate-limiting events on the pathway to colon cancer. In particular, colon cancer among FAP subjects does not appear to fit the retinoblastoma paradigm, *i.e.*, inheritance of the FAP mutation is not equivalent to inheriting one of the steps on the pathway to colon cancer.

Electron microscopic studies have shown that there are approximately 10^8

crypts in the adult human colon. If each crypt develops from 1–10 stem cells, then there are approximately 10^8–10^9 stem cells in the adult human colon. In all my computations, I assume that there are 10^8 stem cells. My general conclusions would remain unchanged if this number were an order of magnitude different. For technical details I refer the reader to (*11*).

Data on the incidence of colon cancer among polyposis subjects are not easy to come by. So far as I know, the only available data are those reported by Veale (*9*). These data have been abstracted by Ashley (*12*). In a recent paper (*11*), Georg Luebeck and I analyzed these data. In order to compare the incidence in a general population that is similar to the population in which the polyposis cases arose, we also analyzed the incidence of colon cancer in Birmingham, United Kingdom. When the Armitage-Doll model $I(t)=ct^k$ is fit to the colon cancer incidence (per 10^5 individuals) among Birmingham males, the estimates of the parameters are $\hat{c}=4\times10^{-2}$, and $\hat{k}=4.54$, suggesting that at most 5 or 6 mutations are required for the genesis of colon cancer among Birmingham males. Assuming that there are 10^8 stem cells and that the mutation rates are equal leads to an estimate of this common mutation rate of $\hat{\lambda}=2.5\times10^{-3}$ per cell per year if there are 5 mutations on the pathway to colon cancer, and $\hat{\lambda}=8.85\times10^{-3}$ if there are 6 mutations. If each stem cell divides 100 times per year, these rates translate into 2.5×10^{-5} and 8.85×10^{-5} mutations per cell division, respectively. These mutations are two orders of magnitude higher than measured rates of specific locus mutation. Thus, if 5 or 6 mutations are involved in colon carcinogenesis, then an early step must confer a mutator phenotype on the cell. The Armitage-Doll model yields very similar results when fit to incidence among females.

A problem with the Armitage-Doll model is that it does not consider cellular proliferation. In fact, as I will discuss below, when cellular proliferation is incorporated into the model, the colon cancer incidence data are consistent, as well, with two or three mutations on the carcinogenic pathway. Thus, age-specific incidence data should not be used to *infer* the number of rate-limiting steps required for malignant transformation, and do not offer evidence in favor of the notion that many steps must be involved in carcinogenesis. The estimate of the number of steps obtained by fitting the Armitage-Doll model can be viewed as upper bounds for the number of rate-limiting steps in multistage carcinogenesis.

Both the two-mutation and three-mutation models were also fit to the Birmingham population incidence data. Both models described the data well. In these models, polyps are identified with clones of cells in the intermediate compartments. With the assumptions that the number of stem cells is 10^8, that each stem cell divides 100 times annually, and that the mutation rates are equal, the estimated mutation rates are 3×10^{-10} per cell division and 4.7×10^{-8} per cell division, respectively, for the two- and three-mutation models. The net proliferation rate ($\alpha-\beta$) of intermediate cells in the two-mutation model was estimated to be 0.107 per cell per year. This quantity is a measure of the net rate of cell divisions of type 2, which results in clonal expansion of intermediate cells. This estimate indicates that, on average, a stem cell undergoes an effective division of this type approximately once every ten years. With the three-mutation model, $\alpha_1-\beta_1$ is estimated to be close to zero and $\alpha_2-\beta_2$ is estimated to be 0.1 per cell per year. Thus, most of the promotion in

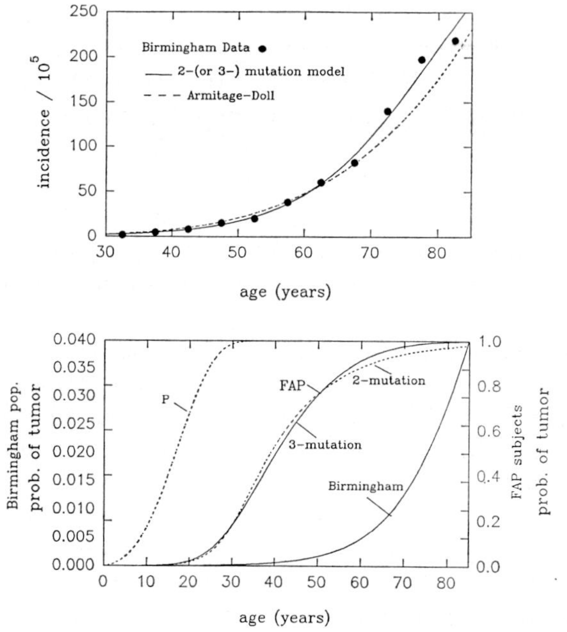

FIG. 2. Upper panel: age-specific incidence of colon cancer among Birmingham males, and the age-specific incidence curves generated by the Armitage-Doll and the two- and three-mutation models. The curves generated by the latter two models are indistinguishable. Lower panel: probability of tumor by a given age plotted against age for colon cancer among Birmingham males and polyposis subjects. Curves generated by the two- and three-mutation models. Note that the probability among Birmingham males Prob(t) is related to the incidence I(t) shown in the upper panel by the relationship Prob$(t) = 1 - \exp(-\int h(s)ds)$, where $h(s) = I(s)/10^5$. The curve labelled P denotes the predicted probability of cancer among polyposis subjects if inheritance of the polyposis gene were equivalent to inheriting one of the necessary mutations in a three-mutation model.

this model appears to occur in intermediate compartment 2. However, the standard error of the estimate of $\alpha_1 - \beta_1$ is large and some clonal expansion of cells in this compartment cannot be ruled out.

Both models describe the incidence of colon cancer well (Fig. 2). However, the estimated mutation rates of the two-mutation model appear to be far too small. Laboratory measurements of specific locus mutation rates are based on assays that measure inactivation of the locus in question. These measurements indicate that specific locus inactivations occur at a rate of about 10^{-7} per cell division (*13*). However, inactivation of a gene can be brought about in a number of ways. Activation of a gene, on the other hand, may require a very specific alteration at one of a few codons in the gene. Thus, an activation event may be very rare. Loeb (*13*) has estimated the mutation rate per base pair to be approximately 10^{-10} per cell generation. Thus, the estimated mutation rates for a two-mutation model are compatible with activation events. This observation is interesting in light of Weinberg's suggestion (*14*) that activation of two oncogenes, a nuclear oncogene and a cytoplasmic oncogene, are required for malignant transformation. There is little laboratory evidence, however, that oncogene activations are important in colon carcinogenesis.

The estimated mutation rates for a three-mutation model are much more in line with laboratory-measured rates. A three-mutation model is more consistent, as well, with the genetic alterations that have been observed to be associated with colon cancer. I shall present a comprehensive working model of colon cancer below. But before doing so, I would like to discuss FAP briefly.

FAP

FAP, a dominantly inherited condition, is characterized by the appearance at an early age of a large number of adenomatous polyps in the colon. Individuals with the condition are at enormously increased risk of colon cancer, and a prophylactic colectomy is considered to be the procedure of choice once polyps begin to appear. The locus for FAP was mapped to chromosome 5q in 1987 (*15*). Very recently, two genes of importance to colon cancer have been cloned from this locus (*16, 17*). Germeline mutations of one of these genes, the adenomatous polyposis coli (APC) gene, appear to be responsible for FAP. The other gene, the mutated in colon cancer (MCC) gene, is mutated in some sporadic cases of colon cancer. An interesting ques-

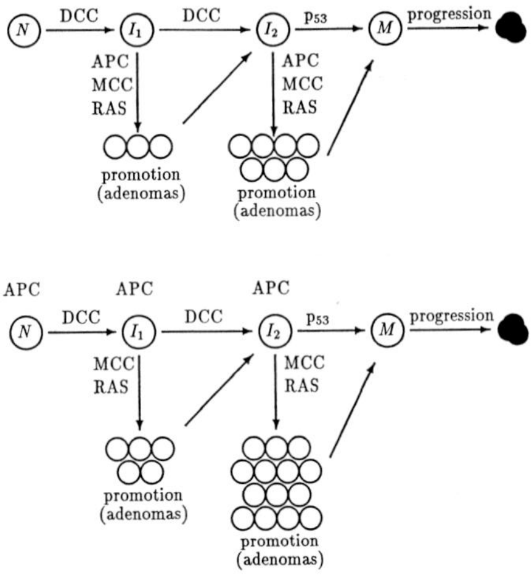

FIG. 3. Schema for colon carcinogenesis. Upper panel: in the general population. N=normal stem cell. Lower panel: among polyposis cases. N=stem cell carrying a mutation of the APC gene. Mutation at both DCC loci and a dominant negative mutation at p53 locus are required for malignant transformation. Mutations at the FAP locus and activation of the Ras gene are considered to be promoter mutations leading to enhanced growth of cells in the intermediate stages. Promotion greatly increases the efficiency of malignant transformation by increasing the population of target cells. However, promotion is not a *necessary* event on the pathway to malignancy. Thus, for example, increasing the number of target cells in intermediate compartments one and two increases the probability that one of these cells sustains the next mutation (either at the DCC locus or the p53 locus) on the pathway to malignancy. Thus, the arrows from I_1 to I_2 and from I_2 to M indicate that promotion is not required for these transformations. However, if the population of these cells is enlarged by clonal expansion, then transformations are brought about much more efficiently. Although we have presented the mutations as occurring in a specific order, accumulation of the events rather than the order in which they occur is probably important (*8*).

TABLE 1. Results of Fitting the Two- and Three-mutation Models to Colon Cancer Incidence among Polyposis Subjects

Age group	Males			Females		
	Observed	Expected		Observed	Expected	
		A	B		A	B
0– 9	0	0.4	0.1	1	0.3	0.9
11–14	1	0.9	0.6	0	0.7	0.4
15–19	0	2.4	2.4	2	1.7	1.7
20–24	6	5.9	6.8	5	3.9	4.5
25–29	14	11.4	12.3	8	6.9	7.5
30–34	17	15.2	14.5	10	6.2	9.4
35–39	8	14.2	13.4	7	9.8	9.3
40–44	14	12.1	12.2	6	8.3	8.4
45–49	6	6.2	7.1	10	6.2	7.1
50–54	3	3.6	4.7	3	2.4	3.1
55–59	2	2.4	3.5	1	1.1	1.5
60–64	1	1.6	2.5	0	0.3	0.6
65–69	1	1.0	1.9	1	0.3	0.6
70–74	2	0.7	1.3	—	—	—

The data were taken from the table in Ashley (*12*). The table shows the observed number of colon cancer cases among polyposis subjects and the expected number generated by the two-mutation (A) and the three-mutation (B) models.
Two-mutation model: Estimated mutation rates $=4.5\times10^{-9}$ / cell generation. Estimated α-$\beta=0.207$.
Three-mutation model: Estimated mutation rates $=2.6\times10^{-7}$ / cell generation. Estimated α_1-$\beta_1=0$. Estimated α_2-$\beta_2=0.307$.

tion is whether the gene for FAP acts in the same way as the gene for retinoblastoma, *i.e.*, whether inheriting the gene for FAP is equivalent to inheriting one of the essential steps on the pathway to colon cancer. I shall argue below that this is not so.

I report the results of analyses of the incidence of colon cancer among polyposis subjects within the framework of the two- and three-mutation models. The data, which were collected by Veale, are taken from Ashley's paper. Since cell proliferation kinetics are clearly important in FAP, and because the Armitage-Doll model does not consider these, the data were not analyzed within the framework of the Armitage-Doll model. As can be seen from Table 1 and Fig. 2, both models describe the data well, and yield virtually identical results for the probability of malignant tumor as a function of age among polyposis subjects. One hundred percent of FAP subjects can be expected to develop colon cancer by the age of 80 if a prophylactic colectomy is not performed.

Table 1 shows also the parameter estimates obtained by fitting the two- and three-mutation models to the Veale data. As expected, the estimated mutation rates are higher than those estimated by fitting the corresponding models to incidence in the Birmingham population. The increase in mutation rates may be attributable, in large part, to the increased cell proliferation in the colons of individuals with FAP. The parameter estimates indicate, as well, that there is an increase in the net rate of type 2 cell division of intermediate cells. That is, inheritance of the gene for FAP appears to have a strong promotional effect in the colon.

Concluding Remarks

The incidence of colon cancer in the general population appears to be most consistent with a model postulating 3 rate-limiting events on the pathway to malignancy. Although a two-mutation model describes the data well, the estimated mutation rates appear to be far too small. If 4 or more mutations are required, the estimated mutation rates appear to be too high, requiring that an early step confer a mutator phenotype on the cell.

Models postulating two and three rate-limiting events describe the occurrence of colon cancer among polyposis subjects equally well. However, the estimated mutation rates (Table 1) are still too small with the two-mutation model. The main effect of inheritance of the polyposis gene appears to be a promotional effect, *i.e.*, an increase in the net rate of type 2 proliferation of intermediate cells. Thus, the incidence data are consistent with the notion that the FAP gene causes a slight shift in homeostasis, away from differentiation and towards stem cell proliferation.

Is it possible that inheritance of the FAP gene is equivalent to inheritance of one of the essential steps on the pathway to malignancy? This appears to be unlikely for the following reason. For concreteness, let me assume that sporadic colon cancer requires three rate-limiting steps for its genesis. If inheritance of the FAP gene is equivalent to inheriting one of these steps, then colon cancer among polyposis cases would be a two-mutation tumor. A two-mutation model describes colon cancer among polyposis cases well. However, as can be seen from Table 1, the estimated mutation rates are much lower than the mutation rates estimated by fitting the three-mutation model to sporadic colon cancer. Thus, one would have to conclude that the FAP gene *decreases* mutation rates and *increases* type 2 cell division rates. This seems highly implausible. Another way to view the situation is to ask the following question. If sporadic colon cancer is a three-mutation tumor, what would the risk of colon cancer be among individuals inheriting one of these mutations? The curve labelled P in the lower panel of Fig. 2 illustrates this hypothetical situation. The risk of developing colon cancer would be much higher than that observed among polyposis subjects. Indeed, 100% of individuals inheriting one of the essential steps on the pathway to colon cancer would be expected to develop the disease by the age of 30.

Note from Fig. 2 that approximately 95% of polyposis cases have developed cancer by age 70. By contrast, 95% of retinoblastoma gene carriers develop malignant tumors by age 5. This contrast is all the more striking when we note that the colon has many more cells at risk than the retina, and the number of stem cell divisions also seems to be much larger in the colon. Hethcote and Knudson have estimated that there are approximately 10^7 stem cell divisions in the retina before the organ is fully differentiated. If, on the other hand, our estimates of 10^8 stem cells in the colon, and a division rate of 100 per cell per year are reasonable, then there are approximately 10^{10} stem cell divisions in the colon per year in adult life. Thus, the polyposis gene is "weaker" than the retinoblastoma gene in conferring the cancer phenotype. This observation suggests the possibility that these genes act by very different mechanisms. Further support for this notion is provided by the recent finding that the APC gene is a new kind of gene.

The laboratory findings in colon cancer can be readily accommodated within the framework of a three-mutation model. The most consistently found genetic alterations are at the Deleted in Colon Cancer (DCC) locus on 18q and the p53 locus on 17p. In addition, alterations at the FAP locus (mutations of either APC or MCC) and mutations of the *ras* gene are also found (*8*). For reasons discussed above, inheritance of the gene for FAP is not equivalent to inheritance of one of the necessary steps on the pathway to malignancy. This suggests that mutation of the APC gene is not required for malignant transformation. Further *ras* gene activation is found only in 50% of tumors suggesting that this event is not required either. Based on these observations, one model for colon carcinogenesis would postulate that homozygous losses of gene function at both the DCC and p53 loci are required for colon carcinogenesis. Such a model would appear to require four mutations. However, it is now known that many p53 mutations are dominant negative (*8*), *i.e.*, mutation at one allele leads to loss of function of both alleles (trans-dominant loss of function). Thus, in the model shown in Fig. 3 mutations at the two DCC loci and a (dominant negative) mutation at the p53 locus are required for malignant transformation. Although clonal expansion of intermediate cells, especially in compartment 2, can occur without mutations at the FAP locus or of the *ras* gene, such mutations are postulated to stimulate clonal growth of these cells. Thus, mutations at the FAP locus or of the *ras* gene are regarded as "promoter" mutations that increase the efficiency of malignant transformation by increasing the population of target cells. However, these mutations are not required for malignant transformation. In summary, this model postulates that there is a common pathway to cancer among polyposis cases and in the general population, and that the polyposis gene increases the risk of colon cancer by increasing the rate of type 2 cell division.

The Li-Fraumeni syndrome is a dominantly inherited cancer syndrome in which the risk of divers tumor types is increased (*18*). However, the risk of colon cancer appears to be only slightly elevated, if at all. Recently a germline mutation of the p53 gene has been described in Li-Fraumeni families. If mutation of the p53 gene is important in colon carcinogenesis, then the observation that the incidence of colon cancer is apparently not increased in the Li-Fraumeni families is puzzling. If homozygous loss of p53 function is required for colon carcinogenesis, then an explanation may be provided by the finding that the germline p53 mutations in these families do not produce protein in large enough quantity to exert a trans-dominant loss of function of the wild-type allele (*18*). If most somatic mutations of the p53 gene are dominant negative, then a three-mutation model involving homozygous loss of function at the DCC locus together with a (dominant negative) mutation of p53 would be consistent with the population incidence data and also with the observation that the risk of colon cancer is not elevated in the Li-Fraumeni syndrome.

REFERENCES

1. Foulds, L. The experimental study of tumor progression: A review. Cancer Res., *14*: 317–339, 1954.
2. Armitage, P. and Doll, R. The age distribution of cancer and a multi-stage theory

of carcinogenesis. Br. J. Cancer, *8*: 1–12, 1954.
3. Knudson, A. G. Mutation and cancer: Statistical study of retinoblastoma. Proc. Natl. Acad. Sci. U.S.A., *68*: 820–823, 1971.
4. Knudson, A. G., Hethcote, H. W., and Brown, B. W. Mutation and childhood cancer: A probabilistic model for the incidence of retinoblastoma. Proc. Natl. Acad. Sci. U.S.A., *72*: 5116–5120, 1975.
5. Hethcote, H. W. and Knudson, A. G. Model for the incidence of embryonal cancer: Application to retinoblastoma. Proc. Natl. Acad. Sci. U.S.A., *75*: 2453–2457, 1978.
6. Moolgavkar, S. H. and Venzon, D. J. Two-event models for carcinogenesis: incidence curves for childhood and adult tumors. Math. Biosci., *47*: 55–77, 1979.
7. Moolgavkar, S. H. and Knudson, A. G. Mutation and cancer: a model for human carcinogenesis. J. Natl. Cancer Inst., *66*: 1037–1052, 1981.
8. Fearon, E. R. and Vogelstein, B. A genetic model for colorectal tumorigenesis. Cell, *61*: 759–767, 1990.
9. Veale, A. M. O. Intestinal Polyposis. Eugenics Laboratory Memoirs, No. 40, Cambridge University Press, Cambridge, 1965.
10. Lipkin, M. Biomarkers of increased susceptibility to gastrointestinal cancer: new application to studies of cancer prevention in human subjects. Cancer Res., *48*: 235–245, 1988.
11. Moolgavkar, S. H. and Luebeck, E. G. Multistage carcinogenesis: population-based model for colon cancer. J. Natl. Cancer Inst., *84*: 610–618, 1992.
12. Ashley, D. J. B. Colonic cancer arising in polyposis coli. J. Med. Gen., *6*: 376–378, 1969.
13. Loeb, L. A. A mutator phenotype may be required for multistage carcinogenesis. Cancer Res., *51*: 3075–3079, 1991.
14. Weinberg, R. A. Oncogenes, antioncogenes, and the molecular bases of multistep carcinogenesis. Cancer Res., *49*: 3713–3721, 1989.
15. Bodmer, W. F., Bailey, C. J., Bodmer, J. *et al.* Localization of the gene for familial adenomatous polyposis on chromosome 5. Nature, *328*: 614–616, 1987.
16. Kinzler, L. W., Nilbert, M. C., Su, L. K. *et al.* Identification of FAP locus genes from chromosome 5q21. Science, *253*: 661–664, 1991.
17. Nishisho, I., Nakamura, Y., Miyoshi, Y. *et al.* Mutations of chromosome 5q21 genes in FAP colorectal cancer patients. Science, *253*: 665–669, 1991.
18. Malkin, D., Li, F. P., Strong, L. C. *et al.* Germ line p53 mutations in a familial syndrome of breast cancer, sarcomas, and other neoplasms. Science, *250*: 1233–1238, 1990.

Overview and Future Directions

I. Bernard Weinstein

I want to thank the organizers for the opportunity to participate in this exciting symposium, but I do not know why such good friends gave me the impossible task of summarizing the wealth of data and ideas presented at this exciting meeting.

When the famous nuclear physicist Isidore Rabi won the Nobel prize a journalist asked him, "Who had the greatest influence on your career in science?" Rabi answered "My mother". The journalist asked, "Was she also a scientist?" Rabi answered "No". The journalist asked, "So how did she influence your career?" Rabi answered, "As a child, when my friends came home from school their mothers asked them, "Did you answer correctly all of the questions the teacher asked you"? But my mother always asked me "Well, Isidore, today did *you* ask the teacher a good question?" Thus, Rabi emphasized the importance in science of formulating the right question.

This meeting has focused largely on two questions, and has provided important answers to both: 1) what types of mutations accumulate during the multistage carcinogenic process, and 2) what is the functional significance of some of these mutations, *i.e.* what are the normal biochemical functions of the target genes, and how are these functions distorted by the mutations that occur? At the same time, at least two new questions have arisen from the results of these studies: 1) why do we find so many mutations in a given fully malignant tumor? and 2) what mechanisms drive the evolving tumor cell to accumulate these multiple mutations? These questions have become an important focus for future research in the field of multistage carcinogenesis. The second question is of particular importance because if we could identify the factors responsible for driving the occurrence of these mutations then we could design more rational approaches to interrupt the process of tumor progression.

At the end of this overview I want to raise a third question which was only briefly mentioned at this meeting, namely to what extent does the multistage carcinogenic process also involve nonmutational (epigenetic) distortions in mechanisms that control gene expression during normal cellular differentiation?

As Drs. Sugimura, Harris, and Pitot emphasized in their talks, early evidence for the multistage and multifactor nature of the carcinogenic process was first revealed by the experimental studies of Yamagiwa and Ichikawa at the beginning of this century. This evidence was extended by Peyton Rous, Isaac Berenblum, Leslie Fould, and others in the middle decades of this century. Now, in the final decade of this century, studies on the molecular biology of cancer have revealed that these multiple steps appear to reflect at least in part, the progressive accumulation of mutations in cellular oncogenes and growth suppressor genes. A number of these mutations were revealed at this meeting. This year the p53 gene is the champion target for mutations, since over 50% of many of the common tumors show p53 mutations and the specific mutations have been pinpointed in over 500 individual tumors. I suspect that in future years other genes, yet to be discovered, will turn out to also be major targets for mutations in the multistage carcinogenic process. We now know that a single human tumor, for example a colon cancer, can carry 5–10 mutations and this number will probably increase as research proceeds. As mentioned, we do not know what drives the occurrence of these mutational events, and whether all of them are critical to the establishment and maintenance of the phenotype of malignant tumors.

The complex networks of signal transduction described at this meeting suggest that in normal cells there is considerable redundancy and cross talk, thus assuring a high fidelity in regulating gene expression, growth and differentiation. Therefore, several mutations may be required before tumor cells can escape from the tight controls normally operative in the parent cells. We have heard evidence that adds to the growing and unifying theme, that many of these target genes code for components of agonist-induced signal transduction pathways (growth factors, receptors, protein kinases, transcription factors), or negative regulators of such functions (the tumor suppressor genes). Distortion in these pathways can apparently lead to autonomy of growth control, autocrine loops, and escape from hormone dependence.

Another group of genes that appears to be emerging as critical targets involved in multistage carcinogenesis are genes involved in cell cycle control—the cyclins and related protein kinases and protein phosphatases. At least two examples emerged at this meeting: 1) amplification and overexpression of the cyclin D or PRAD-1 gene on chromosome 11 in human esophageal cancer (rearrangement or amplification of this gene also occurs in other human cancers), and 2) evidence that overexpression of the CD25 Hu2 gene is associated with aneuploidy in tumors. These and other findings suggest that the cellular repertoire of potential oncogenes and growth suppressor genes is even larger than previously anticipated. Given the central importance of cell cycle control, it is reasonable to predict that mutations in additional genes that control the cell cycle will be discovered in tumors and found to play a critical role in multistage carcinogenesis.

A question repeatedly raised at this meeting, and one that has implications in terms of cancer prevention, is "What drives the numerous mutations that accumulate during the process of tumor progression?" We have heard evidence that the driving forces might include: external genotoxic agents, endogenous mutagenic events (O_2 radicals, deamination of 5-methyl cytidine, *etc.*) and genomic instability. I suspect that all three mechanisms are involved, and that in some situations their interaction has multiplicative effects. Tumors can display abnormalities in every conceivable function. It seems reasonable, therefore, that this will include aberrations in the normal mechanisms that control the fidelity of DNA synthesis, the efficiency of DNA repair, the fidelity of replicon firing, and/or the fidelity of chromosome replication and segregation.

We have heard several examples of mutational spectra in target genes (especially the p53 gene) which provide a "fossil record" or a 'fingerprint" of the types of muta-

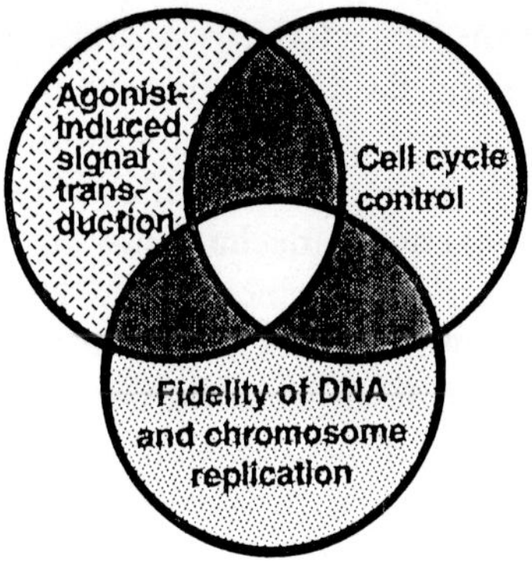

FIG. 1

genic agents and mechanisms responsible for producing point mutations in tumor cells. On the other hand, we have few or no insights into the driving forces and molecular mechanisms responsible for the more complex genetic changes frequently seen in tumors, including allelic deletion, recombination, insertion and amplification. This subject needs much more research and new model systems. Hopefully, further studies in yeast on mechanisms of genetic recombination, replicon firing cell cycle control, and genes that monitor the overall fidelity of cell replication (for example, the phenomenon of "check point control" exercised by the RAD9 gene), will provide insights into the basis for these more complex genomic changes.

Figure 1 displays a holistic view of multistage carcinogenesis. The diagram emphasizes potential interactions between three types of circuitry or control systems in eukaryotic cells: 1) agonist-induced signal transduction, 2) cell cycle control, and 3) control of the fidelity of DNA and chromosome replication. All three of these systems interact with each other through complex cascades of protein phosphorylation and dephosphorylation, and cascades of gene expression. Distortions in any one of these systems can, therefore, be transmitted to the other two systems. For example, distortions in signal transduction might drive cells through G_1 and into persistent cell cycling. Excessive expression of early response genes might also place certain genes or chromosomes in jeopardy of mutational changes, because of the relationships between transcription, DNA repair and DNA replication. Abnormalities in protein kinases that normally regulate signal transduction might also impair later steps in cell cycle control, for example, by aberrant protein phosphorylation. Abnormalities in cell cycle control during DNA replication, G_2 and metaphase could produce DNA amplification, genetic recombination or chromosomal aberrations, thus impairing the function of genes involved in either the positive or negative control of signal transduction pathways, or in cyclin-related functions that control various stages of the cell cycle. These combined events could result in error cascade, genomic instability, tumor progression, and tumor heterogeneity. The resulting disorders in gene expression would disrupt not only the internal machinery of the cell but also the expression of cell surface molecules and molecules destined for secretion, thus enhancing tumor invasion, metastasis and angiogenesis. This scheme is hypothetical but seems reasonable in terms of all of the new information that we have heard at this meeting.

Finally, I want to turn to a subject that was frequently alluded to but not discussed in detail at this meeting, *i.e.* the likelihood that multistage carcinogenesis involves not only mutational changes but also aberrations in epigenetic mechanisms that normally control gene expression and cell differentiation. There are several lines of evidence for implicating epigenetic mechanisms, in addition to gene mutations and chromosomal abnormalities, in carcinogenesis. 1) A variety of non-genotoxic agents can enhance tumor formation apparently by acting through epigenetic mechanisms. 2) Tumors can be induced to differentiate or undergo reversion at very high frequency by non-genotoxic agents, indicating that a major portion of their phenotype is under epigenetic control. 3) Normal differentiation does not involve mutational changes (except in the immune system) and yet produces stable lineages and cell phenotypes. Although the biochemical mechanisms are not well understood, it seems reasonable to assume that distortions in these mechanisms could also produce abnormalities in cell phenotypes that are heritable in somatic cells. 4) The high frequency of cell transformation induced by carcinogens in cell culture also suggests that epigenetic mechanisms might play an important role in carcinogenesis. These ideas are not new, but I think that in the intense race to identify the mutational changes in tumor cells we should not ignore fundamental processes of cell determination and differentiation, and their potential contribution to multistage carcinogenesis.

As the last speaker in this Symposium I would like to express, on behalf of all the foreign participants, our gratitude to the organizing committee, the Princess Takamatsu Research Fund, and the supporting staff, for providing us with a very stimulating conference and a very pleasant stay in Japan. We trust that this exchange of information will catalyze further advances in cancer research, and thus lead to new and more effective strategies for cancer prevention, diagnosis and treatment.

Author Index

Subject Index